University Ho   ibrary

OSTEOPOROSIS AND THE OSTEOPOROSIS OF RHEUMATIC DISEASES

Other companion titles in the *Rheumatology* series

Ankylosing Spondylitis and the Spondyloarthropathies

Psoriatic and Reactive Arthritis

Osteoarthritis

Systemic Lupus Erythematosus

OSTEOPOROSIS AND THE OSTEOPOROSIS OF RHEUMATIC DISEASES

A Companion to *Rheumatology*

First Edition

Nancy E. Lane, MD
Director and Distinguished Professor Aging Center
Medicine and Rheumatology
University of California at Davis Medical Center,
Sacramento, CA

Philip N. Sambrook, MD, FRACP
Florance and Cope Professor of Rheumatology
University of Sydney
Head, Department of Rheumatology
Royal North Shore Hospital
St. Leonard's, Sydney, Australia

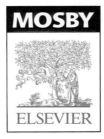

MOSBY

ELSEVIER

1600 John F. Kennedy Boulevard
Suite 1800
Philadelphia, PA 19103-2899

OSTEOPOROSIS AND THE OSTEOPOROSIS OF RHEUMATIC DISEASES   ISBN-13: 9780323 034371
A COMPANION TO RHEUMATOLOGY   ISBN-10: 0-323-03437-3

Notice

Knowledge and best practice in this field are constantly changing. As new research and experience broaden our knowledge, changes in practice, treatment, and drug therapy may become necessary or appropriate. Readers are advised to check the most current information provided (i) on procedures featured or (ii) by the manufacturer of each product to be administered, to verify the recommended dose or formula, the method and duration of administration, and contraindications. It is the responsibility of the practitioner, relying on his or her own experience and knowledge of the patient, to make diagnoses, to determine dosages and the best treatment for each individual patient, and to take all appropriate safety precautions. To the fullest extent of the law, neither the Publisher nor the Authors assume any liability for any injury and/or damage to persons or property arising out of or related to any use of the material contained in this book.

Library of Congress Cataloging-in-Publication Data
Osteoporosis and the osteoporosis of rheumatic diseases: a companion to Rheumatology /
  [editors] Nancy E. Lane, Philip N. Sambrook.–1st
     p. ; cm.
  Includes bibliographical references and index.
  ISBN 0-323-03437-3
   1. Osteoporosis. 2. Rheumatism–Complications. I. Lane, Nancy E. II. Sambrook, Philip N. III.
Rheumatology.
   [DNLM: 1. Osteoporosis. 2. Rheumatic Diseases–complications. WE 250 085116 2006]
  RC931.O73O88 2006
  616.7'16–dc22

                                        2005058428

Acquisitions Editor: Kimberly Murphy
Developmental Editor: Denise Lemelledo
Publishing Services Manager: Frank Polizzano
Senior Project Manager: Natalie Ware
Design Direction: Gene Harris

Printed in the United States of America.

Last digit is the print number: 9   8   7   6   5   4   3   2   1

We would like to dedicate this text to our parents (living or blessed memory), our wives or husbands, and children:

Fred. M. Tileston, Jr., Trevor Lane Tileston, and Reid Lane Tileston.
Brenda L. Sambrook, Andrew M. Sambrook, and Kate L. Sambrook

Contributors

Jonathan (Rick) Adachi, MD
Professor of Medicine, Alliance for Better Bone
Health; Chair in Rheumatology, McMaster
University, Hamilton; Director, Hamilton Arthritis
Center; Head of Rheumatology, St. Joseph's
Healthcare, Hamilton, Ontario, Canada
*The Use of Calcium Supplementation in the
Management and Prevention of Osteoporosis*

Kristina Åkesson, MD, PhD
Associate Professor, Senior Lecturer, Faculty of
Medicine, Lund University, Department of Clinical
Sciences, Malmo; Senior Consultant, Department of
Orthopedics, Malmo University Hospital, Malmo,
Sweden
The Patient with Osteoporosis

Yves Boutsen, MD
Professor, Louvain University, Yvoir, Head,
Department of Rheumatology, University Hospital in
Mont-Godinne, Yvoir, Belgium
The Pathogenesis of Glucocorticoid-Induced Bone Loss

David B. Burr, PhD
Professor and Chairman of Anatomy; Professor of
Orthopedic Surgery and Biomedical Engineering,
Indiana University-Purdue University, Indianapolis,
Indiana
Principles of Bone Biomechanics

Cyrus Cooper, MA, DM, FRCP, FMedSci
Professor of Rheumatology, The MRC Epidemiology
Resource Centre, University of Southampton,
Southampton General Hospital, Southampton,
United Kingdom
The Epidemiology of Osteoporotic Fractures

Elaine Dennison, MA, MB, B.Chir, MSc, PhD
Senior Lecturer, The MRC Epidemiology Resource
Centre, University of Southampton, Southampton
General Hospital, Southampton, United Kingdom
The Epidemiology of Osteoporotic Fractures

Jean-Pierre Devogelaer, MD
Professor of Rheumatology, Université Catholique
de Louvain; Associate Head, Department of
Rheumatology, Saint-Luc University Hospital,
Brussels, Belgium
*The Pathogenesis of Glucocorticoid-Induced
Bone Loss*

Kenneth G. Faulkner, PhD
Vice President of Business Development, Synarc, Inc.,
San Francisco, California
Investigations of Bone: Densitometry

Patrick Garnero, PhD, DSC
Vice President, Molecular Markers, Synarc, and
Senior Research Scientist INSERM 403, Lyon,
France
Biochemical Markers of Bone Turnover

Piet P.M.M. Geusens, MD, PhD
Professor, Department of Rheumatology, University
Hospital, Maastricht, The Netherlands; Professor,
Biomedical Research Institute, Limburgs Universitair
Centrum, Diepenbeek, Belgium
*The Evaluation of the Patient for Osteoporosis: Case
Finding Using Diagnostic Tests for Treatment
Interventions*

David J. Handelsman, MB, BS, PhD, FRACP
Director, ANZAC Research Institute; Head,
Department of Andrology, Concord
Hospital, University of Sydney, Sydney,
Australia
Sex Steroids and Skeletal Health in Men

Nicholas Harvey, MAMB, B.Chir, MRCP
Clinical Research Fellow, The MRC Epidemiology
Resource Centre, University of Southampton,
Southampton General Hospital, Southampton,
United Kingdom
The Epidemiology of Osteoporotic Fractures

Marc C. Hochberg, MD, MPH
Professor of Medicine and Epidemiology and Preventive Medicine; Head Division of Rheumatology and Clinical Immunology, University of Maryland School of Medicine, Baltimore, Maryland
Recommendations for Performing Bone Densitometry to Diagnose Osteoporosis and Identify Persons to Be Treated for Osteoporosis

Mary Beth Humphrey, MD, PhD
Assistant Professor, Department of Medicine and Microbiology and Immunology, University of California San Francisco, San Francisco, California
Pathogenesis of Inflammation-induced Bone Loss

Graeme Jones, MBBS, FRACP, MD, MmedSc, FAFPHM
Professor of Rheumatology and Epidemiology, Menzies Research Institute, University of Tasmania, Hobart, Tasmania
Relevance of Peak Bone Mass to Osteoporosis and Fracture Risk in Later Life

Dina Kulik
Student in MD Programme, McMaster University, Hamilton, Ontario, Canada
The Use of Calcium Supplementation in the Management and Prevention of Osteoporosis

Nancy E. Lane, MD
Director and Distinguished Professor Aging Center, Medicine and Rheumatology, University of California at Davis Medical Center, Sacramento, California
Parathyroid Hormone for the Treatment of Osteoporosis: The Science and the Therapy; Corticosteroid-Induced Osteoporosis

Peter Y. Liu, MBBS, PhD
Postdoctoral Research Fellow, Department of Andrology, Concord Hospital and ANZAC Research Institute, University of Sydney, Sydney, Australia
Sex Steroids and Skeletal Health in Men

Sharmila Majumdar, PhD
Professor, Department of Radiology, University of California San Francisco, San Francisco, California
Imaging Bone Structure and Osteoporosis Using MRI

Naim M. Maalouf, MD
Assistant Professor of Internal Medicine, University of Texas Southwestern Medical Center, Dallas, Texas
Osteoporosis After Solid Organ Transplantation

Daniel Henri Manicourt, MD, PhD
Professor, School of Medicine, Université Catholique de Louvain, Brussels; Head of Clinic in Rheumatology, Saint-Luc University Hospital, Department of Rheumatology, Brussels, Belgium
The Pathogenesis of Glucocorticoid-Induced Bone Loss

Christian Meier, MD
Clinic for Endocrinology, Diabetology, and Clinical Nutrition, University of Basel, Basel, Switzerland
Sex Steroids and Skeletal Health in Men

Paul D. Miller, MD
Clinical Professor of Medicine, University of Colorado Health Sciences Center, Denver; Medical Director, Colorado Center for Bone Research, Lakewood, Colorado
Combination Therapy for Osteoporosis: What Do the Data Show Us?

Mary C. Nakamura, MD
Associate Professor of Medicine, in residence, Division of Rheumatology, Department of Medicine, University of California San Francisco; Staff Physician, San Francisco Veterans Affairs Medical Center, San Francisco, California
Pathogenesis of Inflammation-induced Bone Loss

Ian R. Reid, MD
Professor of Medicine and Endocrinology, University of Auckland, Auckland, New Zealand
Bisphosphonates in the Prevention and Treatment of Postmenopausal Osteoporosis

Evange Romas, MBBS, FRACP, PhD
Senior Lecturer, University of Melbourne; Senior Consultant, Department of Rheumatology, St. Vincent's Hospital, Melbourne, Australia
The Prevention and Treatment of Inflammation-induced Bone Loss: Can It Be Done?

Graham Russell, PhD, DM, FRCP, PRC Path, F Med Sci
Norman Collisson Professor of Musculoskeletal Sciences, Institute Director and Head of Department, The Botnar Research Centre and Oxford University Institute of Musculoskeletal Sciences, Nuffield Department of Orthopedic Surgery, Nuffield Orthopedic Centre, Headington, United Kingdom
Pathogenesis of Osteoporosis

Philip N. Sambrook, MD FRACP
Florance and Cope Professor of Rheumatology,
University of Sydney; Head, Department of
Rheumatology, Royal North Shore Hospital,
St. Leonard's, Sydney, Australia
*Vitamin D and Its Metabolites in the Prevention and
Treatment of Osteoporosis; Selective Estrogen Receptor
Modulators (SERMs); Corticosteroid-Induced
Osteoporosis*

Ego Seeman, BSc, FRACP, MD
Professor of Medicine and Endocrinology, Austin and
Repatriatian Medical Center, University of
Melbourne, Melbourne, Australia
Exercise and the Prevention of Bone Fragility

Markus J. Seibel, MD, PhD
Professor and Chair of Endocrinology; Director, Bone
Research Program, ANZAC Research Institute,
University of Sydney; Head, Department of
Endocrinology, Concord Hospital, Sydney, Australia
Sex Steroids and Skeletal Health in Men

Elizabeth Shane, MD
Professor of Clinical Medicine, College of Physicians
and Surgeons, Columbia University; Attending
Physician in Medicine, Columbia University Medical
Center, New York, New York
Osteoporosis After Solid Organ Transplantation

Sandra J. Shefelbine, BSE, MPhil, PhD
Lecturer, Department of Bioengineering, Imperial
College of London, London, United Kingdom
Imaging Bone Structure and Osteoporosis Using MRI

Stuart L. Silverman, MD, FACP, FACR
Clinical Professor of Medicine and Rheumatology,
Cedars-Sinai Medical Center, University of California
Los Angeles, Greater Los Angeles VA Medical Center,
and the OMC Clinical Research Center; Medical
Director, Fibromyalgia Rehabilitation Program,
Cedars-Sinai Medical Center, Los Angeles, California
Calcitonin in the Treatment of Osteoporosis

Luigi Sinigaglia, MD
Chair, Department of Rheumatology, Gaetano Pini
Institute, University of Milan, Milan, Italy
Epidemiology of Osteoporosis in Rheumatic Diseases

Tim D. Spector, MD, MSc, FRCP
Consultant Rheumatologist, Twin Research and
Genetic Epidemiology Unit, St. Thomas' Hospital;
Honorary Professor in Genetic Epidemiology,
St. Geroge's Medical School, London, United Kingdom
The Genetics of Osteoporosis

Charles H. Turner, PhD
Professor of Biomedical Engineering and Orthopedic
Surgery, Indiana University-Purdue University
Indianapolis, Indianapolis, Indiana
Principles of Bone Biomechanics

Massimo Varenna, MD
Professor, Department of Rheumatology, Istituto
Ortopedicao Gaetano Pini, University of Milan,
Milan, Italy
Epidemiology of Osteoporosis in Rheumatic Diseases

Sarah Westlake, BM, MRCP
Specialist Registrar, The MRC Epidemiology
Resource Centre, University of Southampton,
Southampton General Hospital, Southampton,
United Kingdom
The Epidemiology of Osteoporotic Fractures

Frances M.K. Williams, MBBS, MRCP
Honorary Senior Research Fellow, Twin Research and
Genetic Epidemiology Unit, St. Thomas' Hospital,
London, United Kingdom
The Genetics of Osteoporosis

Anthony D. Woolf, BSc, MB, BS, FRCP
Professor of Rheumatology, Institute of Health and
Social Care Research, Peninsula Medical School,
Universities of Exeter and Plymouth; Consultant
Rheumatologist, Duke of Cornwall Department of
Rheumatology, Royal Cornwall Hospital, Truro,
Cornwall, United Kingdom
The Patient with Osteoporosis

Preface

This monograph takes a very in-depth look at the key aspects of osteoporosis and presents significant advances that have occurred in the field over the past five years. Specifically, this book gathers the works of the top practitioners in the field to discuss the epidemiology, pathogenetic mechanisms, clinical aspects of the disease, treatment options, and secondary osteoporosis and the osteoporosis of the rheumatic diseases.

We discuss bone biology and the new emerging field of osteoimmunology, that connects the field of immunology with inflammatory bone loss. In addition, we carefully provide up-to-date reviews on the epidemiology, pathogenesis, diagnosis, and management of osteoporosis. The epidemiology of osteoporosis and the role of bone mineral density in the definition and prediction of fractures are reviewed, as well as the most current information on the geographical distribution of the disease. The role of peak bone mass acquisition in the prevention of osteoporosis, and a thoughtful review on who should be treated for osteoporosis are included in the first section.

Section II covers the pathogenesis of osteoporosis, and the biomechanics of bone - information any clinician needs to know on what makes bone strong and why it fractures.

The section on the clinical aspects of the disease covers the latest technologies for imaging bone structure and biomechanical markers of bone metabolism. This part of the text is unique in that we review not only the use of DXA and QCT, but also the latest technologies being applied in clinical research, including MRI, that can assess bone structure and apply sophisticated non-invasive modeling to assess bone strength. There has also been a tremendous increase in the number of biochemical tests that measure proteins associated with both bone formation and resorption. In some studies, these biochemical markers of bone turnover appear to be surrogate markers for increased risk of fracture. Also, in some studies, the reduction in thee markers with anti-resorptive therapies, is associated with a reduction in incident fracture risk. These detailed reviews also emphasize how these markers can be used in combination with bone mineral density measurements to educate patients about their potential risk for fracture and their responses to different osteoporosis therapies.

In the next section we present the available modalities for the prevention and treatment of osteoporosis. Among them are the most important aspect of any treatment program, e.g., calcium and vitamin D supplementation, followed by the anti-resorptive agents, including the selective estrogen receptor modulators (SERMs), androgens, gonadal steroids, and calcitonin, and lastly, bisphosphonates. Anabolic agents, such as PTH, and the use of combination and sequential therapies are also discussed in depth.

Lastly, we offer a broad and informative discussion of the newest area of intense investigation: osteoimmunology and the bone loss that is so prevalent in inflammatory conditions like rheumatoid arthritis (RA) and systemic lupus erythematosus (SLE). We begin with a review on the epidemiology of osteoporosis in RA, SLE, and ankylosing spondolytic (AS) patients. The pathogenesis of inflammation-induced bone loss and the treatment of inflammation-induced bone loss are also covered.

Throughout this book, there has been an emphasis on the advances in scientific knowledge as they relate to the biology of postmenopausal bone loss and inflammation-induced bone loss in both women and men, and on the diagnosis and therapy for the prevention and treatment of established disease. Although this book presents major advances in the understanding and treatment of osteoporosis, many outstanding questions remain to be addressed. We hope that the next edition of this monograph will answer some of these questions.

Nancy E. Lane, MD
Philip N. Sambrook, MD

Acknowledgments

The editors would like to acknowledge all of the authors who contributed to this monograph on osteoporosis. In addition, we thank Mollie McGee for her editorial assistance.

Contents

Colour Plates immediately follow the frontmatter.

OSTEOPOROSIS SELF-ASSESSMENT TABLE FOR MEN*

Age (years)	90	100	110	120	130	140	150	160	170	180	190	200	210	220	230	240	250	260	270
30	2	3	3	4	5	6	7	8	9	10	11	12	13	13	14	15	16	17	18
33	1	2	3	4	5	6	7	7	8	9	10	11	12	13	14	15	16	16	17
36	0	1	2	3	4	5	6	7	8	9	10	10	11	12	13	14	15	16	17
39	0	1	2	3	3	4	5	6	7	8	9	10	11	12	13	13	14	15	16
41	0	0	1	2	3	4	5	6	7	8	9	9	10	11	12	13	14	15	16
44	0	0	1	2	2	3	4	5	6	7	8	9	10	11	12	12	13	14	15
47	−1	0	0	1	2	3	4	5	6	6	7	8	9	10	11	12	13	14	15
50	−1	0	0	0	1	2	3	4	5	6	7	8	9	9	10	11	12	13	14
53	−2	−1	0	0	1	2	3	3	4	5	6	7	8	9	10	11	12	12	13
56	−3	−2	−1	0	0	1	2	3	4	5	6	6	7	8	9	10	11	12	13
59	−3	−2	−1	0	0	0	1	2	3	4	5	6	7	8	9	9	10	11	12
61	−4	−3	−2	−1	0	0	1	2	3	4	5	5	6	7	8	9	10	11	12
64	−4	−3	−2	−1	−1	0	0	1	2	3	4	5	6	7	8	8	9	10	11
67	−5	−4	−3	−2	−1	0	0	1	2	2	3	4	5	6	7	8	9	10	11
70	−5	−4	−4	−3	−2	−1	0	0	1	2	3	4	5	5	6	7	8	9	10
73	−6	−5	−4	−3	−2	−1	0	0	0	1	2	3	4	5	6	7	8	8	9
76	−7	−6	−5	−4	−3	−2	−1	0	0	1	2	2	3	4	5	6	7	8	9
79	−7	−6	−5	−4	−4	−3	−2	−1	0	0	1	2	3	4	5	5	6	7	8
81	−8	−7	−6	−5	−4	−3	−2	−1	0	0	1	1	2	3	4	5	6	7	8
84	−8	−7	−6	−5	−5	−4	−3	−2	−1	0	0	1	2	3	4	4	5	6	7
87	−9	−8	−7	−6	−5	−4	−3	−2	−1	−1	0	0	1	2	3	4	5	6	7
90	−9	−8	−8	−7	−6	−5	−4	−3	−2	−1	0	0	1	1	2	3	4	5	6
93	−10	−9	−8	−7	−6	−5	−4	−4	−3	−2	−1	0	0	1	2	3	4	4	5
96	−11	−10	−9	−8	−7	−6	−5	−4	−3	−2	−1	−1	0	0	1	2	3	4	5
99	−11	−10	−9	−8	−8	−7	−6	−5	−4	−3	−2	−1	0	0	1	1	2	3	4

Weight (pounds)

High risk −2 or less	Moderate risk −1 to 3	Low risk 4 or greater

*Based on Osteoporosis Self-assessment tool (OST) formula:
OST index = (Weight in kg−age in years) multiply by 0.2 and truncate to integer

B

Figure 4-1. **B**. The Osteoporosis Self-assessment Table for men.

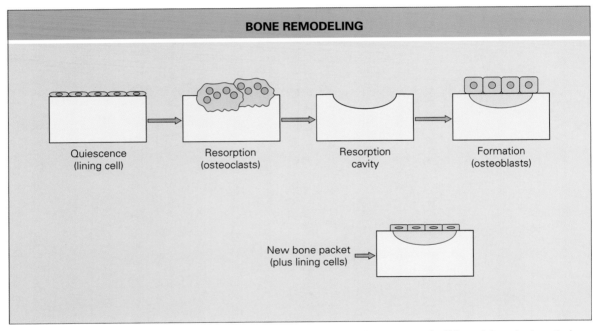

Figure 5-1. Bone remodeling. The remodeling cycle within bone involves a similar sequence of cellular activity at both cortical and trabecular sites. Trabecular surfaces are shown here. An initial phase of osteoclastic resorption is followed by a more prolonged phase of bone formation mediated by osteoblasts. Under normal conditions, the amount of bone removed during resorption is replaced completely. (From Hochberg et al, Rheumatology, 3rd ed, 2003.)

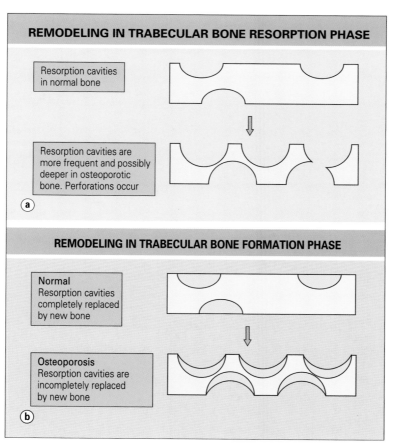

Figure 5-2. Remodeling in trabecular bone. These figures show remodeling under normal conditions and in osteoporosis. (a) Resorption phase. (b) Formation phase. There may be subtle differences between the sexes, with bone thinning predominating in men because of reduced bone formation. Loss of connectivity and complete trabeculae predominates in women. (From Hochberg et al, Rheumatology, 3rd ed, 2003.)

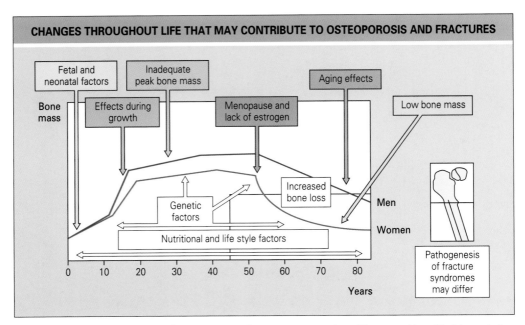

Figure 5-3. Changes throughout life that may contribute to osteoporosis and fractures. (From Hochberg et al, Rheumatology, 3rd ed, 2003.)

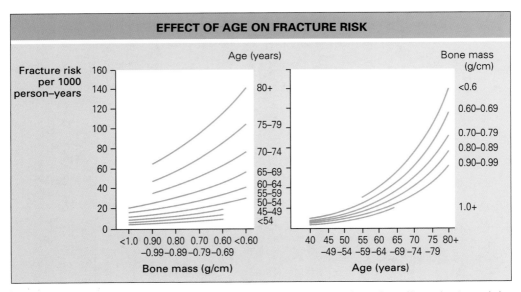

Figure 5-4. Effect of age on fracture risk. Fracture risk increases with age, independent of bone density, and also increases with declining bone density irrespective of age. (Adapted with permission from Hui et al.[14]; from Hochberg et al, Rheumatology, 3rd ed, 2003.)

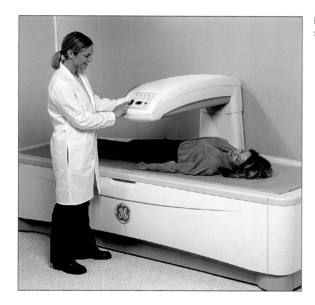

Figure 8-2. Full table dual X-ray absorptiometry system. (From Hochberg: Rheumatology, 3rd ed, 2003.)

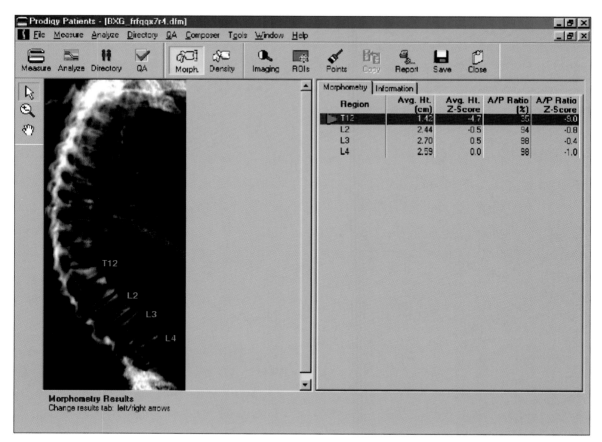

Figure 8-3. Vertebral fracture assessment from a dual x-ray absorptiometry image of the spine. Use of dual-energy images facilitates the visualization of the lumbar and thoracic spine in a single image. In this example, a fracture has been identified at T12. (From Hochberg: Rheumatology, 3rd ed, 2003.)

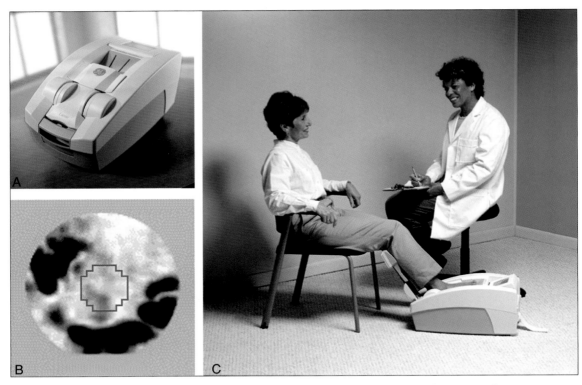

Figure 8-6. **A**, Quantitative ultrasound device for measuring the heel, which incorporates a real-time image for more accurate assessment. **B**, Region of interest (ROI) (*red*) over calcaneus. **C**, Patient undergoing scan of calcaneus. (From Hochberg: Rheumatology, 3rd ed, 2003.)

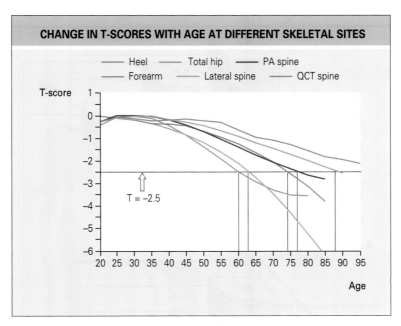

Figure 8-7. Change in T-scores with age at different skeletal sites. (From Hochberg: Rheumatology, 3rd ed, 2003.)

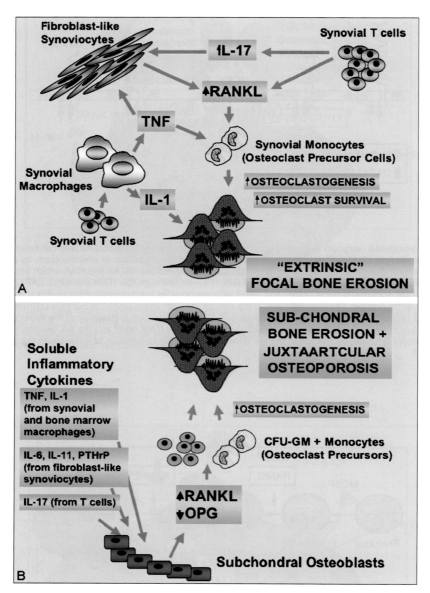

Figure 26-1. A. Cellular and molecular interactions in the synovial compartment facilitate osteoclast differentiation and focal bone erosion at the synovial/bone interface. The main stromal support cell is the activated fibroblast-like synoviocytes, which express membrane-bound macrophage colony-stimulating factor (M-CSF) (not shown) and RANKL. These processes lead to an imbalance in bone resorption relative to bone formation, exhibited as "extrinsic" focal bone erosion. **B.** Cellular and molecular interactions in the subchondral bone marrow compartment facilitate osteoclast differentiation and subchondral bone erosion. The main stromal support cell is the stromal-osteoblasts which express membrane-bound M-CSF (not shown) and RANKL. These processes lead to an imbalance in bone resorption relative to formation, exhibited as subchondral bone erosion and juxta-articular osteoporosis.

1

The Epidemiology of Osteoporotic Fractures

Nicholas Harvey, Sarah Westlake, Elaine Dennison, and Cyrus Cooper

SUMMARY

Osteoporosis is a skeletal disease characterized by low bone mass and microarchitectural deterioration of bone tissue with a consequent increase in bone fragility and susceptibility to fracture. It causes a great burden on public health due to morbidity, reduced survival, and economic costs associated with fragility fractures. Vertebral, hip, and wrist fractures are the most common of these, and the incidence of the first two increase exponentially with age, being more frequent in women than men in older age groups. Recent studies of radiographically defined vertebral fracture have indicated that only around 30% of these fractures present clinically, and that the true incidence is greater than that for hip fracture. There are differences in fracture propensity between populations of different ethnicity and geographical locations. Season also influences fracture incidence, with hip fractures being more frequent in winter months. There has been a secular increase in hip fracture incidence over the last 50 years, which may be plateauing in Western populations. However, incidence is set to rise worldwide, mainly as a result of increases in developing countries, as Western lifestyles are adopted. Recent work has shown that prevalent fracture is a strong predictor of incident fracture, and that this increased risk occurs rapidly. Understanding the epidemiology of osteoporosis is an essential step in developing strategies to reduce the burden of osteoporotic fracture in the population.

Osteoporosis is a major public health problem. The main contributors to this burden are associated fragility fractures. The increased rates of morbidity and mortality consequent to these fractures have a massive impact on both the health of the population and the economy. There were an estimated 1.66 million hip fractures worldwide in 1990,[1] 1,197,000 in women and 463,000 in men. The estimated annual cost in Europe is 13 billion euros, mainly accounted for by hospitalization after fracture. Understanding the epidemiology of osteoporosis is an essential step in developing strategies to reduce the burden of osteoporotic fractures in the population.

DEFINITION OF OSTEOPOROSIS

Osteoporosis is a skeletal disease characterized by low bone mass and microarchitectural deterioration of bone tissue with a consequent increase in bone fragility and susceptibility to fracture.[2] The term *osteoporosis* was first introduced in France and Germany during the last century. It means "porous bone" and initially implied a histological diagnosis, but the term was later refined to mean bone that had normal mineralization but was reduced in quantity.

Historically, the definition of osteoporosis has been difficult. A definition based on bone mineral density (BMD) may not encompass all the risk factors for fracture, whereas a fracture-based definition will not enable identification of at-risk populations. The World Health Organization[3] recently resolved this issue by defining osteoporosis in terms of BMD and previous fracture, as shown in Table 1-1. Thus, the World Health Organization definition does not take into account microarchitectural changes that may weaken bone independently of any effect on BMD.

If this definition is applied to a female population sample in the United Kingdom, the prevalence of osteoporosis at the femoral neck rises from 5.1% at 50

TABLE 1-1 CLASSIFICATION OF OSTEOPOROSIS	
Normal	BMC or BMD value greater than 0.1 SD below young normal adult mean
Osteopenia	BMC or BMD 1-2.5 SD below young normal adult mean
Osteoporosis	BMC or BMD >2.5 SD below the young normal adult mean
Established osteoporosis	Osteoporosis with one or more fragility fractures

BMC = bone mineral density, BMD = bone mineral content, SD = standard deviation.
Data derived from World Health Organization Study Group, 1994.[3]

to 54 years to over 60% at age 85 and above. The corresponding estimates for men are 0.4% and 29.1%.

FRACTURE EPIDEMIOLOGY

All Fractures

Data from the United Kingdom suggest that there is an overall fracture incidence of 21.1 in 1000 per year (23.5/1000 men and 18.8/1000 women),[4] and that there is a bimodal distribution, with peaks in youth and in the very elderly.[5] Any bone will fracture if sufficient force is applied. Fractures of long bones predominate in young people, usually as a result of substantial trauma, and males are involved more frequently than females. Thus, it is the magnitude of the trauma, rather than deficient bone strength, that leads to the fracture in this group. In the elderly, low bone mass is the critical factor, with most fractures occurring as a result of minimal force. The rate of fracture in women increases steeply after the age of 35 years and becomes twice that in men (Figure 1-1).[6,7]

Only around one-third of vertebral fractures reach clinical attention,[8] and until the advent of studies based on radiographic assessment of vertebral deformity, it was thought that hip and distal forearm fractures were the main contributors to this peak. Figure 1-1 demonstrates that the picture is rather different, with the incidence of radiographically defined vertebral deformity being higher than for hip and wrist fractures at all ages. A recent study from Denmark showed that 60-year-old women, expected to live until the age of 81 years, had an estimated residual lifetime risk of radial, humeral, or hip fracture of 17%, 8%, and 14%, respectively. The lifetime risk to those women surviving to the age of 88 years was increased to 32%.[9] Data from the General Practice Research Database (GPRD), which includes the general practitioner records of 6% of the UK population, have given the lifetime risks of any fracture at age 50 years as 53.2% in women and 20.7% in men.[6] The following sections will detail the site-specific epidemiology.

Hip Fracture

Hip fractures are the most devastating consequence of osteoporosis, invariably requiring hospitalization. Typically, they result from a fall from standing height or lower, but they can occur spontaneously.[10] The diagnosis is usually suggested by characteristic clinical features and confirmed by a plain radiograph.

Impact

Hip fractures have major consequences; 5% to 20% of people affected will die within 1 year after a hip fracture, and more than 50% of survivors will be incapacitated, many needing nursing home care.[11] Table 1-2 shows the observed and expected survival rates for men and women aged 65 years and older in the GPRD study.

Mortality

The majority of excess deaths occur within 6 months of the fracture, and the risk of death diminishes with time, so that after 2 years survival probability is comparable with that of similarly aged men and women in the general population. The mortality risk differs, however, according to the age and gender of the person experiencing the hip fracture. In a population-based study, a relative survival rate of 92% was found for white hip fracture victims younger than 75 years of age, as compared with 83% in those 75 years of age and older at the time of the fracture.[12] Despite their greater age at the time of fracture, survival was better among

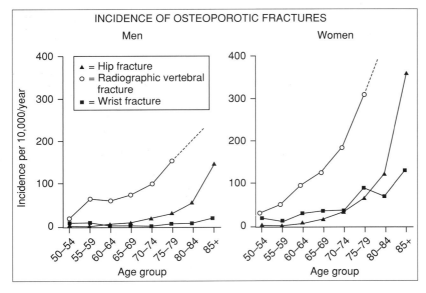

Figure 1-1. Radiographic vertebral, hip, and wrist fracture incidence by age and gender. (Data derived from van Staa TP et al.[6] and EPOS Study Group.[7])

TABLE 1-2 OBSERVED AND EXPECTED SURVIVAL AFTER FRACTURE AMONG MEN AND WOMEN AGED ≥ 65 YEARS						
	Radius/Ulna, %		Femur/Hip, %		Vertebra, %	
	Observed	Expected	Observed	Expected	Observed	Expected
Women						
At 3 months	98.2	98.6	85.6	97.7	94.3	98.4
At 12 months	94.0	94.4	74.9	91.1	86.5	93.6
At 5 years	75.5	73.8	41.7	60.9	56.5	69.6
Men						
At 3 months	97.3	98.0	77.7	97.3	87.8	97.9
At 12 months	89.6	92.4	63.3	90.0	74.3	91.8
At 5 years	62.8	66.4	32.2	58.2	42.1	64.4

Data derived from van Staa TP et al.[6]

women. In the GPRD study (see Table 1-2), observed survival in women 65 years of age and older was 74.9% at 12 months versus 91.1% expected. For men, these figures were 63.3% and 90.0%, respectively.[6] This gender difference has been confirmed in other hospital-based studies and appears to be due to the greater frequency of other chronic diseases in men who sustain hip fractures. The majority of deaths after hip fracture are due to preexisting comorbidity, such as ischemic heart disease, with the minority a direct result of complications or management of the fracture itself.

Morbidity

In the United States, 7% of survivors of all types of fracture have some degree of permanent disability, and 8% require long-term nursing home care. Overall, a 50-year-old white American woman has a 13% chance of experiencing functional decline after any fracture.[13] As with mortality, hip fractures contribute most to osteoporosis-associated disability. Patients are prone to developing acute complications such as pressure sores, bronchopneumonia, and urinary tract infections. Perhaps the most important long-term outcome is impairment of the ability to walk. Fifty percent of people who were ambulatory before the fracture are unable to walk independently afterward. Age is an important determinant of outcome, with 14% of 50- to 55-year-old hip fracture victims being discharged to nursing homes, versus 55% of those more than 90 years old.[13]

Determinants

Age

There is an exponential increase in hip fracture with aging (see Figure 1-1). This is due to an age-related increase in the risk of falling and reduction in bone strength. The majority of fractures occur after a fall from standing height or lower; 90% occur in people older than 50 years and 80% are in women.[14] Much of the lifetime risk of fracture for a 50-year-old

woman is accrued as she reaches 80 years old. Data from the GPRD (Table 1-3) show that the lifetime risk of hip fracture for women aged 50 years is 11.4%, but the risk over the next 10 years is 0.3% at age 50 and 8.7% at age 80 years.[6] This has implications for targeting of treatment. Among postmenopausal women in the United States, the likelihood of experiencing at least one fall annually rises from about one in five women 60 to 64 years old, to one in three women 80 to 84 years old.[10] Comparable data were found in the United Kingdom, with one in three women 80 to 84 years old having fallen in the previous year; this statistic rose to nearly one in two (50%) among women aged 85 years and older.[15] However, only about 1% of all falls lead to a hip fracture. This is because the amount of trauma delivered to the proximal femur depends on various protective responses and the direction of the fall: falling sideways onto the hip is more likely to result in fracture than falling forward onto it.[16]

Femoral neck strength is weaker in women than in men and declines with age in both sexes. Many factors contribute to bone strength, for example BMD and microarchitecture, but all are closely correlated with absolute bone mass. Over a lifetime, the BMD of the femoral neck declines an estimated 58% in women and 39% in men, whereas bone density of the intertrochanteric region of the proximal femur falls by about 53% and 35%, respectively. Each one standard deviation decline in bone mineral density is associated with a 1.8- to 2.6-fold increase in the age-adjusted risk of hip fracture, depending on the exact site that is measured.[17]

Gender

The incidence of osteoporotic hip fractures is lower in men than in women; in 1990, only about 30% of 1.66 million hip fractures worldwide occurred in men.[18] In the United Kingdom, the lifetime risk of hip fracture in men is 3.1% at age 50 (compared with 11.4%

TABLE 1-3 ESTIMATED RISKS OF FRACTURES AT VARIOUS AGES					
	Current Age (years)	Any Fractures (%)	Radius/Ulna (%)	Femur/Hip (%)	Vertebra (%)
Lifetime risk					
Women	50	53.2	16.6	11.4	3.1
	60	45.5	14.0	11.6	2.9
	70	36.9	10.4	12.1	2.6
	80	28.6	6.9	12.3	1.9
Men	50	20.7	2.9	3.1	1.2
	60	14.7	2.0	3.1	1.1
	70	11.4	1.4	3.3	1.0
	80	9.6	1.1	3.7	0.8
10-year risk					
Women	50	9.8	3.2	0.3	0.3
	60	13.3	4.9	1.1	0.6
	70	17.0	5.6	3.4	1.3
	80	21.7	5.5	8.7	1.6
Men	50	7.1	1.1	0.2	0.2
	60	5.7	0.9	0.4	0.3
	70	6.2	0.9	1.4	0.5
	80	8.0	0.9	2.9	0.7

Data derived from van Staa TP et al.[6]

in women), and the 10-year risk is 0.2% at age 50, rising to 2.9% at 80 years of age.[6] Men are relatively protected for several reasons: they have a higher peak bone density, they lose less bone during aging, they do not normally become hypogonadal, they sustain fewer falls, and they have a shorter lifespan. However, this relationship is not true for all populations: in black and Asian groups, the incidence in men is slightly higher.[19]

Ethnicity

Hip fractures are much more frequent among whites than among non-whites. This has been explained by the higher bone mass observed in blacks compared with whites (Figure 1-2).[20]

There is also some evidence that the rate of bone loss is lower in blacks. However, the Bantu people of South Africa have a lower bone mass and a lower fracture rate than whites.[21] Likewise, the incidence of hip fractures among women of Japanese ancestry is about one half that of their white counterparts, even though their bone mass is somewhat lower.[22] These discrepancies may be related to the reported lower risk of falling of black women compared with white women.[23] Asian women have shorter femoral necks than white women, and this shape seems inherently less likely to fracture, despite a lower bone mineral density.[24]

Geography

There is variation in the incidence of hip fracture within populations of a given race and gender.[25-27] Thus, age-adjusted hip fracture incidence rates are higher among white residents of Scandinavia than comparable subjects in the United States or Oceania. In 1986, the Mediterranean Osteoporosis Study (MEDOS) was set up to investigate the incidence of hip fracture in the Mediterranean region. It was discovered that the incidence of hip fracture varied markedly from country to country, and even within countries. Within Europe, the range of variation was approximately 11-fold.[25] These differences were not explained by variation in activity levels, smoking, obesity, alcohol consumption, or migration status.[26] In the United Kingdom, the geographical differences were not associated with differences in water fluoridation or with dietary calcium intake, as assessed by a national food survey.[28] A more recent comparison of studies from several areas of United Kingdom gives an annual incidence of all fractures between 159 and 288 per 10,000 population for men older than 85 years, and between 281 and 810 per 10,000 population for women older than 85 years.[6] Studies in the United States confirm this complex pattern. In more than 2000 counties nationwide, the age-adjusted incidence of hip fracture in white women older than 65 years of age was negatively associated with

Figure 1-2. Hip fracture incidence around the world. (Data derived from Kanis JA et al.[20])

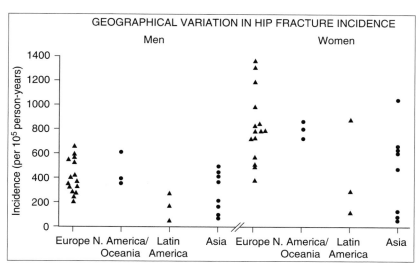

latitude (higher in the south), water hardness, and hours of January sunlight, and positively associated with poverty levels, proportion of the land in farms, and proportion of the population with fluoridated water.[29]

Season

Hip fractures are seasonal, occurring more frequently, in both sexes, during the winter in temperate countries. However, the majority of hip fractures follow falls indoors and are not related to slipping on icy surfaces. Explanations for this include abnormal neuromuscular function at lower temperatures and vitamin D deficiency as a result of the winter-time reduction in sunlight exposure.

Time trends

Life expectancy is increasing around the globe and the number of elderly individuals is rising in every geographical region. The world population is expected to rise from the current 323 million individuals aged 65 years or older, to 1555 million by the year 2050. These demographic changes alone can be expected to increase the number of hip fractures occurring among people 35 years of age and older worldwide: the incidence is estimated to rise from 1.66 million in 1990 to 6.26 million in 2050. Assuming a constant age-specific rate of fracture, as the number of people older than 65 increases from 32 million in 1990 to 69 million in 2050, the number of hip fractures in the United States will increase threefold.[1] In the United Kingdom, the number of hip fractures may increase from 46,000 in 1985 to 117,000 in 2016.[30]

An increasingly elderly population in Latin America and Asia could lead to a shift in the geographical distribution of hip fractures, with only one quarter occurring in Europe and North America (Figure 1-3).[1]

Such projections are almost certainly optimistic considering that increases in the incidence of hip fractures

have been observed even after adjusting for the growth in the elderly population. Although the age-adjusted rate of hip fracture appears to have leveled off in the northern regions of the United States, in parts of Sweden, and the United Kingdom, the rates in Hong Kong rose substantially between 1966 and 1985. Thus, the above figures potentially represent a significant underestimate of the number of hip fractures in the next half-century.

There are three broad explanations for these trends:

Firstly, they might represent some increasingly prevalent current risk factor for osteoporosis or falling; physical activity is the most likely candidate. There is ample evidence linking inactivity to the risk of hip fracture, whether this effect is mediated through bone density, the risk of falls, or both. Furthermore, some of the steepest secular trends have been observed in Asian countries, such as Hong Kong, which have witnessed dramatic reductions in the customary activity levels of their populations in recent decades.

Secondly, the elderly population is becoming increasingly frail. As many of the disorders leading to frailty are independently associated with osteoporosis and the risk of falling, this tendency might have contributed to the secular increases in Western nations during earlier decades of this century.

Finally, the trends could arise from a cohort phenomenon—some adverse influence on bone mass or the risk of falling that acted at an earlier time and is now manifesting as a rising incidence of fractures in successive generations of the elderly.

Vertebral Fracture

Definition

Vertebral fractures have been synonymous with the diagnosis of osteoporosis since its earliest description as a metabolic bone disorder.[31] However, their epidemiology remains less well characterized than that of

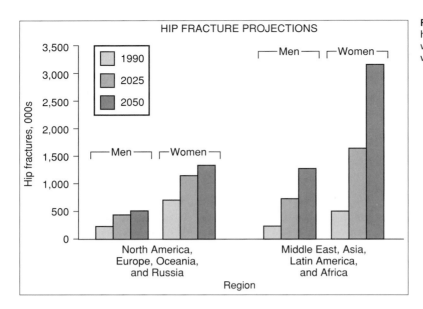

Figure 1-3. Estimated numbers of hip fractures among men and women in different regions of the world in 1990 and 2050.

hip or wrist fractures, because there is no universally accepted definition of a vertebral fracture from thoracolumbar radiographs, and because a substantial proportion of vertebral deformities are asymptomatic.

There is significant variation in vertebral body shape, both within the spine and between individuals. This results in considerable difficulty in deciding whether a vertebral body is deformed. Early epidemiological studies of vertebral fractures used subjective radiological assessments of wedge, crush, and biconcave deformities, but these were poorly reproducible. These methods gave way to morphometric measurements of vertebral height, with fractures defined according to fixed cut-off values.[32]

Each vertebral body in the spinal column has unique dimensions, however, and recent analyses have focused on determining the distribution of vertebral dimensions at each spinal level and calculating cut-off values from these.[32,33] The most widely adopted thresholds for defining and grading deformities are as follows: moderate (or grade 1) fractures are deformities that fall between three and four standard deviations from the mean value specific to each vertebra; severe (or grade 2) fractures are those that fall four standard deviations or more from this mean. When morphometric studies are performed without reference to clinical presentation, the abnormalities found are usually referred to as deformities rather than fractures. Three broad categories of vertebral fracture have been described: compression (or crush) fractures, in which there is loss of both anterior and posterior vertebral height; wedge (or partial) fractures, in which anterior height tends to be lost; and biconcave (balloon) fractures, in which loss of central bony tissue leads to concavity of both vertebral end plates.

Incidence

The application of recently developed morphometric techniques to various population samples in the United States has permitted the estimation of the incidence of new vertebral fractures in the general population (Figure 1-4).

Using the data shown, the age-adjusted incidence among white US women aged 50 years and older was found to be 18 per 1000 person-years.[34] This is more than twice the corresponding incidence of hip fracture (6.2 per 1000 person-years). The corresponding figure for vertebral fracture from the European Vertebral Osteoporosis Study (EVOS, a large pan-European longitudinal study) was 10.7 per 1000 person-years.[7] In the GPRD study, the overall incidence standardized to the UK population was 3.2 per 1000 person-years for men and 5.6 per 1000 person-years for women. This population included all ages from 20 years, hence the lower overall incidence. It is important to note the disparity between the incidence of vertebral fractures identified on radiographs and those reported clinically. In Rochester, Minnesota, the incidence of clinically diagnosed vertebral deformities was 30% of that expected from a study using radiographic diagnosis. This implies that as few as one in three vertebral fractures comes to medical attention.[8]

Prevalence

The prevalence of vertebral deformity was investigated in an age-stratified random sample of the population of Rochester, Minnesota, USA. The prevalence was estimated at 25.3 per 100 Rochester women aged 50 years and older (95% confidence interval, 22.3–28.2).[35] More recent data from the EVOS group suggested the age-standardized prevalence across

Figure 1-4. The incidence of vertebral deformities in a population sample of women from the United States. (Data derived from Cooper C et al.[8])

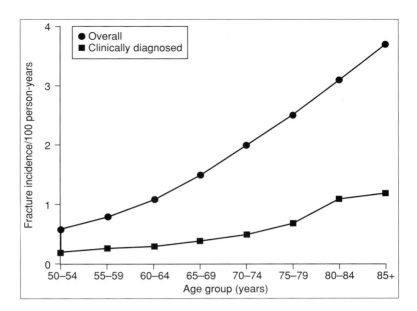

Europe was 12.2% for men and 12.0% for women aged 50 to 79 years.[36] The higher Rochester figure represents the inclusion of women older than 80 years, up to older than 90 years. Because people in this age range have a greatly increased prevalence of vertebral fracture when compared with people in the the 50- to 79-year-old age range, the overall figure is significantly higher.

Impact

Spine fractures cause significant pain, deformity, and long-term disability. Data from the Study of Osteoporotic Fractures,[37] a population-based US study of 9606 women 65 years of age and older, showed that women who had grade 2 deformities were 2.6 times more likely to suffer disability and 1.9 times more likely to report moderate or severe back pain than those with no deformity. Women with grade 1 deformities did not have significantly elevated risks of these clinical sequelae. Cross-sectional data from out-patients also support this notion, with severe vertebral deformity being much more closely associated with adverse outcomes than moderate deformity.[38]

Mortality

Examination of the survival of patients after a clinically diagnosed vertebral fracture rather surprisingly reveals a similar excess mortality rate at 5 years to that found with hip fractures (Figure 1-5).[34]

This excess is observed in patients with vertebral fractures caused by moderate or minimal trauma, but not in those whose fractures follow severe trauma. The impairment of survival after vertebral fracture also markedly worsens as time from diagnosis of the fracture increases. This is in contrast to the pattern of survival for hip frac-

ture patients. In the United Kingdom (GPRD study; see Table 1-2), the observed survival rate in women 12 months after vertebral fracture was 86.5%, versus 93.6% expected. At 5 years, the survival rate was 56.5% observed and 69.9% expected.[6] Furthermore, there does not appear to be any particular cause of death that explains this finding. This accords with the observations of recent US and Swedish studies that low bone density per se is associated with premature death.[39,40] These data suggest that the association might be due to a number of factors, such as smoking, alcohol consumption, and immobility: these predispose independently to both bone loss and increased mortality risk.

Morbidity

The health impact of vertebral fractures has proved considerably difficult to quantify. Despite only a minority of vertebral fractures coming to clinical attention, vertebral fractures account for 52,000 hospital admissions in the United States and 2188 in England and Wales each year among patients aged 45 years and older. The major clinical consequences of vertebral fracture are back pain, kyphosis, and height loss. The pain associated with a new compression fracture is typically severe and tends to decrease in severity over several weeks or months. This pain is associated with exquisite localized tenderness and paravertebral muscle spasm, which markedly limits spinal movements. Figure 1-6 shows quality-of-life score against age and number of vertebral fractures,[41] clearly illustrating the impact of age and number of fractures, with higher quality-of-life scores indicating lower health-related quality of life.

A proportion of patients may develop chronic pain experienced while standing and during physical stress, particularly bending. For example, in the control

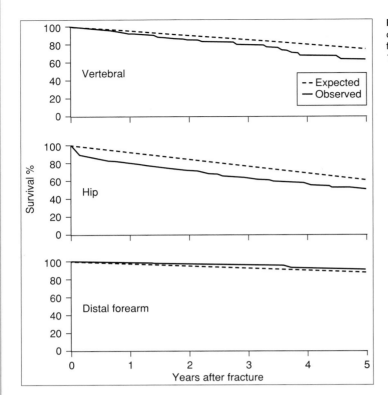

Figure 1-5. Five-year survival following a clinically diagnosed hip, vertebral or distal forearm fracture in Rochester, MN, USA, 1985-1989.

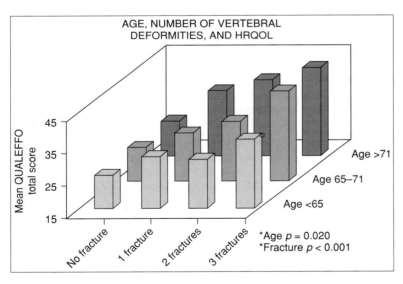

Figure 1-6. Health-related quality of life related to age and number of vertebral deformities.

group of one treatment study, patients were noted to have persistent pain for 6 months after fracture.[42] This chronic pain is believed to arise from spinal extensor muscle weakness and the altered spinal biomechanics that result from vertebral deformation. A number of indices of physical function, self-esteem, body image, and mood also appear to be adversely affected in patients with vertebral fractures. Whenever self-report scales of functional status or quality of life have been applied to patients with vertebral fractures, scores have

been found to be worse for patients with more severe or multiple deformities.[43]

Determinants

Age

Most studies agree that the prevalence of vertebral fractures rises with age among women. In an age-stratified random sample of 762 Rochester women who underwent thoracolumbar radiography, the prevalence of one or more deformities increased from 7.6% at

50 to 54 years to 64.3% in those 90 years of age and older. In Europe, the prevalence for men and women, respectively, was 9.9% and 5.0% at 50 to 54 years of age, rising to 18.1% and 24.7% at 75 to 79 years of age (Figure 1-7).[36]

Gender

Although it is generally believed that vertebral fractures are much more common in women than in men, historically there has been little epidemiological evidence to support this notion. However, more recent evidence from EVOS has shown a twofold greater incidence of vertebral fractures in women than men (relative risk 2.3 at age 50-54 years and 2.9 at age 70-74 years).[7] In this population, the incidence of vertebral fracture in men was 1.7 per 1000 person-years at 50 to 54 years of age and rose to 14.6 per 1000 person years at 75 to 79 years of age. In the GPRD data, overall incidence in men was 3.2 per 10,000 person-years versus 5.6 per 10,000 person-years for women.[6] Overall, however, the picture for prevalence differs: men aged 50 to 64 years had a higher prevalence of deformity compared with similarly aged women, with the reverse being the case for those aged 65 years.[36] Whereas 90% of vertebral fractures in women occurred as a result of moderate or minimal trauma in this study, an appreciable proportion of fractures in men (37%) occurred as a result of severe trauma, for example, road traffic accidents.

The most frequent vertebral levels involved are L1, T12, and T8. These correspond with the most biomechanically compromised regions of the thoracolumbar spine: the midthoracic region, where dorsal kyphosis is most pronounced, and the thoracolumbar junction, where the relatively rigid thoracic spine meets the freely moving lumbar segment.

Ethnicity

There are few studies assessing the influence of ethnicity on vertebral fracture prevalence, although one study found vertebral deformities in around 5% of selected white women aged 45 years and older but in none of the 137 black women studied.[44] This finding is in accord with the often-replicated observation that hip fracture incidence rates are markedly higher among whites. However, recent data from Japan suggest that prevalence rates for vertebral deformity in Asian women may be similar to those observed in white populations.[45]

Previous fracture

Previous fracture is increasingly recognized as an important determinant of future fracture risk, independent of BMD. A previous hip fracture increases the odds of an incident hip fracture by six- to eightfold,[46] and a forearm fracture increases the risk of subsequent hip fracture by 1.4 and 2.7 times in women and men, respectively.[47] The corresponding figures for subsequent vertebral fracture are 5.2 and 10.7. Prevalent vertebral deformity predicts incident hip fracture with a rate ratio of 2.8 to 4.5, and this increases with the number of vertebral deformities.[48] Previous hip fracture strongly predicts multiple (more than two) vertebral deformities in men (odds ratio 10.2), and incident vertebral fracture is predicted by the morphometry and number of the baseline deformities (Table 1-4).[49] The incidence of new vertebral fracture within a year of an incident vertebral fracture is 19.2%,[50] which reinforces the importance of prompt therapeutic action on discovering vertebral deformities. Figure 1-8 summarizes the cumulative incidence of a subsequent vertebral fracture over time after a baseline event.[51,52]

Figure 1-7. Prevalence of vertebral deformity, European Vertebral Osteoporosis Study (EVOS).

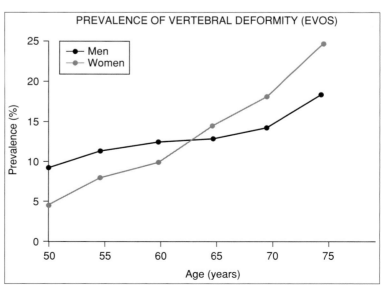

PREVALENCE OF VERTEBRAL DEFORMITY (EVOS)

TABLE 1-4 VERTEBRAL DEFORMITY AND RISK OF VERTEBRAL FRACTURE		
	Relative Risk of Subsequent Fracture	95% CI
Number of Deformities	3.2	2.1-4.8
1	9.8	23.3
2	6.1-15.8	15.3-35.4
≥3		
Position of height loss		
Anterior/middle	5.9	4.1-8.6
Posterior/middle	1.6	0.8-3.2

Data derived from Lunt M et al.[51]

Time trends

The impact of osteoporotic fractures is set to rise in the future, commensurate with the increasing number of elderly people in the population. Little is known about secular increases in the age-adjusted incidence of vertebral fractures. In Rochester, Minnesota, there was no significant increase in the incidence of clinically diagnosed vertebral fractures between 1950 and 1989.[53] However, when categorized into subgroups, a significant increase in the incidence of fractures after moderate or minimal trauma in postmenopausal women is revealed. This increase occurred between 1950 and 1964, with a plateau in age-adjusted incidence thereafter. Rates for severe trauma fractures and for vertebral fractures from any cause among younger men and women remained stable. This rise in the incidence of moderate trauma fractures in women paralleled that for hip fractures in Rochester. An increase in the prevalence of osteoporosis over this period is consistent with these trends.

Two European studies have also investigated secular trends in the incidence of vertebral fractures. Men and women, aged 60 years and older, presenting with thoracic and lumbar vertebral fractures between 1950 and 1952 and between 1982 and 1983, in Malmö, Sweden, were studied.[54] Among women, the incidence rates during the 1982 to 1983 period were higher than those during the 1950 to 1952 period at all ages over 60 years. Among men, the increase was only apparent above the age of 80 years. The prevalence of radiographic vertebral deformities in two samples of 70-year-old Danish women studied in 1979 and 1989 were found to be virtually identical.[55] The secular tendency reported from Rochester, with a rise in incidence between 1950 and 1964, followed by a plateau, is consistent with both these reports.

Geographical

The EVOS study found a threefold difference in the prevalence of vertebral deformities between countries, with the highest rates in Scandinavia. The prevalence range between centers was 7.5% to 19.8% for men and 6.2% to 20.7% for women. The differences were not as great as those seen for hip fracture in Europe, and some of the differences could be explained by levels of physical activity and body mass index.[36] More recent data from EVOS showed a correspondingly higher incidence of vertebral fracture in Scandinavia (age-standardized incidence 17.7 per 1000 person-years) than in Western Europe (age-standardized incidence 10.2 per 1000 person-years[7]).

Distal Forearm Fracture

Definition

The most common distal forearm fracture is Colles fracture. This fracture lies within 1 inch of the wrist joint margin and is associated with dorsal angulation and

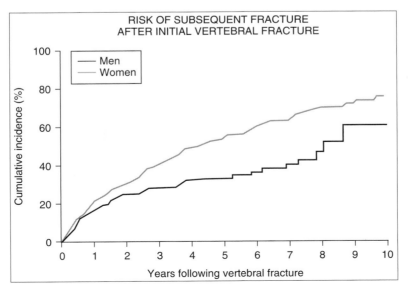

Figure 1-8. Cumulative incidence of a subsequent vertebral fracture over time after a baseline event.

RISK OF SUBSEQUENT FRACTURE AFTER INITIAL VERTEBRAL FRACTURE

— Men
— Women

Cumulative incidence (%)

Years following vertebral fracture

displacement of the distal fragment of the radius and with a fracture of the ulnar styloid. Distal forearm fractures nearly always follow a fall on an outstretched arm.

Impact
Despite the fact that only around one-fifth of all patients with distal forearm fractures are hospitalized, they account for some 50,000 hospital admissions and more than 400,000 physician visits in the United States each year, and 10,000 hospital admissions in the United Kingdom. Admission rates appear to vary markedly with age, such that only 16% of those occurring in women 45 to 54 years old require in-patient care as compared with 76% of those occurring in women 85 years old and older. There is a 30% increase of algodystrophy after these fractures, as well as a risk of neuropathies and post-traumatic arthritis. Wrist fractures do not appear to increase mortality risk. Although wrist fractures may affect some activities such as writing or meal preparation, overall, few patients are completely disabled, despite more than one half reporting only fair to poor function at 6 months.[13,56-58]

Determinants
Age
Distal forearm fractures display a different pattern of incidence from that of the other osteoporotic fractures (see Figure 1-1). In white women, incidence rates increase linearly between 40 and 65 years of age and then stabilize. In men, the incidence remains constant between 20 and 80 years of age. The reason for the plateau in female incidence remains obscure but may relate to a change in the pattern of falling with advancing age. The slower gait and impaired neuromuscular coordination of elderly women make them more likely to fall on their hip rather than on their wrist. However, more recent studies have shown a gentle progressive increase in incidence after menopause,[59] suggesting that there has been a change in the pattern of incidence with age, the explanation for which is not clear.

Gender
The age-adjusted female-to-male ratio of 4:1 for distal forearm fractures is more marked than that of either hip or vertebral fractures. Fifty percent occur in women older than 65 years. After the age of 35 years, the age-adjusted incidence of wrist fracture is 36.8 per 10,000 person-years in women and 9.0 per 10,000 person-years in men. The incidence in men is low and does not rise much with aging.[60]

Season
There is a winter peak in the incidence of Colles fracture that is more pronounced than the peak observed in hip fracture and also is more closely related to falls outdoors during episodes of icy weather. This seasonal variation has been found to exist in northern Europe but is not apparent in southern Europe.

COST OF OSTEOPOROTIC FRACTURES

The total cost of osteoporosis is difficult to assess because it includes the costs of in-patient and out-patient medical care, loss of working days, chronic nursing home care, and medication. The direct costs of osteoporosis stem mainly from the management of patients with hip fractures.

In the United Kingdom, hip fracture patients occupy one-fifth of all orthopedic beds. In 1994, the direct cost in England and Wales was £750 million,[61] and a more recent estimate puts the figure at £942 million.[62] In France, an estimated 56,000 hip fractures annually cost about 3.5 billion francs. The cost of fractures in the United States may be as much as $20 billion per year, with hip fractures accounting for more than one-third of the total. Table 1-5 summarizes the impact of osteoporotic fractures in Europe in the 1990s, reaching a total cost of around €13 billion.[63]

The greatest expense is incurred by the in-patient, out-patient, and nursing home care of patients with hip fractures. About 10% of women who sustain a hip fracture become functionally dependent in the activities of daily living (taking prefracture functional status into account), and 19% require long-term nursing home care because of the fracture.[13] Nursing home care is extremely expensive, accounting for more than one-half of the total annual cost of hip fractures. At least 60,000 nursing home admissions are attributed to hip fractures each year in the United States. As many as 8% of all nursing home residents have had a hip fracture.

FRACTURES IN CHILDREN

There has been much less investigation of the role of bone fragility in childhood fractures, probably because of the perception that the primary determinant of fracture in this age group is trauma. Most evidence

TABLE 1-5 IMPACT OF OSTEOPOROSIS-RELATED FRACTURES IN UNITED KINGDOM			
	Hip	Spine	Wrist
Lifetime risk (%)			
Women	14	28	13
Men	3	6	2
Cases/year (n)	70,000	120,000	50,000
Hospitalization (%)	100	2-10	5
Relative survival	0.83	0.82	1.00
Costs	All sites combined ~ £1.7 billion		

comes from two large studies, based in the United Kingdom and Sweden, which describe the epidemiology of fractures in childhood.[64-66] In the series from Malmö, Sweden, data were collected over 30 years on all childhood fractures by radiograph retrieval. Based on 8500 incident fractures, the overall incidence of fracture was 212 per 10,000 girls and 257 per 10,000 boys, with 27% of girls and 42% of boys sustaining a fracture between birth and 16 years of age. Fractures of the distal radius occurred most commonly, followed by fractures of the phalanges of the hand.[65] A follow-up study in Malmö between 1993 and 1994 found the incidence of fracture had decreased by almost 10% since the original study.[67]

In the United Kingdom, the GPRD was used to investigate the epidemiology of fracture in childhood between 1988 and 1998.[64] The overall incidence of fracture was 133.1 per 10,000 children. The gender differences were similar to those found in the Malmö study, with fractures being more common among boys than girls, with an incidence of 161.6 per 10,000 and 102.9 per 10,000, respectively. Again, the most common fracture site in children of both sexes was the radius/ulna, with a total of 39.3 per 10,000 per year.

Historically, most work has focused on the impact of trauma in the etiology of childhood fractures, contrasting with the role of bone fragility in the elderly. However, several recent studies have documented lower area and volumetric bone mineral density in children with distal forearm fractures than age- and sex-matched control subjects.[68] The age and sex distribution of fractures may also suggest an influence of bone fragility. In the GPRD, fracture incidence peaked at 14 years in boys and 11 years in girls. Thus, peak fracture rate was found to be highest in both sexes at the start of puberty, when the discordance between height gain and accrual of volumetric bone density is greatest.[64]

As with fractures in the elderly, there appears to be a geographical variation in childhood fracture incidence. There was an almost 50% increased incidence in Northern Ireland, Scotland, Wales, and the north of England when compared with London and the southeast of England. This could be due to socioeconomic fractures, with a greater risk of accidents in lower social classes.[64]

Childhood fractures are a significant problem, and evidence is accumulating to suggest that bone fragility, as well as propensity to trauma, play an important role in their pathogenesis. Further work in this area may allow children with low bone mass to be identified in childhood and strategies put in place to reduce their risk of further fractures in later life.

CONCLUSION

Osteoporosis is a disease that has a huge effect on public health. The impact of osteoporotic fracture is massive, not just for individuals, but also for the health service, the economy, and the population as a whole. Strategies to reduce the burden of this widespread disease are thus urgently needed.

ACKNOWLEDGMENTS

We are grateful to the Medical Research Council, the Wellcome Trust, the Arthritis Research Campaign, the National Osteoporosis Society, and the Cohen Trust for support of our research program into the developmental origins of osteoporotic fracture. The manuscript was prepared by Mrs. G. Strange.

REFERENCES

1. Cooper C, Campion G, Melton LJ: Hip fractures in the elderly: a world-wide projection. Osteoporos Int 1992;2:285-289.
2. Anon: Consensus development conference: diagnosis, prophylaxis and treatment of osteoporosis. Am J Med 1993;941:646-650.
3. World Health Organization Study Group: Assessment of fracture risk and its application to screening for postmenopausal osteoporosis. 1994.
4. Johansen A, et al: Fracture incidence in England and Wales: a study based on the population of Cardiff. Injury 1997;28:655-660.
5. Cooper C, O'Neill T, Silman A: The epidemiology of vertebral fractures. Bone 1993;14:S89-S97.
6. van Staa TP, Dennison EM, Leufkens HG, Cooper C: Epidemiology of fractures in England and Wales. Bone 2001;29:517-522.
7. Incidence of vertebral fracture in Europe: results from the European Prospective Osteoporosis Study (EPOS). J Bone Miner Res 2002;17:716-724.
8. Cooper C, Atkinson EJ, O'Fallon WM, Melton LJ III: Incidence of clinically diagnosed vertebral fractures: a population-based study in Rochester, Minnesota, 1985-1989. J Bone Miner Res 1992;7:221-227.
9. Lauritzen JB, Schwarz P, Lund B, et al: Changing incidence and residual lifetime risk of common osteoporosis-related fractures. Osteoporos Int 1993;3:127-132.
10. Nevitt MC, Cummings SR: Type of fall and risk of hip and wrist fractures: the study of osteoporotic fractures. The Study of Osteoporotic Fractures Research Group. J Am Geriatr Soc 1993;41:1226-1234.
11. Melton LJ, Cooper C: Magnitude and impact of osteoporosis and fractures. In Marcus R, Feldman D, Kelsey J, eds: Osteoporosis, 2nd ed (Vol 1). San Diego, Academic Press, 2001:557-567.
12. Melton LJ: Epidemiology of fractures. In: Riggs BL, Melton LJ, eds: Osteoporosis: etiology, diagnosis and management. New York: Raven Press, 1995:133-154.
13. Chrischilles EA, Butler CD, Davis CS, Wallace RB: A model of lifetime osteoporosis impact. Arch Intern Med 1991;151:2026-2032.
14. Gallagher JC, Melton LJ, Riggs BL, Bergstrath E: Epidemiology of fractures of the proximal femur in Rochester, Minnesota. Clin Orthop 1980;150:163-171.
15. Winner SJ, Morgan CA, Evans JG: Perimenopausal risk of falling and incidence of distal forearm fracture. BMJ 1989;298:1486-1488.
16. Melton LJ III, Riggs BL: Risk factors for injury after a fall. Clin Geriatr Med 1985;1:525-539.

17. Marshall D, Johnell O, Wedel H: Meta-analysis of how well measures of bone mineral density predict occurrence of osteoporotic fractures. BMJ 1996;312:1254-1259.

18. Anderson DC: Osteoporosis in men. BMJ 1992;305:489-490.

19. Garton MJ, Reid DM: Osteoporosis in the 1990's: investigation and management. Hospital Update 1993;363-367.

20. Kanis JA, et al: International variations in hip fracture probabilities: implications for risk assessment. J Bone Miner Res 2002;17:1237-1244.

21. Solomon L: Bone density in ageing Caucasian and African populations. Lancet 1979;2:1326-1330.

22. Ross PD, Johnell O, De Laet C, et al: A comparison of hip fracture incidence among native Japanese, Japanese Americans, and American Caucasians. Am J Epidemiol 1991;133:801-809.

23. Tinetti ME, Speechley M, Ginter SF: Risk factors for falls among elderly persons living in the community. N Engl J Med 1988;319:1701-1707.

24. Cummings SR, Cauley JA, Palermo L, et al: Racial differences in hip axis lengths might explain racial differences in rates of hip fracture. Study of Osteoporotic Fractures Research Group. Osteoporos Int 1994;4:226-229.

25. Elffors I, Allander E, Kanis JA, et al: The variable incidence of hip fracture in southern Europe: the MEDOS Study. Osteoporos Int 1994;4:253-263.

26. Johnell O, Gullberg B, Allander E, Kanis JA: The apparent incidence of hip fracture in Europe: a study of national register sources. MEDOS Study Group. Osteoporos Int 1992;2:298-302.

27. Nagant DD, Devogelaer JP: Increase in the incidence of hip fractures and of the ratio of trochanteric to cervical hip fractures in Belgium. Calcif Tissue Int 1988;42:201-203.

28. Cooper C, Wickham C, Lacey RF, Barker DJ: Water fluoride concentration and fracture of the proximal femur. J Epidemiol Community Health 1990;44:17-19.

29. Jacobsen SJ, Goldberg J, Miles TP, et al: Regional variation in the incidence of hip fracture: US white women aged 65 years and older. JAMA 1990;264:500-502.

30. Royal College of Physicians: Fractured neck of femur: prevention and management. Summary and report of the Royal College of Physicians. J Roy Coll Physicians Lond 1989;23:8-12.

31. Albright F, Smith PH, Richardson AM: Postmenopausal osteoporosis: its clinical features. JAMA 1941;116:2465-2474.

32. Eastell R, Cedel SL, Wahner HW, et al: Classification of vertebral fractures. J Bone Miner Res 1991;6:207-215.

33. Black DM, Cummings SR, Stone K, et al: A new approach to defining normal vertebral dimensions. J Bone Miner Res 1991;6:883-892.

34. Cooper C, Atkinson EJ, Jacobsen SJ, et al: Population-based study of survival after osteoporotic fractures. Am J Epidemiol 1993;137:1001-1005.

35. Melton LJ III, Lane AW, Cooper C, et al: Prevalence and incidence of vertebral deformities. Osteoporos Int 1993;3:113-119.

36. O'Neill TW, et al: The prevalence of vertebral deformity in European men and women: the European Vertebral Osteoporosis Study. J Bone Miner Res 1996;11:1010-1018.

37. Ettinger B, et al: An examination of the association between vertebral deformities, physical disabilities and psychosocial problems. Maturitas 1988;10:283-296.

38. Ross PD, Ettinger B, Davis JW, et al: Evaluation of adverse health outcomes associated with vertebral fractures. Osteoporos Int 1991;1:134-140.

39. Browner WS, Seeley DG, Vogt TM, Cummings SR: Non-trauma mortality in elderly women with low bone mineral density. Study of Osteoporotic Fractures Research Group. Lancet 1991;338:355-358.

40. Johansson SJ, Gardsell P, Mellstrom,D, et al: Bone mineral measurment is a predictor of survival. Bone Miner 1992;17:166.

41. Oleksik A, et al: Health-related quality of life in postmenopausal women with low BMD with or without prevalent vertebral fractures. J Bone Miner Res 2000;15:1384-1392.

42. Ringe JD: Proceedings of the International Symposium on Osteoporosis Vol 2. Christiansen C, Johansen JS, Riggs BJ, eds. Copenhagen: Osteopress; 1987:1262-1264.

43. Kanis JA, McCloskey EV: Epidemiology of vertebral osteoporosis. Bone 1992;13(Suppl 2):S1-10.

44. Smith RW Jr, Rizek J: Epidemiologic studies of osteoporosis in women of Puerto Rico and southeastern Michigan with special reference to age, race, national origin and to other related or associated findings. Clin Orthop 1966;45:31-48.

45. Orimo H, Fujiwara S: Epidemiology of vertebral fracture in Asia. Spine 1994;8:13-21.

46. Schroder HM, Petersen KK, Erlandsen M: Occurrence and incidence of the second hip fracture. Clin Orthop 1993;289:166-169.

47. Cuddihy MT, Gabriel SE, Crowson CS, et al: Forearm fractures as predictors of subsequent osteoporotic fractures. Osteoporos Int 1999;9:469-475.

48. Ismail AA, Cockerell W, Cooper C, et al: Prevalent vertebral deformity predicts incident hip though not distal forearm fracture: results from the European Prospective Osteoporosis Study. Osteoporos Int 2001;12:85-90.

49. Lunt M, O'Neill TW, Felsenberg D: European Prospective Osteoporosis Study Group. Characteristics of prevalent vertebral deformity predict subsequent vertebral fracture: results from the European Prospective Osteoporosis Study (EPOS). Bone. 2003 Oct;33(4):505-513.

50. Lindsay R, Silverman SL, Cooper C, et al: Risk of new vertebral fracture in the year following a fracture. JAMA 2001;285:320-323.

51. Lunt M, O'Neil TW, Felsenberg D, et al: Characteristics of a prevalent vertebral deformity predict subsequent vertebral fracture: results from the European Prospective Osteoporosis Study (EPOS). Bone 2003;33:505-513.

52. Melton LJ III, Atkinson EJ, Cooper C, et al: Vertebral fractures predict subsequent fractures. Osteoporos Int 1999;10:214-221.

53. Cooper C, Atkinson EJ, Kotowicz M, et al: Secular trends in the incidence of postmenopausal vertebral fractures. Calcif Tissue Int 1992;51:100-104.

54. Bengner U, Johnell O, Redlund-Johnell I: Changes in incidence and prevalence of vertebral fractures during 30 years. Calcif Tissue Int 1988;42:293-296.

55. Hansen MA, Overgaard K, Goffredson A, Christiansen C: In: Christiansen C, Overgaard K, eds: Osteoporosis. Copenhagen: Osteopress, 1990:95.

56. Kaukonen JP, Karaharju EO, Porras M, et al: Functional recovery after fractures of the distal forearm: analysis of radiographic and other factors affecting the outcome. Ann Chir Gynaecol 1988;77:27-31.

57. Greendale GA, Silverman SL, Hays RD, et al: Health-related quality of life in osteoporosis clinical trials. The Osteoporosis Quality of Life Study Group. Calcif Tissue Int 1993;53:75-77.

58. Kaukonen JP, Karaharju EO, Porras M: Functional recovery after fractures of the distal forearm: analysis of radiographic and other factors affecting outcome. Ann Chir Gynaecol 1988;77:27-31.

59. O'Neill TW, Cooper C, Finn JD, et al: Incidence of distal forearm fracture in British men and women. Osteoporos Int 2001;12:555-558.

60. Melton LJ, Cooper C: Magnitude and impact of osteoporosis and fractures. In: Marcus R, Feldman D, Kelsey J, eds: Osteoporosis, 2nd ed (Vol 1). San Diego: Academic Press, 2001:557-567.

61. Department of Health: Advisory group on osteoporosis. Rockville, MD: US Department of Health, 1994.

62. Royal College of Physicians: Osteoporosis: clinical guidelines for prevention and treatment. London: Royal College of Physicians, 1999.

63. Cooper C: An overview of osteoporosis epidemiology. In: Kleerekoper M, ed. Drug therapy for osteoporosis. Oxon, Taylor & Francis, 2005:1-18.

64. Cooper C, Dennison EM, Leufkens HG, et al: Epidemiology of childhood fractures in Britain: a study using the general practice research database. J Bone Miner Res 2004;19: 1976-1981.

65. Landin LA: Epidemiology of children's fractures. J Pediatr Orthop B 1997;6:79-83.

66. Landin LA: Fracture patterns in children: analysis of 8,682 fractures with special reference to incidence, etiology and secular changes in a Swedish urban population 1950-1979. Acta Orthop Scand Suppl 1983;202:1-109.

67. Tiderius CJ, Landin L, Duppe H: Decreasing incidence of fractures in children: an epidemiological analysis of 1,673 fractures in Malmö, Sweden, 1993-1994. Acta Orthop Scand 1999;70:622-626.

68. Jones IE, Taylor RW, Williams SM, et al: Four-year gain in bone mineral in girls with and without past forearm fractures: a DXA study. Dual energy X-ray absorptiometry. J Bone Miner Res 2002;17:1065-1072.

2 The Genetics of Osteoporosis

Frances M.K. Williams and Tim D. Spector

SUMMARY

Osteoporosis is well known to be highly influenced by genetic factors. Bone mineral density (BMD)—its main risk factor—has also been shown to be highly heritable. Other known risk factors for osteoporotic fractures, such as reduced bone quality, femoral neck geometry, and bone turnover, are now also known to be heritable. Different approaches are currently being used to identify the many genes responsible, including linkage studies in humans and experimental animals as well as candidate gene studies and alterations in gene expression. Linkage studies have identified multiple quantitative trait loci (QTLs) for regulation of BMD and, along with twin studies, have indicated that the QTL effects are dependent both on the sex of the subject and on the site of osteoporosis. For the most part, the genes responsible for BMD regulation in these QTLs have not been identified. Many studies have used the candidate gene approach. The vitamin D receptor gene (*VDR*), the collagen type I alpha I gene (*COLIA1*), and the estrogen receptor gene alpha (*ER*) have been widely investigated and found to play roles in regulating BMD. Their effects, however, are modest and probably account together for less than 5% of the heritable contribution to BMD. The low-density lipoprotein receptor-related protein-5 (*LRP-5*) gene was identified by linkage and confirmed in association studies and has been shown to be physiologically important in the Wnt signaling pathway. Genes vary in their influence of particular intermediate phenotypes, and we know that not all genes influencing BMD will be important in fractures. Susceptibility to osteoporosis is mediated, in all likelihood, by multiple genes each having small effect. The number of genes involved in osteoporosis may be too great for us to understand precisely how they all work together, but their identification leads to greater understanding of the physiological pathways involved, pathways that could yield novel therapeutic targets.

OSTEOPOROSIS GENES AND THEIR IDENTIFICATION

Osteoporosis is a skeletal condition characterized by diminished bone mineral density and deterioration in bone microarchitecture. The main clinical endpoint is fracture. Genetic factors have long been recognized to play an important role in both osteoporosis and its associated phenotypes, which include bone mineral density (BMD), bone mass, broadband ultrasound attenuation, and velocity of sound, to name but a few. Twin and family studies have estimated that 50% to 85% of the variance in bone mass is genetically determined.[1-4] Similar studies have shown evidence of significant genetic effects on other determinants of fracture risk, including quantitative ultrasonographic properties of bone,[5] several aspects of femoral neck geometry,[5] muscle strength,[6] bone turnover markers,[7,8] body mass index,[9] and age at menopause.[10]

Unfortunately, there are few data describing the heritability of osteoporotic fracture, mainly because recruiting adequate numbers of subjects with fracture is difficult and expensive. Several studies have shown that a family history of fracture is a risk factor for fracture, independent of BMD.[11-14] One small twin study from Finland found identical twins to have only slightly higher rates of concordance for fracture than nonidentical twins,[15] suggesting that environmental factors are important. This illustrates the important difference between associated phenotypes, osteoporosis, and fracture: associated phenotypes have been found to be highly heritable but identifying the genes responsible does not necessarily identify genes for other associated phenotypes or, indeed, those influencing fracture. Another such example is that of genes influencing bone density and wrist fracture. A larger UK twin study than previously performed recently reported both wrist BMD and wrist fracture to be independently heritable. However, only a modest genetic overlap was found between BMD and velocity of sound properties of bone and genes influencing fracture.[16]

Several approaches are being employed currently in the search for genes that contribute to osteoporosis in the general population.[17] Rare monogenic conditions affecting bone have already been used to cast light on

Study	Locus	BMD	Affected Bone
Devoto et al. (1998)[31]	1p36	3.51	Hip
	2p23	2.29	Hip
	4q33	2.95	Hip
Nui et al. (1999)[33]	2p21	2.15	Wrist
Koller et al. (2000)[34]; Econs et al. (2004)[68]	1q21	3.86	Spine
	1q	3.6	Spine
	5q33	2.23	Hip
Karasik et al. (2002)[42]	6p21	2.93	Spine
	21q22	3.14	Hip
Wilson et al. (2003)[38]	3p21	2.7	Spine
	1p36	2.4	Hip
Styrkarsdottir et al. (2003)[39]	20p12	3.18	Hip
	20p12	2.89	Spine
Ralston et al. (2005)[40]	10q21	4.4	Hip in young men
	20q13	3.2	Spine in young women

TABLE 2-1 MAIN QUANTITATIVE TRAIT LOCI FINDINGS FOR BONE MINERAL DENSITY (BMD) IN HUMANS

genes that may influence population osteoporosis. Looking to the future, the most important approaches include candidate gene association studies and linkage studies. All three methods are discussed here (Table 2-1).

GENES OF RARE MONOGENIC DISEASES

Osteoporosis and fragility fractures are features of several rare monogenic diseases and provide an obvious place to start the search for genes influencing osteoporosis in the general population. Such conditions are not always informative, however. They include osteogenesis imperfecta, the osteoporosis-pseudoglioma syndrome, and syndromes associated with inactivating mutations of the estrogen receptor alpha and aromatase genes (Figure 2-1).

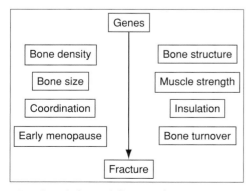

Figure 2-1. Genetic factors influencing fracture.

Osteogenesis imperfecta describes a heterogeneous group of monogenic disorders characterized by multiple bone fractures. Most forms of osteogenesis imperfecta are caused by mutations in the type I collagen genes COLIA1 and COLIA2. The genes that encode type I collagen have many different mutations, hence the heterogeneous nature of the disorder from mild to extremely severe. Osteoporosis-pseudoglioma syndrome is a rare, autosomal recessive disorder characterized by juvenile-onset osteoporosis and blindness due to persistent vascularization of the eye. Initial linkage studies mapped osteoporosis-pseudoglioma syndrome to chromosome 11q12-13.[18] Subsequent work showed the disease to be caused by inactivating mutations in the low-density lipoprotein-related receptor-5 (Lrp-5).[19] Another phenotype, autosomal dominant high-bone-mass, maps to the same region[20] and was reported independently to be caused by an activating mutation of the same receptor.[21] Osteoporosis has been reported in association with homozygous inactivating mutations of the estrogen receptor and aromatase genes, emphasizing the importance of estrogen in the attainment and maintenance of peak bone mass. Mutations in the latency-activating peptide domain of the transforming growth factor beta-1 gene are associated with Camurati-Engelmann disease, a condition characterized by increased BMD in the diaphysis of long bones.[22] Mutations of the TCIRG1 gene, which encodes a subunit of the osteoclast proton pump, have been shown to be responsible for the autosomal recessive condition osteopetrosis.[23]

The important question is whether the genetic clues obtained from these rare disorders cast any light on the problem of osteoporosis in the normal population. There is evidence that some do contribute to regulation of "normal" BMD. For example, lipoxygenase LRP-5 gene polymorphisms have been shown recently to be associated with bone mineral content, bone area, and stature, particularly in males.[24] Several groups have reported polymorphisms in the transforming growth factor beta gene to be associated with BMD and osteoporotic fracture,[25,26] and polymorphisms of the TCIRG1 genes (subunit of osteoclast proton pump) have been found to be associated with BMD in normal subjects.[27]

OTHER METHODS OF IDENTIFYING GENES IN OSTEOPOROSIS

Linkage Studies

Linkage disequilibrium refers to the phenomenon whereby genes lying close together tend to be inherited together. Evidence suggests that linkage disequilibrium is influenced greatly and variably by both the chromosomal region and the human population studied. It can extend to 350 Kb or further.[28] Using this effect, linkage studies are a well-validated method for the identification of genes responsible for monogenic diseases and have been used to identify chromosomal regions that harbor genes regulating quantitative traits such as bone mass. These regions are called quantitative trait loci (QTLs). An advantage of linkage-based studies is that they offer a way of identifying new molecular pathways that regulate bone metabolism. In addition, they are not influenced by population admixture. One disadvantage is that they have low statistical power to detect genes having modest effects on BMD. Studies thus require family samples of considerable size (several thousand) as well as an independent validation group.

Linkage Studies in Animals

Linkage studies in experimental animals have long been used in the identification of genes responsible for complex traits. This approach has several advantages: optimal control over the environment can be exercised, thereby minimizing the influence of confounding factors, and large numbers of progeny can be generated, providing suitable power. In addition, fine mapping of loci identified can be achieved using a technique known as *back-crossing*. The single most obvious disadvantage of such an approach is that the genes/loci regulating BMD in mice may not be influential in humans.

A recent study has combined genetic and genomic approaches in mice to provide evidence of a role for the *Alox15* gene. Previous studies by the same group had identified a region on mouse chromosome 11 as influencing peak BMD.[29] In the recent work, a congenic mouse model was constructed using the area of interest on chromosome 11 and shown to have increased BMD.[30] Microarray analysis identified *Alox15* as the differentially expressed gene that encodes 12/15 lipoxygenase (12/15-LO), and other studies confirmed that this overexpression had biological impact (increased expression of CD36 and reduced osteocalcin). A 12/15-LO knockout mouse model also confirmed the findings, as did pharmacological inhibitors of 15-lipoxygenase.[30] Work in humans has also shown linkage to a region on human chromosome 17 containing the genes for 12 and 15 lipoxygenase, raising hope that the findings in mice may be of direct relevance to human BMD regulation.[31]

Linkage Studies in Humans

Linkage studies in sibling pairs and extended families with osteoporosis have also been used to identify loci linked to BMD. Early studies identified loci on chromosomes 1p36, 2p23-p24, and 4q32-34,[31] with subsequent work in a second sample confirming linkage to the 1p36 locus.[32] Using a Chinese sample, a genome-wide search in for loci regulating forearm BMD[33] also revealed the highest LOD score at 2p23-24. Koller and coworkers conducted a whole genome search in a series of 595 healthy white and African-American female sibling pairs, finding LOD equal to +3.86 at chromosome 1q21-23[34] and an area suggestive of linkage at 5q33-35. Linkage studies in the same population identified multiple loci for regulation of femoral neck geometry on chromosomes 5q and 4q and 17q.[35] Karasik and colleagues[36] have reported a genome scan on 330 families (Framingham study) and identified several QTLs suggestive of linkage on chromosomes 6 and 20. Of interest, a subsequent analysis using the same population suggested that QTL-regulation of BMD differs between men and women, and different QTLs were found for the phenotypes peak bone mass and bone loss.[37] More recently, Wilson and colleagues[38] performed one of the largest linkage studies with 1100 dizygous UK twin pairs, defining two regions of suggestive linkage on chromosomes 1p36 and 3p21. Linkage to the 3p21 region was confirmed in a validation sample of 254 extreme discordant or concordant affected sibling pairs with low BMD.

Most linkage studies have used BMD as the associated phenotype of interest. In a recent study of Icelandic families, however, Styrkarsdottir and colleagues[39] used a novel classification system and detected significant linkage (LOD = 5.1) of osteoporosis to chromosome 20p12. They scored study participants as "affected" if they had reduced BMD (Z-score less than −1.0 at spine or hip) or if they had a history of fragility fractures, or if they were undergoing bisphosphonate treatment for osteoporosis. This Icelandic study also suggested linkage of spine and hip BMD to chromosome 20p12, with LOD scores of around +3.0 on the genome-wide scan and LOD scores of between +3.4 and +4.0 on fine mapping. Further analysis showed that part of the linkage signal was due to an association between osteoporosis and a polymorphism in the *BMP2* gene, which results in a serine-alanine amino acid change at codon 37. One of the largest studies to date was in a collection of 715 European families having probands with low BMD (The Famos study). Overall analysis revealed no significant linkage, but when age and gender subgroups were studied, several promising regions were identified including, in men, linkage to 10q21.[40] These now require independent replication in another sample.

Non-bone Mineral Density Linkage Studies

Other osteoporosis risk phenotypes have also been examined. Using ultrasonography to generate two associated phenotypes, broadband ultrasound attenuation, and velocity of sound, Wilson and associates[41] have performed a genome-wide screening of dizygous twin pairs using 737 highly polymorphic microsatellite markers. Evidence was found of linkage to chromosome 2q33-37 (broadband ultrasound attenuation, LOD 2.1-5.1) and 4q12-21 (velocity of sound, LOD 2.2-3.4). LOD scores greater than 2 were also identified on chromosomes 1, 2, 13, 14, and X. Similar work using the Framingham study sample showed quantitative ultrasonographic findings to be linked to chromosomal regions 1p36.1.[42] Subsequently, this group has used combined bone phenotypes to see if more information can be obtained. Using BMD and quantitative ultrasonography, they performed principal components analyses: linkage to 1q21.3 and 8q24.3 was found with the first prinicipal component (LODs 2.5, 2.4) and 1p36 was found with the second (LOD 2.1).[43]

Biochemical markers of bone turnover have previously been shown to be heritable and have recently been the subject of a large twin study.[44] A genome-wide scan was performed on levels of markers of bone formation (alkaline phosphatase, osteocalcin), bone resorption (urinary deoxypyridinoline corrected for urine creatinine), and calcium metabolism (parathyroid hormone). This revealed an area of significant linkage (LOD = 3.9) on chromosome 1 and area of suggestive linkage on chromosome 4 (LOD = 2.5). Of particular interest, the QTL on chromosome 1 had pleiotropic effects, acting to lower urinary deoxypyridinoline and increase serum parathyroid hormone. This study of 932 nonidentical female twin pairs has the advantage over other sibling pair studies of matching for age and sex. Both are important factors in bone metabolism and osteoporosis.

Given the polygenic nature of BMD regulation and osteoporosis susceptibility, most linkage studies performed to date have probably been underpowered, although the two large studies mentioned each included more than 1000 subjects.[38,39] Overall, results from different linkage studies show more discrepancy than agreement, probably because of the effects of using different study populations and differing criteria for subject enrollment. It is partly for these reasons and because of relatively easy access to clinical samples that association studies are becoming more widely used.

Candidate Gene Studies

Candidate gene studies are among the most widely used methods at present. Candidate gene association studies are fairly simple to perform and may have sufficient power to detect small allelic effects. They may be disadvantaged, however, by the effects of confounding factors and genetic heterogeneity as well as population stratification. Furthermore, demonstration of an association between a candidate gene and BMD does not necessarily mean that the gene is responsible for the effect observed, as there may be linkage disequilibrium with a nearby causal gene. The transmission disequilibrium test can help by testing candidate genes for both association and linkage.

Candidate genes investigated thus far have included genes influencing cytokines and growth factors that regulate bone turnover; genes that encode components of bone matrix; and genes that encode receptors for calciotropic hormones. Individual candidate genes that have been implicated in the regulation of bone mass or osteoporotic fractures have been reviewed elsewhere.[45] Recent advances in our knowledge are discussed in more detail here.

Vitamin D receptor

Vitamin D interacts with its receptor (VDR) to play an important role in calcium homeostasis by regulating bone cell growth and differentiation, intestinal calcium absorption, and parathyroid hormone secretion. The VDR was therefore a natural place to begin looking for genetic variation that might account for osteoporosis. The original finding that VDR alleles played a role in BMD is now more than 10 years old.[46] Since then, studies of VDR in relation to bone mass have been conflicting, and it is likely that the VDR genotype is associated with relatively modest effects on bone mass. Of interest, the relationship between VDR genotype and BMD is believed to be modulated by both calcium intake and vitamin D intake. Various different polymorphisms have been described, in different populations,[47,48] although the mechanisms by which these polymorphisms modulate VDR function remain unclear: Some 3′ polymorphisms may influence RNA stability, and isoforms of VDR encoded by different alleles may possess different functions.[47] In addition, there are data to suggest that an interaction between 5′ and 3′ polymorphisms is involved in regulating VDR function.

Type I collagen

The genes encoding type I collagen (COLIA1 and COLIA2) are important, well-studied candidates for the pathogenesis of osteoporosis. A common polymorphism affecting the transcription factor Sp1 binding site has been shown to have increased prevalence in osteoporosis patients.[49] Positive associations between the COLIA1 Sp1 polymorphism and bone mass or osteoporotic fractures were subsequently reported in several populations, and meta-analysis confirmed that the COLIA1 genotype conferred differences in BMD.[50] Ethnic differences have been reported in population prevalence of COLIA1 Sp1 alleles, with the polymorphism being common in white populations, but rare in Africans and Chinese.[51] Overall, the data suggest that the COLIA1 Sp1 polymorphism is a functional variant that has adverse effects on bone composition and mechanical strength. Haplotype analysis has shown that susceptibility to fracture is driven by the Sp1 polymorphism rather than other known polymorphisms at the *COLIA1* locus,[52] although it remains possible that hitherto unidentified polymorphisms in linkage disequilibrium with the Sp1 polymorphism contribute to the observed effects. From a clinical viewpoint, the *COLIA1* polymorphism may be of value, not as a therapeutic target but as a marker of osteoporotic fracture risk, because it predicts fractures independently of BMD as well as interacting with BMD to enhance fracture prediction.[53]

Estrogen receptors and aromatase genes

In view of the strong relationship between estrogen deficiency and bone loss, the estrogen receptor alpha (*ER*) gene has long been a strong candidate gene for osteoporosis. An association has been reported between a TA repeat polymorphism in the *ER* promoter and bone mass in both Japanese and US populations. Other investigators have reported positive associations between haplotypes defined by *PvuII* and *XbaI* polymorphisms in intron 1 of the *ER* gene and bone mass[54] as well as age at menopause.[55] The molecular mechanism by which these polymorphisms influence bone mass are as yet unclear, but a meta-analysis of the intron 1 polymorphisms indicated that the association with BMD and fracture is attributable mainly to variation at the *XbaI* site.[56] More recently, a large-scale study comprising eight European centers has attempted to answer the question more definitively using almost 19,000 subjects. Three common *ER* gene polymorphisms were studied, and none of the polymorphisms was shown to be associated with BMD. The absence of a Xba1 polymorphism recognition site conferred a risk reduction in all fractures of 19%, whereas the risk reduction for vertebral fractures was 35%. The effects on fracture were independent of BMD. Polymorphisms in *PvuII* and TA repeats did not appear to have any influence.[57]

Aromatase is the enzyme that converts androgens into estrogens, so it is likely to be of importance in bone metabolism in men and postmenopausal women. It is encoded by the *CYP19* gene. A recent study from Australia has shown the TTTA repeat polymorphism of *CYP19* to be associated with higher circulating estrodiol, higher BMD at the hip and lumbar spine, and lower markers of bone turnover in more than 1200 women aged 70 years or older.[58] Similar findings have also been reported in elderly Italian men.[59]

Other genes

Polymorphisms in several other candidate genes have been associated with bone mass and/or osteoporotic fracture including transforming growth factor beta-1 and the interleukin-6 locus. The effects of these polymorphisms on interleukin-6 function are yet to be determined. Two studies have looked at the possible associations between apolipoprotein E alleles and

osteoporosis, but again the mechanisms by which apolipoprotein E alleles influence susceptibility to osteoporosis are also unclear. Two groups have reported an association between a coding polymorphism of the calcitonin receptor gene and BMD. The osteocalcin gene has been found to be associated and linked to BMD and bone quality.[60] Other candidate genes that have been studied in relation to BMD include parathyroid hormone, the androgen receptor, aromatase, osteoprotegerin, Klotho, and the interleukin-1 receptor antagonist. Most of these have not been consistently replicated. A list of recent associations is given in Table 2-2.

TABLE 2-2 CANDIDATE GENES IMPLICATED IN OSTEOPOROSIS		
Biological Classification	Candidate Gene	Chromosome Location
Calciotropic hormones and receptors	VDR	12q12-14
	ER-α	6q25
	ER-β	14q22-24
	CT	11p15
	CTR	7q21
	PTH	11p15
	PTHR1	3p22-21
	CYP19	15q21
	GCCR	5q31
	CASR	3q13-21
	AR	Xq11-12
Cytokines, growth factors, and receptors	TGF-β1	19q13
	IL-6	7p21
	IGF-1	12q22-24
	IL-1RA	2q14
	OPG	8q24
	TNF-α	6p21
	TNFR2	1p36
Bone matrix proteins	COL1A1	17q21-22
	COL1A2	7q22
	BGP	1q25-31
	MGP	12p13-12
	AHSG	3q27
Miscellaneous	ApoE	19q13
	MTHFR	1p36
	P57(KIP2)	11p15
	HLA-A	6p21
	PPAR-γ	3p25
	FRA-1	11q13
	RUNX-2	6p21
	Klotho gene	13q12
	WRN (Werner syndrome gene)	8p12-11
	LRP-5	11q12-13

Adapted from Lui et al.,[45] with acknowledgments and thanks to Drs Lui and Deng.

Gene-Gene and Gene-Environment Interactions

In addition to the study of single genes or polymorphisms in isolation, it has been realized that both gene-gene and gene-environment interactions play an important role in the variation of expression of complex traits such as osteoporosis.

A Dutch study of 1000 postmenopausal women looked at the effects of a combination of both the G-to-A polymorphism in the *COL1A1* Sp1 binding site and the "baT" haplotype of VDR. The investigators found a significant interaction between the genotypes, both being independent of the effect of BMD.[61] The Danish Osteoporosis Prevention Study recently reported the influence of polymorphisms within the *CYP19* and androgen receptor genes in almost 1800 newly postmenopausal women who were randomized to receive estrogen replacement therapy or no treatment.[62] Although perimenopausal bone loss was not associated with either gene's polymorphisms, the BMD response over 5 years to estrogen was influenced by genotype: one *CYP19* allele was associated with significantly greater response. Although the androgen receptor genotype was not related to BMD, a modifying effect of sex hormone–binding globulin was observed. Thus, in the highest quartile of sex hormone–binding globulin, androgen receptor genotype was associated with baseline BMD.

These types of study emphasize the importance of both gene-gene and gene-environment interactions and highlight once again the need for large, usually multicenter, studies to recruit sufficient numbers of subjects to enable well-powered studies to be performed. They also raise the issue of multiple testing, which may give rise to spurious positive findings unless it is taken into account in the interpretation of the data.

Gene Expression Studies

A novel approach to the question of osteoporosis genes is that involving gene expression studies. In this type of study, differences in gene expression are explored in tissues derived from subjects having and not having the trait of interest. Very much greater power is obtained if the genetic background of the trait-discordant subjects is similar, or the same as in the case of identical twins. One small study has used osteoblast-like cultures from two pairs of monozygotic twins discordant for BMD and one concordant pair. Genome-wide gene expression of the cell culture derived from bone marrow aspirates suggests that the following genes were differentially expressed: chondroitin beta 1,4 *N*-acetylgalactosaminyltransferase, inhibin beta A, IL-1β, and colony stimulating factor 1 macrophage.[63] These genes are known to play a part in bone physiology. Although the numbers studied were small, this study highlights both the potential of the emerging new technology for examining gene expression and the further benefits that may be derived from the twin registers in a number of countries, by providing informative subjects willing to take part in such studies.

Pooling Studies

Another newer method being used to increase the power and cost-effectiveness of studies of osteoporosis is that of pooling. This type of association study contrasts DNA pools from several hundred subjects with and without the trait of interest, for example BMD. One such study has examined 25,000 SNPs in 16,000 genes from women with high and low BMD. To compensate for the loss of power with multiple testing, the findings were verified by individual genotyping in two further case control groups. The differences in allele frequency between the two trait expression groups suggested a candidate locus in the phosphodiesterase 4D gene (*PDE4D*) on chromosome 5q12. This was fine-mapped using 80 SNPs within 50 kB of the marker SNP.[64] This study also produced evidence in support of the association with the Ser37Val polymorphism in *BMP2,* a gene known to interact with *PDE4D* (and implicated in Icelandic studies). These data illustrate the potential of these methods, particularly when used in conjunction, and also highlight the need for replication in at least two further independent samples.

Overlapping Phenotypes

In addition to the associated phenotypes and traits that can be used as surrogates of the main clinical outcome of interest, other bone diseases may also shed light on genes of importance in osteoporosis. Studies have shown that perhaps 30% of genes involved in bone metabolism overlap with those influencing osteoarthritis, a condition affecting bone as well as cartilage. Genes believed to be common to both include the *VDR*, the *COL1A1*, and possibly the *ER* genes.[65] A recent example of an association study of osteoarthritis progression by Valdes and colleagues[66] implicated several bone genes such as *BMP2* and genes involved in inflammation. Cytokines have been found, somewhat surprisingly, to be associated with chronic diseases such as disc degeneration[67] that hitherto have been considered noninflammatory. With the finding that the *LRP-5* gene is associated with osteoporosis comes the realization that genes controlling pathways such as lipid metabolism and inflammation may be important in so-called noninflammatory bone conditions. Thus, the range of potential candidate genes is growing considerably larger, and genetic researchers increasingly need to cross traditional disease boundaries.

FUTURE WORK

What direction is work into identification of osteoporosis genes likely to take? At present, some argue, lines of investigation are driven not by scientific rationale but by technology and the increasing availability of new assay techniques handling ever larger numbers of polymorphisms. Although the estimated number of human genes continues to fall (currently around 23,000), the number of recognized SNPs is increasing, with more than 30,000 known nonsynonymous SNPs. The possibility of testing samples for more than 500,000 validated SNPs at a future cost of less than 1 US cent per SNP beckons. The new technology will enable increasingly large panels of polymorphisms, as well as gene expression levels and, in the future, proteins and metabolic profiles, to be studied simultaneously. Funding for future work should be prioritized for those studies that have sufficient power to answer the question being addressed, although the increasing problems of multiple testing and the difficulties in having large numbers of replicate clinical cohorts will make the task no less difficult.[17]

In conclusion, osteoporosis is a good example of a complex genetic trait. The associated phenotypes studied thus far have heritabilities of 50% to 80% and a large number of genes are likely to be involved in its pathogenesis. Several candidate genes have been identified, but their individual effects are small. Many genome-wide linkage scans have been performed, but other than for *LRP-5*, the results are inconsistent, highlighting some of the difficulties in pinpointing the genes and suggesting that to maximize the chances of gene discovery, a full range of phenotypes and methods will need to be utilized.

REFERENCES

1. Pocock NA, Eisman JA, Hopper JL, et al: Genetic determinants of bone mass in adults: a twin study. J Clin Invest 1987;80:706-10.
2. Smith DM, Nance WE, Kang KW, et al: Genetic factors in determining bone mass. J Clin Invest 1973;52:2800-8.
3. Gueguen R, Jouanny P, Guillemin F, et al: Segregation analysis and variance components analysis of bone mineral density in healthy families. J Bone Miner Res 1995;12:2017-22.
4. Krall EA, Dawson-Hughes B: Heritable and life-style determinants of bone mineral density. J Bone Miner Res 1993;8:1-9.
5. Arden NK, Baker J, Hogg C, et al: The heritability of bone mineral density, ultrasound of the calcaneus and hip axis length: a study of postmenopausal twins. J Bone Miner Res 1996;11:530-34.
6. Arden NK, Spector TD: Genetic influences on muscle strength, lean body mass, and bone mineral density: a twin study. J Bone Miner Res 1997;12:2076-81.
7. Hunter D, de Lange M, Snieder H, et al: Genetic contribution to bone metabolism, calcium excretion, and vitamin D and parathyroid hormone regulation. J Bone Miner Res 2001;16:371-78.
8. Garnero P, Arden NK, Griffiths G, et al: Genetic influence on bone turnover in postmenopausal twins. J Clin Endocrinol Metab 1996;81:140-46.
9. Kaprio J, Rimpela A, Winter T, et al: Common genetic influences on BMI and age at menarche. Hum Biol 1995;67:739-53.
10. Snieder H, MacGregor AJ, Spector TD: Genes control the cessation of a woman's reproductive life: a twin study of hysterectomy and age at menopause. J Clin Endocrinol Metab 1998;83:1875-80.
11. Torgerson DJ, Campbell MK, Thomas RE, Reid DM: Prediction of perimenopausal fractures by bone mineral density and other risk factors. J Bone Miner Res 1996;11:293-97.
12. Cummings SR, Nevitt MC, Browner WS, et al: Risk factors for hip fracture in white women. Study of Osteoporotic Fractures Research Group. N Engl J Med 1995;332:767-73.
13. Keen RW, Hart DJ, Arden NK, et al: Family history of appendicular fracture and risk of osteoporosis: a population-based study. Osteoporosis Int 1999;10:161-66.
14. Deng HW, Chen WM, Recker S, et al: Genetic determination of Colles' fracture and differential bone mass in women with and without Colles' fracture. J Bone Miner Res 2000;15:1243-52.
15. Kannus P, Palvanen M, Kaprio J, et al: Genetic factors and osteoporotic fractures in elderly people: prospective 25 year follow up of a nationwide cohort of elderly Finnish twins. Br Med J 1999;319:1334-37.
16. Knapp KM, Andrew T, MacGregor AJ, et al: An investigation of unique and shared gene effects on speed of sound and bone density using axial transmission quantitative ultrasound and DXA in twins. J Bone Miner Res 2003;18:1525-30.
17. Huang Q-Y, Recker RR, Deng H-W: Searching for osteoporosis genes in the post-genome era: progress and challenges. Osteoporos Int 2003;14:701-715.
18. Gong Y, Vikkula M, Boon L, et al: Osteoporosis-pseudoglioma syndrome, a disorder affecting skeletal strength and vision, is assigned to chromosome region 11q12-13. Am J Hum Genet 1998;1996:146-51.
19. Gong Y, Slee RB, Fukai N, et al: LDL receptor-related protein 5 (LRP5) affects bone accrual and eye development. Cell 2001;107:513-23.
20. Johnson ML, Gong G, Kimberling W, et al: Linkage of a gene causing high bone mass to human chromosome 11 (11q12-13). Am J Hum Genet 1997;60:1326-32.
21. Little RD, Carulli JP, Del Mastro RG, et al: A mutation in the LDL receptor-related protein 5 gene results in the autosomal dominant high-bone-mass trait. Am J Hum Genet 2002;70:11-9.
22. Janssens K, Gershoni-Baruch R, Guanabens N, et al: Mutations in the gene encoding the latency-associated peptide of TGF-beta 1 cause Camurati-Engelmann disease. Nat Genet 2000;26:273-75.
23. Sobacchi C, Frattini A, Orchard P, et al: The mutational spectrum of human malignant autosomal recessive osteopetrosis. Hum Mol Genet 2001;10:1767-73.
24. Ferrari SL, Deutsch S, Choudhury U, et al: Polymorphisms in the low-density lipoprotein receptor-related protein-5 (LRP5) gene are associated with variation in vertebral bone mass, vertebral bone size and stature in whites. Am J Hum Genet 2004;74:866-875.
25. Langdahl BL, Carstens M, Stenkjaer L, Eriksen EF: Polymorphisms in the transforming growth factor beta 1 gene and osteoporosis. Bone 2003;32:297-310.
26. Keen RW, Snieder H, Molloy H, et al: Evidence of association and linkage disequilibrium between a novel polymorphism in the transforming growth factor beta 1 gene and hip bone mineral density: a study of female twins. Rheumatology (Oxford) 2001;40:48-54.
27. Sobacchi C, Vezzoni P, Reid DM, et al: Association between a polymorphism affecting an AP1 binding site in the promoter of the TCIRG1 gene and bone mass in women. Calcif Tissue Int 2004;74:35-41.
28. Reich DE, Cargill M, Bolk S, et al: Linkage disequilibrium in the human genome. Nature 2001;411:199-204.
29. Klein RF, Mitchell SR, Phillips TJ, et al: Genetic analysis of bone mass in mice. J Bone Miner Res 1998;13:1648-56.

30. Klein RF, Allard J, Avnur Z, et al: Regulation of bone mass in mice by the lipoxygenase gene Alox15. Science 2004;303:229-232.

31. Devoto M, Shimoya K, Caminis J, et al: First-stage autosomal genome screen in extended pedigrees suggests genes predisposing to low bone mineral density on chromosomes 1p, 2p and 4q. Eur J Hum Genet 1998;6:151-57.

32. Devoto M, Specchia C, Li HH, et al: Variance component linkage analysis indicates a QTL for femoral neck bone mineral density on chromosome 1p36. Hum Mol Genet 2001;10:2447-52.

33. Nui T, Chen C, Cordell H, et al: A genome-wide scan for loci linked to forearm bone mineral density. Human Genetics 1999;104:226-33.

34. Koller DL, Econs MJ, Morin PA, et al: Genome screen for QTLs contributing to normal variation in bone mineral density and osteoporosis. J Clin Endocrinol Metab 2000;85:3116-20.

35. Koller DL, Liu G, Econs MJ, et al: Genome screen for quantitative trait loci underlying normal variation in femoral structure. J Bone Miner Res 2001;16:985-91.

36. Karasik D, Myers RH, Cupples LA, et al: Genome screen for quantitative trait loci contributing to normal variation in bone mineral density: the Framingham Study. J Bone Miner Res 2002;17:1718-27.

37. Karasik D, Cupples LA, Hannan MT, Kiel DP: Age, gender, and body mass effects on quantitative trait loci for bone mineral density: the Framingham Study. Bone 2003;33:308-16.

38. Wilson SG, Reed PW, Bansal A, et al: Comparison of genome screens for two independent cohorts provides replication of suggestive linkage of bone mineral density to 3p21 and 1p36. Am J Hum Genet 2003;72:144-55.

39. Styrkarsdottir U, Cazier J-B, Kong A, et al: Linkage of osteoporosis to chromosome 20p12 and association to BMP2. Public Library Sci Biol 2003;1:1-9.

40. Ralston SH, Galwey N, MacKay I, et al: Loci for regulation of bone mineral density in men and women identified by genome wide linkage scan: the FAMOS study. Hum Mol Genet 2005;14:943-51.

41. Wilson SG, Reed PW, Andrew T, et al: A genome-screen of a large twin cohort reveals linkage for quantitative ultrasound of the calcaneus to 2q33-37 and 4q12-21. J Bone Miner Res 2004;19:270-77.

42. Karasik D, Myers RH, Hannan MT, et al: Mapping of quantitative ultrasound of the calcaneus bone to chromosome 1 by genome-wide linkage analysis. Osteoporos Int 2002;13:796-802.

43. Karasik D, Cupples LA, Hannan MT, Kiel DP: Genome screen for a combined bone phenotype using principal component analysis: the Framingham study. Bone 2004;34:547-56.

44 Andrew T, Wilson S, Swaminathan R, Spector TD: A genome-wide screen for the genetic regulation of bone turnover and calcium metabolism in healthy dizygotic female twins shows evidence for linkage on chromosomes 1 and 4. J Bone Miner Res 2005; Jan; 20(1):67-74.

45. Liu YZ, Liu YJ, Recker RR, Deng HW: Molecular studies of identification of genes for osteoporosis: the 2002 update. J Endocrinol 2003;177:147-96.

46. Morrison NA, Qi JC, Tokita A, et al: Prediction of bone density from vitamin D receptor alleles. Nature 1994;367:284-87.

47. Arai H, Miyamoto K-I, Taketani Y, et al: A vitamin D receptor gene polymorphism in the translation initiation codon: effect on protein activity and relation to bone mineral density in Japanese women. J Bone Miner Res 1997;12:915-21.

48. Arai H, Miyamoto KI, Yoshida M, et al: The polymorphism in the caudal-related homeodomain protein Cdx-2 binding element in the human vitamin D receptor gene. J Bone Miner Res 2001;16:1256-64.

49. Grant SFA, Reid DM, Blake G, et al: Reduced bone density and osteoporosis associated with a polymorphic Sp1 site in the collagen type I alpha 1 gene. Nat Genet 1996;14:203-5.

50. Mann V, Hobson EE, Li B, et al: A COL1A1 Sp1 binding site polymorphism predisposes to osteoporotic fracture by affecting bone density and quality. J Clin Invest 2001;107:899-907.

51. Beavan S, Prentice A, Dibba B, et al: Polymorphism of the collagen type I alpha 1 gene and ethnic differences in hip-fracture rates. N Engl J Med 1998;339:351-52.

52. McGuigan FE, Reid DM, Ralston SH: Susceptibility to osteoporotic fracture is determined by allelic variation at the Sp1 site, rather than other polymorphic sites at the COL1A1 locus. Osteoporos Int 2000;11:338-43.

53. McGuigan FEA, Armbrecht G, Smith R, et al: Prediction of osteoporotic fractures by bone densitometry and COLIA1 genotyping: a prospective, population-based study in men and women. Osteoporos Int 2001;12:91-96.

54. Kobayashi S, Inoue S, Hosoi T, et al: Association of bone mineral density with polymorphism of the estrogen receptor gene. J Bone Miner Res 1996;11:306-11.

55. Weel AE, Uitterlinden AG, Westendorp IC, et al: Estrogen receptor polymorphism predicts the onset of natural and surgical menopause. J Clin Endocrinol Metab 1999;84:3146-50.

56. Ioannidis JP, Stavrou I, Trikalinos TA, et al: Association of polymorphisms of the estrogen receptor alpha gene with bone mineral density and fracture risk in women: a meta-analysis. J Bone Miner Res 2002;17:2048-60.

57. Ioannidis JP, Ralston SH, Bennett ST, et al: Differential genetic effects of ESR1 gene polymorphisms on osteoporosis outcomes. JAMA 2004;292:2105-14.

58. Dick IM, Devine A, Prince RL: Association of an aromatase TTTA repeat polymorphism with circulating estrogen, bone structure and biochemistry in older women. Am J Physiol Endocrinol Metab 2004; Epub ahead of print.

59. Gennari L, Masi L, Merlotti D, et al: A polymorphic CYP19 TTTA repeat influences aromatase activity and estrogen levels in elderly men: effects on bone metabolism. J Clin Endocrinol Metab 2004;89:2803-10.

60. Andrew T, Mak YT, Reed P, et al: Linkage and association for bone mineral density and heel ultrasound measurements with a simple tandem repeat polymorphism near the osteocalcin gene in female dizygotic twins. Osteoporos Int 2002;13:745-54.

61. Uitterlinden AG, Weel AE, Burger H, et al: Interaction between the vitamin D receptor gene and collagen type I alpha 1 gene in susceptibility for fracture. J Bone Miner Res 2001;16:379-85.

62. Tofteng CL, Kindmark A, Brandstrom H, et al: Polymorphisms in the CYP19 and AR genes: relation to bone mass and longitudinal bone changes in postmenopausal women with or without hormone replacement therapy. The Danish Osteoporosis Prevention Study. Calcif Tissue Int 2004;74:25-34.

63. Mak YT, Hampson G, Beresford JN, Spector TD: Variations in genome-wide gene expression in identical twins: a study of primary osteoblast-like culture from female twins discordant for osteoporosis. BMC Genetics 2004;5:14.

64. Reneland RH, Mah S, Kammerer S, et al: Association between a variation in the phosphodiesterase 4D gene and bone mineral density. BMC Genetics 2005;Mar 7;6:9.

65. Spector TD, MacGregor AJ: Risk factors for osteoarthritis: genetics. Osteoarthritis Cartilage 2004;12(Suppl A):S39-44.

66. Valdes AM, Hart DJ, Jones KA, et al: Association study of candidate genes for the prevalence and progression of knee osteoarthritis. Arthritis Rheum 2004;50:2497-507.

67. Valdes AM, Hassett G, Hart DJ, Spector TD: Radiographic progression of lumbar spine disc degeneration is influenced by variation at inflammatory genes: a candidate SNP association study in the Chingford cohort. Spine 2005;30:2445-2451.

68. Econs MJ, Koller DL, Hui SL, et al: Confirmation of linkage to chromosome 1q for peak vertebral bone mineral density in premenopausal white women. Am J Hum Genet 2004;74:223-28.

3 Relevance of Peak Bone Mass to Osteoporosis and Fracture Risk in Later Life

Graeme Jones

OSTEOPOROSIS AND FRACTURES

Fractures in later life due to osteoporosis are a significant public health problem. Bone mass assessed by densitometry has consistently been identified as a major predictor of these fractures.[1] Bone mass in later life is a function of bone mass developed in younger life and bone loss in later life. Certainly, prevention of fractures in later life by increasing peak bone mass is an attractive concept from a public health viewpoint. This chapter reviews the evidence relating peak bone mass to osteoporosis and fracture in later life.

DEFINITION AND TIMING OF PEAK BONE MASS

Peak bone mass is a difficult concept to define. Conceptually, peak bone "strength" is the time at which skeletal strength is maximal during life. However, strength can be estimated only in living subjects. Bone mass assessed by densitometry is a reasonable surrogate for bone strength, as it explains a large percentage of the variation in bone breaking strength.[2] The timing of peak bone mass varies by site and sex. The best estimates suggest age 16 in females and age 20 in males for the hip and spine, with a peak sometime during the third decade for the total body.[3] Bone loss appears to start premenopausally in women, but studies are lacking in men. In contrast, different estimates apply for bone size, which appears to increase throughout life at a number of sites.

In 1973, Dent stated that senile osteoporosis is a pediatric disease.[4] There is no direct high-quality evidence to support this statement, as such a study would need to be at least 50 years in duration with good measures of bone mass, which will not be feasible for many years given that dual x-ray absorptiometry scanners only became available in the late 1980s. There is, however, indirect evidence from a number of studies to support this proposition in a number of areas (Figure 3-1).

1. The genetic effect on bone mass is primarily on bone development.
2. Bone mass tracks throughout life.
3. Exposures during childhood have been related to bone development, and some of these have an ongoing effect on either bone mass or fractures in later life.

It should be noted that these studies are largely observational, and the cross-sectional data, in particular, are subject to potential bias. Their conclusions need to be confirmed in longitudinal studies.

Direct Studies of Contribution of Peak Bone Mass to Bone Mass and Fracture in Later Life

Shorter term studies have estimated the contribution of peak bone mass to bone mass in later life. There have been five studies of this issue.[5-9] One studied

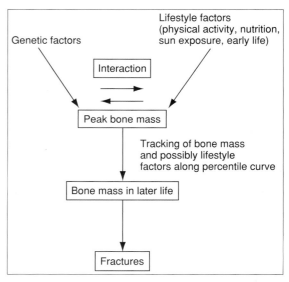

Figure 3-1. Conceptual pathways illustrating importance of peak bone mass for osteoporosis and fracture in later life.

women at the time of menopause and followed them for 12 years for bone mass[5] and 15 years for fracture.[6] From these studies, it can be estimated that bone mass prior to menopause contributed about three-quarters of bone mass 12 years after menopause and that bone mass and bone loss over 15 years contributed equally and significantly to fracture risk. In the second study, Hui and colleagues[7] modeled the contribution of bone mass and bone loss from a population-based cross-sectional and longitudinal dataset and concluded that bone mass prior to age 70 and subsequent bone loss contributed equally to bone mass in later life, implying a much smaller contribution from peak bone mass. The other two studies used computer modeling rather than actual datasets. Horsman and Burkinshaw[8] estimated that two-thirds of fracture risk in later life was related to variation in peak bone mass, whereas Hernandez and colleagues[9] concluded that peak bone mass was the major contributor to bone mass in later life when compared with menopausal and age-related bone loss. Thus, although these studies are consistent with regard to peak bone mass having a substantial influence on bone mass and fracture risk in later life, they conflict with regard to the magnitude of this effect. The observational studies are likely to underestimate the contribution of peak bone mass because of the relatively short follow-up period, suggesting that computer modeling approaches may be more robust even though such exercises are prone to a number of biases, particularly in terms of assumptions.

Genetic Effect on Bone Development as It Affects Bone Mass

There are many studies documenting a strong genetic contribution to bone mass.[10-15] Estimates are generally higher for twin studies as compared with family studies, which may reflect some well-documented limitations of the twin model in regard to shared environment.[10] Clearly, this effect is most marked for peak bone mass and appears to peak at age 26.[14] There are lesser contributions to bone loss, which may again reflect the dilutional effect of measurement error on heritability from short-term studies. Given this finding, the genetic effect on fracture should be strong, but twin studies have been inconclusive to date.[13] This may partly be due to methodological issues such as power and fracture definition or may reflect the strong additional contribution of falls to fracture risk. Interestingly, in a novel family study, Seeman and colleagues[11] described a deficit in femoral (but not spine) bone mass in the daughters of women with hip fractures, which directly implicates peak bone mass in fracture etiology through genetic mechanisms.

Evidence that Bone Mass Tracks Throughout Life

The hypothesis that bone mass tracks throughout life stems from the original observation that the population variance of bone mass does not increase in later life.[16] If bone loss were independent of bone acquisition, then the variance should increase over time. Many short-term studies over 1 to 2 years have documented very high correlations between initial and follow-up bone mass. The longest studies have confirmed this in women over 15 years[6] and children over 2 years.[17]

Furthermore, a single bone density reading (measured by technology that is now regarded as outdated) has good predictive value for fracture up to 25 years later.[18] The strength of association did decrease over time but was similar to that obtained in studies with much shorter follow-up,[1] which is intriguing given the radial site of measurement and the higher measurement error. The concept of fast and slow losers appears conceptually opposite to these findings, as tracking would imply that each person closely follows their percentile band throughout life. However, most studies suggest that bone loss is normally distributed and a substantial amount of the variation can be explained by measurement error and regression to the mean rather than crossing of percentile curves. Lastly, low bone mass in childhood is linked with an increased risk for fractures of the distal forearm,[19,20] and women who report these fractures also have a deficit in bone mass in later life,[21] supporting the tracking concept.

Childhood Exposures Related to Bone Development and Ongoing Effect on Bone Mass and Fractures in Later Life

Physical activity

There is no doubt that physical activity in younger life is associated with substantial gains in bone mass, especially in the prepubertal years.[22] However, the evidence that this protects against fracture in later life is much less convincing. In part, this is due to issues of the design of the studies, which are generally retrospective, prone to recall and survivor bias, and use measurement tools of uncertain and questionable validity. The effects of these factors will be to decrease the magnitude of association. Only some of the gain in bone mass is retained after cessation of the activity,[23,24] suggesting that physical activity may need to be a lifelong pattern to lead to fracture protection. A number of observational studies have documented that physical activity during younger life does seem to confer protection against hip fracture in particular, with less convincing evidence for vertebral and wrist fractures.[25] No studies have had sufficient sample size to assess whether the effect of early life exercise is independent of later life exercise or represents lifelong behavior. Most authorities would accept that lifelong physical activity will protect against fractures in later life even if it increases fracture risk in younger life,[26,27] and a randomized controlled trial of this question is not feasible.

Nutrition

There have been numerous trials of calcium supplementation in children. These have consistently shown a beneficial effect that is generally small in magnitude. This benefit is mostly lost on cessation of calcium supplementation,[28,29] implying that lifetime continuation of high intakes is required for any potential benefit. Milk intake has also been shown to be beneficial in adolescent girls and may be associated with a long-term gain in bone mass based on observational evidence.[30,31] The Medos study reported that calcium intake in earlier life was less important for hip fracture risk than calcium intake in later life.[32,33] The role of other nutrients is uncertain at this time, although maternal diet during pregnancy (specifically phosphorus, protein, magnesium, and fat) and breastfeeding for up to three months have been linked to gains in bone mass in the breastfed children 8 years later.[34,35] There has been recent interest in fruit and vegetables and bone health in children, but research is at a very early stage.[36]

Hormonal factors

Anorexia nervosa has been associated with a long-term increase in fracture risk.[37] This is likely to be due to impaired menstruation, low body weight, and poor nutrition. There have also been a number of studies linking late menarche and/or years of menstruation to bone mass and fracture risk in later life.[38]

Sunlight and vitamin D

Relatively few studies have been undertaken in the area of sunlight and vitamin D as related to bone mass and fracture risk. The MEDOS study reported quite strong associations between sun exposure and hip fracture risk in both men and women in later life.[32,33] In women, but not in men, the odds ratios were stronger for childhood and young adulthood than later life, which is surprising given the likely diluting effect of variations in long-term recall and strongly suggests exposure at early life is more important. This effect may be through bone mass or falls risk. The available studies support the former. Vitamin D levels in cord blood have been linked with bone mass in the children 9 years later, whereas vitamin D supplementation in the first year of life also is associated with higher bone mass at age 8,[39] and winter sun exposure is associated with bone mass in prepubertal children in Tasmania, especially females.[40] Furthermore, vitamin D levels have been linked with bone turnover and density in both male and female children.[41,42] Vitamin D deficiency may also explain the association between growth velocity during childhood and hip fracture risk in later life in a Finnish cohort.[43] There have been many recent studies documenting low levels of vitamin D in children and ensuring sufficiency would appear to be a safe and desirable current health priority.

Other early life exposures

Birth weight has been linked to later bone mass in a number of studies.[44-46] This has also been linked positively to fracture risk in childhood[47] but not in later life to date. This effect may be mediated by genetic factors.[46] Smoking in utero has been reported to reduce bone mass in neonates[48] and in 8-year-old children.[49] This effect was mediated through placental function, suggesting that smoking may program later bone responses. Smoking in utero has not been associated with fracture risk in children,[47,50] but there have been no studies relating it to peak bone mass or fractures in later life.

Injury

Fractures in childhood have been associated with a deficit in bone mass in later life. This may be due to immobilization associated with the fracture event, such as femoral shaft fractures,[51] or may reflect an increased risk of fracture in childhood associated with lower bone mass, such as for wrist and forearm fractures,[21] even though the deficit in later life was somewhat larger than that observed around the time of the fracture event.

CONCLUSIONS

Taken as a whole, the current observational data make a compelling case that peak bone mass is of major relevance to osteoporosis and risk for fractures in later life. A better understanding of peak bone strength, its determinants, and how to measure it are research priorities.

REFERENCES

1. Marshall D, Johnell O, Wedel H: Meta-analysis of how well measures of bone mineral density predict occurrence of osteoporotic fracture. BMJ 1996;312:1254-59.
2. Jarvinen TL, Sievanen H, Kannus P, et al: Dual-energy X-ray absorptiometry in predicting mechanical characteristics of rat femur. Bone 1998;22:551-58.
3. Bonjour JP, Theintz G, Law F, et al: Peak bone mass. Osteoporos Int 4 1994;S1:7-13.
4. Dent CE: Keynote address: problems in metabolic bone disease. In: Frame B, Parfitt MA, Duncan H, eds: Clinical aspects of metabolic bone disease. Amsterdam: Excerpta Medica, 1973:1-6.
5. Hansen MA, Overgaard K, Riis BJ, et al: Role of peak bone mass and bone loss in postmenopausal osteoporosis: 12 year study. BMJ 1991;303:961-64.
6. Riis BJ, Hansen MA, Jensen AM, et al: Low bone mass and fast rate of bone loss at menopause: equal risk factors for future fracture: a 15-year follow-up study. Bone 1996;19:9-12.
7. Hui SL, Slemenda CW, Johnston CC Jr: The contribution of bone loss to postmenopausal osteoporosis. Osteoporos Int 1990;1:30-4.
8. Horsman A, Burkinshaw L: Stochastic models of femoral bone loss and hip fracture risk. In Kleerekoper MJ, Krane SM, eds. Clinical disorders of bone and mineral metabolism. New York: Mary Ann Liebert, 1989:253-63.
9. Hernandez CJ, Beaupre GS, Carter DR: A theoretical analysis of the relative influences of peak BMD, age-related bone loss and menopause on the development of osteoporosis. Osteoporos Int 2003;14:843-47.
10. Slemenda CW, Christian JC, Williams CJ, et al: Genetic determinants of bone mass in adult women: a reevaluation of the twin model and the potential importance of gene interaction on heritability estimates. J Bone Min Res 1991;6:561-67.
11. Seeman E, Tsalamandris C, Formica C, et al. Reduced femoral neck bone density in the daughters of women with hip fractures: the role of low peak bone density in the pathogenesis of osteoporosis. J Bone Miner Res 1994;9:739-43.
12. Danielson ME, Cauley JA, Baker CE, et al: Familial resemblance of bone mineral density (BMD) and calcaneal ultrasound attenuation: the BMD in mothers and daughters study. J Bone Min Res 1999;14:102-110.
13. Kannus P, Palvanen M, Kaprio J, et al: Genetic factors and osteoporotic fractures in elderly people: prospective 25 year follow up of a nationwide cohort of elderly Finnish twins. BMJ 1999;319:1334-37.
14. Gueguen R, Jouanny P, Guillemin F, et al: Segregation analysis and variance components analysis of bone mineral density in healthy families. J Bone Min Res 1995;10:2017-22.
15. Hopper JL, Green RM, Nowson CA, et al: Genetic, common environment, and individual specific components of variance for bone mineral density in 10- to 26-year-old females: a twin study. Am J Epidemiol 1998;147:17-29.
16. Newton-John HF, Morgan DB: The loss of bone with age, osteoporosis, and fractures. Clin Orthop 1970;71:229-52.
17. Ferrari S, Rizzoli R, Slosman D, et al: Familial resemblance for bone mineral mass is expressed before puberty. J Clin Endocrinol Metab 1998;83:358-61.
18. Duppe H, Gardsell P, Nilsson B, et al: A single bone density measurement can predict fractures over 25 years. Calcif Tissue Int 1997;60:171-74.
19. Ma D, Jones G: The association between bone mineral density, metacarpal morphometry and upper limb fractures in children: a population based case-control study. J Clin Endocrinol Metab 2003;88:1486-91.
20. Goulding A, Cannan R, Williams SM, et al: Bone mineral density in girls with forearm fractures. J Bone Miner Res 1998;13:143-48.
21. Fiorano-Charlier C, Ostertag A, Aquino JP, et al: Reduced bone mineral density in postmenopausal women self-reporting premenopausal wrist fractures. Bone 2002;31:102-6.
22. Seeman E: The Achilles' heel of exercise-induced bone mass increments: cessation of exercise. J Bone Miner Res 2001;16:1370-73.
23. Bass S, Pearce G, Bradney M, et al: Exercise before puberty may confer residual benefits in bone density in adulthood: studies in active prepubertal and retired gymnasts. J Bone Min Res 1998;13:500-8.
24. Khan K, Bennell KL, Hopper JL, et al: Self-reported ballet classes undertaken at age 10-12 years and hip bone mineral density in later life. Osteoporosis Int 1998;8:165-73.
25. Gregg EW, Pereira MA, Caspersen CJ: Physical activity, falls, and fractures among older adults: a review of the epidemiologic evidence. J Am Geriatr Soc 2000;48:883-93.
26. Wyshak G, Frisch RE, Albright TE, et al: Bone fractures among former college athletes compared with nonathletes in the menopausal and postmenopausal years. Obstet Gynecol 1987;69:121-26.
27. Ma D, Jones G: Television, computer and video viewing, physical activity and upper limb fracture risk in children: a population based case-control study. J Bone Min Res 2003; 18:1970-77.
28. Lee WT, Leung SS, Leung DM, et al: A follow-up study on the effects of calcium-supplement withdrawal and puberty on bone acquisition of children. Am J Clin Nutr 1996;64:71-7.
29. Bonjour JP, Chevalley T, Ammann P, et al: Gain in bone mineral mass in prepubertal girls 3.5 years after discontinuation of calcium supplementation: a follow-up study. Lancet 2001;358:1208-12.
30. Sandler RB, Slemenda CW, LaPorte RE, et al: Postmenopausal bone density and milk consumption in childhood and adolescence. Am J Clin Nutr 1985;42:270-4.
31. Murphy S, Khaw KT, May H, et al: Milk consumption and bone mineral density in middle aged and elderly women. BMJ 1994;308:939-41.
32. Kanis J, Johnell O, Gullberg B, et al: Risk factors for hip fracture in men from southern Europe: the MEDOS study. Osteoporos Int 1999;9:45-54.
33. Johnell O, Gullberg B, Kanis JA, et al: Risk factors for hip fracture in European women: the MEDOS Study. Mediterranean Osteoporosis Study. J Bone Miner Res 1995;10:1802-15.
34. Jones G, Riley M, Dwyer T: Breastfeeding in early life and prepubertal bone mass: a longitudinal study. Osteoporos Int 2000;2:146-52.
35. Jones G, Riley M, Dwyer T: Maternal diet during pregnancy is associated with bone mass in prepubertal children: a longitudinal study. Eur J Clin Nutr 2000;54:749-56.
36. Jones G, Riley MD, Whiting S: The association between urinary potassium, urinary sodium, current diet and bone density in prepubertal children. Am J Clin Nutr 2001;73:839-44.
37. Lucas AR, Melton LJ 3rd, Crowson CS, et al: Long-term fracture risk among women with anorexia nervosa: a population-based cohort study. Mayo Clin Proc 1999;74:972-77.
38. Nguyen T, Jones G, Sambrook PN, et al: Effects of estrogen exposure and reproductive factors on bone mineral density and osteoporotic fractures. J Clin Endocrinol Metab 1995;80:2709-14.
39. Zamora SA, Rizzoli R, Belli DC, et al: Vitamin D supplementation during infancy is associated with higher bone mineral mass in prepubertal girls. J Clin Endocrinol Metab 1999;84: 4541-44.
40. Jones G, Dwyer T: Bone mass in prepubertal children: gender differences and the role of physical activity and sunlight exposure. J Clin Endocrinol Metab 1998;83:4274-79.
41. Cheng S, Tylavsky F, Kroger H, et al. Association of low 25-hydroxyvitamin D concentrations with elevated parathyroid hormone concentrations and low cortical bone density in early pubertal and prepubertal Finnish girls. Am J Clin Nutr 2003;78:485-92.
42. Jones G, Dwyer T, Hynes K, et al: Vitamin D insufficiency in adolescent boys in Northwest Tasmania: prevalence, determinants and relationship to bone turnover markers. Osteoporos Int 2005;16:636-41.
43. Cooper C, Eriksson JG, Forsen T, et al: Maternal height, childhood growth and risk of hip fracture in later life: a longitudinal study. Osteoporos Int 2001;12:623-29.
44. Cooper C, Cawley M, Bhalla A, et al: Childhood growth, physical activity and peak bone mass in women. J Bone Min Res 1995;10:940-47.

45. Cooper C, Fall C, Egger P, et al: Growth in infancy and bone mass in later life. Ann Rheum Dis 1997;56:17-21.

46. Jones G, Dwyer T: Birth weight, birth length and bone density in prepubertal children: evidence for an association that may be mediated by genetic factors. Calcif Tiss Int 2000;67:304-8.

47. Jones IE, Williams SM, Goulding A: Associations of birth weight and length, childhood size, and smoking with bone fractures during growth: evidence from a birth cohort study. Am J Epidemiol 2004;159:343-50.

48. Godfrey K, Walker-Bone K, Robinson S, et al: Neonatal bone mass: influence of parental birthweight, maternal smoking, body composition, and activity during pregnancy. J Bone Miner Res 2001;16:1694-703.

49. Jones G, Riley M, Dwyer T: Maternal smoking during pregnancy, growth and bone mass in prepubertal children. J Bone Min Res 1999;14:147-52.

50. Ma D, Jones G: Clinical risk factors but not bone density are associated with prevalent fractures in prepubertal children. J Paed Child Hth 2002;38:497-500.

51. Leppala J, Kannus P, Niemi S et al. An early-life femoral shaft fracture and bone mineral density at adulthood. Osteoporos Int 1999;10:337-42.

4

Recommendations for Performing Bone Densitometry to Diagnose Osteoporosis and Identify Persons to Be Treated for Osteoporosis

Marc C. Hochberg

Osteoporosis has been defined as a systemic skeletal disorder characterized by compromised bone strength predisposing to an increased risk of fracture.[1] Bone strength is determined by many factors, including primarily bone mass. Bone mass is estimated in clinical practice by bone mineral density (BMD), the quantity of mineral (grams of calcium) divided by the area of the bone. There is a strong nonlinear relationship between BMD and the risk of fracture, such that for every decrease in one standard deviation below the age-adjusted mean for total hip BMD the risk of hip fracture increases by a factor of greater than 2.[2] The World Health Organization defined osteoporosis in white women as a BMD measured at the femoral neck of 2.5 or more standard deviations below the mean of young white women aged 20 to 39 years.[3] This definition has been generalized to women of other ethnicities and to men with the proviso that normative data for young persons be sex and race specific.

The most important osteoporotic fractures, from the standpoints of both incidence and consequences, are vertebral and hip fractures.[4-6] Results of randomized placebo-controlled clinical trials have demonstrated that treatment of postmenopausal women with either prevalent vertebral fractures or low BMD (T-score of −2.0 or below) can reduce the risk of vertebral, nonvertebral, and hip fractures.[7-9] Similarly, treatment of men with low BMD can reduce the risk of vertebral fractures.[10,11]

This chapter reviews recommendations and algorithms for identifying persons who should undergo measurement of BMD in an attempt to identify women and men with low BMD who should undergo treatment to reduce their risk of fracture.

WHO SHOULD HAVE BONE MINERAL DENSITY MEASURED?

Lewiecki[12] recently reviewed guidelines for BMD testing. He performed a systematic review of MEDLINE and the National Guideline Clearinghouse to identify clinical practice guidelines that were written in English and had been published, updated, or endorsed since 2000. A total of 78 publications were identified; of these, there were five unique published BMD testing guidelines (Table 4-1).[13-17] The most widely recognized guidelines are those of the National Osteoporosis Foundation (NOF).[13] The NOF recommends BMD testing in all postmenopausal women aged 65 and older as well as in younger postmenopausal women with one or more of the following risk factors: personal history of low-trauma clinical fracture, history of osteoporotic fracture in a first-degree relative, low body weight (127 lbs or less), or current smoking. These recommendations apply directly to white women; however, they have been liberally expanded for all women. The NOF currently is developing recommendations for men.

The American Association of Clinical Endocrinologists (AACE) also recommends that postmenopausal women aged 65 and older should undergo BMD testing.[14] In addition, younger postmenopausal women with a history of a clinical fracture not caused by major trauma (e.g., motor vehicle accident) as well as those with other risk factors for fracture should undergo BMD

TABLE 4-1 GUIDELINES FOR MEASUREMENT OF BONE MINERAL DENSITY (WEBSITES)

American Association of Clinical Endocrinologists (www.aace.org/clin/guidelines)
International Society for Clinical Densitometry (www.iscd.org/Visitors/positions/OfficialPositionsText.cfm)
National Osteoporosis Foundation (www.nof.org/professionals/clinical.htm)
North American Menopause Society (www.menopause.org/edumaterials/cliniciansguide)
United States Preventive Services Task Force (www.ahrq.gov/clinic/uspstf/uspsoste.htm)

testing. This includes not only diseases but also drugs that are associated with secondary osteoporosis (Tables 4-2 and 4-3).

The North American Menopause Society's (NAMS') recommendations are similar to those of the AACE but

TABLE 4-2 DISEASES ASSOCIATED WITH SECONDARY OSTEOPOROSIS
Endocrine diseases
Hypogonadism
Hyperparathyroidism
Hyperthyroidism
Hypercortisolism
Hyperprolactinemia
Diabetes mellitus, type I
Gastrointestinal diseases
Inflammatory bowel disease
Malabsorption syndromes
Celiac disease
Chronic liver disease
Gastric bypass operations
Other chronic diseases
Chronic rheumatic disorders
Rheumatoid arthritis
Ankylosing spondylitis
Chronic obstructive pulmonary disease
Renal disorders
Renal tubular acidosis
Idiopathic hypercalciuria
Malignancy
Multiple myeloma
Metastatic disease
Infiltrative disorders
Systemic mastocytosis
Hereditary disorders of connective tissue
Osteogenesis imperfecta
Organ transplantation
Dietary disorders
Vitamin D deficiency and insufficiency
Calcium deficiency
Excessive alcohol intake
Anorexia nervosa
Total parenteral nutrition

TABLE 4-3 DRUGS ASSOCIATED WITH SECONDARY OSTEOPOROSIS
Glucocorticoids
Anticonvulsants
Excessive thyroid hormone replacement
Immunosuppressive agents
Heparin
GnRH antagonists
Depo-Provera
Drugs used to treat breast cancer
Tamoxifen (premenopausal women)
Aromatase inhibitors (postmenopausal women)

also include testing of premenopausal women with low-trauma osteoporotic fractures or secondary causes of osteoporosis.[15] Testing of premenopausal women results in a conundrum, as no medications are approved for treatment of osteoporosis in premenopausal women.

The International Society for Clinical Densitometry (ISCD) recommends BMD testing in all postmenopausal women aged 65 and older and all men aged 70 and older.[16] The ISCD also recommends BMD testing in younger postmenopausal women and men aged 50 with not only diseases but also taking drugs that are associated with secondary osteoporosis. The ISCD is the only organization that has proposed recommendations for BMD testing in men.

Finally, the US Preventive Services Task Force has the most restricted guidelines, recommending BMD testing in all postmenopausal women aged 65 and older and women aged 60 to 64 with risk factors for fracture.[17]

Several algorithms have been published that can be used to identify women who should undergo BMD testing; these complement the recommendations listed in Table 4-1 and briefly reviewed above.[18-21] These algorithms include the Osteoporosis Risk Assessment Index, the Simple Calculated Osteoporosis Risk Equation (SCORE), and the Osteoporosis Self-Assessment Tool (OST); the OST has also been used in men.[22] The Osteoporosis Risk Assessment Index includes five questions and the SCORE includes six questions; both of these require calculation of a score that leads to identification of individuals who should be referred for testing for osteoporosis. The OST uses a formula based solely on age and body weight and has been adopted by the State of Maryland's Osteoporosis Task Force for identifying women and men who are at low, medium, or high risk for osteoporosis based on a BMD T-score of −2.5 or lower (Figure 4-1).[23]

Raisz, in reviewing these recommendations and algorithms, concluded that BMD measurements should be obtained routinely in all women older than 65 years and in men and younger women who have had a fragility fracture or have medical conditions or are taking medications that are associated with secondary osteoporosis; in addition, he recommends measurement of BMD with dual energy x-ray absorptiometry in women who have a T-score of −1.0 or lower based on a peripheral densitometry measurement.[24]

There is now evidence that universal testing of women aged 60 and older is associated with a reduced rate of fractures.[25,26] LaCroix and colleagues randomized more than 9000 women aged 60 to 80 years who were not taking hormone therapy or other osteoporosis medications to one of three groups: universal testing (n = 1986), testing based on results of the SCORE (n = 1940), and testing based on results of a 17-item

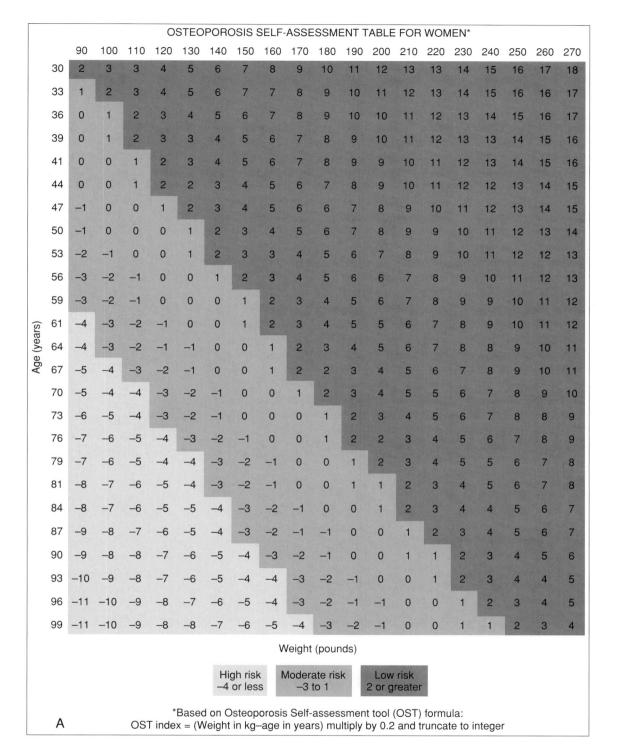

OSTEOPOROSIS SELF-ASSESSMENT TABLE FOR WOMEN*

Weight (pounds)

Age (years)	90	100	110	120	130	140	150	160	170	180	190	200	210	220	230	240	250	260	270
30	2	3	3	4	5	6	7	8	9	10	11	12	13	13	14	15	16	17	18
33	1	2	3	4	5	6	7	7	8	9	10	11	12	13	14	15	16	16	17
36	0	1	2	3	4	5	6	7	8	9	10	10	11	12	13	14	15	16	17
39	0	1	2	3	3	4	5	6	7	8	9	10	11	12	13	13	14	15	16
41	0	0	1	2	3	4	5	6	7	8	9	9	10	11	12	13	14	15	16
44	0	0	1	2	2	3	4	5	6	7	8	9	10	11	12	12	13	14	15
47	−1	0	0	1	2	3	4	5	6	6	7	8	9	10	11	12	13	14	15
50	−1	0	0	0	1	2	3	4	5	6	7	8	9	9	10	11	12	13	14
53	−2	−1	0	0	1	2	3	3	4	5	6	7	8	9	10	11	12	12	13
56	−3	−2	−1	0	0	1	2	3	4	5	6	6	7	8	9	10	11	12	13
59	−3	−2	−1	0	0	0	1	2	3	4	5	6	7	8	9	9	10	11	12
61	−4	−3	−2	−1	0	0	1	2	3	4	5	5	6	7	8	9	10	11	12
64	−4	−3	−2	−1	−1	0	0	1	2	3	4	5	6	7	8	8	9	10	11
67	−5	−4	−3	−2	−1	0	0	1	2	2	3	4	5	6	7	8	9	10	11
70	−5	−4	−4	−3	−2	−1	0	0	1	2	3	4	5	5	6	7	8	9	10
73	−6	−5	−4	−3	−2	−1	0	0	0	1	2	3	4	5	6	7	8	8	9
76	−7	−6	−5	−4	−3	−2	−1	0	0	1	2	2	3	4	5	6	7	8	9
79	−7	−6	−5	−4	−4	−3	−2	−1	0	0	1	2	3	4	5	5	6	7	8
81	−8	−7	−6	−5	−4	−3	−2	−1	0	0	1	1	2	3	4	5	6	7	8
84	−8	−7	−6	−5	−5	−4	−3	−2	−1	0	0	1	2	3	4	4	5	6	7
87	−9	−8	−7	−6	−5	−4	−3	−2	−1	−1	0	0	1	2	3	4	5	6	7
90	−9	−8	−8	−7	−6	−5	−4	−3	−2	−1	0	0	1	1	2	3	4	5	6
93	−10	−9	−8	−7	−6	−5	−4	−4	−3	−2	−1	0	0	1	2	3	4	4	5
96	−11	−10	−9	−8	−7	−6	−5	−4	−3	−2	−1	−1	0	0	1	2	3	4	5
99	−11	−10	−9	−8	−8	−7	−6	−5	−4	−3	−2	−1	0	0	1	1	2	3	4

High risk	Moderate risk	Low risk
−4 or less	−3 to 1	2 or greater

*Based on Osteoporosis Self-assessment tool (OST) formula:
OST index = (Weight in kg–age in years) multiply by 0.2 and truncate to integer

A

Figure 4-1. The Osteoporosis Self-assessment Tool index tables for women and men. *A,* The Osteoporosis Self-assessment Table for Women. (See Color Plates.)

Continued

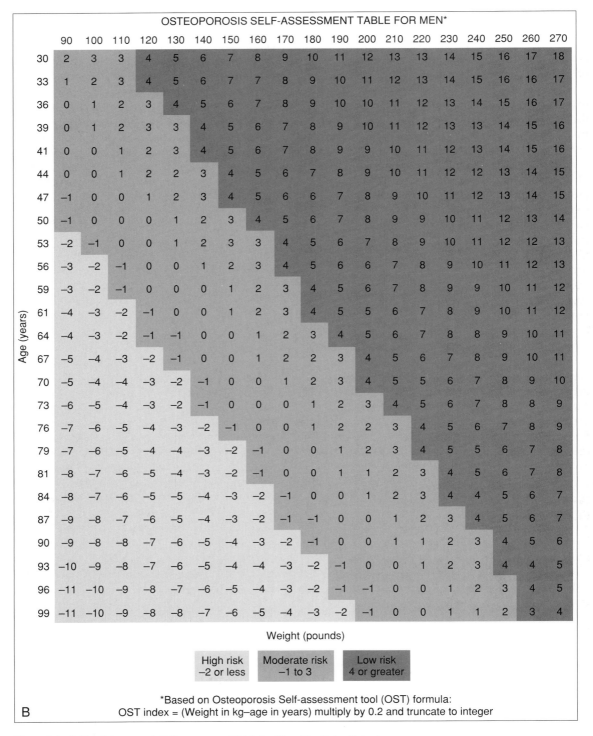

Figure 4-1. *B,* The Osteoporosis Self-assessment Table for Men. (See Color Plates.)

questionnaire adapted from known risk factors for hip fracture (n = 5342).[25] BMD measurements were performed in 415, 425, and 150 women in each of the groups, respectively. During a mean follow-up period of 33 months, the rate of osteoporotic fractures was 74.11, 99.44, and 91.77 per 1000 woman-years, respectively ($P < .05$ comparing the other two groups with the universal screening group). The rate of hip fractures was also lower in the universal screening group, but differences were not statistically significant (8.54, 9.04, and 13.31 per 1000 woman-years, respectively). These results were extended by an analysis of data from the Cardiovascular Health Study.[26] In this population-based observational cohort study, 1378 eligible participants enrolled in the Sacramento County (California) and Allegheny County (Pennsylvania) sites completed measurement of BMD at the hip whereas 1685 participants enrolled in the Washington County (Maryland) and Forsyth County (North Carolina) sites received usual care; mean age was 76 years, the majority of subjects were women, and more than 80% were white. The incidence of hip fractures over a mean of 4.9 years of follow-up was 8.2 and 4.8 per 1000 person-years in the usual care and screened group, respectively (multiple variable adjusted relative hazard = 0.64; 95% confidence interval, 0.41-0.99). There was no evidence of a statistical interaction between screening and sex, age group, or race; however, there were only four hip fractures among the 532 black participants. Hence, these two studies support the recommendations for universal BMD testing summarized earlier.

WHO SHOULD BE TREATED TO REDUCE FRACTURE RISK?

Lewiecki identified three unique guidelines that address treatment: the AACE, NAMS, and NOF.[12] All three are focused on treating postmenopausal women. The AACE and NAMS guidelines recommend treating women with a T-score derived from BMD testing at a central site of −2.5 or below, whereas the NOF guidelines recommend treatment at a T-score cutpoint of −2.0 or lower. All guidelines modify the T-score cut-point in the presence of other risk factors for fracture, including a prior history of a low-trauma symptomatic fracture or prior radiographic vertebral fracture. Hence, the NOF recommends treatment at a T-score cutpoint of −1.5 or lower in the presence of one or more risk factors, including a prior clinical fracture or radiographic vertebral fracture.

Solomon and colleagues[27] also performed a systematic review of the English-language literature using MEDLINE and HealthStar for the period between January 1992 and December 2003 to identify osteoporosis treatment guidelines. They identified 18 unique guidelines; 17 provided recommendations for postmenopausal women and 13 provided recommendations for men.[26] The majority of guidelines that included treatment recommendations for postmenopausal women also suggested that treatment should be provided to patients with BMD T-scores higher than −2.5 if other risk factors for fracture were present. Delmas and colleagues,[28] in outlining the position of the International Osteoporosis Foundation, concluded that treatment of postmenopausal women with established osteoporosis is always cost-effective and that additional scenarios exist in which treatment is cost-effective. These additional scenarios depend upon the crossing of an "intervention threshold," where the future morbidity from osteoporotic fractures, largely derived from the risk and costs of hip fracture, exceeds the costs of interventions that have been shown to reduce the risk of these fractures, largely bisphosphonates.[29] Additional risk factors, over and above BMD, that contribute to the estimate of this risk include age, sex, prior history of fragility fracture, parental history of hip fracture, current smoking, use of systemic glucocorticoids, excess alcohol intake, and presence of rheumatoid arthritis.[29] Algorithms are currently being developed to allow calculation of person-specific risk that can then be applied on a country-specific basis to determine whether treatment is warranted. The impact of this policy will become apparent over the next decade.

REFERENCES

1. NIH Consensus Development Panel on Osteoporosis: Osteoporosis prevention, diagnosis and therapy. JAMA 2001;285:785-95.
2. Cummings SR, Black DM, Nevitt MC, et al: Bone density at various sites for prediction of hip fractures. Lancet 1993;341:72-5.
3. World Health Organization Study Group: Assessment of fracture risk and its application to screening for postmenopausal osteoporosis. World Health Organ Tech Rep Ser 1994;843:1-129.
4. Kado KM, Browner WS, Palermo L, et al: Vertebral fractures and mortality in older women: a prospective study. Arch Intern Med 1999;159:1215-20.
5. Ensrud KE, Thompson DE, Cauley JA, et al: Prevalent vertebral deformities predict mortality and hospitalization in older women with low bone mass: Fracture Intervention Trial Research Group. J Am Geriatr Soc 2000;48:241-49.
6. Department of Health and Human Services: Bone health and osteoporosis: a report of the Surgeon General. Rockville, MD: Office of the Surgeon General, 2004.
7. Cranney A, Guyatt G, Griffith L, et al: Meta-analyses of therapies for postmenopausal osteoporosis: IX. Summary of meta-analyses of therapies for postmenopausal osteoporosis. Endocr Rev 2002;23:570-78.

8. Neer RM, Arnaud CD, Zanchetta JR, et al: Effect of parathyroid hormone (1-34) on fractures and bone mineral density in postmenopausal women with osteoporosis. N Engl J Med 2001;344:1434-41.

9. Chesnut CH III, Skag A, Christiansen C, et al: Effects of oral ibandronate administered daily or intermittently on fracture risk in postmenopausal osteoporosis. J Bone Miner Res 2004;19:1241-49.

10. Orwoll E, Ettinger M, Weiss S, et al: Alendronate for the treatment of osteoporosis in men. N Engl J Med 2000;31:343:604-10.

11. Kaufman JM, Orwoll E, Goemaere S, et al: Teriparatide effects on vertebral fractures and bone mineral density in men with osteoporosis: treatment and discontinuation of therapy. Osteoporos Int 2005;16:510-16.

12. Lewiecki EM: Review of guidelines for bone mineral density testing and treatment of osteoporosis. Curr Osteoporos Rep 2005;3:75-8.

13. National Osteoporosis Foundation: Osteoporosis: review of the evidence for prevention, diagnosis and treatment and cost-effectiveness analysis. Osteoporos Int 1998;8(Suppl 4):S7-S80.

14. Hodgson SF, Watts NB, Bilezikian JP, et al: American Association of Clinical Endocrinologists medical guidelines for clinical practice for the prevention and treatment of postmenopausal osteoporosis: 2001 edition, with selected updates for 2003. Endocrin Prac 2003;9:544-64.

15. Management of postmenopausal osteoporosis: position statement of the North American Menopause Society. Menopause 2002;9:84-101.

16. Writing Group for the International Society for Clinical Densitometry: International Society for Clinical Densitometry Position Development Conference: indications and reporting for dual-energy x-ray absorptiometry. J Clin Densitom 2004;7:37-44.

17. U.S. Preventive Services Task Force: Screening for osteoporosis in postmenopausal women: recommendations and rationale. Ann Intern Med 2002;137:526-28.

18. Cadarette SM, Jaglal SB, Krieger N, et al: Development and validation of the Osteoporosis Risk Assessment Instrument to facilitate selection of women for bone densitometry. CMAJ 2000;162:1289-94.

19. Lydick E, Cook K, Turpin J, et al: Development and validation of a simple questionnaire to facilitate identification of women likely to have low bone density. Am J Managed Care 1998;4:37-48.

20. Geusens P, Hochberg MC, van der Voort DJ, et al: Performance of risk indices for identifying low bone density in post-menopausal women. Mayo Clin Proc 2002;77:629-37.

21. Cadarette SM, McIsaac WJ, Hawker GA, et al: The validity of decision rules for selecting women with primary osteo-porosis for bone mineral density testing. Osteoporos Int 2004;15:361-66.

22. Adler R, Tran MT, Petkov VI: Performance of the osteoporosis self-assessment screening tool for osteoporosis in American men. Mayo Clin Proc 2003;78:723-27.

23. Maryland Department of Health and Mental Hygiene Family Health Administration: Osteoporosis Risk Assessment in Maryland: Maryland Osteoporosis Prevention and Education Task Force Risk Assessment Workgroup Recommendations, 2004. Available at http://www.strongerbones.org/tfworkgroups.html (Accessed August 22, 2005).

24. Raisz LG: Screening for osteoporosis. N Engl J Med 2005;353:164-71.

25. LaCroix AZ, Buist DSM, Brenneman SK, Abbott TA: Evaluation of three population-based strategies for fracture prevention: results of the Osteoporosis Population-Based Risk Assessment (OPRA) Trial. Med Care 2005;43:293-302.

26. Kern LM, Powe NR, Levine MA, et al: Association between screening for osteoporosis and the incidence of hip fracture. Ann Intern Med 2005;142:173-81.

27. Solomon DH, Morris C, Cheng H, et al: Medication use patterns for osteoporosis: an assessment of guidelines, treatment rates, and quality improvement interventions. Mayo Clin Proc 2005;80:194-202.

28. Delmas PD, Rizzoli R, Cooper C, Reginster J-Y: Treatment of patients with postmenopausal osteoporosis is worthwhile: the position of the International Osteoporosis Foundation. Osteoporos Int 2005;16:1-5.

29. Kanis JA, Borgstrom F, De Laet C, et al: Assessment of fracture risk. Osteoporos Int 2005;16:581-89.

5 Pathogenesis of Osteoporosis

Graham Russell

SUMMARY

The pathogenesis of osteoporosis reflects the complex interplay among genetic, metabolic, and environmental factors that determine

- bone growth
- peak bone mass
- calcium homeostasis
- bone loss

These factors are influenced by

- aging
- physical inactivity
- sex hormone deficiency
- nutritional status

Osteoporosis is the most common clinical disorder of bone metabolism. Its pathophysiological basis includes a genetic predisposition to low peak bone mass and subtle alterations in bone remodeling due to changes in systemic and local hormones, coupled with environmental influences.

The remarkable advances in the study of osteoporosis and its treatment have occurred mainly since the early 1990s. The published literature is vast, and this chapter can only deal with highlights. Readers are referred to recent reviews for further information.[1-4]

THE FEATURES OF OSTEOPOROSIS

Osteoporosis literally means "holes in bones." Tunnels created by bone resorption but not refilled with new bone characteristically occur in cortical bone, whereas in trabecular bone there is thinning of the bony plates so that they eventually perforate.

These changes occur progressively and are present in almost everyone in later decades of life. Fractures are the clinical endpoint of this loss of bone. The relationship between the decline in bone mass and the occurrence of fractures in osteoporosis is therefore analogous to the relationships that exist between risk factors and other diseases, such as elevated serum cholesterol and myocardial infarction, and hypertension and stroke. In fact, the relationship between bone mass, measured as bone mineral density (BMD), and fractures is the strongest of these three examples.

There are therefore problems in defining osteoporosis in a precise manner. A definition that relies solely on the presence of fracture impedes the clinical identification of individuals at high risk whose bones have not yet fractured. Conversely, a definition based on bone mass will include individuals who never experience fractures and exclude patients who sustain fractures despite having a bone mass above the defined threshold.

The single most important advance that has allowed the spectacular progress in this field over the past decade has been the development of reproducible and accurate methods of measuring bone mass by noninvasive techniques. The technical advances in bone densitometry based in particular on dual energy x-ray absorptiometry were key to this.

In 1994, the World Health Organization produced a definition of osteoporosis based on low BMD. Osteoporosis was defined by a BMD of 2.5 SD or more below the mean for young adults (i.e., a T-score of less than −2.5). Severe osteoporosis was defined by a T-score of less than −2.5 plus one or more fracture. Individuals with T-scores between −1.0 and −2.5 were defined as having osteopenia. These definitions are important because they have, perhaps unintentionally, become related to thresholds for therapeutic intervention, since entry to drug trials is usually based on these values. They are also important in discussions of pathogenesis, in which causative associations are identified from epidemiological studies based on T-score definitions of osteoporosis.

It is increasingly appreciated that better predictors of fracture risk than BMD alone are needed. BMD is only one of several factors that predict fractures. Moreover, changes in BMD only partially account for responses to treatment. The definition of osteoporosis and risk of fracture needs to evolve to include not only the traditional measures of bone quantity, such as mass, but also measures of bone quality, which contributes to bone strength.

The most recent definition of osteoporosis issued by a Consensus Development Conference[5] sponsored by the National Institutes of Health now refers to decreased bone strength instead of just low BMD and is worded as follows: "Osteoporosis is a skeletal disorder characterized by compromised bone strength predisposing a person to an increased risk of fracture."

The Pathogenesis of Fracture: Bone Fragility and Falls

Fractures occur when bones are too fragile to resist relatively minor degrees of trauma that should not normally result in fracture. The conventional definition of osteoporotic fracture in terms of being "nontraumatic" poses problems of defining the degree of trauma. Practically, the occurrence of any fracture in an elderly person is often considered to be osteoporotic, especially if it was related to a fall from no more than a standing height, or if there was little or no recognized trauma.

Although not the focus of this chapter, one must remember that an increased susceptibility to falls contributes to an increased risk of fracture, and reducing falls might be expected to reduce fractures in the elderly.[6] The wearing of hip-protecting devices has been shown to reduce rates of fracture in controlled trials.[7]

Usually, osteoporotic fractures heal quite normally, unlike fractures associated with other pathological conditions such as bone metastases.

THE PATHOGENESIS OF OSTEOPOROSIS AND FRACTURES

The pathogenesis of osteoporosis involves many different factors. It results from a complex interaction among genetic, hormonal, and environmental influences. Factors that contribute to osteoporosis and fractures that have been identified from epidemiological[8] and other studies are listed in Table 5-1.

It is helpful to define the contributory processes at multiple biological levels as well as in terms of known risk factors, and to identify their functional inter-relationships. The biological levels include molecular, biochemical, and cellular changes. Effects of these changes are on bone as a tissue and on the altered physiology of mineral metabolism in osteoporosis.

Bone Growth and Development: Modeling and Remodeling

A consideration of the normal process of bone modeling and remodeling is fundamental to the understanding of the pathogenesis of osteoporosis. During growth, the skeleton enlarges in size. In long bones this is achieved by the epiphysial growth plates, which produce increases in length, whereas increases in diameter result from deposition of new bone on the periosteal

TABLE 5-1 FACTORS ASSOCIATED WITH OSTEOPOROSIS (LOW BONE MINERAL DENSITY) IN EPIDEMIOLOGICAL STUDIES
Sex (women > men)
Age
Ethnicity (especially white and Asian)
Low body weight and body mass index
High bone turnover
Maternal history of fracture
Sex hormone deficiency (especially estrogen)
Early menopause, ovariectomy, amenorrhea
Previous low-trauma fracture
Physical inactivity
Drugs, especially glucocorticosteroids, anticonvulsants
Endocrine disorders (hyperthyroidism)
Neoplastic disorders (multiple myeloma)
Gastrointestinal disease (e.g., celiac disease)
Rheumatoid arthritis, ankylosing spondylitis
Vitamin D deficiency
Cigarette smoking
Excessive alcohol consumption

From Hochberg et al, Rheumatology, 3rd ed, 2003.

surfaces, accompanied by resorption from the endosteal surfaces.

During development and growth, bone is produced by two main processes, intramembranous ossification, as occurs in skull bones, and endochondral ossification involving the growth plate, as occurs in limb bones. Modeling is the process that results in bones achieving their characteristic shape and overall structure.

Bone is metabolically active throughout life. Growth in utero can influence bone mass in later life.[9] After skeletal growth is complete, remodeling of both cortical and trabecular bone continues. The remodeling of both cortical and trabecular bone requires the sequential and coordinated actions of osteoclasts to remove bone and osteoblasts to replace it (Figure 5-1). These processes can be monitored by histological means. Cortical bone is replaced at a lower rate (approximately 2% per annum) than trabecular bone (approximately 10% per annum).

The purpose of remodeling is to allow the bone to adapt to changes in distribution of mechanical forces and to repair microdamage, which can occur in response to repeated loading.[10] The amount of bone made under normal conditions corresponds very closely to the amount removed, so that, in any remodeling cycle within bone, the total amount of bone tends to remain constant.

Bone loss in osteoporosis results from an imbalance between the two components of the bone renewal process, bone resorption and bone formation.[11] This is the fundamental basis of osteoporosis. Specifically, the numbers of sites of bone remodeling increase, and the

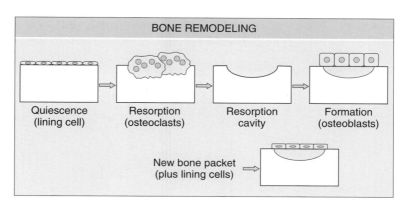

Figure 5-1. Bone remodeling. The remodeling cycle within bone involves a similar sequence of cellular activity at both cortical and trabecular sites. Trabecular surfaces are shown here. An initial phase of osteoclastic resorption is followed by a more prolonged phase of bone formation mediated by osteoblasts. Under normal conditions, the amount of bone removed during resorption is replaced completely. (From Hochberg et al, Rheumatology, 3rd ed, 2003.) (See Color Plates.)

extent of resorption may be greater and the amount of bone replaced smaller (Figure 5-2).[12]

In cortical bone, incomplete replacement of osteons creates tunnels, which may coalesce to create points of weakness.[13]

Peak Bone Mineral Mass and Bone Loss in Later Life

Peak bone mass is defined as the amount of bone that can be accumulated by early to middle adult life, when it is greater than at other times of life.

Peak bone mass is determined by many factors, only some of which are alterable. Inherited factors are probably the most important and may set the potential upper limit. A wide variety of lifestyle, nutritional, environmental, and medical factors modify this genetic potential.

Bone mass at any time in later life is the net sum of this peak achieved in earlier life and subsequent loss, particularly after the menopause in women (Figure 5-3).

Postmenopausal bone loss is the single most important cause of bone loss. The rate of loss is greatest early after menopause. Age-related bone loss starts before menopause and continues from 30 to 50 years of age onward in both men and women. Loss from different bone sites occurs at different ages and at different rates.

Changes in Bone Mass and Effects of Age on Fracture Risk

Bone mass declines with age and this is a major contributor to the susceptibility to fracture. The relationship between BMD and fracture is such that fracture rates approximately double for every standard deviation reduction in BMD.

Changes in bone mass are measured as decreases in BMD (see Chapter 8). Although this is very useful in clinical practice, BMD is calculated in two dimensions, so that the important effects on strength of bone size and dimensions are not assessed. Age itself is a very important risk factor for osteoporotic fractures that is independent of but obviously closely related to low BMD (Figure 5-4).[14]

Age may also be a surrogate measure for falls. In common with other structures, the tissues of the musculoskeletal system undergo many changes with aging.

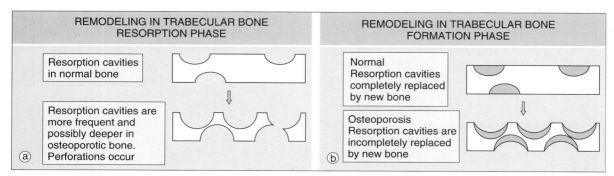

Figure 5-2. Remodeling in trabecular bone. These figures show remodeling under normal conditions and in osteoporosis. **A,** Resorption phase. **B,** Formation phase. There may be subtle differences between the sexes, with bone thinning predominating in men because of reduced bone formation. Loss of connectivity and complete trabeculae predominates in women. (From Hochberg et al, Rheumatology, 3rd ed, 2003.) (See Color Plates.)

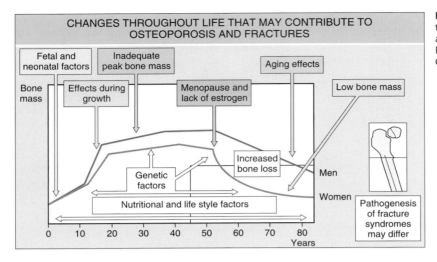

Figure 5-3. Changes throughout life that may contribute to osteoporosis and fractures. (From Hochberg et al, Rheumatology, 3rd ed, 2003.) (See Color Plates.)

In addition to the changes in bone that lead to osteoporosis and fractures, muscle changes (sarcopenia) contribute to frailty.

THE CELLULAR BASIS OF OSTEOPOROSIS

Osteoblasts[15] within trabecular bone differentiate from stromal cell precursors in bone marrow and manufacture a complex extracellular matrix, which subsequently mineralizes. The older concept that the bone matrix is entirely normal in osteoporosis is undergoing revision as knowledge increases. For example, there may be subtle but significant changes in the type I collagen matrix due to the Sp1 polymorphism (see below), and also in cross-linking within collagen.

Many growth factors affect bone formation. These include insulin-like growth factors, fibroblast growth factors, and especially members of the transforming growth factor beta family, particularly the bone morphogenetic proteins. Many of these factors are produced by bone cells themselves and can be deposited in bone matrix. Changes in the production and action of these many regulatory factors are clearly potentially important in the pathogenesis of osteoporosis, but detailed knowledge is very limited at present.

Osteoclasts are the major cells involved in bone resorption.[16] Osteoclasts differentiate from hematopoietic stem cell precursors under the direction of factors that include cytokines such as the RANK/RANK-ligand system, colony-stimulating factors (especially macrophage colony-stimulating factor), interleukins (e.g., IL-1, IL-11) and other factors. Prostaglandins and nitric oxide are other endogenous mediators that have complex effects on osteoclast function.

Bone loss is a feature of several inflammatory diseases. This loss may be systemic, leading to fractures, as

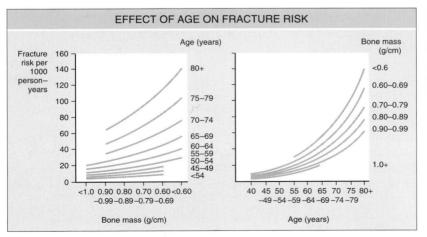

Figure 5-4. Effect of age on fracture risk. Fracture risk increases with age, independent of bone density, and also increases with declining bone density irrespective of age. (Adapted with permission from Hui et al.[14]; from Hochberg et al, Rheumatology, 3rd ed, 2003.) (See Color Plates.)

in rheumatoid arthritis, whereas local erosive lesions occur in bone in osteomyelitis, rheumatoid arthritis, and periodontal disease. The pathogenic mechanisms probably involve proinflammatory cytokines such as IL-1, tumor necrosis factor, and IL-6, and aberrant expression of RANK-ligand.

Apoptosis (programmed cell death) is emerging as a major means of regulating the lifespan of bone cells of all lineages, osteoclasts, osteoblasts, and osteocytes.[17] This may contribute to changes in bone turnover under physiological and pathological conditions. Drugs with adverse effects on bone such as glucocorticoids induce osteoblast and osteocyte apoptosis, whereas therapeutic agents that inhibit bone resorption, including estrogens and bisphosphonates, shorten the lifespan of osteoclasts. Increased apoptosis of osteocytes is a feature seen in fractures of the femoral neck in patients with osteonecrosis.

Rates of Bone Turnover and Bone Loss

There is increasing use of biochemical measurements to assess and monitor rates of bone resorption and formation. High rates of bone turnover predict fractures independently of other factors such as BMD. Evidence exists that rates of bone loss vary, and that patients defined as "fast" losers based on biochemical measurements do lose more bone mass than "slow" losers. Responses to treatment may be greater in those with high turnover.[18]

THE PHYSIOLOGICAL BASIS OF OSTEOPOROSIS

Physiological Regulation of Calcium Metabolism

The physiological regulation of calcium homeostasis involves three main organs: the gut, the kidney, and the skeleton. The fluxes of calcium and phosphate through these organs contribute to the integration of calcium metabolism throughout growth and adult life.

The physiological control of calcium metabolism and of skeletal remodeling is under the regulation of systemic hormones, especially the calcium-regulating hormones, parathyroid hormone, 1,25-dihydroxy vitamin D (calcitriol), and calcitonin, acting in concert with other hormones and local mediators. Many hormones, including thyroid and pituitary hormones and adrenal and gonadal steroids, have major effects on the skeleton, as seen in clinical disorders in which their secretion is abnormally high or low.

The setpoint for plasma calcium concentrations is determined mainly by the renal tubular reabsorption of calcium and the effects of parathyroid hormone on this process.

Intestinal absorption of calcium is enhanced by calcitriol, but the efficiency of absorption may be diminished with age. Production of calcitriol may be impaired, particularly if renal function is reduced. Parathyroid hormone values increase with age, possibly in response to impaired intestinal absorption of calcium, and this may contribute to bone loss.

Interestingly, the challenges of pregnancy and lactation seem to have no lasting adverse effects on bone. Examples of osteoporosis associated with pregnancy are exceedingly rare.

In women, the loss of estrogen at menopause is the major change leading to loss of bone, but many other factors contribute, and there is a strong interplay between genetic and environmental influences.

The Role of Estrogen Deficiency

The effects of estrogen on bone are of particular interest in relation to the loss of bone after menopause in women and the therapeutic use of estrogen to prevent this loss. Estrogen receptors (α and β isoforms) are widely distributed in the body, and there are many ways that estrogens can exert their effects on their various target tissues. Some effects of estrogens are mediated by nongenomic means.

The bone loss associated with estrogen deficiency is accompanied by increased bone resorption. Part of this may be due to loss of direct effects on osteoclasts and their precursors, but indirect actions on the immune system may also be involved. The production of cytokines such as IL-1, tumor necrosis factor alpha, and IL-6, all of which can potentially enhance bone resorption, can be suppressed by physiological doses of estrogen.[19]

It is also possible that estrogens have significant anabolic effects on bone by stimulating osteoblasts or their precursors.

The pathogenesis of osteoporosis in men is less well studied than in women but is clinically important, with secondary causes such as hypogonadism being common. It is now believed that estrogens derived by metabolism from androgens play an important role in protecting against bone loss in men.[20,21]

THE GENETIC BASIS OF OSTEOPOROSIS

The many genetic factors that regulate skeletal development and function are rapidly being identified, and recent examples include the *CBFA1* gene for osteoblast differentiation and the RANK/RANK-ligand system for osteoclasts.

Osteoporosis is common, and there are strong genetic contributors to skeletal size and composition. Comparisons of identical and nonidentical twins have led to estimates that more than 50% of peak bone mass is determined by genetic factors.

Overall, physique affects susceptibility to osteoporosis and may underlie racial differences in prevalence.

Hip fractures typically occur in the thin and frail rather than the fat and robust, and low body weight is a risk factor. Hip axis length is a quantifiable geometric measure related to fracture risk.

Rarely, osteoporosis or unusually high bone mass can occur as the result of mutations in a single gene. Thus, inactivating mutations in the lipoprotein receptor-related protein 5 gene are the cause of the osteoporosis-pseudoglioma syndrome, whereas the high bone mass syndrome is caused by activating mutations of the same gene.[22] In the various forms of osteogenesis imperfecta (brittle bone disease), defects in the synthesis or structure of type I collagen occur because of a range of different mutations in type I collagen genes.

In the more common forms of osteoporosis, genetic factors play an important role in regulating skeletal size and geometry, BMD, ultrasonographic properties of bone, and bone turnover, as well as contributing to the pathogenesis of osteoporotic fracture.[23] These phenotypes are determined by the combined effects of several genes and environmental influences. Genome-wide linkage studies in humans have identified loci on chromosomes 1p36, 1q21, 2p21, 5q33-35, 6p11-12, and 11q12-13 that show definite or probable linkage to BMD, but so far the causative genes remain to be identified. Linkage studies in mice have similarly identified several loci that regulate BMD.

Most research has so far been done on candidate genes. Among the best studied are the vitamin D receptor and the collagen type I a1 gene. Polymorphisms of vitamin D receptor have been associated with bone mass in several studies, and there is evidence to suggest that this association may be modified by dietary calcium and vitamin D intake. A functional polymorphism affecting an Sp1 binding site has been identified in the collagen type I a1 gene that predicts osteoporotic fractures independently of bone mass by influencing collagen gene regulation and bone quality.[24] An important problem with most candidate gene studies is small sample size, and this has led to inconsistent results in different populations. This is also complicated by the multiple clinical endpoints (e.g., BMD, fracture, rates of bone loss) to which genetic factors may contribute in different ways.

There is evidence that genetic variants in various hormones and cytokines and their receptors that are involved in bone remodeling may also contribute to the development of osteoporosis.

NUTRITIONAL FACTORS AND OSTEOPOROSIS

Dietary calcium is obviously a potentially important factor in osteoporosis. Calcium restriction in experimental animals results in osteopenia. In humans, calcium deficiency in childhood leads to rickets. Although low calcium intake might be expected to be associated with osteoporosis, the nature of the relationship between calcium intake and osteoporosis remains controversial.

Results from calcium balance studies suggest that premenopausal women require calcium intakes in excess of about 800 mg per day to avoid net bone loss, whereas postmenopausal women may require as much as 1500 mg per day, perhaps less if they are receiving sex hormone replacement therapy.

Calcium supplementation in many trials in patients with osteoporosis results in gains in bone mass, but to a lesser extent than can be achieved when antiresorptive drugs are given as well.

Dietary calcium intake during growth may play a role in the development and maintenance of peak BMD. It is likely that various other environmental and lifestyle factors, particularly exercise, modulate this effect. Calcium supplementation in growing children produces small increases in BMD, which tend not to be maintained and may represent increased mineralization of existing osteons rather than true and sustained increases in bone mass.

Poor nutrition in pregnancy can affect bone in postnatal life, since low birth weight is associated with low bone mass in later life.

Calcium is not the only component of diet that can affect bone; magnesium also may be important. Vitamin D is vital for optimal absorption of calcium from the diet. In many countries, vitamin D is added to foods; otherwise, adequate skin exposure to ultraviolet light is necessary to maintain vitamin D levels from endogenous synthesis.

There is little evidence that micronutrients such as zinc, copper, and boron have major effects on bone health. Some diets, particularly those rich in soy protein, can provide significant sources of estrogens. Excessive salt and caffeine intake may have adverse effects on bone, perhaps by increasing urinary calcium excretion directly and thus contributing to a negative calcium balance. However, these effects are probably relatively minor. Alcohol is another dietary component that may be quite important, with adverse effects in excess but perhaps beneficial effects at moderate levels of intake.

PHYSICAL ACTIVITY, MECHANICAL LOADING, AND OSTEOPOROSIS

Mechanical forces exert strong influences on bone shape and modeling. At a cellular level, the osteocytes, which lie embedded within individual lacunae in mineralized bone, are believed to be the cellular system that responds to mechanical deformation and loading. Osteocytes connect with each other via the canalicular system and thus form a cellular network, much like a neural network. Early biochemical responses to mechanical loading may include induction of prostaglandin synthesis, increased nitric oxide production and later increases in IGFs, changes in amino acid transporters, and eventually increases in new bone formation. There may be a "mechanostat," so far hypothetical only, that senses and responds to loading. Estrogens may affect the setpoint at which bone responds.[25]

Immobilization, for example after major injury and illness, can be associated with rapid bone loss. If sustained, as in patients with paraplegia or hemiplegia, fractures can occur.

The excessive bone resorption associated with immobility can also result in "immobilization hypercalcemia," particularly in the presence of renal impairment.

Bone loss associated with microgravity may be a limiting factor for long-term space flight.

The positive effects of mechanical loading on bone mass can be seen in weight lifters and other athletes. Sometimes the increased bone density is localized to the loaded side, for example in tennis players' arms.

Physical inactivity correlates with low BMD and fractures in epidemiological studies. However, the potential beneficial effects of exercise programs may only produce limited changes in bone mass and have not yet been shown to reduce fractures.

DRUGS AND OSTEOPOROSIS

Several drugs have adverse effects on the skeleton and thereby reduce bone mass and increase the risk of fracture. Glucocorticoids are among the most important of these and are an important cause of bone loss and fractures.

Anticonvulsant drugs such as phenytoin and various barbiturates have long been believed to modify vitamin D metabolism, but their contribution to osteoporosis is probably not major. Heparin is another agent that reduces bone mass.

Because deficiencies of estrogen and testosterone both contribute to bone loss, drugs that reduce sex hormone levels cause bone loss. Androgen deprivation therapy with agonists of gonadotropin-releasing hormone is now frequently used in the treatment of recurrent and metastatic prostate cancer because it induces medical castration, which renders these men hypogonadal.

This is becoming an important iatrogenic cause of osteoporosis.

The use of tamoxifen appears to cause bone loss by antagonizing estrogen in premenopausal women with breast cancer, whereas it has a weak protective effect against bone loss in postmenopausal women. Depot medroxyprogesterone used as a contraceptive in premenopausal women can result in bone loss.

Epidemiological studies show that tobacco smoking is a risk factor for osteoporotic fracture. The mechanisms are uncertain but may include direct adverse effects on bone, induction of early menopause, changes in acid-base status, and increased falling secondary to cerebrovascular disease.

In contrast, several drugs may increase bone mass and reduce fractures. Thiazide diuretics decrease urinary calcium excretion and have been associated with increased BMD and reduced hip fracture rates.

There has also been much recent interest in the statins. These drugs are used to reduce cholesterol and have been shown experimentally to induce BMP-2 and increase bone mass in rats. A variety of epidemiological studies suggest that statin users have lower rates of hip fracture than nonusers, but it has proved difficult to demonstrate large effects on bone mass and turnover in prospective clinical trials.

Of course, those drugs actually used in the therapy of osteoporosis increase bone mass. They include sex hormone replacement therapy with estrogens, calcitonin, selective estrogen receptor modulators, and the bisphosphonates, all of which reduce bone resorption and decrease the rate of incident vertebral fractures. Only estrogen and the nitrogen-containing bisphosphonates have been shown to reduce the risk of nonvertebral fractures in postmenopausal women. Anabolic agents, such as intermittent parathyroid hormone given as a daily subcutaneous injection, increase bone formation and reduce fracture risk.

CONCLUSION

Osteoporosis is clearly a multifactorial disorder, and much has been learned in recent years about the many pathogenic processes that contribute to bone loss and fragility. Drug treatments are now available to prevent bone loss and reduce fracture, and there are prospects for modifying some of the pathogenic processes themselves.

REFERENCES

1. Seeman E: Pathogenesis of bone fragility in women and men. Lancet 2002;359:1841-50.
2. Melton LJ III, Cooper C: Magnitude and impact of osteoporosis and fractures. In: Marcus R, Feldman D, Kelsey J, eds.
Osteoporosis, 2nd ed (vol 1). San Diego, CA: Academic Press, 2001:557-67.
3. Delmas PD: Treatment of postmenopausal osteoporosis. Lancet 2002;359:2018-26.

4. Favus MJ, ed. Primer of the metabolic bone diseases and disorders of mineral metabolism, 4th ed. Philadelphia: Lippincott Williams & Wilkins, 1999.

5. Consensus Development Conference. JAMA 2001;285:785-95.

6. Francis RM: Falls and fractures. Age Ageing 2001;30(suppl 4):25-8.

7. Royal College of Physicians: Osteoporosis: clinical guidelines for prevention and treatment. Including supplement on resource database of randomised controlled trials in osteoporosis. London: Royal College of Physicians of London, 1999, 2000.

8. Cummings SR, Melton LJ: Epidemiology and outcomes of osteoporotic fractures. Lancet 2002;359:1761-67.

9. Javaid MK, Cooper C: Prenatal and childhood influences on osteoporosis. Best Pract Res Clin Endocrinol Metab 2002;16:349-67.

10. Burr DB, Robling AG, Turner CH: Effects of biomechanical stress on bones in animals. Bone 2002;30:781-86.

11. Parfitt AM: Skeletal heterogeneity and the purposes of bone remodelling: implications for the understanding of osteoporosis. In: Marcus R, Feldman D, Kelsey J, eds. Osteoporosis. San Diego, CA: Academic Press, 2001:433-44.

12. Lips P, Courpron P, Meunier PJ: Mean wall thickness of trabecular bone packets in the human iliac crest: changes with age. Calcif Tissue Res 1978;10:13-17.

13. Jordan GR, Loveridge N, Bell KL, et al: Spatial clustering of remodeling osteons in the femoral neck cortex: a cause of weakness in hip fracture? Bone 2000;26:305-13.

14. Hui S, Slemeda C, Johnston C: Age and bone mass as predictors of fracture in a prospective study. J Clin Invest 1988;81:1804-9.

15. Ducy P, Schinke T, Karsenty G: The osteoblast: a sophisticated fibroblast under central surveillance. Science 2000;289:1501-4.

16. Teitelbaum SL: Bone resorption by osteoclasts. Science 2000;289:1504-08.

17. Manolagas SC: Birth and death of bone cells: basic regulatory mechanisms and implications for the pathogenesis and treatment of osteoporosis. Endocr Rev 2000;21:115-37.

18. Bjarnason NH, Christiansen C: Early response in biochemical markers predicts long-term response in bone mass during hormone replacement therapy in early postmenopausal women. Bone 2000;26:561-69.

19. Pfeilschifter J, Köditz R, Pfohl M, Schatz H: Changes in proinflammatory cytokine activity after menopause. Endocr Rev 2002;23:90-119.

20. Riggs BL, Kholsa S, Melton LJ III: A unitary model for involutional osteoporosis: estrogen deficiency causes both type 1 and type 2 osteoporosis in postmenopausal women and contributes to bone loss in aging men. J Bone Miner Res 1998;13:763-73.

21. Szulc P, Munoz F, Claustrat B, et al: Bioavailable estradiol may be an important determinant of osteoporosis in men: the MINOS study. J Clin Endocrinol Metab 2001;86:192-99.

22. Gong Y, Slee RB, Fukai N, et al: LDL receptor-related protein 5 (LRP5) affects bone accrual and eye development. Cell 2001;107:513-23.

23. Ralston SH: Genetic control of susceptibility to osteoporosis. J Clin Endocrinol Metab 2002;87:2460-66.

24. Mann V, Hobson EE, Li B, et al: A COL1A1 Sp1 binding site polymorphism predisposes to osteoporotic fracture by affecting bone density and quality. J Clin Invest 2001;107:899-907.

25. Lanyon L, Skerry T: Postmenopausal osteoporosis as a failure of bone's adaptation to functional loading: a hypothesis. J Bone Miner Res 2001;16:1937-47.

6 Principles of Bone Biomechanics

Charles H. Turner and David B. Burr

SUMMARY

This chapter covers the fundamentals of skeletal biomechanics. We discuss practical issues concerning the mechanical roles of the skeleton, basic biomechanical concepts, and the ways aging and drug treatments affect bone biomechanics in the first eight sections of the chapter. In addition, we have included a ninth section entitled "Biomechanical Test Methods" that describes protocols for measuring biomechanical properties of bone. This section is intended for researchers who wish to conduct biomechanical measurements.

BIOMECHANICAL ROLES OF THE SKELETON

The skeleton serves several functions.[1] Probably most importantly, it provides a ready source of calcium ions to maintain appropriate serum calcium levels and facilitate proper muscle function. Bones also provide acoustic amplification and impedance matching in the middle ear. But in this chapter, we focus on the skeleton as a structure. There are at least two key biomechanical roles for bones. First, bones shield vital organs from trauma. Many protective bones have a sandwich structure, similar to corrugated cardboard, in which a compliant core separates two stiff plates (Figure 6-1). The porous spongy bone acts as a soft interface between the two bony plates. In the skull, mechanical energy resulting from blunt trauma concentrates mainly in the spongy bone separating the bony plates. Consequently, very little energy is transferred to the innermost bony plate, and the cranial vault is preserved. In addition, bones serve as levers for muscles to contract against (Figure 6-2). Muscles typically operate at negative mechanical advantage ($r/R<1$). This arrangement increases the range of motion over which muscles can operate effectively, but it also increases the muscle force needed to move a limb. Increased muscle force translates to larger forces on the joints. To better distribute joint forces, the ends of long bones are broadened to reduce stress (load/area) and that stress is carried by trabecular bone beneath the joint surface to distribute the force into the long bone cortex.

BASIC BIOMECHANICS

A number of biomechanical parameters can be used to characterize the integrity of bone. The key relationship is between load applied to a structure and displacement in response to the load-displacement curve (Figure 6-3). The slope of the elastic region of the load-displacement curve represents the extrinsic stiffness or rigidity of the structure (S). Besides stiffness, several other biomechanical properties can be derived, including ultimate force (F_u), work to failure (area under the load-displacement curve, U), and ultimate displacement (d_u). Each of these measured parameters reflects a different property of the bone: ultimate force reflects the general integrity of the bone structure, stiffness is closely related to the mineralization of the bone, work to failure is the amount of energy necessary to break the bone, and ultimate displacement is inversely related to the brittleness of the bone. The biomechanical status of bone may be poorly described by just one of these properties. For instance, a bone

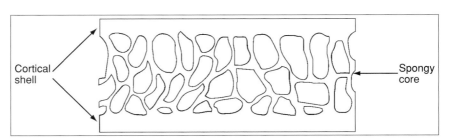

Figure 6-1. Drawing of sandwich bone of the skull. (Reprinted from Bone Formation [F. Bronner and M.C. Farach-Carson, eds.], copyright 2004, with permission from Springer-Verlag.)

Cortical shell

Spongy core

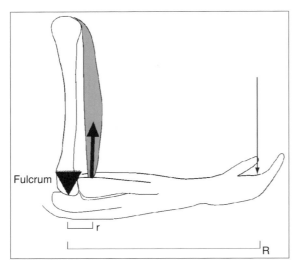

Figure 6-2. Bones as levers.

from an osteoporotic patient will tend to be very stiff but also very brittle, resulting in reduced work to failure and increased risk of fracture (Figure 6-4). On the other hand, a bone from a young child will tend to be poorly mineralized and weak but very ductile (large ultimate displacement), resulting in increased work to failure. Because of these properties, "greenstick" fractures, in which the bone undergoes large deformation but does not completely break, are sometimes observed in children.

When load is converted to stress and deformation converted to strain by engineering formulae, the relationship between stress and strain in bone follows a curve called the *stress-strain curve*. The slope of the stress-strain curve within the elastic region is called the *elastic* or *Young modulus* (E). The Young modulus is a measure of the intrinsic stiffness of the material. The area under the stress-strain curve is a measure of the amount of energy needed to cause material failure. This property of a material is called *energy absorption* or *modulus of toughness* or just *toughness*. The maximum stress and strain the bone can sustain are called the *ultimate strength* and *ultimate strain*, respectively. It should be noted that strength, as it is defined by the stress-strain curve, is an intrinsic property of bone. That is, these strength values are independent of the size and shape of the bone. The force required to break the bone is different from the intrinsic strength, because ultimate load varies with bone size. It is important to keep this distinction in mind, because intrinsic strength and ultimate load can show different trends in drug or genetic studies, especially if the drug or gene affects the size of the bone. Strength measures that are not presented in units of stress do not represent the intrinsic strength of the material but are influenced by extrinsic factors such as specimen size and shape.

The elastic strain region and the plastic strain region of the stress-strain curve are separated by the yield point (Figure 6-5). The yield point represents a gradual

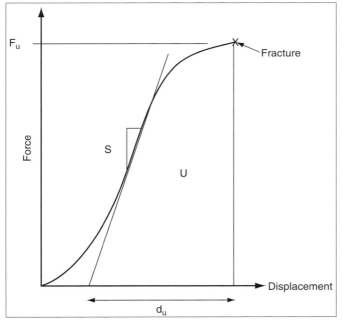

Figure 6-3. Load-displacement curve for bone tissue. The slope of the linear region of the curve represents the extrinsic stiffness or rigidity of the structure (S); the height of the curve denotes ultimate force (F_u); area under the curve is work to failure (U); and total displacement to fracture is ultimate displacement (d_u).

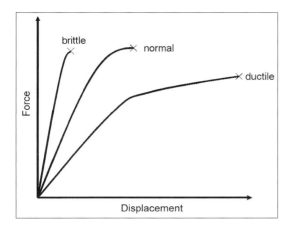

Figure 6-4. Load-displacement curves for different bone conditions. Osteoporotic bone is brittle and thus displays reduced work to failure. On the other hand, a bone from a young child is ductile with larger ultimate displacement, resulting in increased work to failure.

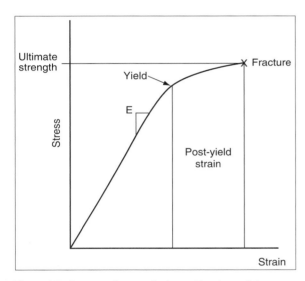

Figure 6-5. Stress-strain curve for bone. The slope of the curve is called Young modulus (E). The height of the curve is the ultimate strength. The yield point represents a transition above which strains begin to cause permanent damage to the bone structure. Post-yield strain is inversely proportional to the brittleness of the bone.

transition, above which stresses begin to cause permanent damage to the bone structure. Post-yield strains (i.e., strains beyond the yield point) represent permanent deformations of bone structure caused by slip at cement lines, trabecular microfracture, crack growth, or combinations of these. The yield point is seldom well-defined when testing bone specimens. Several methods have been proposed to determine the yield point. For instance, the yield point is often defined as the point where the stress-strain curve begins to be nonlinear.[2] Other techniques include offset methods in which a line parallel with the linear portion of the stress-strain curve and offset by 0.03% to 0.2% strain is constructed.[3] The point where this line intersects the stress-strain curve is arbitrarily called the yield point.

THE IMPORTANCE OF BONE SIZE

The mechanical properties of bone tissue are similar among mammals. For instance, the Young modulus of rat femoral bone[4] is similar to that of human femoral bone.[5] The major difference between rats and humans is, of course, size. Likewise, the majority of the variation in skeletal load carrying capacity is due to differences in bone size. Bone fragility could be largely eradicated if bones were massively overstructured. Large, dense bones last a lifetime without developing osteoporosis. A clinical example of skeletal overstructuring is the high bone mass mutation in the *LRP5* gene, which results in bone mass that is about 5 standard deviations above normal.[6] Individuals with this mutation are effectively osteoporosis-free. For most people, however, bones are not designed for extreme longevity, as evidenced by the incidence of age-related bone fractures.

Long bones are for the most part thick, walled tubes. This geometry allows bones to carry loads effectively but remain relatively light. To understand the principle behind this, one must first consider that long bones are loaded mainly in bending.[7] The deflection of a beam in bending is given by $ML^2 8EI$, where M is the bending moment, L is length, E is the Young modulus, and I is the second moment of area. For a given value of M, beam deflection can be reduced by shortening the beam (decrease L), stiffening the beam material (increase E), or increasing I. The last option applies best to bones. For a tubular bone, the second moment of area I equals $\pi/4$ $(r_o^4 - r_i^4$, where r_o is the outer radius and r_i is the inner radius (Figure 6-6). For mammalian long bones, r_o is about 1.8 times r_i, giving $I = 0.71r_o^4$. If the marrow cavity were filled completely, I would be $0.78r_o^4$. Therefore, the presence of a marrow cavity reduces the bending rigidity of the bone by less than 10% but reduces its weight by more than 15% (if we include the weight of the marrow). Flying animals increase the rigidity-to-weight ratio further by increasing r_i (relative to r_o) and removing the bone marrow. Most extraordinary among such animals was the *Pteranodon*, in which the ratio of bone diameter to cortical thickness exceeded 40.[8]

WHY BONES BREAK

Strength and stiffness are typically used to define the "health" of a bone, but they are not as clearly related to risk of fracture as is the amount of energy required to

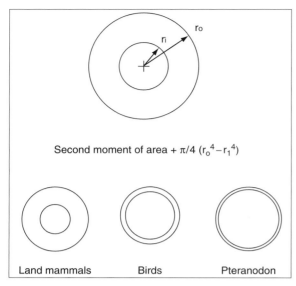

Second moment of area + π/4 ($r_o^4 - r_1^4$)

Land mammals   Birds   Pteranodon

Figure 6-6. The resistance to bending stresses for a long bone is represented by the second moment of area (I). Bones with larger values of I but less bone mass are more structurally efficient. The ratio of the diameter (D) to cortical thickness (t) is a measure of structural efficiency. Land mammals have D/t ratios of 4 to 5; for birds, D/t can be 10 or greater. The values for D/t can exceed 40 in the ancient *Pteranodon*.[8]

cause fracture. Trauma transfers energy into the bone and, if that energy exceeds what the bone can absorb, the bone will break. A bone that is highly mineralized is also stiff and brittle and will require much less energy to fracture (the area under the curve) than a bone that is more compliant. Bone mineral density (BMD) is highly correlated with strength and stiffness, but there is an inverse relationship between bone stiffness (or Young modulus) and ultimate strain (Figure 6-7). Deer antler, which is not highly mineralized, has a very high ulti-

mate strain (ductility) but low Young modulus. This combination of properties makes an antler exceedingly difficult to break.[9] On the other hand, the tympanic bulla of a fin whale has high mineral content and a high Young modulus and is very brittle. The bulla is not as strong as antler or bone due to its brittleness; however, it is not designed for strength, but for acoustic properties. Like the middle ear ossicles, the bulla is highly mineralized to provide proper acoustic impedance. Long bone tissue has intermediate mechanical properties.

Cracks forming in bone tissue provide a means by which energy is released. Energy absorbed by the bone during loading builds up and is released as damage accumulates or when the bone fractures. Bone subjected to high-energy trauma, such as a gunshot wound, will form many cracks because energy accumulates quickly and must be released. High-energy trauma causes the bone to break into fragments. Lower energy trauma causes simple fractures, without fragmentation (Figure 6-8). Bone tissue is weakest in tension or shear and strongest in compression; thus, cracks tend to propagate along tension or shear planes within the bone tissue. Shear planes run at 45-degree angles from compressive stresses and because of this bending forces can create "butterfly" fractures. Fracture lines follow shear planes to create a fragment that resembles a butterfly wing. Likewise, a plane of maximum tension falls 45 degrees from the shear plane, so torsional (shear) loads often cause spiral fractures that propagate along a helical plane of maximum tension.

MATRIX COMPOSITION AND BONE BIOMECHANICS

Bone tissue is a two-phase porous composite material composed primarily of collagen and mineral, with

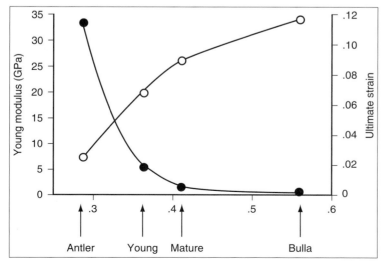

Figure 6-7. Biomechanical properties of mineralized tissues (from Currey 1990). As mineral volume fraction (x-axis) increases, Young modulus (open circles) is improved but ultimate strain (closed circles) decreases. Deer antler is less stiff (lower Young modulus) and less brittle (higher ultimate strain), whereas the tympanic bulla from a fin whale is very brittle and stiff. Bone tissue from a young (1-year-old) cow is less stiff and brittle than tissue taken from mature (9-year-old) cows.

Figure 6-8. Types of bone fractures. A low-energy impact causes a simple fracture, whereas high-energy impact causes a fragmented or comminuted fracture. Bending tends to cause a butterfly fracture with fracture planes following maximum shear and tension lines. Torsion causes a spiral fracture with the fracture plane following a maximum tension plane.

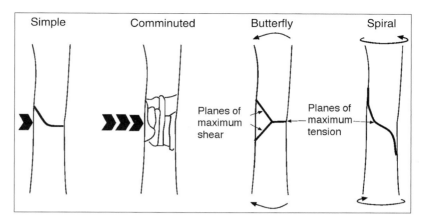

mechanical properties determined primarily by the amounts, arrangement, and molecular structure of these primary constituents. The mineral component confers strength and stiffness to the tissue. The collagen phase is tough and improves bone's work to failure or toughness.

The ratio of mineral to collagen in bone affects both bone strength and brittleness.[10] Excessive mineral content, or a change in the stoichiometry or quality of the mineral[11] increases brittleness and is detrimental. The maturity and perfection of the mineral crystal undoubtedly have effect on biomechanical properties, apart from the amount of mineral, but the specific effect is unknown. Reports using infrared spectrometry[12] suggest that larger crystals are present in bone from older osteoporotic women and that increased crystallinity itself, or changes in the morphology of the mineral crystal, may decrease the amount of post-yield deformation that occurs before ultimate failure.

Collagen has a small influence on the strength and stiffness of bone but mostly improves bone toughness.[13,14] The most obvious clinical example of the mechanical effects of a collagen defect is osteogenesis imperfecta. Osteogenesis imperfecta is a family of heritable disorders that involve mutations in the type I procollagen genes. People with osteogenesis imperfecta have a markedly increased risk of fracture and often present with multiple fractures at a young age. This is likely due to a combination of poor bone tissue properties together with low bone volume and thin long bone cortices. The poor tissue properties are the result of abnormally thin collagen fibers, smaller than normal mineral crystals, with greater extrafibrillar deposition of mineral.[15]

Subtle genetic variation in collagen content and structure can also affect the mechanical properties of bone. The COL1A1 gene polymorphism, which encodes the $\alpha 1(I)$ protein chain of type I collagen and alters the ratio of the α-1 and α-2 chains is associated with a 5.9-fold increase in fracture risk in postmenopausal women and a 4.8-fold increase when prevalence is adjusted for age, body mass index, and BMD.[16,17] There is a stronger association between the COL1A1 Sp1 binding site polymorphism and osteoporotic fracture than between these and BMD or body mass index at both the lumbar spine and the femoral neck.[18,19]

The orientation of collagen fibers within the bone matrix also affects strength. Linear regression analyses have demonstrated that collagen fiber orientation explains 71% of the variation in bone tensile strength,[20] whereas the combination of mineralization and collagen fiber orientation explains up to 88% of the variation in elastic modulus.[21] The orientation of collagen fibers tends to be tightly regulated by the nature of the applied stress on bone.[22,23] An orthogonal alteration of collagen fibers in adjacent lamellae, or multidirectional arrangement ("twisted plywood"),[24] are well suited to resist multidirectional shear and compressive stresses. It has been suggested that reorientation of collagen fibers can maintain strength even in the face of losses in BMD.[25]

INFLUENCE OF AGE AND OSTEOPOROSIS ON BIOMECHANICAL PROPERTIES

The strength of cortical bone declines 2% to 5% per decade of life, and the amount of energy absorbed prior to failure of cortical bone declines 7% to 12% per decade.[26] The decline in cancellous bone strength is between 8% to 10% per decade.

As one ages, there is an inherent fragility in the bone tissue that allows it to be damaged more easily from cyclic loading.[27,28] In addition, with age, bone is less able to sustain further deformation once it is damaged.[29] Reasons for the inherent fragility and reduced ductility are not known but could be related to higher mineralization associated with the greater mean tissue age of older bone, or to changes in collagen structure and cross-linking. This decline in bone's ability to absorb energy is clinically important in making bones in elderly people more prone to failure from any impact load, such as one resulting from a fall.

Decreased fracture toughness in bones from older people is indicative of a change in the quality of bone tissue with age. Tough materials can sustain large amounts of damage without failure. Bone that is highly mineralized or has a high degree of collagen cross-linking tends not to sustain much damage before failure and is not very tough, typical of a more brittle structure. Reduced toughness may partly explain the observation that fracture risk in older people is greater than predicted by the loss of bone mass alone.[30,31]

During the normal aging process, changes in the collagen moiety affect the post-yield deformation of bone, which can alter the manner in which cracks are initiated and grow.[32,33] Increases with age in nonenzymatic collagen cross-links[13] make the bone stiffer and reduce post-yield deformation.[34] This reduces the toughness of the bone for both crack initiation and crack growth.[32] However, the greatest effect of nonenzymatic cross-linking is to reduce the resistance to crack growth, allowing cracks that are initiated to grow more easily.[31,32] Increased nonenzymatic cross-links can lead to a brittle fracture of the tissue even without associated changes in the bone mineral.[35] Changes in collagen may be partly responsible for the changes in toughness associated with aging.[14,36]

Changes to the collagen content or molecular stability with age contribute to either enhance bone strength or impair it. The age-related decline in collagen content is associated nonlinearly with reductions in strength and stiffness, although cause and effect have not been established. In osteoporotic women, fewer reducible collagen cross-links with no change in collagen concentration[37] increases bone fragility.[38] As pointed out earlier, natural increases in nonenzymatic cross-links with age, indicated by an increased concentration of pentosidine, will reduce toughness, particularly for crack growth.[32,33] The increased lysine hydroxylation found in newly synthesized bone matrix from osteoporotic paients is correlated to decreased strength in three-point bending.[39]

Periosteal apposition of bone with age serves a biomechanically important function by compensating for reduced tissue properties (or reduced bone volume) in men (Figure 6-9), but this compensation is not sufficient to offset the larger losses of bone that occur in modern populations of women.[40] Before menopause, women lose bone at the rate of 4% per decade from the femoral neck but maintain strength. Postmenopausally, however, the increased rate of loss (7% per decade) is not compensated for and results in estimated femoral neck stresses that are 4% to 12% higher than in younger women.[41] Similar periosteal compensations have been shown for the vertebral body in men but not in women.[42]

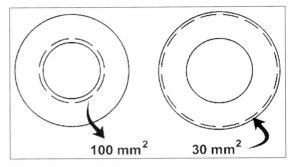

Figure 6-9. Two idealized long bone cross-sections. The section on the left represents a younger person's bone. The right section represents an older person's bone after loss of bone from the endocortical surface and subsequent periosteal apposition. With age, the bone lost 100 units of area from the endocortical surface and added 30 units on the periosteal surface. Despite the net loss of bone in the left section, both sections have equal resistance to bending.

INFLUENCE OF MICRODAMAGE ACCUMULATION ON BIOMECHANICAL PROPERTIES

By definition, accumulation of microdamage in any material reduces its elastic modulus. Stiffness loss occurs before the microscopic appearance of cracks,[43,44] so that histologically visible microdamage in bone presumes a loss of bone stiffness. Animal and postmortem human studies show that microdamage accumulation also reduces bone strength.[45] Importantly, microcrack accumulation has an effect on bone toughness. A two- to threefold elevation of microdamage accumulation in the vertebrae, produced as a consequence of a suppression of remodeling, is associated with a 20% to 40% reduction in bone toughness without a reduction in strength.[46,47]

INFLUENCE OF DRUG THERAPIES ON BIOMECHANICAL PROPERTIES OF BONE

Therapeutic bone active agents have specific effects on bone architecture, matrix properties, mineralization, microdamage accumulation, and bone turnover. The effects on bone quality and fragility can be striking. Examples include high-dose fluoride or etidronate treatments, which impair bone mineralization and can cause severe bone fragility.[48,49]

Other osteoporosis drugs have more subtle effects on bone quality.[50] Each of these drugs affects the mechanical properties of the bone. Often, cortical and cancellous bone compartments are affected differently.

Effects of Antiresorptive Agents

Antiresorptive therapies prevent bone loss by suppressing bone turnover, which in turn increases the tissue age of the bone because old bone is not as readily replaced by new bone.[51] Increased bone tissue age is associated with increased mineral content, increased mineral homogeneity, and increased microdamage accumulation. Also, suppressed bone turnover may decrease the porosity of cortical bone and the number of resorption pits in trabeculae.

Bisphosphonate treatment increases tissue mineralization above that found in osteopenic subjects,[52-54] which makes the bone tissue stiffer and more brittle. This increased mineralization might account for much of the observed increase in BMD and reduced fracture risk found with either alendronate or raloxifene.[55] Reduced fracture risk even after long-term bisphosphonate therapy[56] has been used as an argument against the idea that the increased mineralization consequent to treatment increases bone fragility. Although increased mineralization can cause subtle increases in bone brittleness, these changes appear not to be sufficient to increase fracture rates.

One effect of remodeling suppression is that it increases the homogeneity of the bone tissue as more of the tissue becomes mineralized to the same degree.[57,58] Because the effectiveness of bone in stopping cracks is positively proportional to the stiffness ratio across its internal interfaces, a homogeneous material will be less effective in slowing or stopping cracks initiated in the bone matrix. This would allow cracks to grow more quickly to critical size and ultimately increase fracture risk.

Reduced turnover by antiresorptive treatments may reduce fracture risk more than expected, based on the subsequent BMD increases, by preventing resorption-based weakening of trabecular struts.[59] Rapid turnover accelerates osteoclastic resorption on trabecular surfaces that can reduce the resistance of trabecular struts to failure by buckling.[60] In addition, accelerated resorption will increase the probability for perforation and elimination of trabecular struts.[61]

Bisphosphonates alter three-dimensional trabecular architecture, independent of the change in bone mineral density, making the cancellous bone more platelike and denser, with thicker and more numerous trabeculae compared with that of untreated control subjects.[62] Trabecular architecture becomes more isotropic with bisphosphonate treatment, perhaps providing better protection against fracture risk in falls that load the bone in unusual directions. The combination of architectural changes and reduced trabecular perforation may provide a rationale for the clinical observation that fracture risk decreased by 50% to 60% in the first year of bisphosphonate therapy despite only a 5% increase in bone mineral density.[63]

The impressive fracture risk reduction seen in the first year of treatment with antiresorptive agents appears to be most prominent at trabecular bone sites. Antiresorptive agents have little effect on cortical bone geometry. Consequently, increased strength of cortical bone, if it occurs, must occur through increased tissue mineralization or decreased cortical porosity, or both, rather than through geometric changes.

Effects of Anabolic Agents

The current paradigm for anabolic therapy is intermittent treatment with parathyroid hormone (PTH) or a fragment of this peptide PTH (1-34). The PTH fragment increases bone formation substantially but also accelerates bone turnover. As a consequence, PTH decreases the mean tissue age of bone,[64] which decreases bone mineral content and microdamage accumulation while increasing porosity. PTH increases bone strength primarily through increased bone volume and improved cancellous architecture.

The acceleration of bone turnover increases the amount of bone that is hypomineralized and makes the tissue more compliant. It also increases the heterogeneity of the bone tissue, creating mixed populations of older bone and new bone. This creates stiffness variations that would slow crack growth, increase toughness, and delay or prevent fracture. These effects are likely to remain as long as PTH treatment is continued.

Parathyroid hormone has a beneficial effect on trabecular architecture through a different mechanism than the antiresorptive agents. Treatment with recombinant PTH (1-34) increases cancellous bone volume and improves trabecular architecture by increasing trabecular number. This occurs via longitudinal tunneling, converting thickened trabecular to multiple struts of normal thickness.[65] This change in architecture, in combination with increased net bone formation, is associated with increased bone strength. Clinically, the effect of these changes is to reduce fracture risk by more than 60% with 1 year of treatment.[66]

In cortical bone, PTH (1-34) increases turnover and cortical porosity, but this effect is most apparent close to the marrow cavity. The bone near the marrow cavity carries less stress than does the periosteal bone. Consequently, increased porosity near the endosteal surface has only a small negative effect on bone strength. The small loss of bone consequent to increased turnover is offset by increased periosteal apposition, which maintains or improves bone strength.[67] This is likely the mechanism for the observed reduction in nonvertebral fractures.[66]

BIOMECHANICAL TEST METHODS

Biomechanics has become a standard assay for evaluating the effects of putative osteoporosis treatments on animal bones. There are many different methods for measuring bone biomechanical properties.

Tensile Testing

Tensile testing can be one of the most accurate methods for measuring bone properties, but bone specimens must be relatively large and carefully machined. Strain measurement can be accomplished accurately by attaching a clip-on extensometer to the mid-section of the specimen. Stress is calculated as the applied force divided by the bone cross-sectional area in the mid-section of the specimen. The tensile test is limited in usefulness by the need for relatively large specimens, particularly when testing cancellous bone.[68]

Compressive Testing

Compressive testing of bone specimens is a popular technique, especially for cancellous bone, because relatively small specimens can be used. Compressive tests tend to be less accurate than tensile tests due to end effects imposed on the specimen during the test. Should the faces of the bone specimen be slightly misaligned with the loading plate, large stress concentrations can occur, causing an underestimation of both Young modulus and strength. Although it is more difficult to achieve accurate results using a compressive test than using a tensile test, the compressive test has several advantages. First, the compressive specimens need not be as large as tensile specimens; this is a major advantage when testing cancellous bone. Second, fabrication of compressive specimens may not be as difficult as with tensile test specimens. Finally, in some regions of the skeleton (e.g., the vertebrae) compressive tests more closely simulate the in vivo loading conditions to which the bone is exposed. The compressive test is preferred for measuring mechanical properties of vertebral specimens. There are several issues to consider when testing whole vertebrae in compression. Generally the spinous processes posterior to the spinal canal should be removed, while care is taken not to damage the vertebral body. The precision of the test can be improved by removing the end plates of the vertebral body with parallel cuts using a diamond wafering saw. The final specimen should have parallel faces and its height should be equal to or less than its width. For a specimen in compression, stress is calculated as the applied force divided by the bone specimen's cross-sectional area. However, the calculation of stress is complicated for cancellous bone specimens by the underlying trabecular architecture. For cancellous bone, force divided by cross-sectional area gives an apparent stress, yet less than 30% of the specimen is bone tissue. Consequently, the apparent stress in the specimen and the true stress in the trabecular tissue are quite different quantities. The trabecular stress is more accurately approximated as

$$\sigma = (F/A)(\,1\,/\,A_f) \qquad [1]$$

where σ is stress, F is force, A is the specimen cross-sectional area, and A_f is the area fraction of trabecular tissue.

Bending Tests

Bending tests are useful for measuring the mechanical properties of bones from rodents as well as larger animals. For small bones, it is very difficult to machine tensile or compressive test specimens. In the bending test, the whole long bone is loaded in bending until failure. Bending causes tensile stresses on one side of the bone and compressive stresses on the other. Bone is weaker in tension than compression,[69] so in a bending test, failure usually occurs on the tensile side of the bone. Bending can be applied to the bone using either three-point or four-point loading (Figure 6-10). The span of the specimen that is loaded (shown as L in Figure 6-10) must be sufficiently long to guarantee an accurate test. If L is very short, most of the displacement induced by loading will be due to shear stresses and not bending. For bone specimens, L should be about 20 to 25 times the thickness of the specimen.[70] In bending tests of whole bones, unfortunately, a length-to-width ratio of 20:1 cannot be achieved. The advantage of three-point loading is its simplicity, but it has the disadvantage of creating high shear stresses near the mid-section of the bone. Four-point loading produces pure bending between the two upper loading points, which insures that transverse shear stresses are zero. However, four-point bending requires that the force at each loading point be equal. This requirement is simple to achieve in regularly shaped specimens but difficult to achieve in whole bone tests. Therefore, three-point bending is used more often for measuring the mechanical properties of rodent bones.

Stresses due to bending can be calculated using the beam-bending formulas (equations 2 and 3). These beam-bending formulas are valid for beams with symmetrical cross-sections. For some bones, the tibia for instance, the cross-section is assymmetrical and a more complicated formula is required to accurately calculate stresses.[71] For three-point loading the equation is

$$\sigma = \frac{FLC}{4I}, \varepsilon = \frac{12cd}{L^2}, E = \frac{F}{d}\,\frac{L^3}{48I} \qquad [2]$$

and for four-point loading it is

$$\sigma = \frac{Fac}{2I}, \varepsilon = \frac{6cd}{a(3L-4a)}, \text{ and } E = \frac{F}{d}\,\frac{a^2}{12I}(3L-4a) \qquad [3]$$

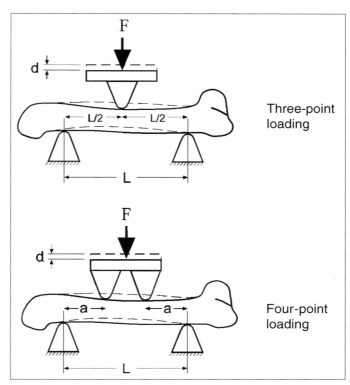

Figure 6-10. Bending can be applied to rodent bones and machined bone specimens using either three-point or four-point loading. F is the applied force and d is the resulting displacement.

Three-point loading

Four-point loading

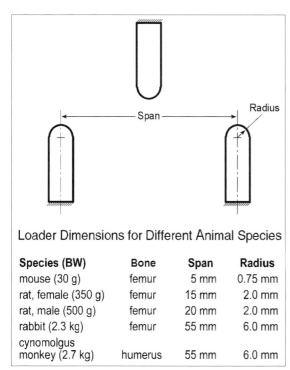

Loader Dimensions for Different Animal Species

Species (BW)	Bone	Span	Radius
mouse (30 g)	femur	5 mm	0.75 mm
rat, female (350 g)	femur	15 mm	2.0 mm
rat, male (500 g)	femur	20 mm	2.0 mm
rabbit (2.3 kg)	femur	55 mm	6.0 mm
cynomolgus monkey (2.7 kg)	humerus	55 mm	6.0 mm

Figure 6-11. The key dimensions for a three-point bending test of a long bone are the span between the lower loaders and the radius of curvature of the loading surfaces. The table shows representative dimensions used successfully in our laboratory.

where σ is stress, ε is strain, c is the distance from the center of mass, F is applied force, d is displacement, and a and L are lengths given in Figure 6-10.[72] Indirect calculation of strain is inaccurate, however, for two reasons. First, substantial deformation of the specimen occurs where the loaders contact the bone. Second, there is always some deformation due to induced shear stresses.[73] These effects cause the measured displacement to be greater than the flexural displacement of the bone. This error causes an overestimation of strain and an underestimation of Young modulus. Keys to a successful three-point bending test for whole bones are the dimensions of the testing fixtures. Of greatest importance are the span between the lower loaders and the radius of curvature of the loading surfaces (Figure 6-11)—the former determines the length-to-width ratio and the latter determines how much bone deformation will occur beneath the loaders. For bending tests, as in tensile tests, it is important to distinguish between intrinsic stiffness and extrinsic stiffness of the bone. Again, the intrinsic stiffness is equal to the Young modulus (E), whereas the extrinsic stiffness or *flexural rigidity* is equal to EI, where I is the cross-sectional moment of inertia. As noted above, bending tests on whole bone specimens give inaccurate values for Young modulus and strain, but accurate results can be obtained by testing a strip of bone machined from the cortical diaphysis. For a machined specimen tested in three-point bending, the stress, strain, and Young modulus are estimated by the following equation:

$$\sigma = (3FL)/(2wt^2), \quad \varepsilon = 6td/L^2, \text{ and}$$

$$E = (FL^3)/(4dwt^3) \qquad [4]$$

where F is applied force, d is loader displacement, L is the span of the loaders, and w and t are the specimen width and thickness. Equation 4 does not account for shear deformation in the specimen, yet the error associated with this simplification is minimal if the ratio of L to t is greater than 20. Spatz and colleagues[70] recommended designing a test for bone tissue with L/t = 25, whereas the American Society for Testing and Materials recommends L/t = 16 for plastics.

Torsional Testing

A torsion test can be used to measure the mechanical properties of bone in shear. When a torque is applied to a circular specimen, shear stress varies from zero at the center of the specimen to a maximum at the surface. The general equations for calculating shear stress and shear modulus of elasticity in a torsion test are

$$\tau = \frac{Tr}{J} \text{ and } G = (TL)/(\theta J) \qquad [5]$$

where τ is shear stress, G is shear modulus, T is applied torque, θ is rotational displacement, r is the radius of the specimen, L is the length of the specimen test region, and J is the polar moment of inertia of the specimen. It should be noted that the general equation for shear stress (equation 5) is inaccurate if the cross-section is not circular. Equations for shear stress in noncircular cross-sections can be found in various references.[74]

For thin-walled cylinders, shear stress can be approximated using the following formula

$$\tau = \frac{T}{2At} \qquad [6]$$

where A is the average of the inner and outer areas of the cylinder, and t is the thickness of the cylinder wall. Equation 6 is sometimes used to approximate the shear stress in whole bone torsion tests. However, the use of equation 6 in bone tests can lead to substantial error. For instance, equation 6 underpredicts the shear stress in the adult rat femur by more than 19%.[68]

Torsion tests are often used to measure the strength of whole bones from rodents.[75,76] The bone is gripped by embedding the ends in blocks of plastic or a metal alloy with a low melting point, and the two blocks are twisted relative to one another. The shear modulus of elasticity can be calculated from slope of the torque-twist curve (the torsion analog to the load-displacement curve):

$$G = \frac{T}{\theta} \frac{L}{K} \qquad [7]$$

where $\frac{T}{\theta}$ is the slope of the torque-twist curve and K is the torsional constant. For circular cross-sections, K is equal to J. Unfortunately, K is difficult to determine for irregularly shaped specimens such as many long bones. The best way to accurately measure shear modulus in irregularly shaped bones (e.g., the tibia) is to divide the applied stress by strain measured directly using a rosette strain gauge bonded to the surface of the midshaft of the bone.[77] Like other tests, torsion tests provide measures of both intrinsic stiffness and extrinsic stiffness. In a torsion test, the intrinsic stiffness is equal to the shear modulus (G), whereas the extrinsic stiffness or *torsional rigidity* is equal to GJ, where J is the polar moment of inertia of the cross-section. A major disadvantage of torsional testing of whole bones is the difficulty of mounting the specimen ends into the testing grips. The bone ends must be embedded to allow rigid fixation with the testing grips. Embedding adds specimen preparation time and expense for each test. There also are potential errors associated with embedding. The specimen must remain perfectly aligned while the embedding resin hardens. Any misalignment could induce a bending moment that would confound the test result. Also, plastic embedding resins have significant compliance and thus allow substantial rotation of the ends of the specimen within the grips, resulting in an overestimation of rotational displacement and an underestimation of torsional rigidity. Consequently, bending rather than torsional testing is the preferred methodology for large-scale screening of long bones for pharmaceutical or genetic effects.

Torsion offers a distinct advantage over bending tests for measuring the biomechanical effects of fracture healing, bone defects, or bone grafts, however. Torsion allows the load to be applied at the ends of the bone, away from the bone defect/graft, whereas three-point bending requires loading near or directly above the defect/graft. Besides torsion, four-point bending is another useful method for testing long bones with grafts or defects.

Indentation tests are used to map the biomechanical properties of subchondral bone and the underlying trabecular bone near diarthrodial joints or bone adjacent to implants. The biomechanical properties of bone in these regions are clinically important in studies of osteoarthritis progression and joint replacement arthroplasty. Indentation testing also can be used for measuring Young modulus and strength of trabecular bone specimens.[78,79] As the indentor penetrates the specimen, a load-displacement curve is created. The strength of the bone is estimated as the maximum load divided by the cross-sectional area of the indentor. The Young modulus is calculated as follows:

$$E = S (1 - v2)/d \qquad [8]$$

where S is the slope of the load-displacement curve, v is the Poisson's ratio of the bone (i.e., the ratio of its deformation in two perpendicular planes), and d is the diameter of the indentor.[80]

Bone Fatigue

When a material is repetitively loaded, with loads within the pre-yield region of the stress-strain curve, its mechanical properties gradually degrade over a period of time. This degradation of strength and Young modulus with time is called *fatigue*. In bone, the reduction in mechanical properties is attributed to the formation of small cracks within the bony structure. As loading continues, these cracks grow and coalesce until, ultimately, the bone fails catastrophically. Fatigue properties can be measured using tensile, compressive, bending, or torsional loading. The results of fatigue tests can be summarized on an S-N diagram. The S-N diagram depicts the peak applied stress as a function of the number of fatigue cycles before failure. For instance, a bone specimen cycled between zero and 100 MPa may last for 10 cycles before failure, whereas a specimen cycled between zero and 50 MPa will last longer than 100,000 cycles. Generally, fatigue failure is defined as the number of cycles necessary to cause a specimen to lose 30% of its intrinsic stiffness (i.e., the slope of the linear portion of the stress-strain curve is decreased by 30%). The fatigue properties of bone are very sensitive to testing temperature; specimens tested at room temperature undergo twice as many loading cycles before failure than bone tested at 37°C.[81] Fatigue properties also change substantially if the bone is dehydrated. Fatigue in bone can occur in two ways, creep (slippage at the cement lines)[82] or crack accumulation.[83] Carter and Caler[84] have shown that creep is the major cause of fatigue failure if the bone is loaded in tension or at high stress (>60 MPa), whereas crack accumulation causes fatigue failure if the specimen is loaded in compression at low stress (<60 MPa). Therefore, one must carefully design the parameters of a fatigue test to examine the phenomenon of interest. A major problem in designing a fatigue test is the fact that a cortical bone specimen can undergo as many as 37 million low-stress (24 MPa) loading cycles.[85] This translates to 43 days of fatigue testing at 10 cycles per second. The fatigue life is shortened considerably if the applied stress is raised to 50 MPa—5 days in tension and 45 days in compression at 2 Hz.[86] Raising the applied stress to about 60 MPa (with an applied strain of about 3000 μstrain) reduces fatigue life even further—3 hours in tension and 4 days in compression.[84]

CONCLUSION

We have presented a summary of bone biomechanics and descriptions of several types of biomechanical tests. We recognize that our presentation is incomplete. Instead of a comprehensive treatment of the subject, we limited our discussion to several major issues. It is important to note that biomechanics is not simply a compendium of methods, but a science unto itself. Consequently, biomechanical concepts will continue to evolve and improve. This chapter represents a snapshot of these concepts as they exist today.

REFERENCES

1. Martin RB, Burr DB, Sharkey NA: Skeletal Tissue Mechanics. New York, Springer-Verlag, 1998.
2. Hvid I, Jensen J: Cancellous bone strength at the proximal human tibia. Engng Med 1984;13:21-5.
3. Turner CH: Yield behavior of cancellous bone. J Biomech Eng 1989;111:1-5.
4. Kohles SS, Bowers JR, Vailas AC, Vanderby R Jr: Ultrasonic wave velocity measurement in small polymeric and cortical bone specimens. J Biomech Eng 1997;119:232-36.
5. Ashman RB, Cowin SC, Van Buskirk WC, Rice JC: A continuous wave technique for the measurement of the elastic properties of cortical bone. J Biomech 1984;17:349-61.
6. Little RD, Carulli JP, Del Mastro RG, et al: A mutation in the LDL receptor-related protein 5 gene results in the autosomal dominant high-bone-mass trait. Am J Hum Gen 2002; 70:11-19.
7. Rubin CT, Lanyon LE: Limb mechanics as a function of speed and gait: a study of functional strains in the radius and tibia of horse and dog. J Exp Biol 1982;101:187-211.
8. Currey JD: The Mechanical Adaptations of Bones. Princeton, NJ: Princeton University Press, 1984.
9. Currey JD: Physical characteristics affecting the tensile failure properties of compact bone. J Biomechanics 1990;23:837-44.
10. Currey JD: Bones: Structure and Mechanics. Princeton, NJ: Princeton University Press, 2002.
11. Huang R, Miller LM, Carlson CS, Chance MR: FTIR analysis of tibia bone from ovariectomized cynomolgus monkeys (*Macaca fascicularis*) and the effect of nandrolone decanoate treatment. Bone 2002;30:492-97.
12. Paschalis EP, Betts F, diCarlo E, et al: FTIR microspectroscopic analysis of human iliac crest biopsies from untreated osteoporotic bone. Calcif Tissue Int 1997;61:487-92.
13. Wang X, Shen X, Li X, Agrawal CM: Age-related changes in the collagen network and the toughness of bone. Bone 2002;31:1-7.
14. Zioupos P, Currey JD, Hamer AJ: The role of collagen in the declining mechanical properties of aging human cortical bone. J Biomed Mater Res 1999;45:108-16.
15. Boskey AL, Wright TM, Blank RD: Collagen and bone strength. J Bone Miner Res 1999; 4:330-35.
16. Langdahl BL, Ralston SH, Grant SFA, Eriksen EF: An Sp1 binding site polymorphism in the COL1A1 gene predicts osteoporotic

fractures in both men and women. J Bone Miner Res 1998; 13:1384-89.

17. Bernad M, Martinex MW, Escalona M, et al: Polymorphism in the Type I collagen (COL1A1) gene and risk of fractures in post-menopausal women. Bone 2002; 30:223-28.

18. Mann V, Hobson EE, Li B, et al: A COL1A1 Sp1 binding site polymorphism predisposes to osteoporotic fracture by affecting bone density and quality. J Clin Invest 2001;197:899-907.

19. Mann V, Ralston SH: Meta-analysis of COL1A1 Sp1 polymorphomism in relation to bone mineral density and osteoporotic fracture. Bone 2003;32:711-17.

20. Martin RB, Ishida J: The relative effects of collagen fiber orientation, porosity, density, and mineralization on bone strength. J Biomech 1989;22:419-26.

21. Martin RB, Boardman DL: The effects of collagen fiber orientation, porosity, density and mineralization on bovine cortical bone bending properties. J Biomech 1993;26:1047-54.

22. Riggs CM, Vaughan LC, Evans GP, et al: Mechanical implications of collagen fiber orientation in cortical bone of the equine radius. Anat Embryol 1993;187:239-48.

23. Takano Y, Turner CH, Owan I, et al: Elastic anisotropy and collagen orientation of osteonal bone are dependent on the mechanical strain distribution. J Orthop Res 1999;17:59-66.

24. Giraud-Guille M-M: Liquid crystalline phases of sonicated type I collagen. Biol Cell 1989;67:97-101.

25. Puustjärvi K, Nieminen J, Räsänen T, et al: Do more highly organized collagen fibrils increase bone mechanical strength in loss of mineral density after one-year running training? J Bone Miner Res 1999;14:321-29.

26. Burstein AH, Reilly DT, Martens M: Aging of bone tissue: mechanical properties. J Bone Joint Surg Am 1976;58:82-6.

27. Courtney AC, Hayes WC, Gibson LJ: Age-related differences in post-yield damage in human cortical bone: experiment and model. J Biomech 1996;29:1463-71.

28. Sobelman OS, Gibeling JC, Stover SM, et al: Do microcracks decrease or increase fatigue resistance in cortical bone? J Biomech 2004;37:1295-1303.

29. McCalden RW, McGeough JA, Barker MB, Court-Brown CM: Age-related changes in the tensile properties of cortical bone. J Bone Joint Surg Am 1993;75:1193-1205.

30. Hui S, Slemenda CW, Johnston CC Jr: Age and bone mass as predictors of fracture in a prospective study. J Clin Invest 1988;81:1804-9.

31. DeLaet CEDH, van Hout BA, Burger H, et al: Bone density and risk of hip fracture in men and women: cross-sectional analysis. Br Med J 1997;315:221-25.

32. Vashishth D, Wu PC: Age related loss in bone toughness is explained by non-enzymatic glycation of collagen. Trans Orthop Res Soc 2004;29:497.

33. Nalla RK, Kruzic JJ, Kinney JH, Ritchie RO: Effect of aging on the toughness of human cortical bone: evaluation by R-curves. Bone 2004;35:1240-46.

34. Catanese J III, Iverson EP, Ng RK, Keaveny TM: Heterogeneity of the mechanical properties of demineralized bone. J Biomech 1999;32:1365-69.

35. Wu P, Koharski C, Nonnenmann H, Vashishth D: Loading of non-enzymatically glycated and damaged bone results in an instantaneous fracture. Trans Orthop Res Soc 2003;28.

36. Zioupos P, Currey JD: Changes in the stiffness, strength, and toughness of human cortical bone with age. Bone 1998;22:57-66.

37. Oxlund H, Mosekilde Li, Ørtoft G: Reduced concentration of collagen reducible cross links in human trabecular bone with respect to age and osteoporosis. Bone 1996;19:479-84.

38. Bailey AJ, Wotton SF, Sims TJ, Thompson PW: Biochemical changes in the collagen of human osteoporotic bone matrix. Conn Tiss Res 1993;29:119-32.

39. Knott L, Bailey AJ: Collagen cross links in mineralizing tissues: a review of their chemistry, function and clinical relevance. Bone 1998;22:181-87.

40. Martin RB, Atkinson PJ: Age and sex-related changes in the structure and strength of the human femoral shaft. J Biomech 1977;10:223-31.

41. Beck TJ, Oreskovic TL, Stone KL, et al: Structural adaptation to changing skeletal load in the progression toward hip fragility: the study of osteoporotic fractures. J Bone Miner Res 2001;16:1108-19.

42. Duan Y, Turner CH, Kim B-T, Seeman E: Sexual dimorphism in bone fragility is more the result of gender differences in age-related bone gain than bone loss. J Bone Miner Res 2001;16:2267-75.

43. Schaffler MB, Boyce TM, Fyhrie DP: Tissue and matrix failure modes in human compact bone during tensile fatigue. Trans Orthop Res Soc 1996;21:57.

44. Burr DB, Turner CH, Naick P, et al: Does microdamage accumulation affect the mechanical properties of bone? J Biomech 1998;31:337-45.

45. Burr DB, Forwood MR, Fyhrie DP, et al: Bone microdamage and skeletal fragility in osteoporotic and stress fractures. J Bone Miner Res 1997;12:6-15.

46. Mashiba T, Hirano T, Turner CH, et al: Suppressed bone turnover by bisphosphonates increases microdamage accumulation and reduces some biomechanical properties in dog rib. J Bone Miner Res 2000;15:613-20.

47. Komatsubara S, Mori S, Mashiba T, et al: Long-term treatment of incadronate disocium accumulates microdamage but improves the trabecular bone microarchitecture in dog vertebra. J Bone Miner Res 2003;18:512-20.

48. Lundy MW, Stauffer M, Wergedal JE, et al: Histomorphometric analysis of iliac crest bone biopsies in placebo-treated versus fluoride-treated subjects. Osteoporos Int 1995;5:115-29.

49. Hirano T, Turner CH, Forwood MR, et al: Does suppression of bone turnover impair mechanical properties by allowing microdamage accumulation? Bone 2000;27:13-20.

50. Turner CH: Biomechanics of bone: determinants of skeletal fragility and bone quality. Osteoporosis Int 2002;13:97-104.

51. Burr DB, Miller L, Grynpas M, et al: Tissue mineralization is increased following 1-year treatment with high doses of bisphosphonates in dogs. Bone 2003;33:960-69.

52. Meunier PJ, Boivin G: Bone mineral density reflects bone mass but also the degree of mineralization of bone: therapeutic implications. Bone 1997;21:373-77.

53. Boivin G, Chavassieux PM, Santora AC, et al: Alendronate increases bone strength by increasing the mean degree of mineralization of bone tissue in osteoporotic women. Bone 2000;27:687-94.

54. Nuzzo S, Lafage-Proust MH, Martin-Badosa E, et al: Synchrotron radiation microtomography allows the analysis of three-dimensional microarchitecture and degree of mineralization of human iliac crest biopsy specimens: effects of etidronate treatment. J Bone Miner Res 2002;17:1372-82.

55. Cranney A, Guyatt G, Griffith L, et al: IX: Summary of meta-analyses of therapies for postmenopausal osteoporosis. Endocrine Rev 2002;23:570-78.

56. Bone HG, Hosking D, Devogelaer J-P, et al: Ten years' experience with alendronate for osteoporosis in post-menopausal women. N Engl J Med 2004;350:1189-99.

57. Roschger P, Rinnerthaler S, Yates J, et al: Alendronate increases degree and uniformity of mineralization in cancellous bone and decreases the porosity in cortical bone of osteoporotic women. Bone 2001;29:185-91.

58. Boivin G, Meunier PJ: The degree of mineralization of bone tissue measured by computerized quantitative contact microradiography. Calcif Tiss Int 2002;70:503-11.

59. Heaney RP: Is the paradigm shifting? Bone 2003;33:457-65.

60. Parfitt AM: High bone turnover is intrinsically harmful: two paths to a similar conclusion. J Bone Miner Res 2002;17:1558-59.

61. Riggs BL, Melton LJ III: Bone turnover matters: the raloxifene treatment paradox of dramatic decreases in vertebral fractures without commensurate increases in bone density. J Bone Miner Res 2002;17:11-14.

62. Borah B, Dufresne TE, Chmielewski PA, et al: Risedronate preserves trabecular architecture and increases bone strength in vertebra of ovariectomized minipigs as measured by three-dimensional microcomputed tomography. J Bone Miner Res 2002;17:1139-47.

63. Cummings SR, Karpf DB, Harris F, et al: Improvement in spine bone density and reduction in risk of vertebral fractures during treatment with antiresorptive drugs. Am J Med 2002; 112:281-89.

64. Paschallis E, Burr DB, Mendelsohn R, et al: Bone mineral and collagen quality in humeri of ovariectomized cynomolgus monkeys given rhPTH (1-34) for 18 months. J Bone Miner Res 2003;18:769-75.

65. Jerome CP, Burr DB, Van Bibber T, et al: Treatment with human parathyroid hormone (1-34) for 18 months increases cancellous bone volume and improves trabecular architecture in ovariectomized cynomolgus monkeys (Macaca fascicularis). Bone 2001;28:150-59.

66. Neer RM, Arnaud CD, Zanchetta JR, et al: Effect of parathyroid hormone (1-34) on fractures and bone mineral density in postmenopausal women with osteoporosis. N Engl J Med 2001;344:1434-41.

67. Burr DB, Hirano T, Turner CH, et al: Intermittently administered human parathyroid hormone (1-34) treatment increases intracortical bone turnover and porosity without reducing bone strength in the humerus of ovariectomized cynomolgus monkeys. J Bone Miner Res 2001;16:157-65.

68. Turner CH, Burr DB: Basic biomechanical measurements of bone: a tutorial. Bone 1993;14:595-608.

69. Reilly DT, Burstein AH: The elastic and ultimate properties of compact bone tissue. J Biomech 1975;8:393-405.

70. Spatz H-Ch, O'Leary EJ, Vincent JFV: Young's moduli and shear moduli in cortical bone. Proc R Soc Lond B Biol Sci 1996; 263:287-94.

71. Levenston ME: Periosteal bone formation stimulated by externally induced bending strains. J Bone Miner Res 1995;10:671.

72. Gere JM, Timoshenko S: Mechanics of materials. Boston, MA, PWS-Kent, 1984.

73. Schriefer JL, Robling AG, Warden SJ, Turner CH: Determining the best skeletal sites for measuring bone fragility of mice. J Biomech, in press.

74. Roark RJ, Young WC: Formulas for stress and strain. New York, McGraw-Hill, 1975.

75. Einhorn TA, Wakley GK, Linkhart S, et al: Incorporation of sodium fluoride into cortical bone does not impair the mechanical properties of the appendicular skeleton of rats. Calcif Tissue Int 1992;51:127-31.

76. Forwood MR, Parker AW: Effects of exercise on bone growth: mechanical and physical properties studied in the rat. Clin Biomech 1987;2:185-90.

77. Keller TS, Spengler DM, Carter DR: Geometric, elastic, and structural properties of maturing rat femora. J Orthop Res 1986;4:57-67.

78. Hvid I, Hansen SL: Trabecular bone strength patterns at the proximal tibial epiphysis. J Orthop Res 1985;3:464-72.

79. Sumner DR, Willke TL, Berzins A, Turner TM: Distribution of Young's modulus in the cancellous bone of the proximal canine tibia. J Biomechanics 1994;27:1095-99.

80. Timoshenko SP, Goodier JN: Theory of elasticity, 3rd ed. New York: McGraw-Hill, 1970:380-409.

81. Carter DR, Hayes WC: Fatigue life of compact bone: I. Effects of stress amplitude, temperature and density. J Biomechanics 1976;9:27-34.

82. Lakes RS, Saha S: Cement line motion in bone. Science 1979; 204:501-3.

83. Schaffler MB, Radin EL, Burr DB: Mechanical and morphological effects of strain rate on fatigue of compact bone. Bone 1989;10:207-14.

84. Carter DR, Caler WC: A cumulative damage model for bone fracture. J Orthop Res 1985;3:84-90.

85. Schaffler MB, Radin EL, Burr DB: Long-term fatigue behavior of compact bone at low strain magnitude and rate. Bone 1990;11:321-26.

86. Caler WE, Carter DR: Bone creep-fatigue damage accumulation. J Biomechanics 1989;22:625-35.

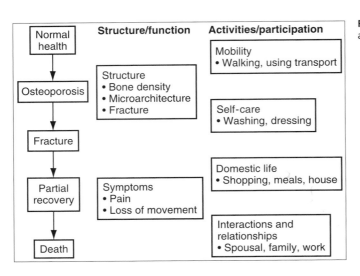

Figure 7-2. A model of the impact of osteoporosis and fracture.

United Kingdom from the age of 50 years has been estimated at 3.1% of women and 1.2% of men.[3] One-third of people older than 50 years with vertebral deformities will have deformities of several vertebrae.[6] The most commonly affected vertebrae are at the thoracolumbar junction and the midthoracic spine (Figure 7-3).[6]

ACUTE SYMPTOMATIC (CLINICAL) VERTEBRAL FRACTURE

Clinical Aspects

Acute clinical vertebral fracture usually manifests with sudden onset of back pain. The pain may be diffuse across the back and is often referred around the body, usually symmetrically. The precipitating trauma is often mild, such as lifting or a sudden jar.

The associated pain with an acute vertebral fracture is often severe, and mobility can be greatly restricted. The pain may be severe for a couple of weeks and then subside, although in many affected people it is persistent. Fractures of the lower thoracic and upper lumbar spine are associated with worse pain. Pain can usually be elicited on percussion, localized to the vertebral fracture; some patients have more diffuse tenderness. The acute pain often precipitates paraspinal muscle spasm and greatly restricted movement of the spine. Rest is preferred to standing or walking. Any movement, in particular coughing, sneezing, or straining, aggravates the pain. Vertebral fractures due to osteoporosis are not typically associated with neurological signs or signs of nerve tension.

Outcome

Acute clinical vertebral fractures affect activities and restrict participation. Between 2% and 10% of affected people are hospitalized,[9] and a great variation has been found between populations of countries in Europe[10] and also between black and white women in the United States.[11] Some patients require long-term care, in particular the more elderly or those with comorbidities. Limitation is mostly due to pain and loss of movement of the spine. The impact of a recent vertebral fracture is greater in people who have already sustained a vertebral fracture.[12] Not all vertebral fractures manifest clinically with pain, but these subclinical fractures are still associated with reduced health-related quality of life affecting physical function and general health perception.[13] Pain and limitation of activities increase with increasing numbers of radiologically identified vertebral fractures.[14,15]

The presenting acute clinical vertebral fracture may be the initial event, but the fracture may be the worsening of a preexisting vertebral fracture or a further vertebral fracture, because those who have already sustained one fracture are at high risk of sustaining further fractures. In a large prospective study, the risk of sustaining a new vertebral fracture was increased fivefold during a year of observation in people who had one or more vertebral fractures at baseline compared with those without vertebral fracture at baseline.[16]

MULTIPLE OR CHRONIC VERTEBRAL FRACTURE

Clinical Aspects

If the person has multiple vertebral deformities, there is an increased risk of chronic back pain and there will be loss of height and stoop. Stoop is associated with symptoms such as loss of spinal mobility, decreased lung capacity and breathlessness, compression of the abdomen with reflux esophagitis, difficulty in eating large meals, constipation, and stress

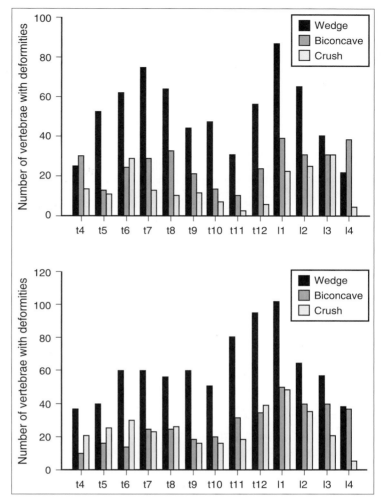

Figure 7-3. Common sites of vertebral fracture. (From Ismail AA, Cooper C, Felsenberg D et al: Number and type of vertebral deformities: epidemiological characteristics and relation to back pain and height loss. European Vetebral Osteoporosis Study Group. Osteoporos Int 1999;9:206-13.)

incontinence. There is typically a protuberant abdomen and sometimes the ribs can impinge on the pelvic brim, causing pain. There may be intertrigo in the abdominal skinfolds. The thoracic kyphosis results in hyperextension of the neck so that the affected people can see where they are going, and this may result in chronic neck pain. There is distress associated with the change in body habitus as well as concern about further fracture.

Outcome

Chronic back pain and impairment of quality of life may accompany these symptoms. Pain and the limitation of activities worsen with each vertebral fracture and with increasing spinal deformity. Although thoracic vertebral fractures result in the most apparent deformity with kyphosis, it is lumbar vertebral fractures that have the greatest impact on quality of life.[14,15] The impact on health-related quality of life has been demonstrated using condition-specific instruments such as QUALEFFO[12-14] and OPAQ[15] and generic health-related quality-of-life instruments.[12,14,17] The domains mainly affected are pain, physical function, and general health status. This has been demonstrated in cross-sectional and longitudinal studies.[12,13,15] The impact has also been shown using measures of functionality such as the Modified Barthel Index and the Timed "Up and Go" test.[17] Vertebral fractures have an impact on health-related quality of life whether or not they are associated with pain. The outcome is worse with age[14] and in the presence of comorbidity.

Vertebral fractures are associated with an increased risk of further vertebral fracture[16,18] and of hip fracture in women,[19] the risk increasing with the number of prevalent vertebral fractures. For two or more prevalent vertebral deformities, the relative risk of hip fracture was increased seven-fold.[19] This is not surprising, as vertebral fractures best indicate the presence of underlying osteoporosis.

Vertebral fractures are associated with a long-term increase in risk for mortality.[20-22] In the Study of Osteoporotic Fractures, as compared with women who did not have a vertebral fracture, women with one or more fractures had a 1.23-fold greater age-adjusted mortality rate, and mortality rose with greater numbers of vertebral fractures, from 19 per 1000 woman-years in women with no fractures to 44 per 1000 woman-years in those with five or more fractures.[22] Excess mortality is largely related to cardiovascular and pulmonary disease and cancer.[21,22] It probably represents the health status of those who sustain vertebral fractures rather than the consequence of the fracture.

The economic impact of vertebral fractures is not as great as for other fractures, as between 2% and 10% necessitate admission to the hospital.[9] They account for about 5% of the direct health care expenditure in the United States related to osteoporosis.[23] Treatment costs should increase as the future risk of these individuals for further fractures is recognized.

HIP FRACTURE

Clinical Aspects

Hip fractures are fractures of the proximal femur, either through the femoral neck (subcapital or transcervical fracture, an intracapsular fracture) or through the trochanteric region (intertrochanteric or subtrochanteric fracture, an extracapsular fracture). The typical age of a person sustaining a hip fracture in Europe is about 80 years. Many affected people are frail with comorbidities and already unable to live independently.

Fractures of the proximal femur usually follow a fall. The acute fracture causes severe pain and immediate loss of mobility and results in hospital admission. In Sweden, such fractures account for 48% of admissions for fracture in men and 49% in women and for 54% and 56% of hospital-bed days, respectively.[24] Virtually all patients with hip fractures in developed countries undergo surgical procedures, either nailing or joint replacement.[25,26]

Outcome

The poor outcome after hip fracture in elderly patients has been shown in several studies. The long-term loss of mobility is a major problem. In a population-based study of all hip fractures in patients 50 years or older in Oslo over a 1-year period, 593 of 1002 subjects completed a questionnaire that demonstrated the impact on activities of daily living and independence.[27] The proportion of patients living in nursing homes increased from 15% before to 30% after the hip fracture, and men were twice as likely to move into a nursing home as women. Of the patients living in their own

homes before the hip fracture, 33% of those older than 85 years and 6% of those younger than 75 years had to move to nursing homes after hip fracture. The proportion of patients walking without any aid decreased from 76% to 36%, and 43% of the patients lost their pre-fracture ability to move outside on their own. More than one-quarter of the patients (28%) lost their ability to cook their own dinner after sustaining hip fracture. The probability of these events increased with increasing age (Figure 7-4). In a prospective study of 102 people 65 years of age and older admitted consecutively after hip fracture to a university and a general hospital,[28] the mean age of the participants was 83 years, 58% of patients came from their own homes, and 42% of patients came from institutions. Nearly 70% of patients had two or more diagnoses other than the hip fracture. Cumulative mortality rate was 20% at 4 months after fracture. Of surviving patients, at 4 months only 57% were back in their original situation for accommodation, 43% reached the same level of walking ability, and 17% achieved the same level of activities of daily living as before fracture.

Outcome is affected by the characteristics of the fracture; age, general health, and functional status of the person sustaining the hip fracture; and the management of their fracture. People living in residential or care homes are much more at risk of having a hip fracture, and this increased risk compared with those living in their own homes has been found to be more marked in the younger elderly.[29]

Formally assessing health-related quality of life after hip fracture is biased by high nonresponse rates in studies due to the age and mental state of many of the subjects.[30] In most older people who sustain a hip fracture, there is some long-term impairment of mobility and sometimes chronic pain. Many lose their independence, in particular those who had some limitation of their activity before the hip fracture, usually related to comorbidity. In a study in France, people living in residential care who sustained a hip fracture had higher subsequent morbidity and mortality than those who had been living in their own homes.[29]

Although those who return to their own homes would appear to have a good outcome, many do not return to their pre-fracture lifestyle and have impaired mobility and balance along with reduced functional and social independence.[31] Function before the fracture[32] and on discharge from the hospital[30] have been found to be the strongest predictors of functional status 1 year after fracture in survivors.

Fear of fracture can alter behavior, and older women place a high marginal value on their health and independence. In a time trade-off study, women older than 75 years who had experienced a fall were prepared to trade off considerable length of life to avoid the

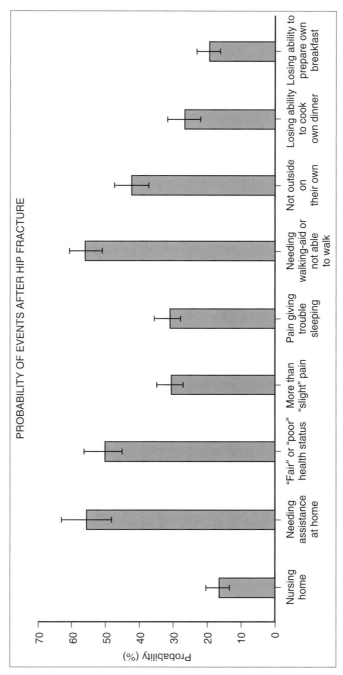

Figure 7-4. Probability of new events after sustaining hip fracture (percent with 95% confidence intervals) (From Osnes EK, Lofthus CM, Meyer HE, et al: Consequences of hip fracture on activities of daily life and residential needs. Osteoporos Int 2004;15:567-74.)

reduction in quality of life that happens after a "bad" hip fracture.[33]

The 1-year mortality rate varies between 12% and 37% in studies, increasing with age, but the greatest excess mortality rate is found among subjects younger than 80 years[34] and in males.[35] Mortality risk is greater for those with coexisting illnesses and poor pre-fracture functional status. Six-month mortality rate has been shown to be highest for patients with displaced femoral neck fractures (15.8%) and lowest for patients with nondisplaced femoral neck fractures (5.7%).[36] Major causes of death are pneumonia, pulmonary embolism, stroke, myocardial infarction, and cardiac failure. Mortality rate is greatest in the first 6 months and returns to the expected level by 2 years.

Hip fractures have the greatest economic impact because of the need for hospitalization[24] and surgery in the acute stage and the loss of independence by those who survive. Only about 45% of those sustaining a hip fracture are discharged home, and 20% require long-stay residential care. Although the health care costs in fracture management are considerable, the indirect costs relating to support in the community are twice as great. These costs, both short- and long-term, relate to the health and social care system and financial incentives of the system. In the United Kingdom, hip fractures account for 87% of the total cost of osteoporotic fractures in women, with the acute hospital cost of a hip fracture estimated at £4808 in 1998 with a total cost per fracture at £12,124.[37] In the European Community, the total hospital costs of hip fracture in 1998 were estimated to be more than 3.5 billion Euros with estimated total care costs of over 9 billion Euros.[38] In a case control study of osteoporotic fractures in Olmsted County, Minnesota, USA, the incremental direct medical costs for the year following an osteoporotic fracture were found to be greatest after distal femur (US$11,756) and hip fractures (US$11,241).[39] Similar figures have been estimated in Europe.[40]

DISTAL RADIUS FRACTURES

Clinical Aspects

Distal radius fracture is one of the most common fractures and is most often a Colles fracture. In women it is considered to be an indicator for osteoporosis and future fracture risk. It is estimated that 16.6% of women and 2.9% of men will suffer a distal radius fracture from the age of 50 years in the United Kingdom.[3] The fracture typically occurs in a person who falls forward reaching out with the hand to break the fall. The fracture is located within the distal 3 to 4 cm of the radius that is rich in trabecular bone but has thin cortices. The most benign type is undisplaced, but dorsal displacement is common, and in more severe fracture

types the fracture continues intra-articularly into the radiocarpal joint. Undisplaced fractures are treated with a stabilizing cast for 4 to 5 weeks, whereas displaced fractures require prior reduction.

Outcome

Distal radius fractures result in pain and loss of function and can result in short-term loss of independence in an older person. Hand function is greatly impaired until the fracture is healed, but long-term weakness of grip and limited activities are common. Most patients are treated as out-patients, but hospitalization rates in the United Kingdom were found to be 23% of men and 19% of women, the proportion being age related.[41] Hospitalization may be less with access to day care facilities. Only 50% of affected people report good functional outcome at 6 months, and up to 30% of individuals may suffer some long-term complication. These problems include algodystrophy (reflex sympathetic dystrophy) and osteoarthritis of the wrist. Many patients exhibit risk factors for osteoporosis,[42] new falls, and fractures.[43]

The direct costs relate to hospital admission, although the economic impact of long-term limitations of upper limb activities is not known. Because these fractures occur in many people of working age, they are likely to have a greater economic impact than is recognized.

The occurrence of distal forearm fracture is an indicator of risk of further fractures in life and is a reason for a full assessment of risk and treatment, if appropriate, to reduce that risk.

PROXIMAL HUMERUS FRACTURE

Clinical Aspects

Fractures of the proximal part of the humerus are common in the elderly and are associated with osteoporosis, whereas proximal humerus fracture in the young often is the result of high-energy trauma. It has been estimated that fractures of the proximal part of the humerus account for 4% to 8% of all fractures.[3,44] In persons older than 40 years of age, fractures of the proximal humerus account for 76% of all fractures of the humerus.[45] Data suggest that fracture of the proximal humerus is the third most common fracture in people older than 65 years.[3,46] Fractures of the proximal humerus have shown a similar pattern of increase as other common fragility fractures,[3,47] and the estimated remaining lifetime risk from age 45 in Sweden is 13.3% in women and 4.4% in men.[48] Fractures of the proximal humerus increase with age in both men and women—with women being somewhat older at the time of fracture, on average around 70 to 74 years versus 65 years in men—when excluding children,[46,49] whereas the highest age-specific incidence is in women between 80 and 89 years of age.[46] Bone mineral density of the femoral neck is a predictor of humerus fracture, doubling the risk,[50] and when combined with risk factors for falls the risk is further increased.[51]

Fracture of the proximal humerus occurs when a person is unable to fully reach out to counteract a fall, and instead falls slightly on the side and hits the shoulder region. Most persons tend to be generally fit and 90% are living at home prior to the fracture.[46] The fracture is most commonly minimally displaced and with a somewhat oblique orientation through the surgical neck of the proximal humerus. A minimally displaced main fracture may be accompanied by avulsion of the greater tuberosity of humerus, that is, the insertion of the supraspinous tendon. According to the study by Court-Brown and colleagues[46] evaluating more than 1000 patients, 66% involved the surgical neck or greater tuberosity. The fracture may also be comminuted with two main fragments or, in severe cases, four fragments, and the severity is associated with increasing age. Multifragmented fractures are often displaced and challenging to treat, whereas the minimally displaced fracture merely requires conservative treatment with a sling for 2 to 3 weeks. The initial period of significant pain even in minimally displaced fractures may last for up to 3 weeks, because conservative treatment provides only limited stability. In addition, bleeding from the fracture may descend through gravity into the soft tissues of the upper arm or even down to the forearm, augmenting the pain because of swelling. It is of utmost importance to start mobility training early, within 2 to 3 weeks, to diminish the functional limitations from decreased range of motion and pain.

Outcome

Fractures of the proximal humerus appear to occur in persons who are relatively fit but less fit than those who sustain distal radius fractures.[52] The immediate problems arise from the shoulder pain, which is continuous but aggravated on motion and when trying to lie down on a bed. Patients often report impaired sleep or the need to sleep in a sitting position. Pain in combination with sleep deprivation affects general well-being, but it normally begins to subside after 2 to 4 weeks. The functional impairment during the rehabilitation period involves problems in preparing food, reaching in cupboards, and personal care such as washing and dressing. Rehabilitation after a proximal humerus fracture often exceeds 3 months of training.

The short- and long-term functional outcomes depend on both fracture-related and patient-related factors. Available reports indicate that functional outcome is associated with age at the time of fracture, the pre-fracture health and functional status of the patient, and the displacement of the fracture. For minimally displaced fractures, the functional outcome was found to be excellent or good in 77% over 12 to 17 months in 104 patients and 88% at 12 months in 507 patients.[46,53] Despite this, the objective range of motion recovery appeared to be lower, about 75% after 1 year, suggesting that patients can cope with a certain limitation of motion, whereas remaining shoulder pain is more disabling. Assessment at 1 year indicated that the clinical status at this time was predictive of long-term outcome, with 55% reporting some shoulder pain and functional limitation up to 13 years after fracture (C. Olsson, PhD Thesis, 2005). Comorbidities significantly affect the results, regardless of fracture type.

Fracture of the proximal humerus is predictive of future fractures in both men and women, with a five times risk increase for subsequent extremity fractures in men.[54] Fracture of the proximal humerus is also associated with increased mortality with an endpoint survival difference of 16% or 3.9 years over 13 years of follow-up (Figure 7-5).[49] The increased mortality risk is most pronounced in men and during the first 3 years after fracture, with cardiovascular disease and malignancy being the most common causes of death.

The economic impact from this type of fracture has not been calculated, but the time in weeks to return to work was 4 to 10 weeks according to Court-Brown and colleagues,[46] with the shortest time for those sustaining a fracture before the age of 40. The time to regain functional capacity for personal care and household chores was between 6 and 21 weeks for patients older than 80 years, suggesting that the costs for social services are not negligible.

PELVIC FRACTURE

Clinical Aspects

Pelvic fractures from high-energy trauma can be life threatening, particularly for an elderly person, but they account for less than 20% of pelvic fractures in the elderly. In total, pelvic fractures account for 2% to 8% of all fractures.[3,55] Pelvic fractures in the elderly occur from minor trauma or from skeletal insufficiency. The low-energy pelvic fracture is a stable fracture passing through either the superior or the inferior pubic ramus or both rami, commonly on the same side. Fractures of the pelvic rami after trauma can be either undisplaced or have varying degrees of displacement, whereas insufficiency fractures are commonly undisplaced and not always detectable on the first x-ray examination. The majority of patients (up to 80%) are women and older than 80 years of age.[56,57] Fractures of the pelvic rami in the elderly are treated symptomatically with adequate pain medications, and mobilization requires walking aids.

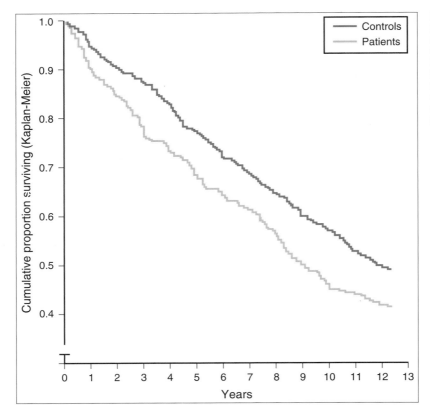

Figure 7-5. Cumulative proportion of patients surviving with fracture of the surgical neck of humerus compared with age- and sex-matched controls. (From Olsson C, Peterson C, Nordquist S: Increased mortality after fracture of the surgical neck of the humerus: a case-control study of 253 patients with a 12-year follow-up. Acta Orthop Scand 2003;74:714-17.)

A pelvic fracture usually occurs after a fall from standing height or from unintentional sliding onto the floor and causes immediate pain located in the groin. Pelvic insufficiency fractures can be identified after a sudden or insidious onset of groin pain and pain on walking. The symptoms from pelvic low-trauma fractures are similar to those of a hip fracture and clinically it is not possible to differentiate a pelvic fracture from a hip fracture with certainty. The fracture needs to be diagnosed using imaging, which may correctly identify a fracture on the initial examination with plain x-ray in 80% of the cases, while additional imaging, preferably magnetic resonance imaging or a bone scan, is necessary to diagnose the remaining especially insufficiency fractures.[57-59]

Outcome

Comorbidities are common in patients with pelvic fractures: 83% had at least two severe disorders and 16% had more than three in a French study.[57] The pre-fracture functional status of the patient had implications for outcome, and furthermore, estimates of dependency are related to the structure of health and social care and thus not exactly comparable. In the study from the United Kingdom, up to 21% of the patients were institutionalized prior to fracture,[56] whereas the majority were living independently in the studies from France and the United States. At discharge, only half of the patients had regained self-sufficiency[57] and half had been transferred to nursing homes.[56]

Most patients with pelvic fractures require hospitalization; patients with pelvic fractures use 6% of the total number of hospital days used by fracture patients in Sweden (hip fracture, 55%), with an average length of stay of 13.4 days for men and 11.5 for women.[24] In addition, owing to the frailty of many of the patients, a number of complicating conditions are common during and after hospitalization. These data indicate that pelvic fracture inflicts a significant burden on the health care system but also on social care, in terms of both economy and personnel.

In relatively healthy and community-dwelling persons, 92% had regained their pre-fracture ambulatory status, and activities of daily living were resumed by 95%[53]; however, in other studies, 24 of 41 previously self-sufficient patients regained their functional status without using a walking aid.[57] Pelvic fracture is clearly a fracture of the frail elderly, and the 1-year mortality rate varies between 12% and 27%.

FRACTURES IN RHEUMATOID ARTHRITIS

Rheumatoid arthritis is associated with osteoporosis, both juxta-articular and generalized, as well as an increased risk of fracture. Vertebral deformities are more prevalent in people with rheumatoid arthritis as compared with control subjects[60,61] and are greater in steroid users.[62] Nonvertebral fractures are also more prevalent, as is most clearly demonstrated for hip fractures.[63] In addition, stress fractures are seen in people with rheumatoid arthritis, which occur without a history of trauma and can be misdiagnosed as an exacerbation of rheumatoid arthritis. They are usually of the lower limbs or pelvis, most commonly the tibia, followed in frequency by the fibula, tibia and fibula, femur, and pubic ramus.[64] Stress fractures of the pelvic ring can be most difficult to diagnose, and scintigraphy or magnetic resonance imaging may be required. Few data are available as to how these fractures affect quality of life, but they almost certainly have a greater impact in people with rheumatoid arthritis than in others because of the cumulative disability.

Impact of Comorbidity

Comorbidity clearly plays an important role for the outcome of fracture. Firstly, comorbidity is a risk factor for fracture, most pronounced for hip fracture and in men.[65] In women, biological age, an indirect measure of frailty and comorbidity, is associated with increased overall fracture incidence and mortality risk[66] and also of falls.[67] Furthermore, comorbidity is a significant factor in the evaluation of a fracture patient upon admission, as it has consequences for both short- and long-term care. The elderly frail individual with several concomitant conditions often suffers complications in the acute phase of a fractures. This is particularly true for fractures severely affecting general mobility, such as hip and pelvic fractures. The complications in this phase include urinary tract infections, pressure sores, pneumonia, myocardial infarctions, cerebrovascular incidents, gastric bleeding, and deep venous thrombosis.[68]

In a longer term perspective, comorbidity affects outcome in terms of general health and functioning. People with worse health at the time of fracture require a longer time to regain functions of daily living, including walking independently, washing, dressing, preparing food, and gripping things, or these abilities are never fully regained. This is again most obvious for patients with hip or pelvic fracture, a large proportion of whom become dependent on partial or full-time care. In this respect, it is pertinent to highlight the importance of adequate fracture treatment for all patients suffering osteoporotic fractures, regardless of pre-fracture status. In a study of hip fracture patients older than 80 years with mental deficiency or institutionalized, a change from pinning to joint replacement improved walking ability and left fewer patients with pain at 1 year, results similar to those of independently living persons undergoing the same treatment and better than previous treatment.[69]

Comorbidity should also be evaluated in patients with vertebral fracture, many of whom have developed osteoporosis secondary to conditions such as chronic obstructive lung disease, gastrointestinal conditions, or other inflammatory conditions including rheumatoid arthritis, or from medication. In an already compromised person, further decline of respiratory function, nutrition, or mobility from spinal deformation and pain necessitates specific considerations and is associated with increased care needs.

CONCLUSION

Fractures in older people caused by underlying osteoporosis have an enormous impact on quality of life in both the short and the long term. They cause pain and loss of function, which may be prolonged. They are also associated with increased mortality risk. The costs to the individual and society are therefore great. The acute management of fracture and subsequent rehabilitation are central to optimizing the outcome, but many people who sustain fractures around the globe do not have access to the necessary level of care. An older person who has sustained a fracture is at increased risk of further fractures and should be assessed and treated as appropriate to reduce that risk.

REFERENCES

1. Assessment of fracture risk and its application to screening for postmenopausal osteoporosis: report of a World Health Organization Study Group. WHO Technical Report Series No. 843. Geneva: World Health Organization, 1994.
2. Osteoporosis prevention, diagnosis, and therapy. NIH Consensus Statement Online 2000;17:1-36. Available at http://consensus.nih.gov/2000/2000Osteoporosis111html.htm.
3. van Staa TP, Dennison EM, Leufkens HG, et al: Epidemiology of fractures in England and Wales. Bone 2001;29:517-22.
4. World Health Organization: International classification of functioning, disability and health: ICF. Geneva: World Health Organization, 2001.
5. Cieza A, Schwarzkopf S, Sigl T, et al: ICF Core Sets for osteoporosis. J Rehabil Med 2004;44 Suppl:81-6.

6. Ismail AA, Cooper C, Felsenberg D, et al: Number and type of vertebral deformities: epidemiological characteristics and relation to back pain and height loss. European Vertebral Osteoporosis Study Group. Osteoporos Int 1999;9:206-13.

7. The European Prospective Osteoporosis Study Group: Incidence of vertebral fractures in Europe: results from the European prospective osteoporosis study (EPOS). J Bone Miner Res 2002;17:716-24.

8. O'Neill TW, Felsenberg D, Varlow J, et al: The prevalence of vertebral deformity in European men and women: the European Vertebral Osteoporosis Study. J Bone Miner Res 1996;11:1010-18.

9. Cooper C: Epidemiology of osteoporosis. Osteoporos Int 1999;9 Suppl 2:S2-S8.

10. Johnell O, Gullberg B, Kanis JA: The hospital burden of vertebral fracture in Europe: a study of national register sources. Osteoporos Int 1997;7:138-44.

11. Jacobsen SJ, Cooper C, Gottlieb MS, et al: Hospitalization with vertebral fracture among the aged: a national population-based study, 1986-1989. Epidemiology 1992;3:515-58.

12. Cockerill W, Lunt M, Silman AJ, et al: Health-related quality of life and radiographic vertebral fracture. Osteoporos Int 2004;15:113-19.

13. Oleksik AM, Ewing S, Shen W, et al: Impact of incident vertebral fractures on health related quality of life (HRQOL) in postmenopausal women with prevalent vertebral fractures. Osteoporos Int 2005;16:861-70.

14. Oleksik A, Lips P, Dawson A, et al: Health-related quality of life in postmenopausal women with low BMD with or without prevalent vertebral fractures. J Bone Miner Res 2000;15:1384-92.

15. Silverman SL, Minshall ME, Shen W, et al: The relationship of health-related quality of life to prevalent and incident vertebral fractures in postmenopausal women with osteoporosis: results from the Multiple Outcomes of Raloxifene Evaluation Study. Arthritis Rheum 2001;44:2611-19.

16. Lindsay R, Silverman SL, Cooper C, et al: Risk of new vertebral fracture in the year following a fracture. JAMA 2001;285:320-23.

17. Hall SE, Criddle RA, Comito TL, et al: A case-control study of quality of life and functional impairment in women with long-standing vertebral osteoporotic fracture. Osteoporos Int 1999;9:508-15.

18. Ross PD, Davis JW, Epstein RS, et al: Pre-existing fractures and bone mass predict vertebral fracture incidence in women. Ann Intern Med 1991;114:919-23.

19. Ismail AA, Cockerill W, Cooper C, et al: Prevalent vertebral deformity predicts incident hip though not distal forearm fracture: results from the European Prospective Osteoporosis Study. Osteoporos Int 2001;12:85-90.

20. Center JR, Nguyen TV, Schneider D, et al: Mortality after all major types of osteoporotic fracture in men and women: an observational study. Lancet 1999;353:878-82.

21. Hasserius R, Karlsson MK, Nilsson BE, et al: Prevalent vertebral deformities predict increased mortality and increased fracture rate in both men and women: a 10-year population-based study of 598 individuals from the Swedish cohort in the European Vertebral Osteoporosis Study. Osteoporos Int 2003;14:61-8.

22. Kado DM, Browner WS, Palermo L, et al: Vertebral fractures and mortality in older women: a prospective study. Study of Osteoporotic Fractures Research Group. Arch Intern Med 1999;159:1215-20.

23. Ray NF, Chan JK, Thamer M, et al: Medical expenditures for the treatment of osteoporotic fractures in the United States in 1995: report from the National Osteoporosis Foundation. J Bone Miner Res 1997;12:24-35.

24. Johnell O, Kanis JA, Jonsson B, et al: The burden of hospitalised fractures in Sweden. Osteoporos Int 2005;16:222-8.

25. Berglund-Roden M, Swierstra BA, Wingstrand H, et al: Prospective comparison of hip fracture treatment: 856 cases followed for 4 months in The Netherlands and Sweden. Acta Orthop Scand 1994;65:287-94.

26. Kitamura S, Hasegawa Y, Suzuki S, et al: Functional outcome after hip fracture in Japan. Clin Orthop Relat Res 1998;348:29-36.

27. Osnes EK, Lofthus CM, Meyer HE, et al: Consequences of hip fracture on activities of daily life and residential needs. Osteoporos Int 2004;15:567-74.

28. van Balen R, Steyerberg EW, Polder JJ, et al: Hip fracture in elderly patients: outcomes for function, quality of life, and type of residence. Clin Orthop Relat Res 2001;390:232-43.

29. Baudoin C, Fardellone P, Bean K, et al: Clinical outcomes and mortality after hip fracture: a 2-year follow-up study. Bone 1996;18:149S-157S.

30. Boonen S, Autier P, Barette M, et al: Functional outcome and quality of life following hip fracture in elderly women: a prospective controlled study. Osteoporos Int 2004;15:87-94.

31. Hall SE, Williams JA, Senior JA, et al: Hip fracture outcomes: quality of life and functional status in older adults living in the community. Aust N Z J Med 2000;30:327-32.

32. Koval KJ, Zuckerman JD: Hip fractures are an increasingly important public health problem. Clin Orthop Relat Res 1998;348:22-8.

33. Salkeld G, Cameron ID, Cumming RG, et al: Quality of life related to fear of falling and hip fracture in older women: a time trade off study. BMJ 2000;320:341-46.

34. Pande I, Pritchard C: Osteoporotic fractures in Cornwall. Lancet 1999;353:1707.

35. Trombetti A, Herrmann F, Hoffmeyer P, et al: Survival and potential years of life lost after hip fracture in men and age-matched women. Osteoporos Int 2002;13:731-37.

36. Cornwall R, Gilbert MS, Koval KJ, et al: Functional outcomes and mortality vary among different types of hip fractures: a function of patient characteristics. Clin Orthop Relat Res 2004;425:64-71.

37. Dolan P, Torgerson DJ: The cost of treating osteoporotic fractures in the United Kingdom female population. Osteoporos Int 1998;8:611-17.

38. Report on Osteoporosis in the European Community: Action for prevention. Luxembourg, European Communities, 1998.

39. Gabriel SE, Tosteson AN, Leibson CL, et al: Direct medical costs attributable to osteoporotic fractures. Osteoporos Int 2002;13:323-30.

40. Autier P, Haentjens P, Bentin J, et al: Costs induced by hip fractures: a prospective controlled study in Belgium. Belgian Hip Fracture Study Group. Osteoporos Int 2000;11:373-80.

41. O'Neill TW, Cooper C, Finn JD, et al: Incidence of distal forearm fracture in British men and women. Osteoporos Int 2001;12:555-58.

42. Peel NF, Barrington NA, Smith TW, et al: Distal forearm fracture as risk factor for vertebral osteoporosis. BMJ 1994;308:1543-44.

43. Nordell E, Kristinsdottir EK, Jarnlo GB, et al: Older patients with distal forearm fracture. A challenge to future fall and fracture prevention. Aging Clin Exp Res 2005;17:90-5.

44. Horak J, Nilsson BE: Epidemiology of fracture of the upper end of the humerus. Clin Orthop Relat Res 1975;112:250-53.

45. Rose SH, Melton LJ III, Morrey BF, et al: Epidemiologic features of humeral fractures. Clin Orthop Relat Res 1982;168:24-30.

46. Court-Brown CM, Garg A, McQueen MM: The epidemiology of proximal humeral fractures. Acta Orthop Scand 2001;72:365-71.

47. Kannus P, Palvanen M, Niemi S, et al: Osteoporotic fractures of the proximal humerus in elderly Finnish persons: sharp increase in 1970-1998 and alarming projections for the new millennium. Acta Orthop Scand 2000;71:465-70.

48. Kanis JA: Assessing the risk of vertebral osteoporosis. Singapore Med J 2002;43:100-105.

49. Olsson C, Petersson C, Nordquist A: Increased mortality after fracture of the surgical neck of the humerus: a case-control study of 253 patients with a 12-year follow-up. Acta Orthop Scand 2003;74:714-17.

50. Nguyen TV, Center JR, Sambrook PN, et al: Risk factors for proximal humerus, forearm, and wrist fractures in elderly men and women: the Dubbo Osteoporosis Epidemiology Study. Am J Epidemiol 2001;153:587-95.

51. Lee SH, Dargent-Molina P, Breart G: Risk factors for fractures of the proximal humerus: results from the EPIDOS prospective study. J Bone Miner Res 2002;17:817-25.

52. Kelsey JL, Browner WS, Seeley DG, et al: Risk factors for fractures of the distal forearm and proximal humerus. The Study of Osteoporotic Fractures Research Group. Am J Epidemiol 1992;135:477-89.

53. Koval KJ, Gallagher MA, Marsicano JG, et al: Functional outcome after minimally displaced fractures of the proximal part of the humerus. J Bone Joint Surg Am 1997;79:203-77.

54. Olsson C, Nordqvist A, Petersson CJ: Increased fragility in patients with fracture of the proximal humerus: a case control study. Bone 2004;34:1072-77.

55. Melton LJ, III, Sampson JM, Morrey BF, et al: Epidemiologic features of pelvic fractures. Clin Orthop Relat Res 1981; 155:43-7.

56. Morris RO, Sonibare A, Green DJ, et al: Closed pelvic fractures: characteristics and outcomes in older patients admitted to medical and geriatric wards. Postgrad Med J 2000;76:646-50.

57. Taillandier J, Langue F, Alemanni M, et al: Mortality and functional outcomes of pelvic insufficiency fractures in older patients. Joint Bone Spine 2003;70:287-89.

58. Koval KJ, Aharonoff GB, Schwartz MC, et al: Pubic rami fracture: a benign pelvic injury? J Orthop Trauma 1997;11:7-9.

59. Samdani S: Pelvic insufficiency fractures. J Am Geriatr Soc 2004;52:854-55.

60. Orstavik RE, Haugeberg G, Mowinckel P, et al: Vertebral deformities in rheumatoid arthritis: a comparison with population-based controls. Arch Intern Med 2004;164:420-25.

61. Spector TD, Hall GM, McCloskey EV, et al: Risk of vertebral fracture in women with rheumatoid arthritis. BMJ 1993;306:558.

62. Peel NF, Moore DJ, Barrington NA, et al: Risk of vertebral fracture and relationship to bone mineral density in steroid treated rheumatoid arthritis. Ann Rheum Dis 1995;54:801-6.

63. Orstavik RE, Haugeberg G, Uhlig T, et al: Self reported non-vertebral fractures in rheumatoid arthritis and population based controls: incidence and relationship with bone mineral density and clinical variables. Ann Rheum Dis 2004;63: 177-82.

64. Kay LJ, Holland TM, Platt PN: Stress fractures in rheumatoid arthritis: a case series and case-control study. Ann Rheum Dis 2004;63:1690-92.

65. Poor G, Atkinson EJ, O'Fallon WM, et al: Predictors of hip fractures in elderly men. J Bone Miner Res 1995;10: 1900-7.

66. Gerdhem P, Ringsberg K, Akesson K, et al: Just one look, and fractures and death can be predicted in elderly ambulatory women. Gerontology 2004;50:309-14.

67. Gerdhem P, Ringsberg KA, Akesson K, et al: Clinical history and biologic age predicted falls better than objective functional tests. J Clin Epidemiol 2005;58:226-32.

68. Obrant K: Prognosis and rehabilitation after hip fracture. Osteoporos Int 6 Suppl 1996;3:52-5.

69. Rogmark C, Carlsson A, Johnell O, et al: Primary hemiarthroplasty in old patients with displaced femoral neck fracture: a 1-year follow-up of 103 patients aged 80 years or more. Acta Orthop Scand 2002;73:605-10.

8 Investigations of Bone: Densitometry

Kenneth G. Faulkner

SUMMARY

- There are several different options for bone density assessment, including dual x-ray absorptiometry (DXA), quantitative computed tomography, and quantitative ultrasonography.

- For the assessment of osteoporosis, estimation of fracture risk, and monitoring of skeletal changes, DXA measurements of the spine and proximal femur are preferred.

- Appropriate subjects for bone density testing include all women older than 65 years, postmenopausal women with risk factors, men and women with low-trauma fractures, and men and women currently taking medications known to have an effect on bone (such as glucocorticoids).

- The most clinically important value from a bone density examination is the T-score, which compares the measured bone density to the young adult average.

DENSITOMETRY TECHNIQUES

Radiographic Techniques

Before the development of bone densitometers, bone mineral density (BMD) was estimated from conventional x-ray images by comparing the brightness of the skeleton with the surrounding tissues. Dense bone appears relatively white on a standard radiograph, whereas demineralized bone has an appearance closer to that of soft tissue. However, this technique is qualitative and does not provide an accurate measure of BMD. It has been suggested that bone mineral losses of at least 30% are required before they may be visually detected on a conventional radiograph.[1]

Because of the insensitivity of x-ray images to bone density changes, several techniques have been developed to improve the accuracy and precision of conventional radiographs for bone mass assessment. Many of these techniques were based on measurements of the hand and forearm, because of easy access for measurement. The primary advantage of these methods is equipment cost, as all medical institutions have standard x-ray units.

The disadvantages, however, include alternations in imaging technique, most notably x-ray energy and type of x-ray film, both of which can cause apparent changes in bone density. To adjust for differences in imaging technique, a calibration wedge is often used during image acquisition as a BMD reference (Figure 8-1).

To analyze the radiographs and produce a BMD value, some techniques require centralized analysis of the radiographs by a third party.[2] Recent improvements include systems that permit local analysis of hand and forearm radiographs, eliminating the need for shipment to a central analysis facility. Results are obtained using custom analysis software for evaluating the digitized images to produce BMD values. Despite these improvements, radiographs are still primarily qualitative images and are not specifically intended for measuring bone density. This has led to the development of devices specifically designed to quantify bone density at various skeletal sites using x-ray and ultrasound technology.

Single-Energy Densitometry

Because of the problems and inaccuracies of using radiographs for measuring bone mass, researchers developed the first dedicated bone densitometer in the 1960s.[3] This device passed a beam of radiation through the forearm and determined the difference between the incoming and the outgoing radiation, called the *attenuation*. The higher the bone mineral content is, the greater the attenuation is. With the introduction of these devices, physicians were able to precisely measure bone density at a very low radiation dose. For the first time, it was possible to accurately and precisely monitor changes in bone density that might occur as the result of aging or treatment.

Single-energy densitometry has important limitations. The technique is limited to measuring peripheral bones such as the heel and forearm, as the measurement site must be immersed in water. Placing the measurement site in water cancels the effect of the overlying soft tissues, so that only the differential attenuation of the bone can be measured. This approach is reasonable for the measurement of the peripheral skeleton, but it is not practical to immerse the entire body in water to

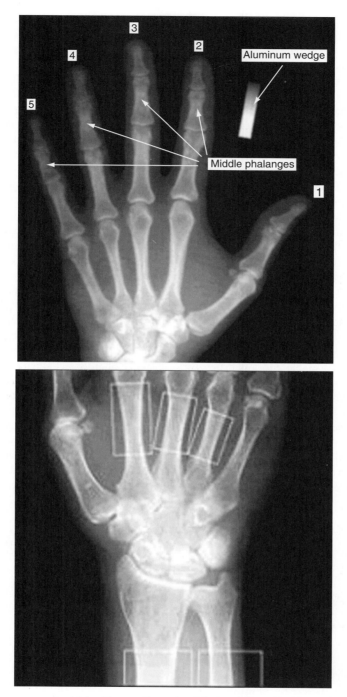

Figure 8-1. Bone density measurements obtained from radiographs of the hand. (From Hochberg: Rheumatology, 3rd ed, 2003.)

obtain measurements of the spine or the hip. Today, virtually all manufacturers of single-energy densitometers have switched to producing dual-energy systems.

Dual-Energy Densitometry

As stated above, the primary limitation of single-energy densitometry is an inability to directly measure

the spine and hip. The challenge was to devise a method that eliminated the need for a water bath so that any skeletal site could be measured. Researchers found that if a dual-energy radiation source was used, the influence of soft tissue could be eliminated without the need for a water bath to equalize soft tissue attenuation. With this technique, it is possible to measure the central skeleton, specifically the lumbar spine and proximal femur. Today, dual x-ray absorptiometry, or DXA (sometimes referred to as DEXA), represents the clinical technique of choice for measuring BMD.

Several different types of DXA systems are available, but they all operate on similar principles. A radiation source is aimed at a radiation detector placed directly opposite the site to be measured. The patient is placed on a table in the path of the radiation beam. The source/detector assembly is then scanned across the measurement region. The attenuation of the radiation beam is determined and is related to the BMD.[4]

Dual x-ray absorptiometry technology can measure virtually any skeletal site, but clinical use has been concentrated on the lumbar spine, proximal femur, forearm, and total body. DXA systems are available as either full-table systems (capable of multiple skeletal measurements, including the spine and hip) or as peripheral systems (limited to measuring the peripheral skeleton). Because of their versatility, and the ability to measure the skeletal sites of greatest clinical interest, full-table DXA systems are the current clinical choice for osteoporosis assessment (Figure 8-2). Peripheral DXA systems, portable and less expensive than full-table systems, are more frequently used as screening and early risk assessment tools.

Spine and proximal femur scans represent the majority of the clinical measurements performed using DXA. Most full-table DXA systems are able to perform additional studies, including lateral spine BMD measurements, evaluation of vertebral fractures, assessment of bone around prosthetic implants, measurements of

children and infants, small-animal studies, and measurements of excised bone specimens.

Early DXA systems used a pencil beam geometry and a single detector, which was scanned across the measurement region. Modern full-table DXA scanners use a fan-beam source and multiple detectors, which are swept across the measurement region. Fan beam provides the advantage of decreased scan times as compared with single-beam systems, but these machines typically cost more because of the need for multiple x-ray detectors. Fan-beam systems use either a single-view or a multiview mode to image the skeleton.

Magnification Error

Single-view systems measure the skeleton with a single pass of the x-ray source and detector across the measurement site. However, single-view fan-beam systems introduce a magnification error to the measurement that depends on the position of the object between the x-ray source and the detectors. By measuring the skeleton from only one angle, the location of the object between the source and detector cannot be determined. This is similar to trying to visually judge the distance of an object when one eye is covered—depth perception is lost when only one view is available. Fortunately, BMD measurements are not significantly affected by this magnification error, so in clinical use, single-view fan beam systems yield accurate BMD results.[5,6]

With the use of a single-view fan beam, area and bone content values must either be corrected for body size or object height, or reported as "estimated" to

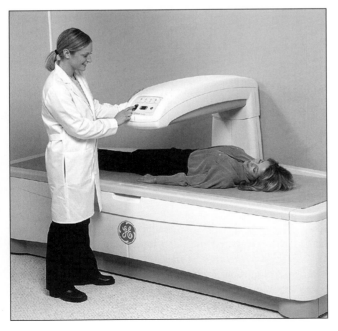

Figure 8-2. Full table dual X-ray absorptiometry system. (From Hochberg: Rheumatology, 3rd ed, 2003.) (See Color Plates.)

allow for some variation in the position of the patient between the source and detector.[6,7] For accurate assessment of bone area and content, multiview fan-beam systems have been developed. By use of overlapping images from different measurement angles, the object plane can be accurately determined. This allows multiview fan-beam systems to accurately determine bone area, content, and geometry. This is of particular importance for evaluating follow-up BMD measurements, in which consistency in area can be used as a gauge of positioning precision. In addition, geometric measurements, such as hip axis length (discussed later), require highly accurate and precise length measurements to be clinically useful.

Vertebral Fracture Assessment

For assessing vertebral heights (also called vertebral morphometry), special software is used to determine vertebral body dimensions.[8,9] The computer (with the help of the technologist) places points on the superior and inferior end-plates of each vertebra. The vertebral heights are calculated and compared with each other as well as to the expected normal dimensions. With the advent of higher-resolution DXA systems, visual assessment of fractures is also possible from DXA-based lateral spine images (Figure 8-3). In this situation, the DXA system essentially functions as a digital x-ray imaging device. Visual assessment is performed from a computer monitor or high-resolution printout. To optimize the assessment, the use of high-definition dual-energy images has been recommended.[10]

Using a DXA system for assessing vertebral fracture status has several advantages. The evaluation of spine fractures can be performed without a conventional lateral spine radiograph. This can be done at the same time and at the same place as the BMD measurement, with much less radiation than a conventional spine radiograph. Despite the apparent advantages, the future of vertebral fracture assessment using DXA remains unclear.

Skeletal radiologists have criticized the technique for being insensitive and inaccurate for detecting vertebral fractures. A DXA image is of lower resolution than a conventional x-ray image and might fail to identify other potential problems or diseases that would be apparent on a spine film. At this time, DXA devices are not generally accepted as a surrogate for spinal radiographs, although they may provide a useful screening tool in higher risk patients when spinal radiographs are unavailable. For example, individuals older than 65, subjects reporting significant height loss, or patients on long-term glucocorticoid therapy who have not had previous vertebral fractures or spinal radiographs could benefit from a vertebral fracture assessment.

Femoral Dual X-Ray Absorptiometry

Newer applications of DXA include sequential measurement of both femurs as well as geometric measurements incorporated into the DXA scanning software. Several studies have shown that left and right femur measurements are highly correlated.[11,12] Yet, for clinical purposes, the relevant question is how often a difference between the left and right femur will change either the diagnosis or the management of an individual patient.

Studies have confirmed that the average BMD difference between left and right femurs is negligible.[11,12] However, the standard error between the left and right measurements is 0.05 g/cm^2, both at the total hip and at the femoral neck. Thus, if only one hip is measured, the

Figure 8-3. Vertebral fracture assessment from a dual x-ray absorptiometry image of the spine. Use of dual-energy images facilitates the visualization of the lumbar and thoracic spine in a single image. In this example, a fracture has been identified at T12. (From Hochberg: Rheumatology, 3rd ed, 2003.) (See Color Plates.)

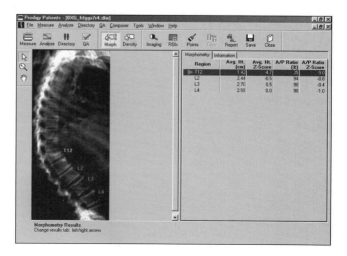

TABLE 8-1 POTENTIAL FOR MISSED DIAGNOSIS OF OSTEOPOROSIS IF ONLY A SINGLE HIP IS MEASURED													
T-score of first hip	0.0	−0.5	−1.0	−1.5	−1.6	−1.7	−1.8	−1.9	−2.0	−2.1	−2.2	−2.3	−2.4
% with second hip at −2.0 or less	0.0	0.1	2.3	15.9	21.2	27.4	34.5	42.1					
% with second hip at −2.5 or less	0.0	0.0	0.1	2.3	3.6	5.5	8.1	11.5	15.9	21.2	27.4	34.5	42.1

In situations where the first hip is within one half of a T-score of a diagnostic or therapeutic criterion, measurement of the second hip is recommended.
From Hochberg, Rheumatology, 3rd ed, 2003.

other hip will differ by an average of ±0.05 g/cm², equivalent to half a T-score. For patients with T-scores approaching the threshold for osteoporosis, the potential for misclassification becomes significant (Table 8-1). For example, if the left femoral neck has a T-score of −1.8, there is a 34% chance that the opposite femoral neck will be −2.0 or less and an 8% chance that it will be −2.5 or less. Thus, the use of the second hip measurement can have an impact on patient management. In addition, the use of both hips greatly reduces precision error and facilitates the evaluation of skeletal response at the femur.

The hip axis length (Figure 8-4) has been identified as an independent indicator of hip fracture risk.[13-19]

This measurement can be obtained from a standard DXA scan of the proximal femur, although on some systems an increased scan field may be required. Each centimeter (10%) increase in hip-axis length doubles the risk for hip fracture. For short-term prediction of hip fracture (within 2 years), hip-axis length was shown to predict hip fractures independent of BMD.

Although hip-axis length cannot be viewed as a stand-alone clinical predictor, it can potentially provide utility in conjunction with BMD to identify high-risk patients. Based on the available data, elderly white women with height- and weight-adjusted hip-axis length more than 1 cm above normal have twice the risk of hip fracture as those with an average hip-axis

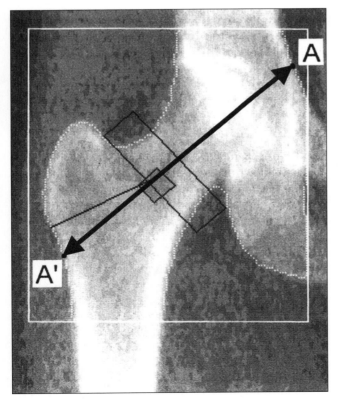

Figure 8-4. The hip-axis length, defined as the length along the femoral neck axis from the base of the greater trochanter to the inner pelvic brim. (From Hochberg: Rheumatology, 3rd ed, 2003.)

length. The use of hip-axis length in younger women, men, and people of other ethnicities has not yet been studied. However, for those with low BMD, hip-axis length can be considered as another factor to help identify those at increased risk for hip fracture.

Quantitative Computed Tomography

Before the advent of DXA, several researchers reported using computed tomography (CT) scanners to obtain bone density measurements.[20-22] This technique is called quantitative CT (QCT) to differentiate it from imaging CT. QCT is the only noninvasive three-dimensional bone mass measurement technique available. QCT reports a volumetric density (in milligrams per cubic centimeter) as opposed to the area density (in grams per square centimeter) obtained using other techniques. Initially, QCT was performed without any special equipment (other than the CT system) by measuring the average CT number of the vertebral body. More advanced procedures have been developed to improve the accuracy and precision of the measurement.

Quantitative computed tomography is used clinically to measure the bone density of the spine. It has the advantage of measuring the central bone of the vertebral body, which is a more sensitive site for detecting bone mineral changes than most other skeletal sites.[23] QCT can be performed on most commercial CT systems with the addition of a bone mineral standard for calibration of the CT measurement (Figure 8-5). Several different types of calibration systems are commercially available from CT manufacturers and third-party vendors.

In the standard QCT protocol, three or four lumbar vertebral bodies are measured using a single 8- to 10-mm slice through the center of each vertebra.[24] The calibration standard must also be measured, either at the same time or immediately after the patient is measured. Low-dose settings are used to reduce radiation exposure to well below that of a standard CT examination but still well above other types of bone density measurement (such as DXA). From the CT images, the average attenuation of the vertebral body bone is determined as well as the attenuation of the calibration standard. Using the known density of each of the standards and the measured CT values of the bone mineral standard, the vertebral CT value is converted to a physical density.

Most QCT studies are limited to the lumbar spine, but specialized QCT systems (called peripheral QCT) have been introduced for measuring the forearm. This technique offers the advantages of measuring the volumetric density of the forearm as well as providing measures of trabecular, cortical, and integral (trabecular plus cortical) bone. These scanners are limited to the forearm and can cost as much as full-table DXA devices capable of density measurements at multiple skeletal sites.

When properly performed, QCT can be a useful clinical tool. The measurement of a purely trabecular bone sample may have some utility for the diagnosis of osteoporosis, assessing fracture risk and monitoring bone changes. There have been relatively few published prospective studies regarding the use of QCT for predicting fracture. The vast majority of prospective studies have been with DXA. For predicting hip

Figure 8-5. Quantitative computed tomography study of the lumbar spine. (From Hochberg: Rheumatology, 3rd ed, 2003.)

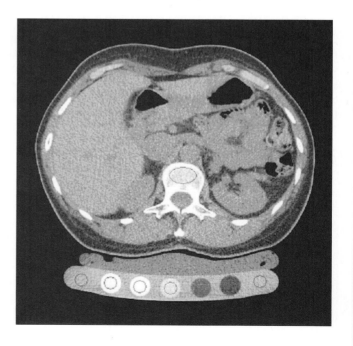

fracture, it is generally agreed that a direct femoral measurement using DXA is the best choice. QCT may offer some advantage in elderly subjects by avoiding artifact introduced in DXA by the degenerative changes typically seen at the spine. On the other hand, it is conceivable that the ability of DXA to measure both cortical and trabecular bone provides some advantage for predicting fracture compared with QCT. Bone strength is influenced by both cortical and trabecular bone, so that measurement of both components by DXA might provide an advantage.

Quantitative computed tomography shows twice to three times the change in BMD seen with DXA, either due to aging or response to therapy. Yet QCT is typically less precise than DXA. Precision errors with QCT are reported to be twice to three times as great as for DXA, because of difficulties with patient positioning, consistent slice location, system stability, and consistent placement of the region of interest. Thus, any increased sensitivity of QCT is offset by the increased precision error of the technique, resulting in no significant advantage for monitoring changes.

As with DXA, it is essential to use proper quality control when monitoring changes with QCT. As CT instruments are designed for imaging and not for quantitative assessment, it is essential that the stability of the system be monitored frequently. Acquisition protocols (tube voltage and current) must be consistent from one examination to another. Daily quality control measures must be maintained to guard against drifts in either the x-ray tube or detectors that might influence the BMD result. All QCT manufacturers provide tools for monitoring system performance that should be followed to ensure consistent results.

An additional consideration with repeated use of QCT is radiation dose (Table 8-2). Compared with most radiological examination techniques, QCT has a very low dose, equivalent to that of a mammogram. Yet a single QCT examination has an effective dose equivalent to 50 to 100 times that of a DXA examination.[25] Improperly performed scans (using imaging protocols

rather than BMD protocols) can increase this dose by another factor of 10. As with all radiological examinations, QCT should be performed only at appropriate intervals to avoid excess or unnecessary exposure.

In addition to the clinical and technical considerations, there are a few practical issues regarding the use of QCT. Foremost is the need for a CT scanner. This limits the use of the technique to radiology facilities with the proper equipment and available scanner time. Often, the lack of scanner time can be the most significant barrier to performing QCT. Daily quality assurance procedures require 15 minutes each day to monitor the QCT system. The examination itself takes 15 to 30 minutes to perform, including time for patient preparation and scan acquisition. With competing pressures for scanner time in many radiology departments, it can be difficult to find time to schedule patients for measurement of bone density.

Quantitative Ultrasonography

Ultrasound has been used for many years to investigate the mechanical properties of various engineering materials. Several commercial ultrasound devices have been introduced for investigating bone status, primarily of the heel (Figure 8-6). This technique is termed quantitative ultrasonography (QUS) to distinguish it from the more commonly known imaging ultrasound techniques. Clinical QUS looks at the transmission of high-frequency sound through bone, whereas pure imaging ultrasound devices employ sound reflection to produce their image. More advanced QUS devices do provide an image, but it is used to identify the measurement region, in much the same way as an image from a DXA system is used (Figure 8-7).

Quantitative ultrasonography offers the advantages of small equipment size, relatively quick and simple measurements, and no need for ionizing radiation. QUS is most easily performed at skeletal sites with minimal and consistent soft tissue covering, such as the calcaneus, radius, tibia, patella, and phalanges. QUS is markedly different from x-ray-based techniques in employing mechanical vibration, rather than electromagnetic waves, to interrogate the bone tissue. The interaction of high-frequency sound with bone, as with any material, uses completely different mechanisms from x-ray techniques.

When measuring the skeleton using QUS, two primary measurements are obtained—the speed of sound and the broadband ultrasound attenuation in the site being measured. Most QUS devices define these parameters in a unique way. In addition, QUS is not standardized in terms of sound frequencies, coupling with the measurement site (water, gel, or a combination), or methods for signal processing and analysis. Yet, despite these inconsistencies in instrumentation and

TABLE 8-2 EFFECTIVE DOSES IN DENSITOMETRY COMPARED WITH OTHER COMMON RADIATION SOURCES	
Radiation Source	Effective Dose (µSv)
Single x-ray absorptiometry	1
Dual x-ray absorptiometry	1-5
Quantitative computed tomography	60
Lateral spine film	700
Natural background (per day)	5-8
Round trip (8-10 h) airplane flight	60

Data from Kalender.[25]
From Hochberg, Rheumatology, 3rd ed, 2003.

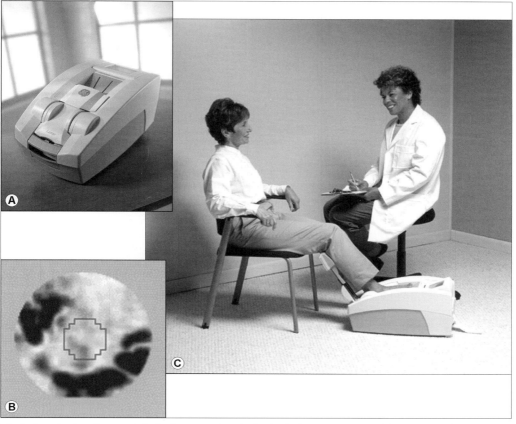

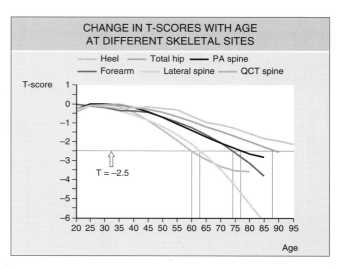

Figure 8-6. *A,* Quantitative ultrasound device for measuring the heel, which incorporates a real-time image for more accurate assessment. *B,* Region of interest (ROI) over calcaneus. *C,* Patient undergoing scan of calcaneus. (From Hochberg: Rheumatology, 3rd ed, 2003.) (See Color Plates.)

Figure 8-7. Change in T-scores with age at different skeletal sites. (From Hochberg: Rheumatology, 3rd ed, 2003.) (See Color Plates.)

physical differences from x-ray-based systems, QUS yields a measurement that is reasonably well correlated with x-ray BMD values at the same skeletal site, particularly at the calcaneus.[26] However, the correlation of calcaneal QUS with density measurements at other skeletal sites is less strong.[27] Much of this discrepancy is due to simple discordance between different skeletal sites and is not related to technical differences between QUS and x-ray technology.[28]

Data from several prospective studies using different QUS devices have shown broadband ultrasound attenuation to be predictive of hip fracture.[29-32]

Furthermore, the predictive ability of QUS appears to be at least partially independent of x-ray-based BMD measurements.[31] This has fueled interest in QUS as a measure of bone quality as well as density. Although the future of QUS appears promising, some questions remain to be answered. For example, researchers are still not certain exactly which parameters of the bone are being measured with QUS.

Comparisons with other BMD techniques indicate that QUS is measuring a combination of bone density and some other property of the bone. It has been speculated that QUS may be measuring a parameter related to bone structure, such as trabecular size and spacing. If this is true, then a QUS measurement would be valuable in combination with bone density to get a better measure of the bone status. It also remains to be determined how QUS can be used to monitor skeletal response to different therapies. However, the compact size and non-radiation-based qualities of QUS make it an attractive choice for population-based screening programs.

CLINICAL USE OF MEASUREMENTS OF BONE MINERAL DENSITY

For BMD measurements to be clinically useful, they must be compared with established normative ranges. All BMD manufacturers provide normative databases for this purpose. These databases are derived from measurements of large groups of men or women of different ages and races. Comparisons are expressed either as a percentage of the expected normal value or as the number of standard deviations (SD) from the expected normal value. The T-score is the most important comparison. The T-score is the number of SD by which the measured BMD differs from the gender-matched young normal (YN) value.

For the diagnosis of osteoporosis, the World Health Organization (WHO) has defined the following criteria for the assessment of osteoporosis based on the T-score:[33,34]

- Normal: A BMD not more than 1 SD below YN (T-score ≥ −1)
- Osteopenia (low bone mass): A BMD between 1 and 2.5 SD below YN (T-score between −1 and −2.5)
- Osteoporosis: A BMD 2.5 or more SD below YN (T-score ≤ −2.5)
- Severe osteoporosis: A BMD 2.5 or more SD below YN (T-score ≤ −2.5) and the presence of one or more fragility fractures.

The WHO definitions were not intended to be used in the diagnosis of osteoporosis in individuals. They

have nevertheless become commonly used for this purpose in clinical practice. Several researchers have pointed out the shortcomings of using T-scores and the WHO criteria for individual diagnosis.[28,35]

Figure 8-7 shows a comparison of the age-related decline in T-scores with different BMD measurements. The central skeleton, particularly the spine, shows the largest T-score decline with age. However, there is considerable variation in the T-scores at different skeletal sites. The normative data cross the −2.5 SD level at age 60 with QCT compared with age 77 for DXA spine measurements. At age 60, the prevalence of osteoporosis using the WHO definition is 50% using QCT compared with 14% with spinal DXA.

It is clear from Figure 8-7 that some techniques, such as spinal QCT and lateral DXA, produce T-scores that are significantly different than those obtained with other measurements. This is predominantly because of differences in the normal data from which the T-scores are derived, resulting in a smaller relative SD for QCT compared with DXA.[28] For this reason, it is now acknowledged that a single T-score criterion cannot be universally applied to all BMD measurements. Specifically, use of the WHO guidelines with lateral DXA or QCT will result in an overestimation of osteoporosis and fracture risk. For the diagnosis of osteoporosis, it is recommended that the lowest T-score from a DXA measurement of the lumbar spine, proximal femur, or total hip be used.

WHO SHOULD RECEIVE A BONE MINERAL DENSITY TEST?

In 1998, the National Osteoporosis Foundation (NOF) in the United States, in collaboration with 10 other professional societies, created a set of guidelines for the use and interpretation of BMD measurements.[36] They recommend BMD measurements for postmenopausal white women who

- are younger than 65 years and have one or more additional risk factors for osteoporosis (besides menopause)
- are 65 and older, regardless of additional risk factors
- present with fractures
- are considering therapy for osteoporosis, if BMD testing would facilitate the decision
- have been on hormone replacement therapy for prolonged periods.

At present, the NOF recommendations are limited to white women because only limited data are available for other populations. However, many physicians are applying these guidelines to postmenopausal women of other ethnicities as well. In addition to the NOF recommendations, other high-risk populations should be considered for measurement. The most evident risk population includes both men and women presenting with low-trauma fracture. BMD should be assessed to confirm the diagnosis of osteoporosis. In addition, individuals on long-term glucocorticoid therapy should have BMD assessed based on recommendations from the American College of Rheumatology.[37] Patients taking 5 mg/day of prednisone (prednisolone) or its equivalent for more than 3 months should receive a BMD test and be considered for antiresorptive therapy to reduce bone loss associated with steroid therapy. In addition, men 65 and older, particularly those with risk factors such as alcoholism or hypogonadism or with radiographic evidence of bone loss, as well as men and women taking drugs known to influence bone density, should be considered for BMD testing.

USE OF BONE MINERAL DENSITY TESTING TO GUIDE TREATMENT

Treatment guidelines were typically developed for use with central DXA measurements.[36] When applied to peripheral measurements, particularly in people younger than 65 years of age, skeletal discordance can cause significant variation in T-scores between sites. Because of differences in skeletal aging and normative data at the different skeletal sites, variations of a full T-score or more can be expected. Usually, it is the central skeleton that will show the first signs of age-related bone loss, so it is recommended that treatment decisions be based on the lowest T-score at the spine, femoral neck, or total hip measured by DXA. In patients with low peripheral T-scores and several additional risk factors, such as age older than 70, the risk may be sufficient to warrant treatment based on this information alone.[36]

If peripheral densitometry is used for screening, the concern is that a normal T-score at the heel, hand, or forearm cannot guarantee that the score at the spine and/or hip would not be low.[38,39] To guard against this situation, a conservative screening approach should be used. If the peripheral skeleton yields a T-score of −1.0 or greater, the patient can be considered to be at low risk. If the T-score at the peripheral skeleton is −2.0 or lower, the central skeleton will typically be as low, if not lower, and the patient should be considered at high risk. For peripheral T-scores between −1.0 and −2.0, additional measurements should be considered, including central densitometry. However, additional risk factors, particularly age and previous fracture history, should be incorporated in any screening program. It is also important to recognize that there is no single BMD measurement, peripheral or central, that will proper identify all patients at risk for fracture.

CONCLUSION

Although all BMD techniques have clinical utility, differences in versatility, specifically the ability to measure both the spine and hip, favor DXA over other methods. As a result, DXA has become the densitometry technique of choice in many clinical departments. Although other methods are still used in some clinics, there is a continued shift to DXA as the clinical standard. DXA has the primary disadvantage of cost, as commercial units typically cost significantly more than peripheral DXA (pDXA) or QUS devices. Because of the advantages of low cost and portability, peripheral densitometry is often used for screening programs or in clinics where central densitometry cannot be accommodated.

The proper clinical use of densitometry requires an understanding of the available techniques, their appropriate application, and the potential sources of measurement error. Clinical guidelines recommend that all women over the age of 65 and all postmenopausal women with risk factors should have their bone density assessed. In addition, BMD measurements should be considered in men 65 years of age and older, individuals with low trauma fractures, and individuals on long-term glucocorticoid therapy.

With the advent of smaller, portable devices, bone density measurements are now widely available. In particular, ultrasound techniques, which do not use radiation, have particular promise for widespread screening applications. Peripheral densitometry alone cannot adequately address all clinical questions, particularly the question of monitoring subtle changes in bone density. Also, although one skeletal site may be found to have normal BMD, it is possible that the density at other skeletal sites could be low. In individuals with multiple risk factors, a moderately low BMD assessment in the peripheral skeleton should be verified by scanning another skeletal site, preferably the spine or hip. For any bone density measurement to be clinically useful, it must be performed with careful attention to detail, particularly with regard to instrument calibration, patient positioning, measurement analysis, and interpretation.

REFERENCES

1. Resnick D: Osteoporosis: radiographic-pathologic correlation. In: Genant HK, ed: Osteoporosis update 1987. San Francisco, CA: Radiology Research and Education Foundation, University of California, 1987:31-39.

2. Cosman F, Herrington B, Himmelstein S, et al: Radiographic absorptiometry: a simple method for determination of bone mass. Osteoporosis Int 1991;2:34-8.

3. Cameron JR, Sorenson G: Measurements of bone mineral in vivo: an improved method. Science 1963;142:230-32.

4. Nord RH: Technical considerations in DPA. In: Genant HK, ed: Osteoporosis update 1987. San Francisco, CA: Radiology Research and Education Foundation, University of California, 1987:203-12.

5. Faulkner KG, Gluer CC, Estilo M, Genant HK: Cross-calibration of DXA equipment: upgrading from a Hologic QDR 1000/w to a QDR 2000. Calcif Tissue Int 1993;52:79-84.

6. Mazess RB, Barden HS: Evaluation of differences between fan-beam and pencil-beam densitometers. Calcif Tissue Int 2000;67:291-6.

7. Young JT, Carter KA, Marion MS, Greendale GA: A simple method for computing hip axis length using fan-beam densitometry and anthropometric measurements. J Clin Densitometry 2000;3:325-31.

8. Steiger P, Cummings SR, Genant HK, Weiss H: Morphometric X-ray absorptiometry of the spine: correlation with morphometric radiography. Osteoporosis Int 1994;4:238-44.

9. Genant HK, Jiao L, Wu CY, Shepherd JA: Vertebral fractures in osteoporosis: a new method for clinical assessment. J Clin Densitometry 2000;3:281-90.

10. Rea JA, Steiger P, Blake GM, Fogelman I: Optimizing data acquisition and analysis of morphometric X-ray absorptiometry. Osteoporosis Int 1998;8:177-83.

11. Faulkner KG, Genant HK, McClung M: Bilateral comparison of femoral bone density and hip axis length from single and fan beam dxa scans. Calcif Tissue Int 1995;56:26-31.

12. Bonnick SL, Nichols DL, Sanborn CF, et al: Right and left proximal femur analyses: is there a need to do both? Calcif Tissue Int 1996;57:340-43.

13. Faulkner KG, Cummings SR, Black D, et al: Simple measurement of femoral geometry predicts hip fracture: the study of osteoporotic fractures. J Bone Miner Res 1993;8:1211-17.

14. Faulkner KG, McClung M, Cummings SR: Automated evaluation of hip axis length for predicting hip fracture. J Bone Miner Res 1994;9:1065-70.

15. Glüer CC, Cummings SR, Pressman A, et al: Prediction of hip fractures from pelvic radiographs: the study of osteoporotic fractures. J Bone Min Res 1994;9:671-77.

16. Boonen S, Koutri R, Dequeker J, et al: Measurement of femoral geometry in type I and type II osteoporosis: differences in hip axis length consistent with heterogeneity in the pathogenesis of osteoporotic fractures. J Bone Miner Res 1995;10:1908-12.

17. Peacock M, Turner CH, Liu G, et al: Better discrimination of hip fracture using bone density, geometry and architecture. Osteoporosis Int 1995;5:167-73.

18. Rosso R, Minisola S: Hip axis length in an Italian osteoporotic population. Br J Radiol 2000;73:969-72.

19. Frisoli A, Paula AP, Szejnfeld V, et al: Comparison between hip axis length of elderly osteoporotic Brazilian women with and without hip fracture. J Bone Min Res 2000;15:S538.

20. Ruegsegger P, Elsasser U, Anliker M, et al: Quantification of bone mineralisation using computed tomography. Radiology 1976;121:93-7.

21. Cann CE, Genant HK: Precise measurement of vertebral mineral content using computed tomography. J Comput Assist Tomogr 1980;4:493-500.

22. Genant HK, Cann CE, Ettinger B, Gorday GS: Quantitative computed tomography of vertebral spongiosa: a sensitive method for detecting early bone loss after oophorectomy. Ann Intern Med 1982;97:699-705.

23. Faulkner KG: Bone densitometry: choosing the proper skeletal site to measure. J Clinical Densitometry 1998;1:279-85.

24. Steiger P, Block J, Steiger S, et al: Spinal bone mineral density measured with quantitative CT: effect of region of interest, vertebral level, and technique. Radiology 1990;175:537-43.

25. Kalender WA: Effective dose values in bone mineral measurements by photon absorptiometry and computed tomography. Osteoporosis Int 1992;2:82-7.

26. Glüer CC, Vahlensieck M, Faulkner KG, et al: Site-matched calcaneal measurements of broadband ultrasound attenuation and single X-ray absorptiometry: do they measure different skeletal properties? J Bone Miner Res 1992;7:1071-79.

27. Faulkner KG, McClung MR, Coleman LJ, Kingston-Sandahl E: Quantitative ultrasound of the heel: correlation with densitometric measurements at different skeletal sites. Osteoporosis Int 1994;4:42-7.

28. Faulkner KG, von Stetten E, Miller P: Discordance in patient classification using T-scores. J Clinical Densitometry 1999;2:343-50.

29. Bauer D, Glüer C, Cauley J, et al: Bone ultrasound predicts fractures strongly and independently of densitometry in older women: a prospective study. Arch Intern Med 1997;157:629-34.

30. Porter R, Miller C, Grainger D, Palmer S: Prediction of hip fracture in elderly women: a prospective study. Br Med J 1990;301:638-41.

31. Hans D, Dargent-Molina P, Schott A, et al: Ultrasonic heel measurements to predict hip fracture in elderly women: the EPIDOS prospective study. Lancet 1996;348:511-4.

32. Marshall D, Johnell O, Wedel H: Meta-analysis of how well measures of bone mineral density predict occurrence of osteoporotic fractures. Br Med J 1996;312:1254-59.

33. The WHO Study Group: Assessment of fracture risk and its application to screening for postmenopausal osteoporosis. Geneva: World Health Organization, 1994.

34. Kanis JA: Assessment of fracture risk and is application to screening for postmenopausal osteoporosis: synopsis of a WHO report. Osteoporosis Int 1994;4:368-81.

35. Greenspan SL, Maitland-Ramsey L, Myers E: Classification of osteoporosis in the elderly is dependent on site-specific analysis. Calcif Tissue Int 1996;58:409-14.

36. National Osteoporosis Foundation: Physician's guide to prevention and treatment of osteoporosis. Washington, DC: National Osteoporosis Foundation, 1998.

37. American College of Rheumatology Ad Hoc Committee on Glucocorticoid-Induced Osteoporosis: recommendations for the prevention and treatment of glucocorticoid-induced osteoporosis: 2001 update. Arthritis Rheum 2001;44:1496-1503. Available at www.rheumatology.org.

38. Baran DT, Faulkner KG, Genant HK, et al: Diagnosis and management of osteoporosis: guidelines for the utilization of bone densitometry. Calcif Tissue Int 1997;61:433-40.

39. Miller PD, Bonnick SL, Johnston CC, et al: The challenges of peripheral bone density testing: which patients need additional central density skeletal measurements? J Clin Densitometry 1998;1:211-17.

9

Imaging Bone Structure and Osteoporosis Using MRI

Sandra J. Shefelbine and Sharmila Majumdar

Osteoporosis is a metabolic disorder that results in a decrease in bone mineral density (BMD) and an alteration in the trabecular architectural structure. Osteoporotic bone has decreased mechanical strength, making it prone to fracture, especially atraumatic vertebral fractures and fall-related hip and radius fractures. Osteoporosis is clinically diagnosed by imaging trabecular bone at peripheral sites, such as the radius, calcaneus, or distal femur, to determine BMD. BMD is usually measured using x-ray or ultrasound imaging techniques. In x-ray imaging (such as dual energy x-ray absorptiometry [DXA] and quantitative computed tomography) the image intensity relates to the tissue mineral density. In ultrasonography, image intensity reflects the change in frequency and amplitude of the sound wave traveling through the tissue. X-ray techniques use ionizing radiation, which can have deleterious effects in sufficient doses. Ultrasonography, though harmless, provides only a small field of view, which may limit the accuracy of the measurement. Recent advances in micro-computed tomography, an x-ray-based three-dimensional technique, has made it possible to obtain images of trabecular bone microarchitecture. Another promising imaging modality for measurement of trabecular bone density and quantification of trabecular architecture is magnetic resonance imaging (MRI). MRI does not use ionizing radiation and can provide three dimensional images of the bone structure. Figure 9-1 illustrates different imaging modalities, such as radiography, DXA, computed tomography (CT), and MRI, used to obtain images of the calcaneus.

MAGNETIC RESONANCE IMAGING BASICS

Nuclei with an odd number of protons and neutrons (such as hydrogen) have a magnetic moment, causing the nucleus to act like a small magnet in the presence of an external magnetic field. The magnetic field of the nucleus aligns in the direction of the external magnetic field. Magnetic resonance imaging (MRI) uses radiofrequency (RF) pulses in a magnetic field to alter the spin of protons in the tissue. Coils detect the change in net magnetization, which after mathematical reconstruction provides spatial and compositional

Figure 9-1. Sagittal images of calcaneus using (a) radiography, (b) MRI, and (c) ultrasonography.[1] Axial CT image of the calcaneus (d) and sagittal reformat from a stack of axial slices (e), as in d. (a-c, From Laugier et al. Calcif Tissue Int 1996;58:328.)

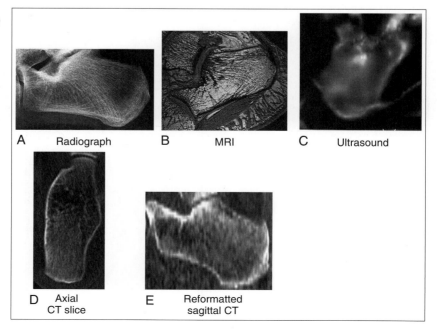

A   Radiograph   B   MRI   C   Ultrasound

D   Axial CT slice   E   Reformatted sagittal CT

77

information of the tissue being imaged. Because clinical MRI usually detects magnetization of hydrogen, compositional information is limited to molecules containing hydrogen, such as water, body fat, and cholesterol.

In a MRI scanner, proton spins in the body align in the direction of the external magnetic field. When an RF pulse is applied, the proton spins change, altering the magnetization. The time it takes for the spin to regain its alignment with the external magnetic field after the RF pulse is turned off depends on the molecule (size and structure) and its surroundings. By altering the sequence of the RF pulses and the gradient of the magnetic field, the location and type of tissue being imaged can be controlled.

The signal received in an MRI reflects intrinsic factors of the tissue, either spin density or relaxation properties of the nuclei. Spin-lattice relaxation time (T1) is the time it takes a tissue to regain longitudinal magnetization after a 90-degree RF pulse that makes the spins perpendicular to the external magnetic field. T1 is a measure of energy transfer to the surroundings (lattice) as the proton recovers its normal spin. T1 relaxation times generally are between 300 and 2000 msec. Spin-spin relaxation time (T2) is a measure of how long the proton spins remain in phase after an RF pulse. Interaction with other molecules (e.g., diffusion) affects the T2 relaxation time. As natural motion of the proton increases, such as in liquids, T2 increases. Water, therefore, has a long T2 and appears white in T2-weighted images (Figure 9-2). T2 relaxation times are shorter than T1 and can range from 30 to 150 msec. Inhomogeneities in the magnetic field can also affect T2. A static internal field (caused by large, slow-moving proteins or rigid trabeculae, for example), may additionally alter the local magnetic environment and affect T2. T2* combines the effects of molecular interactions (T2) and these field imhomegeneities. In addition to relaxation times, more complicated measures may also be obtained from the MRI signal, such as phase analysis, relaxation time distribution, and chemical composition. MR images also can reflect the behavior of tissue water or fat alone. Figures 9-3 and 9-4 show radiographs and MR images of a proximal femur and a vertebral column, respectively. In fat suppression, the signal from the fat in the bone marrow is suppressed, allowing visualization of the bone marrow edema that accompanies trabecular bone fracture.

Bone tissue has low water content, extremely short T2, and thus relatively low MR signal, and therefore appears black in most MR images. The bone marrow in trabecular bone, however, has sufficient water and fat content to provide MR signal. The trabecular bone network may alter the properties of the marrow by creating magnetic inhomogeneities at the bone-marrow interface. Trabecular structure can be imaged by relaxometry, which measures the change in marrow properties due to trabecular structure, or by direct visualization of the black trabecular network. The effect of the trabecular network on marrow magnetic properties are more prominent in T2* than in T1 images.[1] The inhomogeneities at the bone-marrow interface are dependent on the density of the trabecular structure,

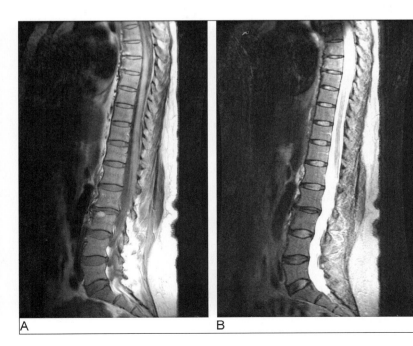

A   B

Figure 9-2. Sagittal images of the spine. *A,* T1-weighted image. *B,* T2-weighted image.

Figure 9-3. Radiograph (a) and fat-suppressed MR image (b) illustrating proximal femur fracture.

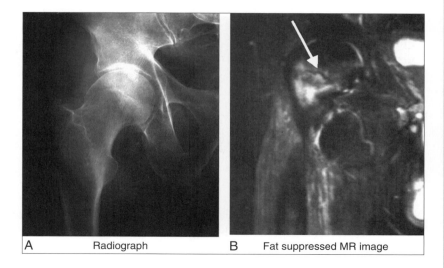

| A | Radiograph | B | Fat suppressed MR image |

Figure 9-4. Images of fractured vertebral column. In the T1-weighted image the fracture appears dark, whereas in the fat suppressed image, the fracture appears white.

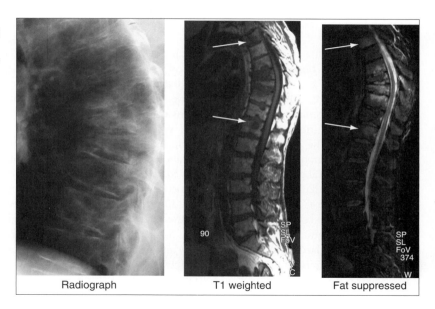

| Radiograph | T1 weighted | Fat suppressed |

the size of the trabeculae and trabecular spaces, and the field strength. In general, a denser network results in shorter T2* relaxation times due to more bone-marrow interfaces and increased inhomogeneities.[2-6]

The sequence and timing of RF pulses determine the image contrast. Common sequences in bone imaging include the spin-echo and gradient-echo sequences. An "echo" reverses the spin, which refocuses the magnetization and in effect cancels out external magnetic field inhomogeneities, which are intrinsic in the magnet of the scanner. In a spin-echo sequence a 90-degree pulse is followed by a 180-degree RF pulse, which produces the echo. In gradient echo sequences, the magnetic field is reversed to create the echo. The echo time (TE) is the time between the original RF pulse and the peak echo

signal. The type of sequence affects the appearance of the trabecular structure. In both spin and gradient echo sequences, the dimensions of the trabeculae may be amplified due to differences in magnetic susceptibility (the amount a material becomes magnetized in a magnetic field) between the marrow and bone.[7,8] The amount of distortion artifact is dependent on TE, with longer TEs resulting in more distortion.[9] In addition, gradient-echo sequences produce more susceptibility artifacts than spin-echo sequences.[3,9] Representative images of the distal radius are shown in Figure 9-5. Spin-echo sequences, however, require a considerably longer scan time and require in vitro samples or smaller fields of view (such as the finger and wrist) because of signal-to-noise and total imaging time considerations.[8]

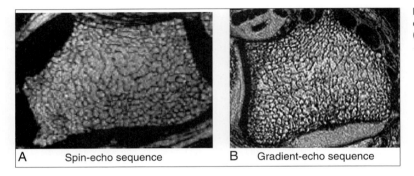

Figure 9-5. Axial images of the calcaneus using (a) spin-echo and (b) gradient-echo sequences.

A   Spin-echo sequence

B   Gradient-echo sequence

Therefore, in vivo imaging of trabecular bone typically is performed using gradient-echo sequences with TEs as short as possible. Alternatively, a fast large-angle spin echo sequence can be used which uses an initial RF pulse greater than 90 degrees. The following 180-degree pulse then partially restores the longitudinal magnetization and reduces the time to repeat, making the spin-echo faster.[10]

Susceptibility artifacts are one of the limitations in imaging trabecular bone with MRI. The typical maximum resolution of a 1.5 T scanner is 78 to 200 μm in-plane and 400 to 1000 μm out-of-plane (slice thickness).[11] Trabeculae are the same dimensions as the in-plane resolution, resulting in partial volume effects, in which the depiction of a trabecula in the image is a projection or average of multiple trabeculae. As a result, the trabecular measures obtained from MRI are different than those obtained with histomorphometry or micro-CT at higher resolutions (20 μm).

The magnetic field strength of the scanner affects the resolution and acquisition time of the scan. A 1.5 T magnet is the standard scanner used clinically and can provide a maximum resolution of approximately $150 \times 150 \times 250$ μm.[12] With high-resolution MRI requiring a stronger magnetic field strength (7-9.4 T) and a small-bore (limited to in vitro scans), resolutions can be improved to $50 \times 50 \times 100$ μm.[8] Nuclear magnetic resonance imaging has even a smaller field of view (2-12 mm) but can obtain isotropic resolutions as high as 10 μm. Nuclear magnetic resonance imaging can additionally determine chemical shift, making it possible to establish distribution of a given chemical.[13] Generally, higher magnetic field strength improves signal-to-noise ratio, scan time, and image quality, but often with limited field of view and other factors such as tissue susceptibility to consider.[14]

IMAGE PROCESSING TECHNIQUES

After obtaining an MR image, preprocessing of the image is usually required to improve the signal-to-noise ratio and image quality and make it possible to differentiate marrow from bone trabeculae. Preprocessing may include coil correction, noise reduction, motion correction, and thresholding. Coil correction is required to correct spatial variations in the sensitivity of the detection coil, as tissue close to the coil usually appears brighter than tissue further away from the coil. Coil correction algorithms depend on the structure of the specific coil. Coils that completely surround the object being scanned (e.g., bird-cage coil) provide sufficient in-plane homogeneity, making longitudinal correction sufficient. In surface coils, which may not provide in-plane homogeneity, a low-pass filter–based coil correction scheme is necessary (Figure 9-6).[15,16]

Noise reduction improves the signal-to-noise ratio and can be accomplished using a median low-pass filter, in which the median of the pixels in a certain kernel size (e.g., 3×3 pixels) surrounding a pixel becomes the new filtered value for the pixel.[11] A low-pass filter removes high-signal noise while preserving the low-signal data. The kernel median allows edge detection, whereas the kernel mean would smooth the data and blur the edges. Hwang and associates[17] proposed a histogram deconvolution method to obtain a noiseless histogram for trabecular bone. In this method, a probability distribution of the noise (e.g., gaussian) and an initial estimate of the noiseless histogram are assumed to predict a histogram. The predicted histogram is iteratively improved by comparing it with the measured histogram. The noiseless histogram and raw image are used to produce a noiseless image. Others have proposed wavelet-based thresholding that allows more local noise reduction while retaining relevant detail information.[18-20]

Imaging trabeculae on the order of 100 μm means that a small amount of motion will affect the image. Various techniques have been devised to correct for motion artifacts. Navigator correction alters the echo sequence, adding echoes to sense small displacements.[21] The data are corrected in k-space by analyzing the phase shift and adjusting for translational motions. Studies have shown that navigator correction improves

Figure 9-6. Effects of coil correction on sagittal images of the calcaneus. Coil correction equalizes the fat and marrow intensities throughout the visible bone.

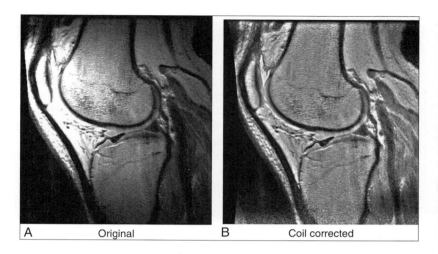

A   Original   B   Coil corrected

reproducibility and accuracy of trabecular bone parameters.[22] Retrospective motion correction can also be performed with autofocusing (Figure 9-7).[23,24] This technique applies trial phase shifts to the data and compares the resulting image with the original. An entropy focusing criterion is applied to minimize the amount of entropy in the image and obtain maximum contrast.

Perhaps the most critical preprocessing step is thresholding, which allows delineation of the trabeculae and the marrow. Because the resolution of in vivo MR images is on the same scale as the trabecular width, partial volume effects occur. In partial voluming, a single voxel may contain signals from multiple tissue types. The voxel intensity is the average signal from the various tissues. The histogram of trabecular bone, therefore, is not bimodal with marrow and bone peaks, but rather monomodal, with a peak intensity between the values of marrow and bone. Various thresholding methods have been established to segment the bone from the marrow where partial volume effects are an issue. Majumdar and associates[11] proposed a dual thresholding method in which the threshold for bone was a mean pixel value taken in the cortical shell and the threshold for marrow was the lower signal intensity at which the histogram reached one-half its peak.

Link and associates[25] compared global and local thresholding methods. Global thresholding applies the same threshold throughout the entire image. The disadvantage of global thresholding is that images of a dense trabecular structure appear completely black, whereas images with a sparse trabecular structure appear white. Using local thresholding, the intensity of a square region surrounding a pixel is averaged. If the central pixel has an intensity lower than the average, it is considered bone; higher than average pixels are considered marrow.

Figure 9-7. Coronal images of the shoulder. *A,* Original image corrupted by motion. *B,* After motion correction.

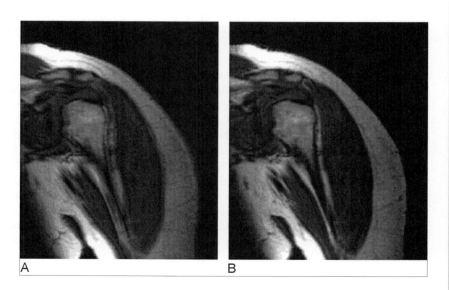

A   B

Local thresholding is not affected by bone density but is dependent on noise in the image. It was found that global thresholding was more accurate in calculating trabecular thickness and local thresholding was more accurate in predicting trabecular spacing.

Wu and colleagues[26] introduced a bayesian approach to segment bone from marrow in which each voxel was divided into subvoxels. The local tissue environment influenced the distribution of bone and marrow within the subvoxels with a Gibbs distribution modeling the interaction between subvoxels. This approach improves segmentation but has only been performed on images from small-bore nuclear magnetic resonance microscopy machines and has yet to be applied to clinical scans. Hwang and colleagues[27] proposed a spatial autocorrelation analysis that also used the local tissue environment to determine the probability of finding bone at specified locations. This method was used to analyze images at in vivo resolution (voxel size of $156 \times 156 \times 391$ µm^3). Similarly, a relaxation labeling process that takes into account the spatial context, in particular local contextual information (as in Markov fields), was used by Antoniadis and colleagues[28] to segment trabecular bone. Each pixel was assigned a probability of being bone or marrow and then iteratively updated according to the local and surrounding segments until the probability of each pixel was either 1 or 0. Thresholding using one of these techniques results in a binarized image that consists of only bone or marrow voxels.

POST-PROCESSING: ARCHITECTURAL PARAMETERS

Bone mineral density and trabecular structure together determine the mechanical strength of trabecular bone. The main objective of imaging trabecular bone structure is to determine morphological parameters of the trabecular architecture. These morphological parameters may help to determine the efficacy of therapeutic treatments for osteoporosis and predict individuals at risk for bone fracture. Standard histomorphometric measures of bone structure include bone volume fraction (BV/TV), trabecular thickness (Tb.Th), trabecular number (Tb.N), and trabecular spacing (Tb.S). These parameters have been adapted to analyze MR images of trabecular structure.

Because the resolution of in vivo MR images is on the same scale as trabecular dimensions, these histomorphometric parameters are the measures of the trabeculae projected across the slice thickness. Majumdar and coworkers[11] introduced "apparent" measures, indicating that the morphometric measures obtained from in vivo MR images may not be exactly equivalent but are related to those obtained from higher resolution

modalities. It was found that trabecular spacing and trabecular number are relatively independent of resolution.[29] Trabecular thickness, however, was strongly dependent on resolution, with lower resolutions resulting in thicker trabeculae.

A three-dimensional distance technique was introduced by Hildebrand and Rüegsegger to determine mean thickness by fitting spheres within the structure.[30] This measure was able to distinguish between trabecular bone composed of a greater percentage of plates or rods.[30] It has also been used to calculate histomorphometric parameters such as app.Tb.Th and app.Tb.Sp from MR images.[14,31] The morphological parameters calculated using the distance technique correlated well with those calculated using the mean intercept length.[14]

Because osteoporosis is believed to result in a thinning of trabeculae and loss of trabecular connectivity, measures of connectivity are important in determining osteoporotic bone quality. Connectivity measures have been established to measure the degree of connectivity of the trabecular network in trabecular bone.[32,33] Connectivity indicates the maximum number of branches that can be broken before the structure is separated into two parts. It is a topological invariant, which means it does not change if the structure is stretched, bent, twisted, or subjected to other rubber-like deformation. Connectivity can be calculated in terms of the Euler characteristic. Previous studies have used the Euler number to analyze MR images of trabecular bone and found that connectivity can vary between regions within a bone[34] and is significantly correlated with bone density and bone volume fraction.[9,35,36]

Fractal dimensions are a measure of the self-similarity of a structure over different scales and have also been used to characterize trabecular architecture. Fractal dimension (D) can be determined using a box-counting technique in which a grid of boxes is superimposed on the trabecular structure.[37-39] The number of boxes (N) that contain trabeculae is determined for various sizes (ε) of grids. Other investigators have used analysis based on brownian motion to estimate the Hurst exponent (H), which indicates whether the structure is random or contains patterns, and derived the fractal dimension from H.[40] Studies found that fractal dimension decreased with age,[11,37] was significantly lower in patients with vertebral compression fracture[37] and hip fracture,[41,42] and was not correlated with BMD.[41,43] Interestingly, it was found that fractal dimension was not different between subjects with osteopenia and those with osteoporosis but was nonetheless an independent predictor of bone failure strength.[43] It has been proposed that a decrease in fractal dimension is related to a disorganization of trabecular architecture and loss of connectivity.[40]

Pothuaud and coworkers[44,45] proposed further classification of the trabecular architecture using a skeleton graph of the trabecular network. The skeleton graph preserved topographical equivalence with the original network, meaning the connectivity did not change as the trabeculae were thinned to 1 pixel width. This method provides further insight into the influence of connectivity on overall trabecular structure. Others went on to classify the connectivity in terms of curves, surfaces, and junctions of the two.[46,47] They found that parameters from this digital topological analysis correlated well with bone volume fraction and measures of mechanical integrity, such as Young modulus.

Trabecular bone structure is anisotropic, and architectural measures may, therefore, differ depending on the orientation. Spatial autocorrelation analysis[48,49] is a method to quantify not only the distance between trabeculae but also how this varies with respect to orientation (i.e., the amount of anisotropy). The autocorrelation function is a measure of the probability of finding bone n pixels away from a certain pixel and is equal to the product of the bone volume fractions for the two pixels. Parameters derived from the autocorrelation function provide measures of the structure's alignment perpendicular to the slice plane (tubularity) and distribution within the slice plane (transverse contiguity). One advantage of autocorrelation analysis is that it does not depend on thresholding or binarizing the images into bone and marrow. It was found that autocorrelation function measures of anisotropy correlate well with Young modulus and are different for normal and osteoporotic trabecular bone.[27,48] The scaling index method has also been used to measure nonlinear structural information from nonbinarized trabecular bone images.[50] The scaling index (α) is a measure of the isotropy of the structure, with larger values of α indicating a more random structure. The scaling index correlated better with mechanical strength and BMD than traditional histomorphometric measures.

COMPARISON WITH OTHER IMAGING MODALITIES

Several studies have explored how MR images compare with other imaging modalities in determining structural parameters (Table 9-1). Hipp and colleagues[51] and Hopper and colleagues[52] used small-bore MRI with resolutions of $92 \times 92 \times 92$ μm^3 and $23 \times 23 \times 39$ μm^3, respectively. All other studies were performed on 1.5 or 3 T scanners with in-plane resolution of 100 to 150 μm and a slice thickness of 300 μm on in vitro bone cubes. Weber and associates[53] compared MR in vivo and in vitro trabecular bone images from mice with histological sections. They found that parameters derived from in vivo images correlated better with histological parameters than did in vitro images and attributed the difference to the better MR signal from bone marrow than formalin. These studies indicate that MR-derived architectural parameters correlate well with measures taken at much higher resolutions. In general, MR tended to overestimate BV/TV and Tb.Th and underestimate Tb.Sp due to partial volume effects.

Architectural parameters have also been compared with BMD and mechanical strength in the radius,[43] lumbar vertebrae,[54] femur,[55] and calcaneus,[56] and among various sites.[36] In these studies, correlation coefficients for BV/TV, Tb.Th, and Tb.N with BMD or mechanical strength were between 0.5 and 0.8. All studies found that Tb.Sp had a correlation coefficient with BMD or mechanical strength of −0.5 to −0.6, indicating that the spacing between the trabeculae increases as BMD and mechanical strength decrease. Studies also found that combining BMD and trabecular structural parameters improved correlations with mechanical strength.

TABLE 9-1 CORRELATION OF MAGNETIC RESONANCE IMAGING–DERIVED TRABECULAR PARAMETERS WITH THOSE DERIVED FROM OTHER IMAGING MODALITIES

Imaging Modality	Bone Type	Correlation Coefficients*				Study
		BV/TV	Tb.Sp	Tb.N	Tb.Th	
X-ray tomographic microscopy (18 μm)	Distal radius	n.s.	n.s.	n.s.	0.87	Majumdar et al[77]
Optical images (23 μm)	Bovine (various)	0.9	0.85	0.73	–	Hipp et al[51]
Optical images (20 μm)	Calcaneus, femur	0.69	0.89	0.78	n.s.	Majumdar et al[36]
Scanning electron microscopy (20 ×)	Rat femur	0.72	0.82	0.91	0.89	Hopper et al[52]
Macro section radiograph (5 μm)	Distal radius	0.67	0.59	n.s.	0.66	Link et al[78]
Macro section radiograph (5 μm)	Calcaneus	0.63	0.58	n.s.	0.68	Vieth et al[79]
CT (247 × 247 × 1000 μm³)	Distal radius	0.72	0.49	0.47	0.57	Link et al[78]
Micro-CT (22 μm)	Femoral head	0.9	0.92	.90	.82	Sell et al[14]

*All values are statistically significant with $P < .05$. See text for definitions of BV/TV, Tb.Sp, Tb.N, and Tb.Th.
CT = computed tomography; n.s. = not statistically significant.

IN VIVO IMAGING IN HUMANS

Dual x-ray absorptiometry is the gold standard for diagnosing osteoporotic bone; however, it only provides an areal measure of bone mineral density. Multi-slice CT can be used for volumetric BMD and structural measurements. Both DXA and CT require ionizing radiation and should be used in limited amounts. Though MRI cannot provide measures of BMD, it can provide trabecular bone structural measures and does not require radiation. Studies have examined the trabecular structure in the calcaneus of normal and osteoporotic women and found that structural parameters (especially BV/TV, Tb.Sp, Tb.N, and connectivity measures) were significantly different between normal samples and osteoporotic trabecular bone (Figure 9-8).[41,57,58] The

same was found to be true in the calcaneus of normal and osteoporotic men.[59] Similar results were obtained in the radius of premenopausal subjects, postmenopausal normal subjects, and postmenopausal patients with hip fractures.[11] Tb.Sp demonstrated the largest change with age, increasing significantly in postmenopausal women with hip fractures. Benito and coworkers[60] detected bone loss in hypogonadal men using MRI. They found that the ratio of plates to rod (surface voxels to curve voxels in their analysis) and bone volume fraction decreased in hypogonadal men. Correspondingly, the erosion index, a combination of topological parameters that increases as bone architecture deteriorates, was higher in men with hypogonadism.

Magnetic resonance imaging has been used to measure structural bone changes in steroid-induced osteoporosis in patients after renal and cardiac transplantation.[61] Structural parameters were significantly lower (except for Tb.Sp, which was higher) after cardiac transplantation due to the altered bone metabolism caused by immunosuppressive drugs. Large pre- and post-transplantation differences in structural parameters were not seen in renal patients, probably because renal failure can alter bone metabolism and trabecular structure before transplantation occurs. Chesnut and coworkers[62] have published the first longitudinal study showing that nasal spray calcitonin preserves trabecular bone microarchitecture in the distal radius.

IMAGING IN ANIMAL STUDIES

Magnetic resonance imaging also has been used to measure structural parameters in animal models of osteoporosis. Jiang and associates[63] treated an ovariectomized sheep model of osteoporosis with salmon calcitonin, an osteoclast inhibitor, to determine whether structural parameters in the neck of the femur could be maintained. It was found that BV/TV and Tb.N decreased and Tb.Sp increased in ovariectomized sheep. Structural parameters of sheep treated with salmon calcitonin were equivalent to sham operated sheep. Small-bore micro-MRI has been used to study osteoporotic bone structure in ovariectomized rats.[64] Analysis of MR images revealed differences in osteoporotic trabecular structure that DXA could not detect.

Takahashi and associates[65] have investigated the effects of corticosteroids on bone structure in rabbit femurs using magnetic resonance microimaging (μMRI). They found that short-term, high-dose administration of corticosteroids resulted in a decrease in trabecular bone volume through trabecular thinning with little change in trabecular network, trabecular number, or trabecular spacing. Using MR spectroscopy, they also determined that hematopoietic bone marrow was converted to fatty marrow in rabbits treated with corticosteroids.

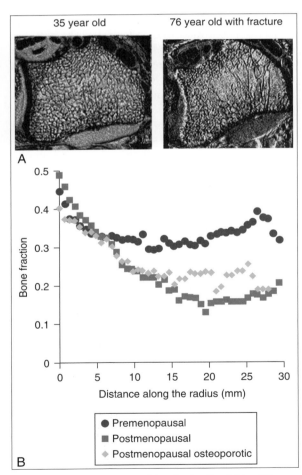

Figure 9-8. Axial MR images of the distal radius (156 × 156 × 500 μm). **A,** Nonosteoporotic 37-year-old subject. **B,** Osteoporotic 76-year-old subject with radial fracture. Note the thinning of the trabeculae and loss of trabecular bone volume. The figure on the right illustrates pre- and postmenopausal decreases in bone fraction in the radius as one moves from the joint line into the shaft.

FUTURE DIRECTIONS

Recent advances in micro-CT imaging in vivo[66,67] make it possible to obtain radius and tibia images using this methodology. However, comparative studies, in vivo case-control studies, and longitudinal studies using micro-CT in vivo in humans have not been undertaken and are clearly warranted. MRI has proved to be a valid method for analyzing trabecular structure and offers distinct advantages over other imaging modalities. Besides being nonionizing and providing the ability to image skeletal sites such as the calcaneus, hip, tibia, and femur, it offers the advantages of characterizing bone and the adjoining soft tissues.

In particular, MRI can visualize soft tissue, such as cartilage, muscle, marrow, and meniscus, which is not possible with x-ray–based imaging modalities. Understanding the relationship between bone and cartilage is critical, particularly in cases of arthritis or injury. It has been found that degradation of cartilage on one compartment of the knee corresponds with a loss of trabecular structure in the other compartment, which is probably linked to mechanical load between the compartments.[54,68]

Most MR images display proton signals from water or fat. It is possible, however, to detect signals from other molecules in a technique called MR spectroscopy.

This technique has been used to a limited degree in bone imaging, in particular to visualize phosphorus in cortical and trabecular bone[69] and lipids in the red bone marrow in hematological diseases.[70] It has also been suggested that MRI can be used to detect the increase in lipid-to-water ratio in the vertebral bodies in patients with osteoporosis.[71]

The combination of MRI and finite element analysis has been used to determine mechanical properties of trabecular bone.[72-74] This allows the in vivo estimation of mechanical properties, which are usually determined by in vitro compression testing. In finite element models derived from MR images, it is possible to incorporate soft tissue structures in the mode, which would be useful not only in mechanobiological models of tissue differentiation and bone remodeling[75] but also in models of fracture healing in which cartilage formation is critical to the process.[76]

Bone quality has been an emerging concept in the area of osteoporosis. Trabecular bone microarchitecture, bone geometry, and associated marrow changes in osteoporosis can all be probed using MRI. Thus, MR techniques have the potential for providing a complete whole-organ assessment of skeletal status in osteoporosis, and further developments in this imaging modality and research studies are clearly warranted.

REFERENCES

1. Davis CA, Genant HK, Dunham JS: The effects of bone on proton NMR relaxation times of surrounding liquids. Invest Radiol 1986;21:472-77.
2. Brismar TB, Hindmarsh T, Ringertz H: Experimental correlation between T2* and ultimate compressive strength in lumbar porcine vertebrae. Acad Radiol 1997;4:426-30.
3. Majumdar S: Quantitative study of the susceptibility difference between trabecular bone and bone marrow: computer simulations. Magn Reson Med 1991;22:101-10.
4. Brismar TB, Karlsson M, Li T, Ringertz H: The correlation between R2' and bone mineral measurements in human vertebrae: an in vitro study. Eur Radiol 1999;9:141-44.
5. Kang C, Paley M, Ordidge R, Speller R: R'2 measured in trabecular bone in vitro: relationship to trabecular separation. Magn Reson Imaging 1999;17:989-95.
6. Majumdar S, Genant HK: In vivo relationship between marrow T2* and trabecular bone density determined with a chemical shift-selective asymmetric spin-echo sequence. J Magn Reson Imaging 1992;2:209-19.
7. Bakker CJ, Bhagwandien R, Moerland MA, Ramos LM: Simulation of susceptibility artifacts in 2D and 3D Fourier transform spin-echo and gradient-echo magnetic resonance imaging. Magn Reson Imaging 1994;12:767-74.
8. Jara H, Wehrli FW, Chung H, Ford JC: High-resolution variable flip angle 3D MR imaging of trabecular microstructure in vivo. Magn Reson Med 1993;29:528-39.
9. Majumdar S, Newitt D, Jergas M, et al: Evaluation of technical factors affecting the quantification of trabecular bone structure using magnetic resonance imaging. Bone 1995;17:417-30.
10. Ma J, Wehrli FW, Song HK: Fast 3D large-angle spin-echo imaging (3D FLASE). Magn Reson Med 1996;35:903-10.
11. Majumdar S, Genant HK, Grampp S, et al: Correlation of trabecular bone structure with age, bone mineral density, and osteoporotic status: in vivo studies in the distal radius using high resolution magnetic resonance imaging. J Bone Miner Res 1997;12:111-18.
12. Link TM, Majumdar S, Grampp S, et al: Imaging of trabecular bone structure in osteoporosis. Eur Radiol 1999;9:1781-88.
13. Timonen J, Alvila L, Hirva P, Pakkanen TT: Nuclear magnetic resonance imaging: a potential method for analysis of bone material. J Mater Sci Mater Med 1998;9:187-90.
14. Sell CA, Masi JN, Burghardt A, et al: Quantification of trabecular bone structure using magnetic resonance imaging at 3 tesla-calibration studies using microcomputed tomography as a standard of reference. Calcif Tissue Int 2005;76:355-64.
15. Newitt D, Majumdar S: Correction for receiver coil inhomogeneity profiles for quantitative analysis of trabecular bone structure from high resolution MRI. Proceedings from 7th ISMRM. Philadelphia: 1999:1046.
16. Newitt DC, van Rietbergen B, Majumdar S: Processing and analysis of in vivo high-resolution MR images of trabecular bone for longitudinal studies: reproducibility of structural measures and micro-finite element analysis derived mechanical properties. Osteoporos Int 2002;13:278-87.
17. Hwang SN, Wehrli FW: Estimating voxel volume fractions of trabecular bone on the basis of magnetic resonance images acquired in vivo. Int J Imaging Syst Technol 1999;10:18-198.
18. Wink AM, Roerdink JB: Denoising functional MR images: a comparison of wavelet denoising and Gaussian smoothing. IEEE Trans Med Imaging 2004;23:374-87.
19. Scheunders P: Wavelet thresholding of multivalued images. IEEE Trans Image Process 2004;13:475-83.

20. Bao P, Zhang L: Noise reduction for magnetic resonance images via adaptive multiscale products thresholding. IEEE Trans Med Imaging 2003;22:1089-99.

21. Ehman RL, Felmlee JP: Adaptive technique for high-definition MR imaging of moving structures. Radiology 1989;173:255-63.

22. Song HK, Wehrli FW: In vivo micro-imaging using alternating navigator echoes with applications to cancellous bone structural analysis. Magn Reson Med 1999;41:947-53.

23. Atkinson D, Hill DL, Stoyle PN, et al: Automatic compensation of motion artifacts in MRI. Magn Reson Med 1999;41:163-70.

24. Atkinson D, Hill DL, Stoyle PN, et al: Automatic correction of motion artifacts in magnetic resonance images using an entropy focus criterion. IEEE Trans Med Imaging 1997;16:903-10.

25. Link TM, Majumdar S, Lin JC, et al: Assessment of trabecular structure using high resolution CT images and texture analysis. J Comput Assist Tomogr 1998;22:15-24.

26. Wu Z, Chung HW, Wehrli FW: A Bayesian approach to subvoxel tissue classification in NMR microscopic images of trabecular bone. Magn Reson Med 1994;31:302-8.

27. Hwang SN, Wehrli FW, Williams JL: Probability-based structural parameters from three-dimensional nuclear magnetic resonance images as predictors of trabecular bone strength. Med Phys 1997;24:1255-61.

28. Antoniadis T, Scarpelli JP, Ruaud JP, et al: Bone labelling on micro-magnetic resonance images. Med Image Anal 1999;3:119-28.

29. Kothari M, Keaveny TM, Lin JC, et al: Impact of spatial resolution on the prediction of trabecular architecture parameters. Bone 1998;22:437-43.

30. Hildebrand T, Rüegsegger P: A new method for the model-independent assessment of thickness in three-dimensional images. J Microsc 1997;185:67-75.

31. Laib A, Newitt DC, Lu Y, Majumdar S: New model-independent measures of trabecular bone structure applied to in vivo high-resolution MR images. Osteoporos Int 2002;13:130-6.

32. Odgaard A, Gundersen HJ: Quantification of connectivity in cancellous bone, with special emphasis on 3-D reconstructions. Bone 1993;14:173-82.

33. Feldkamp LA, Goldstein SA, Parfitt AM, et al: The direct examination of three-dimensional bone architecture in vitro by computed tomography. J Bone Miner Res 1989;4:3-11.

34. Stampa B, Kuhn B, Liess C, et al: Characterization of the integrity of three-dimensional trabecular bone microstructure by connectivity and shape analysis using high-resolution magnetic resonance imaging in vivo. Top Magn Reson Imaging 2002;13:357-63.

35. Majumdar S, Genant HK: Assessment of trabecular structure using high resolution magnetic resonance imaging. Stud Health Technol Inform 1997;40:81-96.

36. Majumdar S, Kothari M, Augat P, et al: High-resolution magnetic resonance imaging: three-dimensional trabecular bone architecture and biomechanical properties. Bone 1998;22:445-54.

37. Weinstein RS, Majumdar S: Fractal geometry and vertebral compression fractures. J Bone Miner Res 1994;9:1797-802.

38. Majumdar S, Weinstein RS, Prasad RR: Application of fractal geometry techniques to the study of trabecular bone. Med Phys 1993;20:1611-19.

39. Chung HW, Chu CC, Underweiser M, Wehrli FW: On the fractal nature of trabecular structure. Med Phys 1994;21:1535-40.

40. Pothuaud L, Benhamou CL, Porion P, et al: Fractal dimension of trabecular bone projection texture is related to three-dimensional microarchitecture. J Bone Miner Res 2000;15:691-99.

41. Link TM, Majumdar S, Augat P, et al: In vivo high resolution MRI of the calcaneus: differences in trabecular structure in osteoporosis patients. J Bone Miner Res 1998;13:1175-82.

42. Majumdar S, Link TM, Millard J, et al: In vivo assessment of trabecular bone structure using fractal analysis of distal radius radiographs. Med Phys 2000;27:2594-99.

43. Hudelmaier M, Kollstedt A, Lochmuller EM, et al: Gender differences in trabecular bone architecture of the distal radius assessed with magnetic resonance imaging and implications for mechanical competence. Osteoporos Int 2005;16:1124-33.

44. Pothuaud L, Porion P, Lespessailles E, et al: A new method for three-dimensional skeleton graph analysis of porous media: application to trabecular bone microarchitecture. J Microsc 2000;199:149-61.

45. Pothuaud L, Newitt DC, Lu Y, et al: In vivo application of 3D-line skeleton graph analysis (LSGA) technique with high-resolution magnetic resonance imaging of trabecular bone structure. Osteoporos Int 2004;15:411-9.

46. Gomberg BR, Saha PK, Song HK, et al: Topological analysis of trabecular bone MR images. IEEE Trans Med Imaging 2000;19:166-74.

47. Wehrli FW, Gomberg BR, Saha PK, et al: Digital topological analysis of in vivo magnetic resonance microimages of trabecular bone reveals structural implications of osteoporosis. J Bone Miner Res 2001;16:1520-31.

48. Rotter M, Berg A, Langenberger H, et al: Autocorrelation analysis of bone structure. J Magn Reson Imaging 2001;14:87-93.

49. Wehrli FW, Saha PK, Gomberg BR, et al: Role of magnetic resonance for assessing structure and function of trabecular bone. Top Magn Reson Imaging 2002;13:335-55.

50. Boehm HF, Raeth C, Monetti RA, et al: Local 3D scaling properties for the analysis of trabecular bone extracted from high-resolution magnetic resonance imaging of human trabecular bone: comparison with bone mineral density in the prediction of biomechanical strength in vitro. Invest Radiol 2003;38:269-80.

51. Hipp JA, Jansujwicz A, Simmons CA, Snyder BD: Trabecular bone morphology from micro-magnetic resonance imaging. J Bone Miner Res 1996;11:286-97.

52. Hopper TA, Meder R, Pope JM: Comparison of high-resolution MRI, optical microscopy and SEM for quantitation of trabecular architecture in the rat femur. Magn Reson Imaging 2004;22:953-61.

53. Weber MH, Sharp JC, Latta P, et al: Magnetic resonance imaging of trabecular and cortical bone in mice: comparison of high resolution in vivo and ex vivo MR images with corresponding histology. Eur J Radiol 2005;53:96-102.

54. Beuf O, Newitt DC, Mosekilde L, Majumdar S: Trabecular structure assessment in lumbar vertebrae specimens using quantitative magnetic resonance imaging and relationship with mechanical competence. J Bone Miner Res 2001;16:1511-19.

55. Link TM, Vieth V, Langenberg R, et al: Structure analysis of high resolution magnetic resonance imaging of the proximal femur: in vitro correlation with biomechanical strength and BMD. Calcif Tissue Int 2003;72:156-65.

56. Ouyang X, Selby K, Lang P, et al: High resolution magnetic resonance imaging of the calcaneus: age-related changes in trabecular structure and comparison with dual X-ray absorptiometry measurements. Calcif Tissue Int 1997;60:139-47.

57. Herlidou S, Grebe R, Grados F, et al: Influence of age and osteoporosis on calcaneus trabecular bone structure: a preliminary in vivo MRI study by quantitative texture analysis. Magn Reson Imaging 2004;22:237-43.

58. Link TM, Bauer J, Kollstedt A, et al: Trabecular bone structure of the distal radius, the calcaneus, and the spine: which site predicts fracture status of the spine best? Invest Radiol 2004;39:487-97.

59. Boutry N, Cortet B, Dubois P, et al: Trabecular bone structure of the calcaneus: preliminary in vivo MR imaging assessment in men with osteoporosis. Radiology 2003;227:708-17.

60. Benito M, Gomberg B, Wehrli FW, et al: Deterioration of trabecular architecture in hypogonadal men. J Clin Endocrinol Metab 2003;88:1497-502.

61. Link TM: High-resolution magnetic resonance imaging to assess trabecular bone structure in patients after transplantation: a review. Top Magn Reson Imaging 2002;13:365-75.

62. Chesnut CHI, Majumdar S, Newitt D, et al: Effects of salmon calcitonin on trabecular microarchitecture as determined by magnetic resonance imaging: results from the Quest study. J Bone Miner Res 2005;20:1548-61.

63. Jiang Y, Zhao J, Geusens P, et al: Femoral neck trabecular microstructure in ovariectomized ewes treated with calcitonin: MRI microscopic evaluation. J Bone Miner Res 2005;20:125-30.

64. Jiang Y, Zhao J, White DL, Genant HK: Micro CT and Micro MR imaging of 3D architecture of animal skeleton. J Musculoskelet Neuronal Interact 2000;1:45-51.

65. Takahashi M, Wehrli FW, Hilaire L, et al: In vivo NMR microscopy allows short-term serial assessment of multiple

skeletal implications of corticosteroid exposure. Proc Natl Acad Sci U S A 2002;99:4574-79.

66. Laib A, Hammerle S, Koller BA: New 100 μm resolution scanner for in vivo 3D-CT of the human forearm and lower leg. Presented at the 16th Annual Bone Densitometry Workshop. Annecy, France, 2004.

67. Boutroy S, Bouxsein M, Munoz F, Delmas P: In vivo assessment of trabecular microarchitecture by high-resolution peripheral quantitative computed tomography. JCEM 2005;90:6508-15.

68. Lindsey CT, Narasimhan A, Adolfo JM, et al: Magnetic resonance evaluation of the interrelationship between articular cartilage and trabecular bone of the osteoarthritic knee. Osteoarthritis Cartilage 2004;12:86-96.

69. Robson MD, Gatehouse PD, Bydder GM, Neubauer S: Human imaging of phosphorus in cortical and trabecular bone in vivo. Magn Reson Med 2004;51:888-92.

70. Schick F, Einsele H, Kost R, et al: Localized MR 1H spectroscopy reveals alterations of susceptibility in bone marrow with hemosiderosis. Magn Reson Med 1994;32:470-5.

71. Lin CS, Fertikh D, Davis B, et al: 2D CSI proton MR spectroscopy of human spinal vertebra: feasibility studies. J Magn Reson Imaging 2000;11:287-93.

72. Pothuaud L, Van Rietbergen B, Mosekilde L, et al: Combination of topological parameters and bone volume fraction better predicts the mechanical properties of trabecular bone. J Biomech 2002;35:1091-9.

73. Newitt DC, Majumdar S, van Rietbergen B, et al: In vivo assessment of architecture and micro-finite element analysis derived indices of mechanical properties of trabecular bone in the radius. Osteoporos Int 2002;13:6-17.

74. van Rietbergen B, Majumdar S, Newitt D, MacDonald B: High-resolution MRI and micro-FE for the evaluation of changes in bone mechanical properties during longitudinal clinical trials: application to calcaneal bone in postmenopausal women after one year of idoxifene treatment. Clin Biomech (Bristol, Avon) 2002;17:81-8.

75. Shefelbine SJ, Augat P, Claes L, Simon U: Trabecular bone fracture healing simulation with finite element analysis and fuzzy logic. J Biomech 2005;38:2440-50.

76. Shefelbine SJ, Simon U, Claes L, et al: Prediction of fracture callus mechanical properties using micro-CT images and voxel-based finite element analysis. Bone 2005;36:480-88.

77. Majumdar S, Newitt D, Mathur A, et al: Magnetic resonance imaging of trabecular bone structure in the distal radius: relationship with X-ray tomographic microscopy and biomechanics. Osteoporos Int 1996;6:376-85.

78. Link TM, Vieth V, Stehling C, et al: High-resolution MRI vs multi-slice spiral CT: which technique depicts the trabecular bone structure best? Eur Radiol 2003;13:663-71.

79. Vieth V, Link TM, Lotter A, et al: Does the trabecular bone structure depicted by high-resolution MRI of the calcaneus reflect the true bone structure? Invest Radiol 2001;36:210-17.

10 Biochemical Markers of Bone Turnover

Patrick Garnero

Osteoporosis is a systemic disease characterized by a low bone mass and microarchitectural deterioration of bone tissue, with a consequent increase in skeletal fragility and susceptibility to fracture.[1] This definition implies that the diagnosis can and probably should be made before any fragility fracture has occurred, which is a real challenge for the clinician. The level of bone mass can be assessed with adequate precision by measuring bone mineral density (BMD) using dual x-ray absorptiometry (DXA). This measurement does not capture all risk factors for fracture, however. Bone fragility also depends on the morphology, the architecture of bone, and the material properties of the bone matrix that cannot be readily assessed, all of these components being regulated by bone turnover (Figure 10-1). Consequently, it has been suggested that bone strength may be reflected, independently of BMD level, by measuring bone turnover using specific serum and urinary markers of bone formation and resorption. Bone turnover markers have also been suggested to be useful to monitor the efficacy of treatment, especially anticatabolic treat-

ments (hormone replacement therapy, bisphosphonates, and calcitonin), but also more recently anabolic therapy, including parathyroid hormone. In this chapter, we briefly review the new developments in biochemical marker biochemistry and technology and then discuss their use for the management of postmenopausal osteoporosis.

BIOCHEMICAL MARKERS OF BONE TURNOVER

Bone remodeling is the result of two opposite activities, the production of new bone matrix by osteoblasts and the destruction of old bone by osteoclasts. The rates of bone production and destruction can be evaluated either by measuring predominantly osteoblastic or osteoclastic enzyme activities or by assaying bone matrix components released in the bloodstream and excreted in the urine (Table 10-1). These have been separated into markers of formation and resorption,

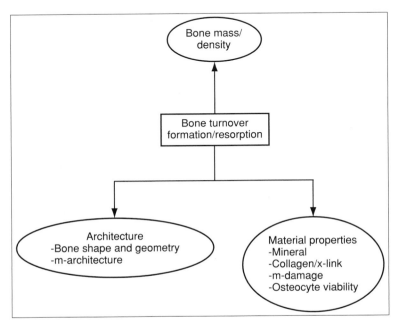

Figure 10-1. The different components of bone strength and the pivotal role of bone turnover in their regulation.

TABLE 10-1 BIOCHEMICAL MARKERS OF BONE TURNOVER*	
Formation	**Resorption**
Total and **bone-specific**	Serum/Plasma Tartrate resistant acid phosphatase (TRAP, 5b isoenzyme)
alkaline **phosphatase** (bone ALP)	*N*-terminal (S-NTX) and *C*-terminal (S-CTX) cross-linking telopeptide of type I collagen
Intact and **total** osteocalcin (OC)	*C*-terminal cross-linking telopeptide of type I collagen generated by MMPs (CTX-MMP) Urine
Type I collagen extension propeptides (PICP, **PINP**)	**Pyridinoline (PYD)** **Deoxypyridinoline (DPD)** **U-NTX** **U-CTX** Type I collagen helicoidal peptide 620-633 Galactosyl-hydroxylysine Hydroxyproline (Hyp) Mid-region osteocalcin fragments

* The markers with the most established performance characteristics in osteoporosis are in bold type.

but it should be kept in mind that in disease states in which both events are coupled and change in the same direction, such as osteoporosis, any marker will reflect the overall rate of bone turnover. Current bone markers cannot discriminate between turnover changes in a specific skeletal envelope, that is, trabecular versus cortical, but reflect whole body net changes. Increasingly specific biochemical markers for bone remodeling have been identified in recent years.[2] At present, in osteoporosis the most sensitive markers for bone formation are serum total osteocalcin, bone alkaline phosphatase, and the procollagen type I *N*-terminal propeptide (PINP). For the evaluation of bone resorption, immunological assays of pyridinium cross-links of collagen (pyridinoline [PYD] and deoxypyridinoline [DPD]) have superseded total pyridinoline assay by high performance liquid chromatography in clinical routine practice, although high performance liquid chromatography or enzyme-linked immunosorbent assays for total DPD remains a valuable marker in clinical research. Immunological assays are now available for PYD and DPD in urine and for *C*-terminal and *N*-terminal cross-linked telopeptides of type I collagen peptides (CTX, ICTP, and NTX, respectively) in serum or urine (Figure 10-2). Most of these biochemical marker assays are now available on automatic platforms with increased precision over manual assays and high throughout, which allow convenient accurate measurements in large number of individuals.

The different collagen-related markers can respond differently with diseases and treatments. It has been shown that although the urinary excretions of cross-linked CTX and NTX peptides markedly decrease after treatments with either estrogen or bisphosphonate treatment, urinary free cross-links (PYD and DPD) show a significant response with estrogens or selective estrogen receptor modulators but do not change or only modestly change after bisphosphonate treatment.[3] Serum and

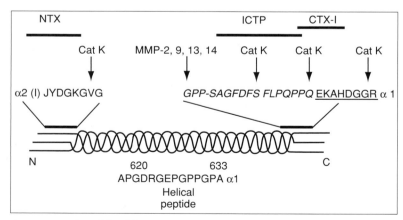

Figure 10-2. Schematic representation of the different type I collagen peptides used as markers of bone resorption and sites of cleavage by cathepsin K (cat K) and matrix metalloproteases (MMPs) on type I collagen. The NTX epitope and CTX epitopes in the *N*- and *C*-telopeptide regions, respectively, are efficiently generated by cat K, the main enzyme responsible for type I collagen degradation in physiological conditions, but not by MMP ,which have been proposed to participate in bone resorption in physiological conditions but also in metastatic processes. In contrast, ICTP epitope is destroyed by the action of cat K and is generated by MMPs, especially MMP 2 and MMP 13.

urine CTX and NTX levels are markedly increased in postmenopausal women with osteoporosis, and their values decrease markedly and rapidly with antiresorptive therapy. This is in contrast with the slight and nonsignificant modifications of another *C*-telopeptide fragment ICTP in these two conditions.[4] In contrast, serum ICTP is a sensitive marker in other pathological conditions, including malignant bone diseases and rheumatoid arthritis.[5-7] These different responses are likely to result from differences in the enzymatic pathways leading to the release of CTX/NTX and ICTP from bone type I collagen (see Figure 10-2). It has been shown that the epitope of ICTP is destroyed by cathepsin K activity,[8] an osteoclastic-specific cysteine protease that is the key enzyme responsible for bone collagen degradation in normal physiological conditions, whereas it is generated by matrix-metalloproteases,[9] whose activity has been suggested to play an important role in collagen degradation associated with pathological bone degradation, including bone metastases and arthritis (see Figure 10-2). In contrast, CTX and NTX epitopes are highly efficiently generated by cathepsin K and not by matrix-metalloproteases.[9,10]

More recently, new biochemical markers and assays have emerged. These include immunoassays for serum tartrate resistant acid phosphate (TRACP), which preferentially detect the isoenzyme 5b, predominantly expressed by the osteoclast.[11,12] In contrast to type I collagen related markers, TRACP 5b isoenzyme is likely to represent mainly the osteoclast number and activity and not directly the rate of bone matrix degradation, although in osteoporosis TRACP 5b was found to correlate with NTX and DPD.[13] Recent studies have also found that plasma TRACP 5b is increased in postmenopausal women, is associated with fracture risk in one study,[14] and was found to decrease with treatment by hormone replacement therapy.[13] TRACP 5b may be of particular interest to evaluate increased osteoclastic activity in women with breast cancer and bone metastases.[15]

Currently, the available markers of type I collagen degradation are based on the measurement of pyridinoline cross-links or associated cross-linked *C*- or *N*-telopeptides, both originating from the telopeptide region. More recently, it has been isolated from urine of patients with Paget disease of the bone, a type I collagen-specific peptide corresponding to residue 620 to 633 of the helicoidal region of $\alpha 1$ chain (see Figure 10-2). The urinary excretion of this peptide is likely to reflect the destruction of the main part of the collagen molecule and could reflect aspects of bone resorption other than the telopeptide derived fragments. We found that the urinary excretion of that helicoidal peptide increased markedly after menopause and was as sensitive as urinary CTX measurements to assess the antiresorptive effects of bisphosphonate and estrogens.[16]

Additional studies are required to fully evaluate the clinical utility of this biochemical marker, especially for fracture risk prediction.

Although most of newly synthesized osteocalcin is captured by bone matrix, a small fraction is released into the blood, where it can be detected by immunoassays and is currently considered as a specific bone formation marker. Circulating osteocalcin is composed of different immunoreactive forms, including the intact molecule but also various fragments.[17] It has been shown that the majority of circulating fragments arises from the in vivo degradation of the intact molecule and thus also reflects bone formation.[17] However, some of these fragments could also be released from the degradation of bone matrix, resistant to the glomeral filtration and accumulated in urine.[18] Using urine samples from patients with Paget disease, a peptide was recently isolated that corresponds to the mid-14-28 molecule sequence of human osteocalcin, and an immunoassay has been developed. Elevated levels of urinary osteocalcin were reported in osteoporotic postmenopausal women.[19] After only 30 days of treatment of osteoporotic women with the bisphosphonate alendronate, urinary osteocalcin levels decreased by 27% ($P = .0059$), a decrease similar to that obtained with the type I collagen resorption markers CTX, NTX, and deoxypyridinoline. This early response of urinary osteocalcin contrasted with the absence of changes in serum osteocalcin and alkaline phosphatase, suggesting that this urinary marker may reflect bone resorption.[19] More recently, antibody-detected isomerized fragments of osteocalcin have also been developed that are believed to reflect the degradation of aged-bone matrix. Urinary excretion of isomerized osteocalcin also decreased 10 days after a single intravenous injection of zoledronate in patients with Paget disease, contrasting with the absence of changes of serum total osteocalcin.[20] From a theoretical point of view, urinary osteocalcin fragments may be more specific for bone resorption than type I collagen related markers, although their clinical value in osteoporosis remains to be more extensively evaluated. Interestingly, a recent study showed that increased urinary osteocalcin, but not serum total osteocalcin, was associated with increased risk of clinical vertebral fracture independent of BMD in a large prospective study of elderly women.[14]

POST-TRANSLATIONAL MODIFICATIONS OF BONE MATRIX PROTEINS

Type I collagen, the main organic component of bone matrix, undergoes a series of enzymatic and nonenzymatic intra- and extracellular post-translational modifications (Figure 10-3). Among the enzymatic

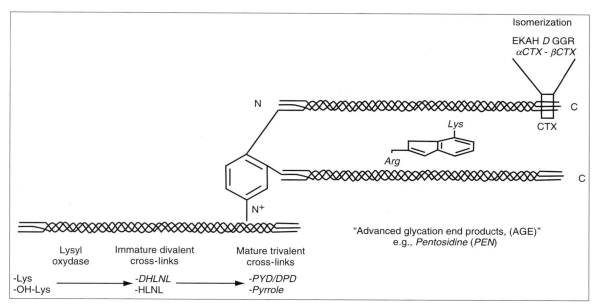

Figure 10-3. Schematic representation of the extracellular post-translational modifications of type I collagen in bone. Type I collagen is constituted by the association in triple helix of two alpha 1 and one alpha 2 chains except of the two ends (*N*- and *C*-telopeptides). In bone matrix, type I collagen is subjected to different post-translational modifications: the mature trivalent cross-links including pyridinoline (PYD), deoxypyridinoline (DPD), and pyrrole, which make bridges between two telopeptides and the helicoidal region of another collagen molecule. These molecules result from the maturation of divalent cross-linking molecules (dihydroxylysinonorleucine [DHLNL] and hydroxylysinonorleucine [HLNL]), whose synthesis requires an enzymatic process (lysil oxydase); the advanced glycation end products (AGEs), which are formed by nonenzymatic glycation involving a sugar such as glucose and amino acid such as lysine. Some AGEs such as pentosine are cross-linking molecules, although their precise location remains to be determined; the nonenzymatic isomerization of aspartic acid (D) occurring in the *C*-telopeptides of alpha 1 chains.

modifications, biochemical studies performed on human bone specimens have shown that overhydroxylation of lysine residues, overglycosylation of hydroxylysine, and a reduction in the concentration of nonreducible cross-links can be associated with reduced bone strength.[19-22] In human vertebral specimens, Banse and colleagues[25] analyzed the content of immature (hydroxylysononorleucine and dihydroxylysinorleucine) and mature cross-links (PYD, DPD, and pyrolle). They showed that the ratio of PYD to DPD was significantly associated with the compressive biomechanical properties of the vertebrae independently of BMD, suggesting that type I collagen cross-linking may be a determinant of bone strength. Nonenzymatic modifications of collagen could also play a role in the mechanical properties of bone tissue. For example, Wang and associates[26] showed that the pentosidine concentration of human femoral bone, an index of nonenzymatic advanced glycation end products, increases with age and that higher levels are associated with decreased bone strength. This suggests that nonenzymatic glycation of collagen could lead to alterations of the biomechanical properties bone that may ultimately result in increased skeletal fragility.

Beta-isomerization of the aspartate (D) residue of the [1209]AHDGGR[1214] sequence (CTX) of the *C*-telopeptide of type I collagen is another nonenzymatic post-translational modification more recently investigated.[27] Histological studies have shown a decreased degree of type I collagen isomerization within the woven pagetic bone, a tissue characterized by increased fragility.[28] Alterations of the degree of bone type I collagen isomerization can be detected in vivo by the differential measurement of native (α) and isomerized (β) CTX fragments in urine. In patients with Paget disease of the bone it has been shown that the urinary excretion of α CTX was markedly increased compared with β CTX, resulting in an abnormal α/β CTX ratio.[28] The relationships between these two isoforms can be normalized after treatment with bisphosphonates,[29,30] (Figure 10-4) a treatment that has been shown to result in the formation of a bone matrix with normal lamellar structure. The investigation of type I collagen isomerization may also be of clinical relevance in cases of postmenopausal osteoporosis. In the OFELY prospective study, we found that the urinary ratio between native and β-isomerized CTX was significantly associated with increased fracture risk, independent of both the level of hip BMD and the bone turnover rate measured by serum bone ALP (Table 10-2).[31,32] It has also been shown that the various antiresorptive treatments, including bisphosphonates and selective estrogen

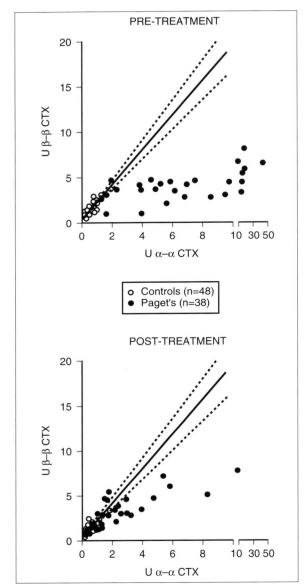

Figure 10-4. Correlation between native (α–α) cross-linked *C*-telopeptide of type I collagen (CTX) and isomerized (β–β) CTX in healthy control subjects and in patients with Paget disease of bone before and after treatment with the bisphosphonate tiludronate. Regression lines and 95% confidence intervals for healthy control subjects are indicated. Note the disproportionately high levels of α–α CTX compared with β–β CTX in patients with Paget disease before treatment. After treatment with bisphosphonate, the relationship between α–α CTX and β–β CTX is similar to that found in healthy control subjects, for most patients. (From Alexandersen P, Peris P, Guanabens N, et al: Non-isomerized C-telopeptide fragments are highly sensitive markers for monitoring disease activity and treatment efficacy in Paget's disease of bone. J Bone Miner Res 2005;20:588-95.)

receptor modulators could influence the urinary α/βCTX ratio differently.[33] In an in vitro model in which the extent of cross-linking can be modified, keeping constant the size and mineral content of the

bone samples, we recently demonstrated that changes in the extent of post-translational modifications of type I collagen (e.g., intermolecular cross-linking such as pyridinoline and pentosidine and CTX isomerization) play a role in determining the mechanical competence of cortical bone, and especially post-yield properties, independently of BMD and porosity.[34] These data indicate that the degree of post-translational modifications of collagen matrix plays an independent role in determining the mechanical competence of cortical bone, and the α/β CTX ratio may provide an in vivo marker of bone collagen quality. The clinical relevance of bone collagen properties as an important independent determinant of skeletal strength has also been suggested by recent studies investigating the relationships between circulating homocysteine levels and the risk of fracture in elderly women and men. Homocysteinuria is a rare autosomal recessive disease that is characterized by generalized osteoporosis. This finding has been attributed to an inhibition of the formation of collagen cross-linking by high homocysteine levels.[35] McLean and coworkers[36] and van Meurs and coworkers[37] found that elderly women and men with plasma levels of homocysteine in the highest quartile had a risk of nonvertebral and hip fracture that was twice the risk in other individuals. It seems, however, that this finding results from the combination of increased homocysteine levels and low serum vitamin B_{12} levels, which provided the highest risk for all fractures in a recent study.[38] Interestingly, in the study from the Netherlands,[38] high homocysteine levels and low vitamin B_{12} were associated with increased bone resorption evaluated by the urinary excretion of DPD.

Bone matrix also contains noncollagenous proteins that can undergo post-translational modifications. Osteocalcin is a noncollagenous protein almost specific for bone matrix that contains three residues of γ-carboxyglutamic acid (GLA). GLA results from the carboxylation of glutamic acid residues, an intracellular post-translational modification that is vitamin K-dependent. It was postulated that impaired γ-carboxylation of osteocalcin could be an index of both vitamin D and vitamin K deficiencies in elderly populations. In two prospective studies performed in a cohort of elderly institutionalized women followed for 3 years[39] and in a population of healthy elderly women (EPIDOS study),[40] levels of undercarboxylated osteocalcin above the premenopausal range was associated with a two- to threefold increase in the risk of hip fracture, although total osteocalcin was not predictive. It has also been shown that a decreased ratio between carboxylated and total osteocalcin, which is an index of increased undercarboxylated osteocalcin, was associated with increased fracture risk in elderly women living at home.[41] The mechanisms relating increased

TABLE 10-2 INCREASED URINARY CTX RATIO AS AN INDEPENDENT PREDICTOR OF THE RISK OF OSTEOPOROTIC FRACTURES*		
Urinary CTX Ratio at Baseline	Relative Risk† (95% CI) of Fracture for Values in the Upper Quartile	
	All Fractures	Nonvertebral Fractures Only
$\alpha L/\beta L$		
Unadjusted	2.0 (1.2-3.5)	2.5 (1.3-4.6)
Adjusted for bone ALP	1.8 (1.1-3.2)	2.2 (1.1-4.2)
Adjusted for femoral neck BMD	1.8 (1.03-3.1)	2.2 (1.2-4.0)
Adjusted for bone ALP + femoral neck BMD	1.7 (0.95-2.9)	2.0 (1.04-3.8)

* Study involved 408 women followed prospectively for 6.8 years; 55 nonvertebral fractures and 16 incident vertebral fractures were recorded.
† Adjusted for age, presence of prevalent fracture, and physical activity
From Garnero P, Cloos P, Sornay-Rendu E, et al: Type I collagen racemization and isomerization and the risk of fracture in postmenopausal women: the OFELY prospective study. J Bone Miner Res 2002; 17:826-33.

undercarboxylation of osteocalcin and fracture risk is unclear. Serum undercarboxylated osteocalcin,[42] but not total osteocalcin, has been found to be associated more strongly with ultrasonic transmitted velocity (which has been suggested to reflect in part changes in bone structure) at the os calcis and tibia than with BMD,[42] suggesting that poor altered bone structure may explain the fracture risk associated with undercarboxylated osteocalcin, possibly as a result of inadequate vitamin K status. Osteocalcin also contains in its sequence five residues of aspartic acid that can undergo age-related isomerization. Although not directly analyzed in bone matrix, isomerized osteocalcin fragments have recently been described in patients with Paget disease of bone.[20] The influence of the isomerization of osteocalcin and other noncollagenous proteins on the mechanical competence of bone matrix remains to be investigated.

Clearly, the above-mentioned studies open new perspectives for the clinical use of bone markers, not only to measure quantitative changes in bone turnover, but also to assess changes in bone matrix properties, an important determinant of bone strength

CLINICAL USES OF BONE MARKERS IN OSTEOPOROSIS

Markers of Bone Turnover and Fracture Risk

With the emergence of effective but rather expensive treatments, it is essential to detect those women at higher risk of fracture. Although several prospective studies have clearly demonstrated a strong association between BMD measurements and the risk of hip, spine, and forearm fractures, as confirmed recently in a meta-analysis that included 29,082 women from 12 different cohorts,[43] about one-half of patients with incident frac-

tures have baseline BMD assessed by DXA above the diagnostic threshold of osteoporosis, defined as a T-score of −2.5 SD or more below the average value of young healthy women.[44-46] Clearly, there is a need for improvement in the identification of patients at risk for fracture. In addition to age, several other clinical risk factors have been shown to contribute to fracture probability independently of BMD in postmenopausal women, including a family history of hip fracture, prior fragility fractures,[47] and low body mass index in some but not all studies, although a recent meta-analysis suggests that the association of body mass index with fracture risk is likely to be mediated by BMD.[48]

Relating baseline bone turnover levels with the subsequent risk of osteoporotic fractures is the valid methodology to assess their clinical utility, because case-control studies can be confounded by the effect of the trauma on biochemical marker levels.[49] Prospective studies investigating the relationships between bone formation markers and fracture risk have yielded conflicting results. In the large multicenter cohort of elderly women in France (EPIDOS), no significant relationships were found between levels of serum osteocalcin and bone alkaline phosphatase and the risk of hip fracture occurring during a 2-year follow-up period.[50] Similar negative findings were recently reported for clinical vertebral and nonvertebral fractures in the elderly women involved in the Malmö study.[14] In contrast, in two prospective studies performed in younger healthy postmenopausal women (OFELY and Hawai'i Osteoporosis Study), a significant positive association between increased levels of bone alkaline phosphatase and the risk of vertebral and nonvertebral fracture was observed.[51,52] The differences between the studies may be related to the type of fracture or to the duration of follow-up, which was 22 months in the EPIDOS study and 5 years in the OFELY study. More recently, we reassessed the OFELY data after a median of 9 years of follow-up in which we recorded 158 incident fractures in 116 women including 50 vertebral and 108 nonvertebral fractures. Over this long follow-up period, we also found a significant association between increased baseline levels of serum osteocalcin, bone alkaline phosphatase, and PINP and the risk of fractures (unpublished data). Melton and coworkers,[53] however, could not find any significant relationship between total alkaline phosphatase levels and serum osteocalcin and the risk of fracture in the following 20 years. The markers that were measured 20 years ago, however, were not the most specific ones and this may have resulted in decreased power to detect a significant association.

More consistent data have been obtained on the relationship between increased levels of bone resorption markers and fracture risk. Five prospective studies (Rotterdam, EPIDOS, OFELY, HOS, and Malmö) found that bone resorption assessed by urinary or serum CTX, urinary free deoxypyridinoline, serum TRACP 5b, or urinary osteocalcin fragments (only one study for these two latter markers) above the premenopausal range were consistently associated with an approximate twofold higher risk of hip, vertebral, non-hip, and nonvertebral fractures over follow-up periods ranging from 1.8 to 5 years.[14,50,51,54,55] It remains to be investigated whether bone resorption markers would predict fracture risk over periods that exceed 5 years. The odds ratio of fracture was not modified after adjusting for potential confounding factors such as mobility status and was only marginally decreased after adjusting for BMD measured by DXA. Thus, the combination of BMD and bone turnover measurement allows the identification of a subgroup of elderly women at much higher risk of hip fracture than those identified by each test alone.[50,51]

It is important to consider the preanalytical variability of biochemical markers of bone resorption when assessing their clinical performance in osteoporosis. Among the potential sources of variability (Table 10-3), circadian variation and food intake play important roles, especially for serum CTX.[56] Because serum CTX levels are markedly affected by food intake,[57,58] an effect that is likely to be mediated mainly by gastrointestinal hormones including glucagon-like peptide 2,[59,60] it should be measured on fasting morning samples to reduce the variability of the measurement. This technical limitation probably explains the lack of significant predictive value of serum CTX levels measured on non-fasting morning serum samples in both the EPIDOS[55] and the SOF[61] studies.

Combined Assessment of Fracture Risk

In the OFELY prospective cohort, we showed that the combination of the strongest single clinical risk factor

TABLE 10-3 SOURCES OF PREANALYTICAL VARIABILITY OF BONE TURNOVER MARKERS

Uncontrollable Factors	Controllable Factors
Age	Diurnal (circadian) variability
Menopausal status	Diet
Gender	Seasonal changes
Ethnicity	Exercise
Recent fractures (up to 1 year)	
Pregnancy and lactation	
Renal and hepatic function	
Drugs	
Antiresorptives	
Bone anabolics	
Glucocorticoids	
Anticonvulsants	
GnRH agonists	
Diseases	
Metabolic bone diseases	
Diabetes	
Thyroid diseases	
Arthritic diseases (e.g., rheumatoid arthritis, osteoarthritis)	
Immobility	

(history of fracture after the age of 45 years) with a low hip BMD and high levels of bone resorption assessed by urinary CTX improve the predictive value of a single test, with relative risk of fracture increasing from the 1.8 to 2.8 range to 5.8.[51] Similarly, in a nested case-control analysis of the EPIDOS study, we compared the ability of history of fracture after the age of 45 years, hip BMD, heel broadband ultrasound attenuation, and urinary CTX to predict the risk of hip fracture and we investigated whether a combination of these parameters could improve the predictive value.[62] In the EPIDOS study, the combination of urinary CTX with either hip BMD or heel broadband ultrasound attenuation increases the specificity by 10% with sensitivity similar to hip BMD or heel broadband ultrasound attenuation alone. Such a combined diagnostic approach might be more cost-effective than BMD measurement alone, as it results in a lower number of patients to be treated to avoid one hip fracture. If DXA or ultrasonography is not available, we found that the combination of a high bone resorption marker and a positive history of any type of fracture gave a predictive value similar to that obtained with BMD or heel broadband ultrasound attenuation alone.[62] As discussed by Johnell and colleagues,[63] the use of odds ratio is not ideal for clinical decision making, because the risk may decrease or remain stable with age, whereas absolute risk increases. Thus, calculating absolute risk such as 10-year probabilities, which depend on knowledge of the fracture and death hazards, is probably more appropriate. Based on the probability of hip fracture in the Swedish population and on the data from the EPIDOS and OFELY studies, it was found that combining urinary CTX with BMD or history of previous fracture results in a 10-year probability of hip fracture that was about 70% to 100% higher than that associated with low BMD alone with a similar pattern for the prediction of all fractures in younger postmenopausal women (Figure 10-5).[63]

The use of bone markers in individual patients may be appropriate in some situations, especially in women who are not found to be at risk by BMD measurements. In the EPIDOS study, we recently reported that urinary free deoxypyridinoline was actually most strongly associated with hip fracture in women who were not classified as having low BMD.[64] In the OFELY study of 671 postmenopausal women followed prospectively over a median of 9 years, we found that among the 116 incident fractures, 48% actually occurred in osteopenic women. Among these women who were not found to be at risk by BMD alone, the combination of lower BMD and/or prior fractures and/or bone alkaline phosphatase in the highest

quartile could detect 85% of incident fractures with an age-adjusted HR of 5.3 (2.3; 11.8).[65] Women at high risk of fracture may benefit from therapeutic intervention, especially if risk factors are amenable to bone-specific agents. Indeed, some BMD-independent risk factors such as falls are particularly important for hip fracture but may not be modified by pharmacological interventions.[66] Conversely, some studies have shown a positive effect of bisphosphonates and raloxifene on fracture risk in osteopenic women[67,68] and a greater reduction in fracture risk has been shown among postmenopausal women with high pretreatment levels of bone turnover with alendronate.[69] Thus, bone markers may be used in the assessment of fracture risk in select cases in which BMD and clinical risk factors are not sufficient to make a treatment decision.

Bone Markers for Monitoring Treatment of Osteoporosis

As with most chronic diseases, monitoring the efficacy of treatment of osteoporosis is a challenge. The goal of treatment is to reduce the occurrence of fragility fractures, but their incidence is low and the absence of

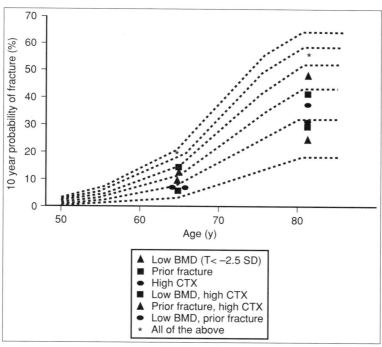

Figure 10-5. Combination of clinical risk factors, bone mineral density, and bone turnover measurements to identify women with the highest risk of fracture. The figure shows the 10-year probability of hip fracture according to age and relative risk. The symbols show the effect of risk factors on fracture probability derived from women aged 65 years (OFELY study) and 80 years (EPIDOS study). The data from the OFELY study are derived from information on all fractures. Low hip BMD was defined as values at -2.5 SD or below the mean of young adults. High urinary CTX corresponds to values above the upper limit of premenopausal women (mean ± -2 SD). (From Johnell O, Oden A, De Laet C, et al: Biochemical markers and the assessment of fracture probability. Osteoporos Int 2002;13:523-26.)

events during the first year or years of therapy does not necessarily imply that treatment is effective. Thus, the use of surrogate markers with a more rapid response is clearly needed for efficient monitoring of treatment in osteoporosis. A surrogate marker can be defined as a laboratory measurement or a physical sign used as a substitute for a clinically meaningful endpoint that measures directly how a patient feels, functions, or survives. Changes induced by therapy on a surrogate endpoint are expected to reflect changes in a clinically meaningful endpoint.

Measurement of BMD by DXA is a surrogate marker of treatment efficacy that has been widely used in clinical trials. Its use in the monitoring of treatment efficacy in the individual patient, however, has not been validated. Given a short-term precision error of 1% to 1.5% of BMD measurement at the spine and hip, the individual change must be greater than 3% to 5% to be seen as significant. With bisphosphonates such as alendronate, repeating BMD measurement 2 years after initiating therapy will allow assessment of whether a patient is responding to therapy, that is, showing a significant increase in BMD, at least at the lumbar spine, which is the most responsive site. With treatments such as raloxifene or nasal calcitonin that induce much smaller increases in BMD, DXA is not appropriate to monitor therapy. With any treatment, DXA does not allow identification of all responders within the first year of therapy. Failure to respond may be due to noncompliance (probably the most important single factor), to poor intestinal absorption (i.e., of oral bisphosphonates), to other factors contributing to bone loss, or to other unidentified factors. Monitoring using bone markers may improve compliance, as has been suggested by recent studies.[70-72]

Several randomized placebo-controlled studies found that resorption-inhibiting therapy is associated with a prompt decrease of bone resorption markers that can be seen as early as 1 month, with a plateau reached within 3 to 6 months. The decrease of bone formation markers is delayed, reflecting the physiological coupling of formation to resorption, and a plateau is usually achieved within 6 to 12 months. The magnitude of the decrease of bone turnover markers under antiresorptive therapy, including hormone replacement therapy and bisphosphonates, usually expressed in percentage of the initial value, is moderately associated with an increase in BMD after 2 to 3 years.[73]

The value of BMD changes to predict the risk of fracture with treatment is debated, especially because treatments such as raloxifene can induce a 30% to 50% reduction in vertebral fracture rate despite a small 2% to 3% increase of BMD at all skeletal sites. Recent re-analyses of placebo-controlled studies suggested that BMD changes under treatment account for only a small part of the efficacy of antiresorptive therapy on fracture risk.[74,75] Thus, BMD changes may not be an adequate surrogate endpoint to analyze the ability of bone markers to predict fracture risk.

Recent studies have investigated the direct relationships between bone marker changes and fracture risk in several large randomized studies of various antiresorptive therapies. It was found that the changes of serum osteocalcin, bone alkaline phosphatase, and PINP with raloxifene treatment were associated with the subsequent risk of vertebral fractures in a large subgroup of osteoporotic women enrolled in the MORE study, whereas changes in hip BMD were not predictive.[76-78] In postmenopausal women with osteoporosis treated with oral risedronate, it has also been shown that changes of urinary CTX and NTX after 3 to 6 months predicted the risk of subsequent incident vertebral fractures after 1 and 3 years (Figure 10-6). These changes explain 50% to 70% of the effect of risedronate on fracture risk.[79] A significant association between changes of bone alkaline phosphatase and vertebral, hip, and nonspine fractures was also found in women treated with alendronate participating in the FIT trial.[80] In the risedronate study, it was shown that the relationships between vertebral fracture risk and changes from baseline in CTX and NTX during 3 to 6 months was not linear and that there may be a level of bone resorption reduction below which there is no further fracture benefit. However, this nonlinear relationship was not observed for nonvertebral fracture in the residronate trials or for vertebral and nonvertebral fractures in the FIT alendronate trial. Ultimately, recommended cut-off values of bone marker changes with treatment should be based on prospective studies with incident fractures as an endpoint.

Bone turnover markers may also be useful to monitor effects of anabolic treatments, including intermittent administration of parathyroid hormone. For example, in the PaTH study with parathyroid hormone 1-84 and with teriparatide in the Fracture Prevention Trial, it was recently shown that parathyroid hormone administered to postmenopausal women with osteoporosis produces a marked and rapid (within a month) increase of markers of bone formation followed by a delayed increase in bone resorption markers (Figure 10-7).[80] In this situation, bone formation markers, especially serum PINP and serum PICP, appear the most promising to monitor efficacy of parathyroid hormone and to predict BMD changes, although these data will need to be confirmed in studies using incident fracture as an endpoint.

Figure 10-6. Relationship between percentage change in bone resorption markers (urinary NTX and CTX) and the incidence of new vertebral fractures. Six hundred ninety-three women with at least one vertebral deformity (mean age, 69 years, SD 7 years) who received placebo or oral risedronate 5 mg daily for 3 years were studied. The relationships between vertebral fracture risk after 1 and 3 years of treatment and changes from baseline in NTX and CTX were not linear ($P < .05$). There was little further improvement in fracture benefit below a decrease of 35% to 40% for NTX and 55% to 60% for CTX. The placebo group is represented by the broken line and the risedronate 5 mg group by the solid line. All patients received calcium supplementation (1000 mg/day) and vitamin D (if levels were low). (From Eastell R, Barton I, Hannon RA, et al: Relationship of early changes in bone resorption to the reduction in fracture risk with risedronate. J Bone Miner Res 2003;18:1051-56.)

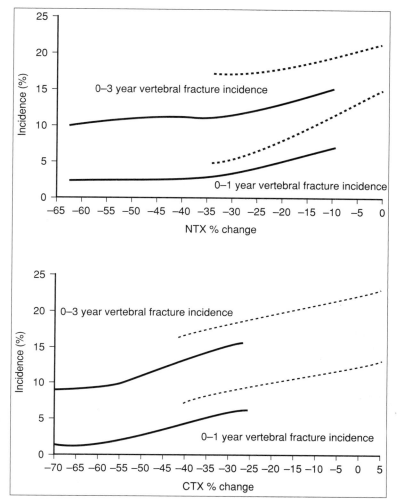

Figure 10-7. Effects of parathyroid hormone (PTH 1-84, 100 μg/d) and oral alendronate (10 mg/day) on bone formation (serum PINP) and bone resorption (serum CTX) markers in postmenopausal with osteoporosis. Results are expressed in median percentage change from baseline (and interquartile range). (From Black DM, Greenspan SL, Ensrud KE, et al: The effects of parathyroid hormone and alendronate alone or in combination in postmenopausal osteoporosis. N Engl J Med 2003;349:1207-15.)

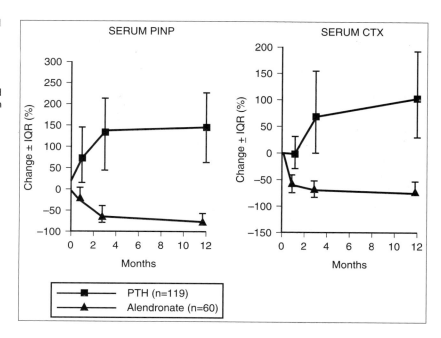

REFERENCES

1. Anonymous: Consensus development conference: diagnosis, prophylaxis and treatment of osteoporosis. Am J Med 1993;94:646-50.
2. Garnero P, Delmas PD: Investigation of bone: bone turnover. In Hochberg MC, Silman AJ, Smolen JS, Weinblatt ME, Weisman MH, eds. Rheumatology, 3rd ed (vol 2). London: Harcourt Health Sciences, 2003:2043-57.
3. Garnero P, Gineyts E, Arbault P, et al: Different effects of bisphosphonate and estrogen therapy on free and peptide-bound bone cross-links excretion. J Bone Miner Res 1995;10:641-49.
4. Garnero P, Shih WJ, Gineyts E, et al: Comparison of new biochemical markers of bone turnover in late postmenopausal osteoporotic women in response to alendronate. J Clin Endocrinol Metab 1994;79:1693-1700.
5. Blomqvist C, Risteli L, Risteli J, et al: Markers of type I collagen degradation and synthesis in the monitoring of treatment responses in bone metastases from breast cancer. Br J Cancer 1996;73:1074-79.
6. Kylmälä T, Tammela TLJ, Risteli L, et al: Type I collagen degradation product (ICTP) gives information about the nature of bone metastases and has prognostic value in prostate cancer. Br J Cancer 1995;71:1061-64.
7. Sassi ML, Aman S, Hakala M, et al: Assay for crosslinked carboxyterminal telopeptide of type I collagen (ICTP) unlike Crosslaps assay reflects increased pathological degradation of type I collagen in rheumatoid arthritis. Clin Chem Lab 2003;41:1038-44.
8. Sassi ML, Eriksen H, Risteli L, et al: Immunochemical characterization of assay for carboxyterminal telopeptide of human type I collagen: loss of antigenicity by treatment with cathepsin K. Bone 2000;26:367-73.
9. Garnero P, Ferreras M, Karsdal MA, et al: The type I collagen fragments ICTP and CTX reveal distinct enzymatic pathways of bone collagen degradation. J Bone Miner Res 2003;18:859-67.
10. Garnero P, Borel O, Byrjalsen I, et al: The collagenolytic activity of cathepsin K is unique amongst mammalian proteinases J Biol Chem 1998;273:32347-52.
11. Oddie GW, Schenk G, Angel N, et al: Structure, function and regulation of tartrate-resistant acid phosphatase. Bone 2000;27:575-84.
12. Yam LT, Janckila AJ: Tartrate-resistant acid phosphatase (TRACP): a personal perspective. J Bone Miner Res 2003;18:1894-96.
13. Hallen JM, Ylipahkala H, Alatalo SL, et al: Serum tartrate resistant acid phosphatase 5b, but not 5a, correlates with other markers of bone turnover and bone mineral density. Calcif Tissue Int 2002;71:20-5.
14. Gerdhem P, Ivaska KK, Alatalo SL, et al: Biochemical markers of bone metabolism and prediction of fracture in elderly women. J Bone Miner Res 2004;19:386-93.
15. Hallen JM: Tartrate-resistant acid phosphatase 5b is a specific and sensitive marker of bone resorption. Anticancer Res 2003;23:1027-29.
16. Garnero P, Delmas PD: An immunoassay for type I collagen alpha 1 helicoidal peptide 620-633, a new marker of bone resorption in osteoporosis. Bone 2003;32:20-6.
17. Garnero P, Grimaux M, Seguin P, Delmas PD: Characterization of immunoreactive forms of human osteocalcin generated in vivo and in vitro. J Bone Miner Res 1994;9:255-64.
18. Taylor AK, Linkhart S, Mohan RA, et al: Multiple osteocalcin fragments in human urine and serum detected by a midmolecule osteocalcin radioimmunoassay. J Clin Endocrinol Metab 1990;70:467-72.
19. Srivastava AK, Mohan FR, Singer FR, Baylink DJ: A urine midmolecule osteocalcin assay shows higher discriminatory power than a serum midmolecule osteocalcin assay during short-term alendronate treatment of osteoporotic patients. Bone 2002;31:62-9.
20. Cloos PAC, Christgau S: Characterization of aged osteocalcin fragments derived from bone resorption. Clin Lab 2004;50:585-98.
21. Batge B, Deibold J, Stein H, et al: Compositional analysis of the collagenous bone matrix: a study on adult normal and osteopenic bone tissue. Eur J Clin Invest 1992;22:805-12.
22. Kowitz J, Knippel M, Schuhr T, Mach J: Alteration in the extent of collagen I hydroxylation, isolated from femoral heads of women with a femoral neck fracture caused by osteoporosis. Calcif Tissue Int 1992;60:501-5.
23. Bailey AJ, Wotton SF, Sims TJ, Thompson PW: Post-translational modifications in the collagen of human osteoporotic femoral head. Biochem Biophys Res Commun 1992;185:801-5.
24. Oxlund H, Moselkilde L, Ortoft G: Reduced concentration of collagen reducible cross-links in human trabecular bone with respect to age and osteoporosis. Bone 1996;19:479-84.
25. Banse X, Sims TJ, Bailey AJ: Mechanical properties of adult vertebral cancellous bone: correlation with collagen intermolecular cross-links. J Bone Miner Res 2002;17:1621-28.
26. Wang X, Shen X, Li X, Agrawal CM: Age-related changes in collagen network and toughness of bone. Bone 2002;31:1-7.
27. Cloos PAC, Fledelius C: Collagen fragments in urine derived from bone resorption are highly racemized and isomerized: a biological clock of protein aging with clinical potential. Biochem J 2000;345:473-80.
28. Garnero P, Fledelius C, Gineyts E, et al: Decreased β-isomerisation of C-telopeptides of type I collagen in Paget's disease of bone. J Bone Miner Res 1997;12:1407-15.
29. Garnero P, Gineyts E, Schaffer AV, et al: Measurement of urinary excretion of nonisomerized and β-isomerized forms of type I collagen breakdown products to monitor the effects of the bisphosphonate zoledronate in Paget's disease. Arthritis Rheum 1998;41:354-60.
30. Alexandersen P, Peris P, Guanabens N, et al: Non-isomerized C-telopeptide fragments are highly sensitive markers for monitoring disease activity and treatment efficacy in Paget's disease of bone. J Bone Miner Res 2005;20:588-95.
31. Garnero P, Cloos P, Sornay-Rendu E, et al: Type I collagen racemization and isomerization and the risk of fracture in postmenopausal women: the OFELY prospective study. J Bone Miner Res 2002;17:826-33.
32. Garnero P, Qvist P, Munoz M, et al: Type I collagen C-telopeptide isomerization predicts the long-term risk of non-vertebral fracture in postmenopausal women, independently of bone mineral density and bone turnover: a non invasive index of bone collagen quality. J Bone Miner Res 2004;19(suppl 1):S19.
33. Byrjalsen I, Cloos PA, Qvist P, Christiansen C: The degree of isomerisation of collagen type I C-telopeptide in postmenopausal women: a potential biochemical index of bone quality. J Bone Miner Res 2004;19(suppl 1):S375.
34. Garnero P, Borel O, Gineyts E, et al: The degree of posttranslational modifications of collagen is an important determinant of the toughness of cortical bone. J Bone Miner Res 2004;19(suppl 1):S220.
35. Kang AH, Trelstad RL: A collagen defect in homocystinuria. J Clin Invest 1971;52:2571-8.
36. McLean RR, Jacques PF, Selhub J, et al: Homocysteine as a predictive factor for hip fracture in older persons. N Engl J Med 2004;350:2042-49.
37. van Meurs JBJ, Dhonukshe-Rutten RAM, Pluijm SMF, et al: Homocysteine levels and the risk of osteoporotic fracture. N Engl J Med 2004;350:2033-41.
38. Dhonukshe-Ruten RAM, Pluijm SMF, de Groot SCGM, et al: Homocysteine and vitamin B12 status relate to bone turnover markers, broadband ultrasound attenuation, and fractures in healthy elderly people. J Bone Miner Res 2005;20:921-29.
39. Szulc P, Chapuy MC, Meunier PJ, Delmas PD: Serum undercarboxylated osteocalcin is a marker of the risk of hip fracture in elderly women. J Clin Invest 1993;91:1769-74.
40. Vergnaud P, Garnero P, Meunier PJ, et al: Undercarboxylated osteocalcin measured with a specific immunoassay predicts hip fracture in elderly women: the EPIDOS study. J Clin Endocrinol Metab 1997;82:719-24.

41. Luukinen H, Kakonen SM, Pettersson K, et al: Strong prediction of fractures among older adults by the ratio of carboxylated to total serum osteocalcin. J Bone Miner Res 2000;15:2473-78.

42. Liu G, Peakcock M: Age-related changes in serum undercarboxylated osteocalcin and its relationships with bone density, bone quality, and hip fracture. Calcif Tissue Int 1998;62:286-89.

43. Johnell O, Kanis JA, Oden A, et al: Predictive value of BMD for hip and other fractures. J Bone Miner Res 2005;20:1185-94.

44. Miller PD, Siris ES, Barret-Connor E, et al: Prediction of fracture risk in postmenopausal white women with peripheral bone densitometry: evidence from the National Osteoporosis Risk Assessment. J Bone Miner Res 2002;17:2222-30.

45. Stone KL, Seeley DG, Lui LY, et al: BMD at multiple sites and risk of fracture of multiple types: long-term results from the Study of Osteoporotic Fractures. J Bone Miner Res 2003;18:1947-54.

46. Schuit SCE, van der Klift M, Weel AEAM, et al: Fracture incidence and association with bone mineral density in elderly men and women: the Rotterdam study. Bone 2004;31:195-202.

47. Kanis JA, Johnell O, De Laet C, et al: A meta-analysis of previous fracture and subsequent fracture risk. Bone 2004;35:375-82.

48. De Laet C, Kanis JA, Oden A, et al: Body mass index as a predictor of fracture risk: a meta-analysis. Osteoporos Int 2005;16:1330-38.

49. Garnero P: Markers of bone turnover for the prediction of fracture risk. Osteoporos Int Suppl 2000;6:S55-S65.

50. Garnero P, Hausherr E, Chapuy MC, et al: Markers of bone resorption predict hip fracture in elderly women: the EPIDOS prospective study. J Bone Miner Res 1996;11:1531-38.

51. Garnero P, Sornay-Rendu E, Claustrat B, Delmas PD: Biochemical markers of bone turnover, endogenous hormones and the risk of fractures in postmenopausal women: the OFELY study. J Bone Miner Res 2000;15:1526-36.

52. Ross PD, Kress BC, Parson RE, et al: Serum bone alkaline phosphatase and calcaneus bone density predict fractures: a prospective study. Osteoporos Int 2000;11:76-82.

53. Melton LJ, Crowson CS, O'Fallon WM, et al: Relative contributions of bone density, bone turnover and clinical risk factors to long-term fracture predictions. J Bone Miner Res 2003;18:312-18.

54. van Daele PLA, Seibel MJ, Burger H, et al: Case-control analysis of bone resorption markers, disability, and hip fracture risk: the Rotterdam study. BMJ 1996;312:482-83.

55. Chapurlat RD, Garnero P, Breart G, et al: Serum type I collagen breakdown product (serum CTX) predicts hip fracture risk in elderly women: the EPIDOS study. Bone 2000;27:283-86.

56. Hannon R, Eastell R: Preanalytical variability of biochemical markers of bone turnover. Osteoporos Int 2000;11(Suppl 6):S30-44.

57. Qvist P, Christgau S, Pedersen BJ, et al: Circadian variation in the serum C-terminal telopeptide of type I collagen (serum CTx): effects of gender, age, menopausal status, posture, daylight, serum cortisol and fasting. Bone 2002;31:57-61.

58. Bjarnason NH, Henriksen EE, Alexandersen P, et al: Mechanism of circadian variation in bone resorption. Bone 2002;30:307-13.

59. Henriksen DB, Alexandersen P, Bjarnason NH, et al: Role of gastrointestinal hormones in postprandial reduction of bone resorption. J Bone Miner Res 2003;18:2180-89.

60. Henriksen DB, Alexandersen P, Byrjalsen I, et al: Reduction of nocturnal rise in bone resorption by subcutaneous GLP-2. Bone 2004;34:140-47.

61. Bauer DC, Black DM, Ensrud K, et al: Serum markers of bone turnover and fractures of the hip and spine: a prospective study. J Bone Miner Res 1999;14(suppl 1):S147.

62. Garnero P, Dargent-Molina P, Hans D, et al: Do markers of bone resorption add to bone mineral density and ultrasonographic heel measurement for the prediction of hip fracture in elderly women? The EPIDOS prospective study. Osteoporos Int 1998;8:563-69.

63. Johnell O, Oden A, De Laet C, et al: Biochemical markers and the assessment of fracture probability. Osteoporos Int 2002;13:523-26.

64. Robbins JA, Schott AM, Garnero P, et al: Risk factors for hip fracture in women with high BMD: EPIDOS study. Osteoporos Int 2005;16:149-54.

65. Sornay-Rendu E, Munoz F, Garnero P, et al: The identification of osteopenic women at high risk of fracture: The OFELY study. J Bone Miner Res 2005;20:1813-9.

66. McClung MR, Geusens P, Miller PD, et al: Hip intervention program study group: effect of risedronate on the risk of hip fracture in elderly women. N Engl J Med 2001;344:333-40.

67. Kanis JA, Johnell O, Black DM, et al: Effect of raloxifene on the risk of new vertebral fracture in post-menopausal women with osteopenia or osteoporosis: a reanalysis of the multiple outcomes of raloxifene evaluation trial. Bone 2003;33:293-300.

68. Black DM, Thompson D, Quandt S, et al: Alendronate reduces the risk of vertebral fracture in women with BMD T-scores above −2.5: results from the Fracture Intervention Trial (FIT). Osteoporos Int 2002;13(suppl 1):S27.

69. Bauer DC, Garnero P, Hochberg MC, et al: Pre-treatment bone turnover and fracture efficacy of alendronate: the Fracture Intervention Trial. J Bone Miner Res 2003;18(suppl 2):S55.

70. Chapurlat RD, Cummings SR: Does follow-up of osteoporotic women treated with antiresorptive therapies improve effectiveness? Osteoporos Int 2002;13:738-44.

71. Clowes JA, Peel NF, Eastell R: The impact of monitoring on adherence and persistence with antiresorptive treatment for postmenopausal osteoporosis: a randomized controlled trial. J Clin Endocrinol Metab 2004;89:1117-23.

72. Delmas PD, Vrijens B, Roux C, et al: Osteoporosis treatment using reinforcement with bone turnover marker data reduces frcature risk: the IMPACT study. J Bone Miner Res 2004;19 (suppl 1):S444.

73. Delmas PD: Markers of bone turnover for monitoring treatment of osteoporosis with antiresorptive drugs. Osteoporos Int 2000;Suppl 6:S66-S76.

74. Cummings SR, Karpf DB, Harris F, et al: Improvement in spine density and reduction in risk of vertebral fractures during treatment with antiresorptive drugs. Am J Med 2002;112:281-89.

75. Delmas PD, Seeman E: Changes in bone mineral density explain little of the reduction in vertebral or nonvertebral fracture risk with anti-resorptive therapy. Bone 2004;4:599-604.

76. Bjarnason NH, Christiansen C, Sarkar S, et al, for the MORE Study Group: 6 months changes in biochemical markers predict 3-year response in vertebral fracture rate in postmenopausal, osteoporotic women: results from the MORE study. Osteoporos Int 2001;12:922-30.

77. Sarkar S, Reginster JY, Crans GG, et al: Relationship between changes in biochemical markers of bone turnover and BMD to predict vertebral fracture risk. J Bone Miner Res 2004;19:394-401.

78. Reginster JY, Sarkar S, Zegels B, et al: Reduction in PINP, a marker of bone metabolism, with raloxifene treatment and its relationship with vertebral fracture risk. Bone 2004;34:344-51.

79. Eastell R, Barton I, Hannon RA, et al: Relationship of early changes in bone resorption to the reduction in fracture risk with risedronate. J Bone Miner Res 2003;18:1051-6.

80. Bauer DC, Black DM, Garnero P, et al: Change in bone turnover and hip, non-spine, and vertebral fracture in alendronate-treated women: the fracture intervention trial. J Bone Miner Res 2004;19:1250-58.

81. Black DM, Greenspan SL, Ensrud KE, et al: The effects of parathyroid hormone and alendronate alone or in combination in postmenopausal osteoporosis. N Engl J Med 2003;349:1207-15.

82. Chen P, Satterwhite JH, Licata AA, et al: Early changes in biochemical markers of bone formation predict BMD response to teriparatide in postmenopausal women with osteoporosis. J Bone Miner Res 2005;20:962-70.

11 The Evaluation of the Patient for Osteoporosis: Case Finding Using Diagnostic Tests for Treatment Interventions

Piet P.M.M. Geusens

SUMMARY

- The clinical significance of osteoporosis rests on the occurrence of fragility fractures, its consequences on morbidity and mortality, and the availability of treatments with proven antifracture efficacy in well-selected patients with a high risk of fragility fractures.

- The risk of fractures is multifactorial. Risk factors are related to bone mineral density (BMD), other determinants that contribute to skeletal fragility, the risk and impact of falling, or a combination of these and are dependent on fracture site.

- The diagnosis of osteoporosis in terms of BMD is based on the measurement by dual x-ray absorptiometry. In addition, combinations of risk factors that are at least partially independent can be integrated to provide information on fracture risk over and above that given by BMD, to enhance calculation of total fracture risk.

- Examples of major clinical risk factors for fragility fractures at the population level are age, low BMD, female gender, history of fragility fracture, history of parenteral hip fracture, low body weight (or low body mass index), severe immobility, and chronic use of glucocorticoids. Other risk factors related to lifestyle, diseases, and drugs, although less frequent and less predictive, can increase fracture risk in the individual patient.

- Guidelines on osteoporosis advocate clinical case finding for identifying patients at the highest risk for fragility fractures based on the presence of risk factors, including selection of patients for bone densitometry.

- Patients with vertebral and nonvertebral fragility fractures require special attention. Only one in three vertebral fractures come to clinical attention, but all are associated with an increased risk for new fractures and increased morbidity and mortality and should therefore be recognized.

- Patients on chronic glucocorticoid treatment deserve attention for increased risk of fractures and the availability of prevention.

   The clinical significance of osteoporosis rests on the occurrence of fragility fractures, its consequences in terms of morbidity and mortality, and the availability of treatments with proven antifracture efficacy in well-selected patients with a high risk of fragility fractures.[1-4]

The risk of fragility fractures is multifactorial and is related to the resistance of bone to fracture and to nonskeletal factors contributing to the incidence and impact of trauma (Figure 11-1). Low bone mineral density (BMD) is part of the definition of osteoporosis and is considered a gold standard for the diagnosis of osteoporosis in all guidelines on osteoporosis.[5] However, there is no justification for screening the whole population using densitometry.[1] The sensitivity of BMD is low (i.e., a proportion of fractures occur in patients with a T-score > -2.5) and fracture risk is also related to components of bone that are not captured by measuring BMD as well as to nonskeletal risk factors. Ten percent to 44% of fractures are attributable to low BMD.[6] This population-attributable risk is 15% on the average for all types of fracture. In untreated individuals, this population-attributable risk is comparable with the population-attributable risk reported for hypertension or lipid profiles and cardiovascular disease.[1]

Although there is no universal validated strategy, case finding is widely accepted as a method of identifying individuals who should be treated for osteoporosis.[5,7] The goal of case finding is to establish the fracture risk based on BMD and BMD-independent risk factors to make decisions regarding the needs for instituting therapy. However, the evaluation for osteoporosis in

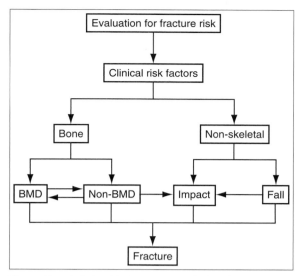

Figure 11-1. Relationship between case finding for risk factors, fracture risk, and available treatments that reduce fracture risk.

daily clinical practice is dependent on the awareness of doctors and patients of risk factors for fractures and available treatment modalities. Recognition of risk factors for osteoporosis before the first fracture has occurred is often lacking.[8] Low awareness for osteoporosis is also found when patients have a history of fragility fracture after the age of 40 to 50 years, many of which are not recognized by doctors and patients as being the result of osteoporosis.[9]

It is the aim of this chapter to review the evaluation for osteoporosis using available tests for identifying patients at highest risk for fracture, in whom fracture risk can be reduced. The focus is on assessing the risk of fractures related to skeletal fragility. Thus, the emphasis is on identifying patients with low BMD or other bone-related risks, including those who have already had a fragility fracture, and using this information to estimate the risk of future fractures and to identify patients, in a timely manner, who could benefit from treatment that has been proven to reduce fracture risk. Although falls are an important factor in increasing the risk of fractures among patients with osteoporosis, the etiology and interventions to prevent falls are generally independent of skeletal fragility and therefore receive less attention here.

RISK FACTORS FOR OSTEOPOROSIS AND FRAGILITY FRACTURES

Many risk factors for osteoporosis (in terms of low BMD) and for fragility fractures in general have been documented in cross-sectional case-controlled studies and in prospective studies with fragility fractures as a primary endpoint.

Major risk factors in postmenopausal women at the population level are increasing age, low body weight (or low body mass index [BMI]), previous fragility fracture, severe immobility, and use of glucocorticoids.[10] Other important risk factors are smoking, excess intake of alcohol, rheumatoid arthritis, and risk factors for falls.[10] However, many more risk factors that are less prevalent in the population or that have less impact on fracture risk have been documented (Table 11-1).

Several attempts have been made to categorize risk factors. Risk factors for osteoporosis and fractures have been grouped in domains such as genetic or constitutional factors, lifestyle and nutritional factors, medical disorders, and drugs (Table 11-2).[1] In some reviews and guidelines, other characteristics of risk factors are also considered, such as the prevalence (high for the main risk factors or low for some forms of secondary osteoporosis) (Table 11-3),[10] the impact (major or minor, based on the relative risk) (Table 11-4),[11] and the timing during life (related to building up peak bone mass or to bone loss once peak bone mass is achieved). Some risk factors are associated with an increased risk for fractures within a short term, such as systemic use of glucocorticoids, after organ transplantation, after anti-androgen therapy in men, and after vertebral and nonvertebral fractures. Risk factors differ between locations of fractures: fall-related risk factors are more frequent for nonvertebral fractures than for vertebral fractures.[12] Risk factors can also be grouped as modifiable (such as lifestyle, certain diseases, and drugs) or not, as proposed by the National Osteoporosis Foundation.[13]

Some risk factors are readily recognizable in clinical practice, such as gender, age, previous fragility fracture, and low body weight. Others require specific attention, as their signs and symptoms can be nonspecific or clinically not readily recognizable, such as diseases that cause secondary osteoporosis (e.g., hyperthyroidism, hyperparathyroidism). Some risk factors require additional technical examination (bone densitometry, x-rays, markers of bone turnover, and laboratory measurements for some diseases). Vertebral fractures are more difficult to diagnose, as two in three occur in the absence of typical signs and symptoms of an acute fracture and as they can occur after a minimal, trivial, or even absent trauma. Some components of the resistance of bone against fractures that have been studied in animal studies and in human biopsies, such as microarchitecture and matrix composition, are currently not measurable in daily practice, although some of those are components of other risk factors, such as age, prevalent fragility fracture, and family history of fractures.

An important characteristic of risk factor is their interrelation.[10] Risk factors can be interdependent or independent. Some are related to BMD and others are related to non-BMD factors that are related to skeletal fragility

TABLE 11-1 FACTORS CONTRIBUTING TO OSTEOPOROSIS AND FRACTURE RISK IN WOMEN

Genetic or constitutional
  Age
  White or Asian ethnicity
  Low body weight (or low body mass index)
  Family (maternal) history of (hip) fracture
  Small body frame
  Long hip axis length
  Premature menopause (<45 years)
  Late menarche
  Genetic polymorphisms (e.g., estrogens receptor, collagen type 1)

Lifestyle and nutritional
  Nulliparity
  Prolonged secondary amenorrhea
  Smoking cigarettes
  Low calcium intake
  Vitamin D status
  Excessive alcohol intake
  Prolonged parenteral nutrition

Medical disorders
  Anorexia nervosa
  Malabsorption syndromes due to gastrointestinal and hepatobiliary diseases
  Primary hyperparathyroidism
  Thyrotoxicosis
  Primary hypogonadism
  Prolactinoma
  Hypercortisolism
  Osteogenesis imperfecta
  Inflammatory rheumatic diseases (rheumatoid arthritis, spondylitis, lupus)
  Chronic obstructive lung disease
  Chronic neurological disorders
  Chronic renal failure
  Mastocytosis
  Type 1 diabetes
  Status post-transplantation

Drugs
  Chronic glucocorticoid therapy
  Excessive thyroid therapy
  Anticoagulants
  Chemotherapy
  Gonadotropin-releasing hormone agonist and antagonist
  Anticonvulsants
  Chronic phosphate binding antacid use

Risk of falls
  Osteoarthritis
  Muscle strength
  Postural instability
  Inactivity
  Prolonged immobilization

Pathophysiology
  Low levels of serum estradiol
  Low serum RANKL
  Homocysteine

TABLE 11-2 RISK FACTORS THAT PROVIDE INDICATIONS FOR THE DIAGNOSTIC USE OF BONE DENSITOMETRY[1]

Presence of strong risk factors
  Estrogen deficiency
    Premature menopause (<45 years)
    Long-term secondary amenorrhea (>1 year)
    Primary hypogonadism
  Glucocorticoid therapy (>7.5 mg/day for >1 year)
  Maternal family history of hip fracture
  Low body mass index
  Other disorders associated with osteoporosis
    Anorexia nervosa
    Malabsorption
    Primary hyperparathyroidism
    Status post-transplantation
    Chronic renal failure
    Hyperthyroidism
    Prolonged immobilization
    Cushing syndrome
Radiographic evidence of osteopenia and/or vertebral deformity
Previous fragility fracture, particularly of the hip, spine, or wrist
Loss of height, thoracic hyperkyphosis (after radiographic confirmation of vertebral deformation)

and to risk and impact of falls, or a combination of these. Risk factors that are at least in part mutually independent have a cumulative effect on fracture risk, as has been found for vertebral fractures[14] and for hip fractures (Figure 11-2).[15] This finding has profound clinical consequences in daily practice. Fracture risk can be substantially higher than when deduced from one risk factor alone. This implies that a distinction has to be made between diagnosis of osteoporosis (which is currently based on BMD, with a T-score < −2.5), and intervention thresholds, which include, besides BMD, assessment of risk of fractures that are not measured by BMD. Many guidelines have therefore adapted a higher T-score as intervention threshold (e.g., a T-score < −1.0 instead of < −2.5) in the presence of risk factors other than low BMD.

The value of case finding is dependent on the availability of treatment. In clinical trials, fracture prevention has been documented in postmenopausal women with low BMD, in postmenopausal women with a prevalent vertebral fracture (independent of BMD), in men and women using systemic glucocorticoids, and in men with osteoporosis.

CASE FINDINGS IN WOMEN

Case Findings in Women with Low Bone Mineral Density

Prior to the occurrence of a vertebral fragility fracture, the diagnosis of osteoporosis and the decision about therapy relied on bone densitometry using dual x-ray

TABLE 11-3 PREVALENCE OF RISK FACTORS FOR OSTEOPOROSIS IN EUROPEAN WOMEN[10]							
Age (years)	Low Body Mass Index (%)	Prior Fracture (%)	Glucocorticoids (%)	Mother with Hip Fracture (%)	Current Smoking (%)	Secondary Osteoporosis (%)	Any (%)
50-59	1.3	17.8	4.5	5.1	16.2	-	33.7
60-69	1.5	25.8	4.5	6.4	18.4	-	45.7
70-79	2.1	31.7	5.8	7.1	10.4	2.4	43.3
80-89	4.0	31.3	4.6	4.9	4.7	2.2	38.5
90+	0.8	22.0	2.2	6.9	3.7	7.9	28.5

TABLE 11-4 CLASSIFICATION OF RISK FACTORS FOR FRACTURE RELATED TO BONE LOSS[11]	
High Risk (RR >2.0)	Moderate Risk (RR 1.0-2.0)
Aging (> 70-80 years)	Female gender
Low body weight	Smoking (active)
Weight loss	Low sunlight exposure (or none)
Physical inactivity	Family history of osteoporotic fracture
Corticosteroids	Surgical menopause
Anticonvulsants	Early menopause (<45 years)
Primary hyperparathyroidism	Short fertile period (<30 years)
Diabetes mellitus type I	Late menarche (>15 years)
Anorexia nervosa	No lactation
Gastrectomy	Low calcium intake (<500-850 mg/day)
Pernicious anemia	Hyperparathyroidism
Prior osteoporotic fracture	Hyperthyroidism Diabetes mellitus type II Rheumatoid arthritis

absorptiometry (DXA). One reason is that, in clinical trials performed in postmenopausal women, fracture prevention has been shown in women with a prevalent vertebral fracture or, in the absence of such fracture, in women with a low BMD (T-score < −2.5) measured by DXA in the spine or hip. Risk factors that provide indications for the diagnostic use of bone densitometry are shown in Table 11-2.[1]

Questionnaires focusing on clinical recognition of patients with low BMD have been studied using combinations of risk factors. The purpose of these indices is to identify women who are more likely to have low BMD, so that individuals can be identified who could then undergo BMD measurement for decision about treatment. The indices are based on the presence of one or more clinical recognizable risk factors, selected on the basis of the available evidence of their relationship to low BMD and fracture risk (Table 11-5).

The simplest questionnaire is the Osteoporosis Self-assessment Tool (OST), which is based on age and weight.[16] A T-score of less than −2.5 in the hip or spine was found in two of three individuals with a high OST (>2), in one of five if OST was intermediate, and in one of 33 if OST was low (<2) (Figure 11-3). With adaptations, it has been shown to be useful for Asian women (OSTA). Other indices, such as the Simple Calculated Osteoporosis Risk Estimation,[17] the Osteoporosis Risk Assessment Index,[18] SOFSURF (derived using data from the Study of Osteoporotic Fractures [SOF]),[19] the DOES-score[20] and OSIRIS,[21] involve one to four other risk factors in addition to age and weight, such as rheumatoid arthritis, history of fracture, smoking, race, and intake of estrogens. Weight was also a useful marker for low BMD in the EPIDOS study.[22] Several studies indicate that OST contributes as well as other indices for selection of patients with low BMD. Such an approach could even be cost-effective for patient selection for bone densitometry.[21] However, such indices are insufficient to identify all women who will have an incident fracture[20] and underscores that low BMD is only one of the factors related to fracture risk.[20]

The ability of the measurement to predict fracture is improved by site-specific measurement, so that for hip fractures, the risk might ideally be measured in the hip.[23] Other techniques of bone measurement are available, such as single-energy x-ray absorptiometry, quantitative computer tomography, and quantitative ultrasonography. They can be helpful in identifying women with low BMD and increased risk of fragility fractures.[1,5] However, they are not considered as a substitute to DXA for selecting women for treatment, except when DXA is not available.[5]

Identifying Women with Fragility Fractures

Women who have already had a fragility fracture after the age of 40 years have twice the risk of subsequent fractures compared with other women.[24] Identifying patients with prior fractures seems so rudimentary that it should not need mention, but the fact is that most fracture patients (even those with recent fractures) are not receiving adequate diagnosis and treatment for osteoporosis in many communities.[8]

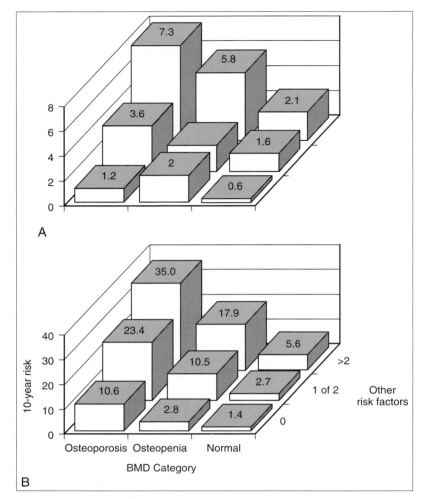

Figure 11-2. A, Cumulative incidence of first incident vertebral fracture.[14] Risk factors are age over 70 years, a prior nonspinal fracture after age 50, body mass index (calculated with knee height) in the lowest 40%, current smoker, low level of physical activity (walks less than 1 block/day and does household chores less than 1 h/day), no moderate- or high-intensity recreational physical activities, fell one or more times in the first 12 months of follow-up, not currently on estrogen replacement therapy, low milk consumption (<1 glass/day) when pregnant (or as a teenager for nulliparous women), ever used aluminum-containing antacids weekly, and paternal history of hip fracture. **B,** Ten-year risk for hip fracture (in percentages) according to the presence of low bone mineral density (BMD) and other risk factors (age >80 years, mother with hip fracture, fracture after 50 years of age, decrease in body length, decreased cognitive functions, slow gait speed, nulliparity, type 2 diabetes, Parkinson disease, disturbed depth vision). Note that the number of risk factors and low BMD increase the risk of hip fracture independently and additively.[15] (See Color Plates.)

TABLE 11-5 CLINICAL RISK FACTORS INCLUDED IN QUESTIONNAIRES						
Risk Factor	**Questionnaire**					
	SCORE[17]	OST/OSTA[16]	SOFSURF[19]	ORAI[18]	OSIRIS[21]	DOES[20]
Age	X	X	X	X	X	X
Weight	X	X	X	X	X	X
History of fracture	X	—	X	—	X	X
Smoking	—	—	—	X	—	—
Race	X	—	—	—	—	—
Rheumatoid arthritis	X	—	—	—	—	—
Estrogen intake	X	—	—	X	X	—
X, Evaluated; —, Not evaluated.						

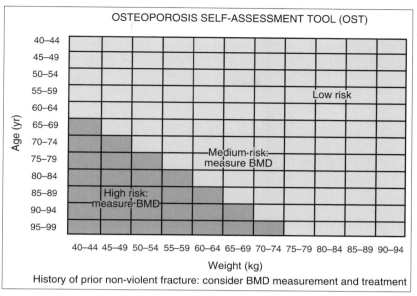

Figure 11-3. The osteoporosis self-assessment tool (OST) is based on age and weight to select postmenopausal women for bone densitometry. A T-score of < –2.5 is found in 2 of 3 patients with high risk, 1 of 5 with intermediate risk, and only 1 of 33 in the low risk patients.

A fragility fracture (or "low-trauma" fracture) is mostly defined as occurring after a fall from standing height or less. However, more severe trauma can also result in fragility fractures and should be interpreted within the global clinical context. On the other hand, many fractures, especially vertebral fractures, can occur after minimal or even without identifiable trauma.[25]

Fragility fractures are associated with an increased risk for new fractures within a short time, and treatments are available that can reduce fracture risk over the short and long term. The increased fracture risk after a fragility fracture is independent of age, gender, and BMD.[26] Therefore, women with a fragility fracture should receive specific attention for osteoporosis as the possible underlying cause and for the presence of other risk factors. They should be evaluated as soon as possible after the fracture has occurred to start treatment in a timely manner with proven antifracture effect at the short term. Furthermore, a question regarding a history of fragility fracture after the age of 40 years should be part of any assessment of fracture risk in women.

Recognizing women with vertebral fractures

Vertebral fractures are the most frequent fractures in women.[27] The risk for subsequent fractures is fourfold after a vertebral fracture, a relative risk that is substantially higher than after nonvertebral fractures.[24] The risk for new fractures is already increased within 1 year: one in five women will suffer a new vertebral fracture and one in four a new fracture.[28] The risk for new fractures is also related to the number and severity of prevalent vertebral fractures.[28,29] Thus, vertebral fractures are considered a major risk factor for new fractures. However, the diagnosis of vertebral fractures in

daily clinical practice is often a diagnostic challenge. Only one in three vertebral fractures comes to clinical attention (so-called "clinical" vertebral fractures), but all vertebral fractures are related to an increased risk for new fractures, morbidity, and mortality.

Typical clinical characteristics for vertebral fractures are the absence of identifiable trauma in many cases, height loss, hyperkyphosis, and acute or chronic back pain.[30]

The circumstances under which vertebral fractures occur are often trivial, even in acute painful clinical cases. In patients with clinically diagnosed vertebral fractures, 14% followed severe trauma and 83% followed moderate or no trauma.[31] Clinical vertebral fractures occurred after an accident at home (such as a fall or stumble) in 13% of cases, after lifting a heavy load in 24% of cases, and without any evident reason in 44% of cases.[32] Thus, the absence of identifiable trauma is no reason to exclude clinical suspicion of a vertebral fracture.

Spontaneous restoration of normal spinal anatomy is not possible after vertebral fracture. Vertebral fractures are associated with varying degrees of height loss,[32,33] thoracic hyperkyphosis in the case of a thoracic vertebral fracture, and flattened lumbar lordosis in the case of a lumbar vertebral fracture.[32,34,35] A self-reported humped back is associated with the presence of vertebral fractures.[36] Lung function progressively decreases with increasing hyperkyphosis.[37] Case findings for vertebral fractures thus include specific questions about changes in body height, changes in kyphosis, and shortness of breath.

Vertebral fractures are associated with varying degrees of back pain. In women with a clinical vertebral fracture, pain onset was sudden in 73% (compared with 21% in women with chronic low back pain without fractures), and 19% of women reported a more gradual beginning of complaints.[32] The pain follows a mechanical pattern (increasing by load and decreasing by rest), with varying frequency, severity, and duration. The acute, severe pain episode after a clinical vertebral fracture gradually subsides within 2 to 6 weeks, but back pain after an acute pain episode can last for many years and decreases over time.[38] In prospective studies using serial radiographs and diagnosing all new vertebral fractures, a single new vertebral fracture, even one not recognized clinically, increased the odds for back pain.[39] Therefore, a vertebral fracture should be considered in the differential diagnosis of any history of acute or chronic back pain in all postmenopausal women.

The clinical consequences of vertebral fractures are well documented, such as with functional disability, decreased activities of daily living, disturbed balance capability, increased dependency, functional limitation, depression, and decreased quality of life.[32] However, these functional repercussions are not specific for vertebral fractures. Therefore, a vertebral fracture should be considered in postmenopausal women with functional limitations.

Clinically, hyperkyphosis can result in the typical clinical presentation of a "dowager's hump." Only limited studies are available on the value of clinical examination for suspicion of vertebral fractures. An occiput-wall distance of greater than 0 cm and a rib-pelvis distance less than 2 fingerbreadths were associated with the presence of thoracic fractures on radiograph (Figure 11-4).[36]

A simple questionnaire has been devised to help identify patients who are more likely to have existing vertebral fractures and who may benefit from spinal radiographs to determine whether vertebral deformity is present. The Prevalent Vertebral Fracture Index (PVFI) is calculated by adding points based on the following five variables: history or diagnosis of a vertebral or nonvertebral fracture, height loss since age 25, history or diagnosis of osteoporosis, and age (Figure 11-5).[40] For example, a 73-year-old woman (2 points) with a previous wrist fracture (1 point) would have a PVFI of 3; if she had also lost 3 cm of height (1 point), her PVFI would be 4. In the original report, the prevalence of women with vertebral fracture was 3.8% among women with a PVFI of 0 and 62% among women with a PVFI greater than 5. A PVFI of 4 or greater identified 66% of women with vertebral fractures (sensitivity), with a specificity of 69%.

A similar algorithm for detecting prevalent vertebral fractures (any vertebral height loss of >25%) was developed based on the European Prospective Osteoporosis Study, based on age, height loss, self-reported history of spinal fracture, other major fracture, and weight.[41]

Once a vertebral fracture is clinically suspected, a radiograph of the spine is indicated. This should include an anteroposterior and a lateral radiograph of the total thoracic and lumbar spine to diagnose all vertebral fractures as well as those without acute symptoms.[4] New devices of DXA offer the opportunity to use DXA for morphometry of the vertebrae.

Currently, there is no gold standard for the diagnosis of a vertebral fracture on radiographs.[42] Several definitions of a vertebral deformity have been developed. These include quantitative and semiquantitative methods. Quantitative methods of vertebral morphometry

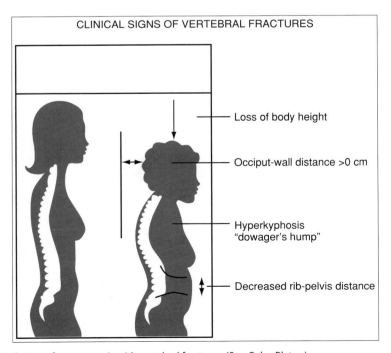

CLINICAL SIGNS OF VERTEBRAL FRACTURES

— Loss of body height

— Occiput-wall distance >0 cm

— Hyperkyphosis "dowager's hump"

— Decreased rib-pelvis distance

Figure 11-4. Clinical signs of osteoporosis with vertebral fractures. (See Color Plates.)

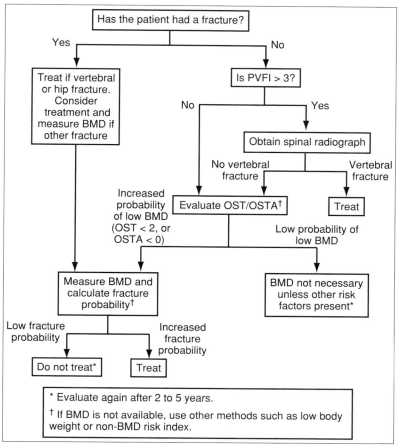

Figure 11-5. The Prevalent Vertebral Fracture Index (PVFI). BMD = bone mineral density; OST = Osteoporosis Self-assessment Tool; OSTA = Osteoporosis Self-assessment Tool with adaptations for Asian women.

include measurements of the anterior, middle, and posterior heights of vertebrae and are merely intended for clinical trials.[42] Semiquantitative methods, such as the Genant score, are more suitable for use in daily practice and are available on the Web.[43]

Even when radiographs of the spine are available, having been taken for medical reasons other than evaluating for osteoporosis, radiographic vertebral fractures are overlooked in daily clinical practice. A survey of 934 hospitalized older women with an available chest radiograph was used to evaluate the frequency with which vertebral fractures were identified and treated by clinicians.[44] Moderate-to-severe vertebral fractures (diminution of >20% in anterior, middle, or posterior height) were identified in 132 (14.1%) of the study subjects, but only 1.7% had a discharge diagnosis of vertebral fracture. Of these, 50% were recorded in the radiology reports and only 17% had a fracture noted in the medical record or discharge summary.[44] Therefore, the diagnosis of vertebral fractures could be enhanced in daily practice by more rigorous measurement and reporting of vertebral deformities with a reduction (e.g., > 20%) in anterior, middle, or posterior height.

Recognizing women with nonvertebral fractures

A nonvertebral fracture is a major risk factor for vertebral and new nonvertebral fractures, also in the short term. In contrast to vertebral fractures, nonvertebral fractures are usually easy to diagnose because of their relation to trauma, typical clinical signs, symptoms, and radiographic findings. Some nonvertebral fractures are more difficult to diagnose clinically, even on radiographs. Typical examples include fractures of the sacrum, fractures of the pedicles of vertebrae, limited cortical fractures without deformation, and stress fractures.

Differential diagnosis in patients with a fragility fracture and/or low bone mineral density

Once a fragility fracture has been diagnosed, its cause remains to be established. In a typical case of a 70-year-old woman with several risk factors for osteoporosis (e.g., low body weight and family history of hip fracture) and an acute painful vertebral fracture after minimal trauma, primary osteoporosis is most likely. However, in the case of a 60-year-old obese woman with an acute painful vertebral fracture after minimal trauma and a moon face and skin striae, secondary osteoporosis (Cushing disease in this case) is more likely. Furthermore, vertebral fractures can be the result of malignant diseases. In one survey of clinical vertebral fractures, 3% were pathological.[31]

Thus, differential diagnosis is necessary in patients with a vertebral fragility fracture. This includes a thorough medical history, general clinical examination, and, according to the clinical context, laboratory examinations. Additional technical examinations, such as magnetic resonance imaging and bone scintigraphy, can be helpful for excluding malignant bone disease in the case of a vertebral fracture. Differential diagnosis of vertebral deformities also includes recognition of Scheuermann disease, osteoarthritis, Paget disease, and osteomalacia.[4]

As for vertebral fractures, differential diagnosis should also be considered after a nonvertebral fragility fracture. Many patients with nonvertebral fractures have correctable underlying disease.[45] It has been shown that patients with a hip fracture have a non-negligible prevalence of vitamin D deficiency, hyperparathyroidism, and malabsorption (coeliac disease).[45,46] Because most nonvertebral fractures occur after falls, fall risk evaluation is advocated in most guidelines.[5]

The same principles of differential diagnosis apply for patients with low BMD without a prevalent fracture. This is especially the case if the Z-score is less than −2.0, as this indicates that the BMD is significantly lower than age-matched controls and could indicate causes of secondary osteoporosis.[47]

Dual X-ray absorptiometry after fragility fracture

In postmenopausal women with a vertebral fragility fracture due to primary osteoporosis (postmenopausal or senile), DXA is not strictly necessary to start treatment.[1] Antifracture effects with several drugs have been shown in clinical trials in patients with a prevalent vertebral fracture, independent of BMD. Many patients in clinical trials in patients with a prevalent vertebral fracture had a T-score greater than −2.5.

After a nonvertebral fracture, DXA has a more prominent role. Nonvertebral fractures increase the risk for new fractures. However, no clinical trials are available that selected patients only on the basis of a prevalent vertebral fracture. Most guidelines therefore advocate bone densitometry after a low-trauma nonvertebral fracture to diagnose osteoporosis in terms of BMD.[5] However, a nonvertebral fragility fracture is a risk factor for new fractures, independent of BMD. Therefore, the level of BMD below which to start treatment is considered higher in the presence of a vertebral fracture (e.g., a T-score of < −1.0) in several guidelines.

To more systematically evaluate patients with a fragility fracture, some institutions have begun referring all patients with a fragility fracture from orthopedic clinics and emergency rooms for evaluation of osteoporosis and fracture risk. One example is the Glasgow fracture program, which has a "fracture nurse" in this capacity.[48] This system has been very successful in improving the diagnosis and treatment of fracture patients with osteoporosis. This clinical approach is now widely supported by the World Orthopaedic Osteoporosis Organization.[49]

It is suggested in several guidelines that DXA could be useful for monitoring response (or lack of response) to therapy and that measuring BMD could enhance compliance, but prospective data to support this last view need further study. The degree of change in BMD during drug therapy does not reflect the degree of risk reduction for vertebral fractures.[50] The relationship between changes in BMD and the risk of nonvertebral fractures during therapy was significant when based on means of trials[51,52] but not when based on individual data.[53] Thus, the value of a follow-up DXA measurement requires special precautions, as discussed elsewhere.

Evaluating Total Fracture Risk in Women

As already mentioned, the predictive value of one risk factor, such as described above for low BMD or a prevalent fragility fracture, can be enhanced by the use of other factors that contribute to fracture risk, as far as they are, at least partially, independent.[10] Such an approach has been successfully applied for predicting death from cardiovascular disease in adults with raised blood pressure.[54]

Measurements that have been shown to enhance the predictive value over and above BMD are age,[10] family history of fractures,[55] markers of bone resorption,[56] hip geometry,[57] fall risks,[15,58] quantitative ultrasonographic findings,[59] self-reported poor health, and poor mobility.[60] In these studies, it has been shown that the combinations were more predictive for fractures than any one measurement alone and could predict patients with high fracture risk in the absence of osteoporosis in terms of low BMD. As an example, in the OFELY study, nearly one-half of fractures occurred in nonosteoporotic women.[56] Among these women, the combination of bone markers and history of previous fracture was highly predictive of fracture risk.

A series of recent meta-analyses from population-based cohorts has shown remarkable international consistency for low BMI, a prior history of fracture, a family history of hip fracture, current smoking, high intake of alcohol, and rheumatoid arthritis.[10] All provide information on fracture risk that is in part independent of BMD.[10]

For any given T-score, fracture risk is much higher in the elderly than in the young. Age is associated with increased fracture risk, over and above BMD. At least one tool for calculating fracture probability of a postmenopausal woman from age, baseline BMD, and bone loss is available on the Internet.[61] This system predicts that high-risk postmenopausal women will have more than one fracture if not treated.

In one study, combining quantitative ultrasonography, BMD, and clinical risk assessment (body weight, age, fall history, balance performance, and gait speed) identified a high-risk group (1 in 10 chance of having a hip fracture over the next 4 years), compared with a low-risk group (1 in 40 chance).[62]

Another proposed strategy includes a stepwise approach based on intervention thresholds. In a first step, based on clinical risk factors, individuals are identified at high, intermediate, and low risk for fractures. BMD measurement would then be restricted to the intermediate risk group to recategorize such individuals to a high- or low-risk group.[7] This approach still needs more formalization before it can be applied in clinical practice. The impact of integrating more risk factors and more combinations is in progress and must be cautiously applied.[10]

Combining of risk factors and antifracture therapy

As discussed, several guidelines have incorporated the view that, in the presence of bone-related risk factors that have been associated with fracture risk over and above BMD, such as age over 65 years, personal or family history of fragility fracture, and use of glucocorticoids, intervention thresholds should be less stringent, such as a T-score of −1.5 SD.

Most clinical trials have been performed using one selection criterion, however, such as low BMD or prevalent fracture independent of BMD. In some studies, post hoc analysis has shown additional value based on additional risk factors. The antifracture effect of raloxifene was independent of the presence of major risk factors at baseline, such as a family history of fractures, but an elevated triglyceride level and low BMD values in the spine at baseline were associated with increased vertebral fracture risk reduction with raloxifene therapy.[63] Risedronate was effective in reducing the risk of vertebral fractures in various subgroups at high risk, such as in women 70 years and older and in patients with more than one vertebral fracture at baseline.[64]

Many patients in clinical trials on fracture prevention had a T-score greater than −2.5.[65] Alendronate prevented nonvertebral fractures in women with a T-score of less than −2.0.[66] In a post hoc analysis, it has been shown that raloxifene decreased the risk of vertebral fractures in women with osteopenia, but the fracture incidence was low.[67] There are thus indications that fracture risk prevention could be achieved in patients with osteopenia.

Age is another major risk factor that has been further analyzed as a contributor to fracture risk reduction with drugs. Data on bone-directed drugs are scarce in elderly people of 80 years and older. Post hoc analyses indicate that the bisphosphonates alendronate and risedronate reduce the risk for vertebral fractures in patients older than 80 years,[68,69] but a reduction in wrist and hip fractures in elderly women of 80 years and older could only be shown with alendronate (in patients with a prevalent vertebral fracture or low BMD).[69] Strontium ranelate did not reduce the risk of hip fractures in the total population studied, but a favorable effect was reported in elderly (>74 years) at the condition they had a low BMD (T-score < −2.4).[70] Thus, when considering age as an enhancer of fracture risk, low BMD still remains an important indicator when it comes to selecting patients in whom bone-directed drugs can reduce fracture risk, when mediated by BMD or other non-BMD-related bone factors. In contrast, raloxifene was significantly more effective in reducing the risk of vertebral fractures in the lowest versus highest age group of the MORE study.[63]

The application of bone turnover is promising in daily practice but depends on well-defined cut-off values. Bone markers could also be of value in women with osteopenia to enhance fracture risk calculation. Currently, the use of bone markers is considered in some guidelines but is not yet advocated for systematic use in daily practice.[5]

The role of falls

Falls contribute to the occurrence of fractures, especially nonvertebral fractures. It is likely that preventing falls would reduce the incidence of fractures. Several fall-preventing strategies have been shown to reduce the risk of falls in older adults.[71] However, no studies have demonstrated a reduction in fracture risk by reducing the incidence of falls. Thus, although evaluating fall risk and prevention of falls is indicated in elderly women and men, there is insufficient evidence that this reduces the risk of fractures.

To what extent fall-related risk factors, which also have been associated with fracture risk over and above BMD, can be used to alter intervention thresholds is less clear. Intervention studies have shown that bone-directed drugs, such as risedronate, reduced the risk of hip fractures in patients with proven osteoporosis (low BMD, with or without prevalent vertebral fracture), but were not effective in reducing the risk of hip fracture in patients who were selected mainly on the basis of risk of falling without proven low BMD.[72] Thus, low BMD remains an important determinant of patient selection for therapy with bone-directed drugs in patients with risk of falls.

One intriguing finding is that there seems to be interaction between fall risk and low BMD in the occurrence of fragility fractures.[73,74] It has been shown that, compared with women with normal BMD, the risk of fractures is increased not only in patients with osteoporosis but also in patients with osteopenia who had a fall, but not in these same patients when they did not fall. This could indicate that patients with osteopenia should have fall prevention if they are fallers, and that fallers with osteopenia should have prevention of bone loss. Studies are underway to further analyze this interaction.

The effect of treatment according to the presence of two or more risk factors is still a matter of debate.[65] One reason is that many of the available data are based on post hoc analyses, which should be interpreted with caution, as they were not the basis of randomization. Further studies will be necessary to further ameliorate such approaches. The finding that fractures can be prevented in populations in whom no BMD was available opens new avenues for case finding.

Fracture risk in the absence of bone densitometry by dual X-ray absorptiometry

When BMD measurements are not available, it appears that patients with increased fracture risk can also be identified using other risk factors (Table 11-6). The large prospective epidemiological study, the SOF, reported that low body weight predicts the risk of hip, pelvis, and rib fractures in elderly (age ≥65) women.[75] Fracture risk among women in the lowest quartile was two or more times greater than for those in the highest quartile. The increase in risk appears to be due to low BMD; there was no difference in risk among weight quartiles after adjusting for hip BMD. Thus, low body weight can be used as an approximation to identify patients with low BMD. The authors concluded that body weight is useful for assessing the risk of hip, pelvis, and rib fractures when BMD has not been measured. In the EPIDOS study, the use of weight to select women for bone densitometry, and then the use of clinical risk factors to enhance the predictive value of BMD, had the same discriminant value for hip fractures as BMD measurement as a population screening tool.[76]

Other methods of identifying high-risk patients, when BMD measurements are not available, have been reported. One technique derived from the SOF is calculated by adding points as follows: age, a fracture after age 50, patient's mother had a hip fracture after age 50, patient currently smokes, weight is 57 kg or less, and patient cannot rise from a chair without using her arms (Fracture Index).[77] In this study, the 5-year risk rate of nonverteberal fractures increased progressively from 11% for women with a score of 1, to 26% for women with scores above 4. The corresponding 5-year risks were 1% (score = 1) to 10% (score >4) for vertebral fractures, and 0.6% (score = 1) to 8% (score >4) for hip fractures. Adding information from BMD measurements did not substantially improve the fracture estimates. Thus, this tool effectively identified large differences in fracture risk without measuring BMD.

In the Rotterdam study, BMD measurement had only a modestly better performance than a score based on age, gender, height, the use of a walking aide, cigarette smoking, and weight.[78]

Almost all patients with vertebral fractures or hip fractures have low BMD and a high risk of subsequent fractures. Furthermore, patients with a T-score less than −1.6 and existing vertebral fracture have a fracture risk similar to that of patients with osteoporosis (T-score <−2.5) but without existing vertebral fractures, and treatment to reduce fracture risk is effective in both types of patients. Thus, it is reasonable to treat patients with vertebral or hip fractures even if BMD measurements are not available.

Other risk factors to consider in the context of case finding for osteoporosis and fragility fractures

This review focused on case finding for diagnosis and treatment of osteoporotic fractures. In addition, several guidelines draw attention to other risks. All guidelines advocate checking reversible risk factors, such as lifestyle (smoking), diet (calcium intake), vitamin D exposure (sun exposure and diet), and exercise.[5] These risks should thus be checked and corrected when possible. However, such measures are mostly quoted as "good for bone health," as proof of the antifracture effects of these measures is limited.[5]

Figure 11-6 gives an overview of the approach of case finding in women, based on the above review.

TABLE 11-6 RISK RATIO FOR HIP FRACTURE ASSOCIATED WITH RISK FACTORS ADJUSTED FOR AGE. WITH AND WITHOUT ADJUSTMENT FOR BONE MINERAL DENSITY (BMD)[10]					
Risk Indicator		**Without BMD**		**With BMD**	
		RR	95% CI	RR	95% CI
Body mass index	20 vs 25	1.95	1.71-2.22	1.42	1.23-1.65
	30 vs 25	0.83	0.69-0.99	1.00	0.82-1.21
Prior fracture after 50 years		1.85	1.58-2.17	1.62	1.30-2.01
Parental history of hip fracture		2.27	1.47-3.49	2.28	1.48-3.51
Current smoking		1.84	1.52-2.22	1.60	1.27-2.02
Ever use of systemic corticosteroids		2.31	1.67-3.20	2.25	1.60-3.15
Alcohol intake >2 units daily		1.68	1.19-2.36	1.70	1.20-2.42
Rheumatoid arthritis		1.95	1.11-3.42	1.73	0.94-3.20

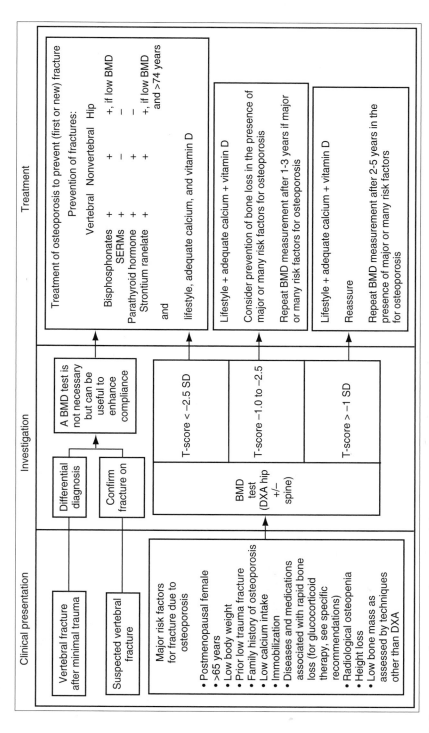

Figure 11-6. Assessment and treatment of osteoporosis in postmenopausal women. BMD = bone mineral density; DXA = dual x-ray absorptiometry; SD = standard deviation.

Future developments

There is a trend for calculating the individual absolute risk for fractures, which brings together the relative risk of several independent risk factors and the timing for fractures and enables prediction of 5- or 10-year fracture risk.[10] Such fracture risk prediction is then adapted to the individual risk profile based on clinical risk factors, BMD, markers of bone turnover, other skeletal risk factors (e.g., genetics) and extraskeletal factors. This should result in the determination of intervention thresholds based on 10-year probability of fracture and decisions about interventions that are cost-effective. The cost-effectiveness of interventions has been shown in men and women in whom hip fracture probability over 10 years ranges from 1% to 10% depending on age.[10] Against this background, evaluation of individual fracture risk is increasingly considered the best basis for treatment decisions.[10] An example of such an approach will be discussed in the section on glucocorticoid-induced osteoporosis.

CASE FINDINGS IN MEN

Osteoporotic fractures in men are less common than in women but their incidence is far from negligible.[79] Risk factors for osteoporosis (in terms of low BMD) and fragility fractures in general are identified for men but are less well documented than in women. Although there is a paucity of clinical trials with fracture prevention as the primary endpoint in men, post hoc analysis indicates that vertebral fractures could be prevented by bisphosphonates in men with osteoporosis.[80]

The principles of case finding are similar for men and women, but less documentation is available for men. Major risk factors are in general similar in women and in men.

Hip fracture risk in men is associated with reduced bone mass and trauma (Table 11-7). In a population survey, an increased risk for hip fracture in men was associated with metabolic disease and disorders of movement or balance.[81] The risk for hip fracture was higher in individuals with a history of thyroidectomy, gastric resection, pernicious anemia, chronic bronchitis, or emphysema.[81] Movement and balance disorders associated with an increased risk for hip fracture include neurological disorders (hemiplegia, parkinsonism, dementia), vertigo, alcoholism, anemia, blindness, and use of a cane or walker.[81] In addition, many more risk factors are described in cross-sectional studies.

Among men with fractures, only 21% were found to have a T-score less than −2.5.[82] In prospective studies, risk factors for vertebral fractures include age, self-reported spine fracture or other major fracture, and low body weight.[41,84] Low BMD was an additional risk factor

TABLE 11-7 CAUSES OF OSTEOPOROSIS IN MEN
Endocrine diseases
Hypogonadism*
Cushing syndrome
Hyperthyroidism
Primary hyperparathyroidism
Hyperprolactinemia
Idiopathic renal hypercalciuria*
Accompanying osteomalacia
Neoplastic disease
Multiple myeloma
Myelo- and lymphoproliferative diseases
Systemic mastocytosis
Diffuse bony metastases*
Vertebral metastasis
Drugs/toxins
Glucocorticoids*
Antiandrogen therapy for prostate cancer
Alcohol abuse*
Excessive thyroid hormone replacement
Heparin
Anticonvulsants*
Genetic collagen disorders
Osteogenesis imperfecta
Ehlers-Danlos syndrome
Marfan syndrome
Homocystinuria
Hemochromatosis
Other disorders
Skeletal sarcoidosis
Gaucher disease
Adult hypophosphatasia
Hemoglobulinopathies
Other factors
Chronic illness (rheumatoid arthritis, liver/renal disease)
Prolonged immobilization
Malnutrition (including calcium deficiency and scurvy)
Gastrectomy*
Aging*
Idiopathic
Juvenile
Adult*
*Most frequent causes.

for incident vertebral fractures.[83] Risk factors for hip fracture also included the use of a walking aid and cigarette smoking.[78] In an extensive meta-analyses of cohorts from different countries, previous fractures and a parental history of hip fracture were associated with fracture risk in men, independent of age and BMD.[26,55]

In men with clinical vertebral fractures, height loss of more than 2.5 cm is common (>50%).[85] In radiographic surveys, however, radiographic vertebral fractures have not been related to back pain.[86] Many men with clinical vertebral fractures have decreased quality of life.[85]

Differential Diagnosis

In contrast to women, 50% of men with clinical vertebral fractures have secondary osteoporosis in some surveys.[87,88] Men with symptomatic vertebral fracture are usually younger than women.[87] Therefore, causes of secondary osteoporosis should always be evaluated in men with vertebral fracture, in addition to measurement of BMD.

GLUCOCORTICOID-INDUCED OSTEOPOROSIS

As always, the patient's individual risk factors should be carefully reviewed when initiating glucocorticoid therapy. All guidelines on osteoporosis advocate that patients treated with glucocorticoids deserve special attention for increased fracture risk.[5]

Factors that influence bone loss and fracture risk include the dose of glucocorticoids, the underlying condition, and the presence of other risk factors such as age, sex, BMI, previous personal and familial fractures, diet, physical activity, smoking, alcohol consumption, menopausal status, general health status, and BMD (Table 11-8).[89-91] Intermittent oral pulse

---

TABLE 11-8 RISK FACTOR EVALUATION FOR PREVENTION AND TREATMENT OF GLUCOCORTICOID-INDUCED OSTEOPOROSIS

Lifestyle
  Smoking
  Alcohol consumption
  Physical activity
  Calcium intake
  Vitamin D status

Underlying disease
Major risk factors
  Age
  Gender
  Menopausal status and gonadal status in men
  Low body weight
  Personal and familial history of fractures
  Other medications

Bone mineral density measurement: at baseline and during follow-up

Laboratory
  Complete blood cell count
  Serum calcium, phosphate, creatinine, alkaline
    phosphatase
  If >65 years: protein electrophoresis, lipids, urinary
    calcium

Figure 11-7. Algorithm for prevention and therapy of glucocorticoid-induced osteoporosis.

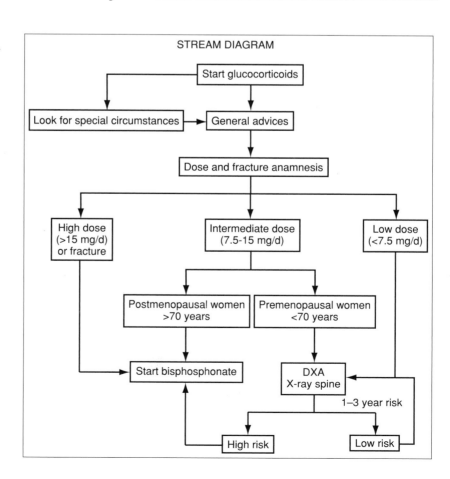

therapy (in men) and inhaled glucocorticoids have been shown to increase vertebral fracture risk to a greater degree than in control subjects, but patients on the intermittent therapy were not as likely to sustain fractures as those on continuous therapy.[92]

These factors should thus be considered in all patients who are anticipated to have treatment with glucocorticoids. An example of a case finding is shown in Figure 11-7, based on the Dutch guidelines.[93]

In one study, risk calculation in glucocorticoid-induced osteoporosis was based on age, sex, BMI, dose of glucocorticoids, smoking, past fracture, past fall, and underlying disease.[94] This allowed calculation of the individual fracture risk. A woman aged 65 years with rheumatoid arthritis, low BMI, and a previous history of fracture and falls who used 15 mg glucocorticoid daily (total risk score 54) had a 5-year fracture risk of 47%, as compared with a man with a similar history whose risk was 30.1%.[94]

REFERENCES

1. Kanis J: Diagnosis of osteoporosis and assessment of fracture risk. Lancet 2002;359:1929-36.
2. Slemenda CW, Johnston CC, Hui SL: Assessing fracture risk. In: Osteoporosis. Marcus R, Feldman D, Kelsey J (eds): Osteoporosis. Academic Press, San Diego. 2001; 1:809-818.
3. Chapuy MC, Meunier PJ: Pathophysiology and prevention of hip fractures in elderly people. In: Dunitz M: Osteoporosis. Diagnosis and management. London. 1998, pp 191-210.
4. Eastell R: Practical management of the patient with osteoporotic vertebral fracture. In: Dunitz M: Osteoporosis. Diagnosis and management. London. 1998, pp 175-190.
5. Geusens P: Review of guidelines for osteoporosis. Curr Osteoporos Rep 2003;I:59-65.
6. Stone KL, Seeley DG, Lui L, et al, for the Study of Osteoporotic Fractures Research Group: BMD at multiple sites and risk of fracture of multiple types: long-term results from the study of osteoporotic fractures. J Bone Miner Res 2003;18:1947-1954
7. Johansson H, Oden A, Johnell O, et al: Optimization of BMD measurements to identify high risk groups for treatment: a test analysis. J Bone Miner Res 2004;19:906-913.
8. Eisman J, Clapham S, Kehoe L: Osteoporosis prevalence and levels of treatment in primary care: the Australian bone care study. J Bone Miner Res 2004;19:1969-1975.
9. Kamel HK, Hussain MS, Tariq S, et al: Failure to diagnose and treat osteoporosis in elderly patients hospitalized with hip fracture. Am J Med 2000;109:326-328.
10. Kanis J, Borgstrom F, De Laet C, et al: Assessment of fracture risk: review. Osteoporos Int 2005;16:581-589.
11. Espallargues M, Sampietro-Colom L, Estrada MD, et al: Identifying bone-mass-related risk factors for fracture to guide bone densitometry measurements: a systematic review of the literature. Osteoporos Int 2001;12:811-22.
12. Nguyen TV, Center JR, Sambrook PN, Eisman JA: Risk factors for proximal humerus, forearm, and wrist fractures in elderly men and women: the Dubbo Osteoporosis Epidemiology Study. Am J Epidemiol 2001;153:587-95.
13. Anonymous report of the National Osteoporosis Foundation. Osteoporos Int 1998;8(suppl 4):1-88.
14. Nevitt MC, Cummings SR, Stone KL, et al: Risk factors for a first-incident radiographic vertebral fracture in women > or = 65 years of age: the study of osteoporotic fractures. J Bone Miner Res 2005;20:131-40.
15. Taylor BC, Schreiner PJ, Stone KL, et al: Long-term prediction of incident hip fracture risk in elderly white women: study of osteoporotic fractures. J Am Geriatr Soc 2004;52:1479-86.
16. Geusens P, Hochberg MC, van der Voort DJ, et al: Performance of risk indices for identifying low bone density in post-menopausal women. Mayo Clin Proc 2002;77:629-37.
17. Lydick E, Cook K, Turpin J, et al: Development and validation of a simple questionnaire to facilitate identification of women likely to have low bone mass. Am J Man Care 1998;4:37-48.
18. Cadarette SM, Jaglal SB, Kreiger N, et al: Development and validation of the osteoporosis risk assessment instrument to facilitate selection of women for bone densitometry. Can Med Ass J 2000;162:1289-94.
19. Black DM, Palermo L, Abbott T, Johnell O: SOFSURF: A simple, useful risk factor system can identify the large majority of women with osteoporosis. Bone 1998;23:S605.
20. Nguyen TV, Center JR, Pocock NA, Eisman JA: Limited utility of clinical indices for the prediction of symptomatic fracture risk in postmenopausal women. Osteoporos Int 2004;15:49-55.
21. Richy F, Ethgen O, Bruyere O, et al: Primary prevention of osteoporosis: mass screening scenario or prescreening with questionnaires? An economic perspective. J Bone Miner Res 2004;19:1955-1960.
22. Dargent-Molina P, Poitiers F, Breart G, for the EPIDOS Group: In elderly women weight is the best predictor of a very low bone mineral density: evidence from the EPIDOS study. Osteoporos Int 2000;11:881-888.
23. Marshall D, Johnell O, Wedel H: Meta-analysis of how well measures of bone mineral density predict occurrence of osteoporotic fractures. BMJ 1996;312:1254-1259.
24. Klotzbuecher CM, Ross PD, Landsman PB, et al: Patients with prior fractures have an increased risk of future fractures: a summary of the literature and statistical synthesis. J Bone Miner Res 2000;15:721-739.
25. Leidig G, Minne HW, Sauer P, et al: A study of complaints and their relation to vertebral destruction in patients with osteoporosis. Bone Miner 1990;8:217-29.
26. Kanis JA, Johnell O, De Laet C, et al: A meta-analysis of previous fracture and subsequent fracture risk. Bone 2004;35:375-82.
27. van Staa TP, Dennison EM, Leufkens HG, Cooper C: Epidemiology of fractures in England and Wales. Bone 2001;29:517-22.
28. Lindsay R, Silverman SL, Cooper C, et al: Risk of new vertebral fracture in the year following a fracture. JAMA 2001;285:320-323.
29. Delmas PD, Genant HK, Crans GG, et al: Severity of prevalent vertebral fractures and the risk of subsequent vertebral and nonvertebral fractures: results from the MORE trial. Bone 2003;33:522-32.
30. Geusens P: Clinical features of osteoporosis. In: Hochberg M, Silman A, Smolen J, et al (eds): Rheumatology. 2003, pp 2081-2092.
31. Cooper C, Atkinson EJ, O'Fallon WM, et al: Incidence of clinically diagnosed vertebral fractures: a population-based study in Rochester, Minnesota, 1985-1989. J Bone Miner Res 1992;7:221-27.
32. Leidig-Bruckner G, Minne HW, Schlaich C, et al: Clinical grading of spinal osteoporosis: quality of life components and spinal deformity in women with chronic low back pain and women with vertebral osteoporosis. J Bone Miner Res 1997;12:663-75.
33. Gold DT: The clinical impact of vertebral fractures: quality of life in women with osteoporosis. Bone 1996;18(suppl):185S-9S.
34. Ensrud KE, Black DM, Harris F, et al. Correlates of kyphosis in older women. The Fracture Intervention Trial Research Group. J Am Geriatr Soc 1997; 45: 682-87.
35. Ettinger B, Black DM, et al: Kyphosis in older women and its relation to back pain, disability and osteopenia: the study of osteoporotic fractures. Osteoporos Int 1994;4:55-60.
36. Green AD, Colon-Emeric CS, Bastian L, et al: Does this woman have osteoporosis? JAMA 2004;292:2890-900.
37. Schlaich C, Minne HW, Bruckner T, et al: Reduced pulmonary function in patients with spinal osteoporotic fractures. Osteoporos Int 1998;8:261-67.
38. Ross PD, Davis JW, Epstein RS, Wasnich RD: Pain and disability associated with new vertebral fractures and other spinal conditions. J Clin Epidemiol 1994;47:231-39.

39. Nevitt MC, Ettinger B, Black DM, et al: The association of radiographically detected vertebral fractures with back pain and function: a prospective study. Ann Intern Med 1998;128:793-800.

40. Vogt TM, Ross PD, Palermo L, et al: Vertebral fracture prevalence among women screened for the Fracture Intervention Trial and a simple clinical tool to screen for undiagnosed vertebral fractures. Mayo Clin Proc 2000;75:888-96.

41. Kaptoge S, Armbrecht G, Felsenberg D, et al, for the EPOS Study Group: When should the doctor order a spine X-ray? Identifying vertebral fractures for osteoporosis care: results from the European Prospective Osteoporosis Study (EPOS). J Bone Miner Res 2004;19:1982-93.

42. Genant HK, Jergas M: Assessment of prevalent and incident vertebral fractures in osteoporosis research. Osteoporos Int 2003;14(Suppl 3):S43-55.

43. International Osteoporosis Foundation. Available at: http://www.osteofound.org/health_professionals/vfi/index-flash.html.last visit March 5, 2006.

44. Gehlbach SH, Bigelow C, et al: Recognition of vertebral fracture in a clinical setting. Osteoporos Int 2000;11:577-82.

45. Tannenbaum C, Clark J, Schwartzman K, et al: Yield of laboratory testing to identify secondary contributors to osteoporosis in otherwise healthy women. JCEM 2002;X:4431-37.

46. Greenspan S, Luckey M: In: Primer on the metabolic bone disorders of mineral metabolism, 5th ed. Baltimore: Lippincott Williams & Wilkins, 1999. pp 355-359. Also available on www.jbmr-online.org/ Last visited March 5, 2006.

47. Kleerekoper M: Extensive personal experience: the clinical evaluation and management of osteoporosis. J Clin Endocrinol Metab 1995;3:757-63.

48. McLellan AR, Gallacher SJ, Fraser M, McQuillian C: The fracture liaison service: success of a program for the evaluation and management of patients with osteoporotic fracture. Osteoporos Int 2003;14:1028-34.

49. World Orthopaedic Osteoporosis Organization. Available at: http://www.osteofound.org/press_centre/pr_2003_06_09.html Last visited March 5, 2006.

50. Delmas PD, Seeman E: Changes in bone mineral density explain little of the reduction in vertebral or nonvertebral fracture risk with anti-resorptive therapy. Bone 2004;34:599-604.

51. Hochberg MC, Greenspan S, Wasnich RD, et al: Changes in bone density and turnover explain the reductions in incidence of nonvertebral fractures that occur during treatment with antiresorptive agents. J Clin Endocrinol Metab 2002;87:1586-92.

52. Hochberg MC, Ross PD, Black D, et al, for the Fracture Intervention Trial Research Group: Larger increases in bone mineral density during alendronate therapy are associated with a lower risk of new vertebral fractures in women with postmenopausal osteoporosis. Arthritis Rheum 1999;42:1246-54.

53. Watts NB, Geusens P, Barton IP, Felsenberg D: The relationship between changes in bone mineral density and nonvertebral fracture incidence associated with risedronate: reduction in risk of nonvertebral fracture is not related to change in bone mineral density. J Bone Miner Res 2005;20:2097-104.

54. Pocock SJ, McCormack V, Gueyffier F, et al: A score for predicting risk of death from cardiovascular disease in adults with raised blood pressure, based on individual patient data from randomised controlled trials. BMJ 2001;323:75-81.

55. Kanis JA, Johansson H, Oden A, et al: A family history of fracture and fracture risk: a meta-analysis. Bone 2004;35:1029-37.

56. Garnero P, Delmas PD: Contribution of bone mineral density and bone turnover markers to the estimation of risk of osteoporotic fracture in postmenopausal women. J Musculoskelet Neuronal Interact 2004;4:50-63.

57. Pulkkinen P, Partanen J, Jalovaara P, Jamsa T: Combination of bone mineral density and upper femur geometry improves the prediction of hip fracture. Osteoporos Int 2004;15:274-80.

58. Cummings SR, Nevitt MC, Browner WS, et al: Risk factors for hip fracture in white women. Study of Osteoporotic Fractures Research Group. N Engl J Med 1995;332:767-73.

59. Gluer CC, Eastell R, Reid DM, et al: Association of five quantitative ultrasound devices and bone densitometry with osteoporotic vertebral fractures in a population-based sample: the OPUS Study. J Bone Miner Res 2004;19:782-93.

60. Miller PD, Barlas S, Brenneman SK, et al: An approach to identifying osteopenic women at increased short-term risk of fracture. Arch Intern Med 2004;164:1113-20.

61. Available at: http://www.medsurf.com/newsite/RLFP_home.asp Last visited March 5, 2006.

62. Dargent-Molina P, Piault S, Breart G: A comparison of different screening strategies to identify elderly women at high risk of hip fracture: results from the EPIDOS prospective study. Osteoporos Int 2003;14:969-77.

63. Johnell O, Kanis JA, Black DM, et al: Associations between baseline risk factors and vertebral fracture risk in the Multiple Outcomes of Raloxifene Evaluation (MORE) study. J Bone Miner Res 2004;19:764-72.

64. Watts NB, Josse RG, Hamdy RC, et al: Risedronate prevents new vertebral fractures in postmenopausal women at high risk. J Clin Endocrinol Metab 2003;88:542-49.

65. Miller PD: Greater risk, greater benefit—true or false? [editorial]. J Clin Endocrinol Metab 2003;88:538-41.

66. Pols HA, Felsenberg D, Hanley DA, et al: Multinational, placebo-controlled, randomized trial of the effects of alendronate on bone density and fracture risk in postmenopausal women with low bone mass: results of the FOSIT study. Fosamax International Trial Study Group. Osteoporos Int 1999;9:461-68.

67. Kanis JA, Johnell O, Black DM, et al: Effect of raloxifene on the risk of new vertebral fracture in postmenopausal women with osteopenia or osteoporosis: a reanalysis of the Multiple Outcomes of Raloxifene Evaluation trial. Bone 2003;33:293-300.

68. Boonen S, McClung MR, Eastell R, et al: Safety and efficacy of risedronate in reducing fracture risk in osteoporotic women aged 80 and older: implications for the use of antiresorptive agents in the old and oldest old. J Am Geriatr Soc 2004;11:1832-1839.

69. Hochberg MC, Thompson DE, Black DM, et al, for the FIT Research Group: The effect of alendronate on the age-specific incidence of symptomatic osteoporotic fractures. J Bone Miner Res 2005;20:971-976.

70. EMEA. European Public Assessment Report. Available at: http://www.emea.eu.int/humandocs/Humans/ EPAR/protelos/protelosM.htm Last visited March 5, 2006.

71. Tinetti ME: Preventing falls in the elderly. N Engl J Med 2003;348:42-9.

72. McClung MR, Geusens P, Miller PD, et al, for Hip Intervention Program Study Group: Effect of risedronate on the risk of hip fracture in elderly women. Hip Intervention Program Study Group. N Engl J Med 2001;344:333-40.

73. Geusens P, Autier P, Boonen S, et al: The relationship among history of falls, osteoporosis, and fractures in postmenopausal women. Arch Phys Med Rehabil 2002;83:903-6.

74. Lee SH, Dargent-Molina P, Breart G, for the EPIDOS Group: Epidemiologie de l'Osteoporose Study. Risk factors for fractures of the proximal humerus: results from the EPIDOS prospective study. J Bone Miner Res 2002;17:817-25.

75. Margolis KL, et al: Body size and risk for clinical fractures in older women. Ann Intern Med 2000;133:123-27.

76. Dargent-Molina P, Douchin MN, Cormier C, et al, for the EPIDOS Study Group: Use of clinical risk factors in elderly women with low bone mineral density to identify women at higher risk of hip fracture: The EPIDOS prospective study. Osteoporos Int 2002;13:593-99.

77. Black DM, Steinbuch M, Palermo L, et al: An assessment tool for predicting fracture risk in postmenopausal women. Osteoporos Int 2001;12:519-28.

78. Burger H, de Laet CE, Weel AE, et al: Added value of bone mineral density in hip fracture risk scores. Bone 1999;25:369-74.

79. Seeman E, Bianchi G, Adami S, et al: Osteoporosis in men—consensus is premature. Calcif Tissue Int 2004;75:120-22.

80. Orwoll E, Ettinger M, Weiss S, et al: Alendronate for the treatment of osteoporosis in men. N Engl J Med 2000;343:604-10.

81. Poor G, Atkinson EJ, O'Fallon WM, Melton LJ 3rd: Predictors of hip fractures in elderly men. J Bone Miner Res 1995;10:1900-7.

82. Schuit SC, van der Klift M, Weel AE, et al: Fracture incidence and association with bone mineral density in elderly men and women: the Rotterdam Study. Bone 2004;34:195-202.

83. Van der Klift M, De Laet CE, McCloskey EV, et al: The incidence of vertebral fractures in men and women: the Rotterdam Study. J Bone Miner Res 2002;17:1051-56.

84. Haentjens P, Autier P, Collins J, et al: Colles fracture, spine fracture, and subsequent risk of hip fracture in men and women: a meta-analysis. J Bone Joint Surg Am 2003;85:1936-43.

85. Scane AC, Sutcliffe AM, Francis RM: The sequelae of vertebral crush fractures in men. Osteoporos Int 1994;4:89-92.

86. Johnell O, O'Neill T, Felsenberg D, et al. Anthropometric measurements and vertebral deformities. European Vertebral Osteoporosis Study (EVOS) Group. Am J Epidemiol 1997;146:287-293.

87. Nolla JM, Gomez-Vaquero C, Romero M, et al. Osteoporotic vertebral fracture in clinical practice: 669 patients diagnosed over a 10 year period. J Rheumatol 2001;28:2289-93.

88. Seeman E: Osteoporosis in men. Osteoporos Int 1999;9(suppl 2):S97-110.

89. Van Staa TP, Leufkens HG, Abenhaim L, et al: Use of oral cortico-steroids and risk of fractures. J Bone Miner Res 2000;15:993-1000.

90. Van Staa TP, Leufkens HG, Cooper C: The epidemiology of corti-costeroid-induced osteoporosis: a meta-analysis. Osteoporos Int 2002;13:777-787.

91. Kanis JA, Johansson H, Oden A, et al: A meta-analysis of prior corticosteroid use and fracture risk. J Bone Miner Res 2004;19:893-899.

92. McEvoy CE, Ensrud KE, Bender E, et al: Association between corticosteroid use and vertebral fractures in older men with chronic obstructive pulmonary disease. Am J Respir Crit Care Med 1998;157:704-709.

93. Geusens PP, de Nijs RN, Lems WF, et al: Prevention of glucocorticoid osteoporosis: a consensus document of the Dutch Society for Rheumatology. Ann Rheum Dis 2004;63:324-325.

94. van Staa T-P, Geusens P, Pols HAP, et al: A simple score for estimating the long-term risk of fracture in patients using oral glucocorticoids. QJM, 2005;3:191-198.

12 Exercise and the Prevention of Bone Fragility

Ego Seeman

SUMMARY

Proof that exercise reduces fracture risk requires demonstration of a reduction in spine and hip fractures in well designed and executed, prospective, randomized studies. None exist. Blinded studies cannot be done, whereas unblinded randomized trials are feasible but have not been done. Data from retrospective and prospective observational and case-control studies suggest that physical activity is associated with fewer fractures, but replicated sampling bias is an equally plausible explanation for this desired endpoint. Exercise during growth is likely to build a larger and stronger skeleton. Cessation of exercise appears to erode the structural benefits produced during growth. Changes produced by bone modeling in response to loading during growth may be permanent, but remodeling changes may not be. Exercise after epiphyseal closure (adulthood) produces small increments in bone mineral density (not in bone tissue mass), perhaps by reducing the remodeling space, or may prevent bone loss. The null hypothesis, that exercise has no effect on fracture rates in old age, cannot be rejected.

About 30% to 50% of women and 15% to 30% of men will suffer a fracture.[1] Drugs reduce fracture risk in the most vulnerable high-risk group, but most fractures come from the larger population at modest risk in whom drug therapy is not appropriate, in part, because the number needed to treat to prevent one fracture is very large. Thus, the public health burden of fractures cannot be solved with drug therapy. Interventions targeted to the community are needed that are safe, inexpensive, and available to all persons. Exercise fulfills these requirements, but whether exercise is efficacious, that is, reduces fracture risk, is uncertain. The purpose of this analysis is to critically examine the evidence that exercise in youth or adulthood reduces fracture risk in old age.

ANTIFRACTURE EFFICACY: THE QUALITY OF THE EVIDENCE

There has never been a randomized trial showing that exercise during growth or adulthood reduces fracture risk. Randomized, double-blind, placebo-controlled trials cannot be done. Although randomized unblinded studies with fracture endpoints are feasible, none have been done. Many observational case-control studies and prospective and retrospective cohort studies report an association with fewer fractures, but causality cannot be inferred because these studies are hypothesis generating. Sampling bias may have produced the result: fewer fractures occur in healthier individuals with better coordination and higher musculoskeletal mass, features that may be the reason exercise is taken up rather than its consequence.

For example, several studies report that individuals with a lower prevalence of "past or current physical activity" are at increased risk of hip fracture.[2,3] Other studies suggest that daily standing, climbing stairs, and walking are associated with a lower risk of hip fracture.[4-11] Although the issue of bias cannot be excluded, there does appear to be a dose-response relationship, with the most active people having fewer fractures than the most sedentary.[7] Exercise may be associated with fewer vertebral fractures,[12] whereas some studies report an increased risk for forearm fractures.[13-15]

In men, several studies report an association with lower hip fracture risk and exercise.[4,7,15-21] Karlsson and associates[22] evaluated 284 retired male soccer players. Fracture prevalence was no lower in former soccer players than in control subjects, but the small numbers of events limit the inference that can be made using these data. Wyshak and associates evaluated 2622 former female athletes aged 20 to 80 years. No fewer retired athletes had fractures than control subjects did.[23] In the Leisure World Study, individuals with an activity level of more than 1 hour per day had a reduced risk of hip fracture, an effect that was lost in women and men with reduced activity.[7] Thus, there is evidence of an association between physical activity in youth and adulthood and lower fracture risk, but sampling bias cannot be excluded.

SURROGATES OF ANTIFRACTURE EFFICACY

In lieu of credible evidence of antifracture efficacy, inferences regarding the benefits of exercise are made based on surrogate endpoints such as the effects of exercise on falls and the material and structural determinants of bone strength during growth, adulthood, and old age.

EXERCISE DURING GROWTH

There is little research examining whether exercise influences material properties of bone such as the degree of secondary mineralization of bone tissue or the extent of collagen cross-linking. There is compelling evidence that loading influences the structural properties of bone. Long-term racket players have 10% to 35% greater cortical thickness and higher bone mineral mass in the playing versus the non-playing arm.[24-27] Differences in bone mineral mass appear to be two to four times higher in the players who started training before menarche than in those who started training more than 15 years after menarche.[28] Studies in competitive athletes demonstrate biologically important changes in bone size and architecture achieved by exercise during growth.[29,30] The results of prospective and retrospective cohort and prospective intervention studies are supportive.[31-39]

Periosteal apposition is active during the prepubertal years in boys and girls. During puberty, periosteal expansion continues in boys but ceases in girls.[40-44] Endocortical contraction occurs in girls and not in boys. Effects of exercise may be partly determined by these surface- and gender-specific growth patterns, increasing bone size before puberty in boys and girls to a similar extent. At puberty, as periosteal apposition continues in boys but stops in girls, exercise may increase periosteal apposition in boys but not girls and increase endocortical apposition in girls but not in boys. Experiments addressing these possibilities have not been done.

Prepubertal gymnasts have a larger cross-sectional area of the forearm despite a smaller stature.[29] Bass and collegues[30] and Bradney and colleagues[35] reported that prepubertal gymnasts increased volumetric bone mineral density (BMD) at the midfemoral shaft due to endocortical contraction not periosteal expansion. Using quantitative computed tomography, Bass and colleagues[39] reported that exercise in the pre- and peripubertal tennis players produced a periosteal response, whereas endocortical contraction was the dominant response in the postpubertal players. The surface-specific responses may also depend on the type of sport. In tennis players, a greater proportion of the forces may be torsional, whereas in gymnasts a greater proportion may be axial. Loading after puberty increased volumetric BMD due to thicker trabeculation at the radius and medullary narrowing.[45-47] In a cross-sectional study of young tennis players, endocortical contraction was found distally and expansion proximally at the humerus.[39]

Trabecular numbers are determined at the growth plate in utero and remain constant during growth. Trabeculation of the cortex as endocortical remodeling proceeds also contributes as resorption excavates the marrow cavity during growth. Whether exercise can influence trabecular number by modifying endochondral bone formation and its regulators is unknown.

Trabeculae increase in thickness during growth and probably do so similarly in males and females, perhaps because this process is mediated through the estrogen receptor.[48,49] Loading may also mediate its effects, in part, through the estrogen receptor (ER). In vitro, strain and sex hormones increase osteoblast proliferation. The effects are additive, and the effect of testosterone is estrogen-dependent because aromatase blockers prevent the proliferative effect. In part, the effect may be mediated by insulin-like growth factor (IGF)-1 (antibodies to IGF-1 block the effect) whereas strain effects are IGF-2 dependent (antibodies to IGF-2 block the effect). It is likely that the effects are mediated through ER-α (ER-α knockouts do not respond to strain, IGF-1, or IGF-2 with osteoblast proliferation).

EXERCISE IN ADULTHOOD AND OLD AGE

Moderate exercise in adulthood has little effect in increasing bone mineral mass. Whether there is an anabolic effect on increasing bone tissue mass is not known. Aerobic exercise results in either small increases in BMD (2–3%), no change in BMD, or a decline in BMD.[50-52] Weight training produces changes of 1% to 2% and no change or a loss in BMD.[53-57] High-impact loading has a modest effect. In one study, 56 subjects were randomized to a high- or low-impact exercise group.[58] One side of the body was loaded. Increases of around 1% to 2% were found in the high-impact, low-repetition group at the trochanter, Wards triangle, and ultradistal radial site. Similar small effects (3–4%) are reported in other studies.[59,60] Thus, moderate exercise in young adult women is unlikely to result in large increases in BMD. The benefits are probably the result of changes in the remodeling space and revert once the exercise has stopped.[52,61]

Prospective studies are difficult to evaluate, as the rate of drop-out ranges from 22% to 41% and compliance is 39% to 100%. At best, these studies suggest that impact and nonimpact exercise in the elderly prevents bone loss or increases BMD by a few percentage points.[62-76] In some studies, bone loss occurs.[71,72] In a meta-analysis involving postmenopausal women (120 exercisers, 110 control subjects) from six prospective randomized or nonrandomized studies, activity increased femoral neck (FN) BMD by 2.4% (2.1% in exercisers plus the −0.3% decrease in control subjects). The drop-out rate ranged from 0% to 14%, compliance was 39 to 90%, and 67% of all studies reported significant exercise-induced skeletal benefits.[77]

Little detailed analysis has been done on the mechanisms and structural basis for any prevention of bone loss or increase in BMD in elderly people. At the onset of exercise, if activation frequency falls, sites undergoing remodeling before exercise begun will complete filling of the remodeling space and produce an increase in BMD. After steady state, if exercise suppresses remodeling, bone loss will slow. Whether exercise reduces the volume of bone removed by osteoclasts or increases bone formation by the osteoblast is not known. Does exercise reduce osteoclast generation, motility, adhesion, activity, or lifespan? Does exercise increase osteoblast production, matrix deposition, mineralization rate, or lifespan? If there are effects on periosteal apposition in old age, why are these less than during growth? Studies have not been done to explore the cellular and surface-specific effects of loading during adulthood and old age.

CESSATION OF EXERCISE

It is likely that cessation of exercise results in bone loss. When exercise is undertaken during growth, changes in bone size and shape achieved by loading may be permanent, whereas those derived by remodeling, such as endocortical accrual, or perhaps trabecular thickening, may be lost. Slowing of bone loss or modest increments in BMD induced by exercise started in adulthood are likely to be the result of filling remodeling transients that reverse when exercise is stopped.

If the effects of exercise started in youth or adulthood are lost, then why should one take up exercise? If the effects of exercise during youth can be maintained by lesser levels of exercise in later life, then information is needed defining the level of exercise needed to sustain a biologically worthwhile benefit in bone structure.

Lifetime tennis players aged 70 to 84 years playing at lower levels of intensity than during youth have a 4% to 7% higher radial bone mineral content than control subjects.[25] Retired soccer players have high BMD during the first 10 to 20 years after cessation of sport, but BMD is lower than in active soccer players.[22] Other studies suggest that BMD is maintained by about 0.5 to

1.0 SD above the age-predicted mean in athletes retired for 10 to 20 years.[22,30,78-86] Haapasalo and coworkers suggested that exercise enlarges bone size without a change in volumetric BMD.[47] This benefit was maintained after retirement. The marrow cavity was wider, not more narrow, in the playing arm, suggesting that the players had greater net endocortical resorption during activity or that bone loss occurred on the endocortical surface after retirement.[47] These observations fit with the notion that exercise produces enlargement of bone size that is permanent after retirement but that endocortical changes—maintenance due to reduced resorption or thickening due to bone formation—may be lost.

MUSCLE SIZE, MUSCLE STRENGTH, AND BONE MINERAL DENSITY

Muscle size, strength, neuromuscular fiber recruitment, and balance decrease with advancing age and correlate with the risk of falling.[87-91] Muscle strength is an independent predictor of femoral neck BMD in some, but not all, studies.[92-95] Grip strength correlates with BMD,[96] but the correlation between strength and BMD may be accounted for by muscle size.[95] It is likely that muscle size and bone size share the genetic determinants producing this association.[95] In 56 monozygotic and 56 dizygotic female twin pairs, with a mean age of 45 years (range, 24–67), genetic factors account for 60% to 80% of the variance in femoral neck BMD and lean mass and more than 50% of their covariance. Thus, higher BMD associated with a higher muscle mass does not necessarily mean exercise produced both (or either); the correlation between them may be the result of genetic factors.

EXERCISE AND FALLS

Exercise improves balance, coordination, muscle strength, reaction time, protective responses during fall, lean body mass, and mobility.[97-107] Strength can be increased by 20% to 200% even in octogenarians. This increase is greater than the increase in cross-sectional muscle area of 2% to 20% or BMD.[107-114] Minimal exercise increases muscle strength. Cessation of exercise results in loss of muscle size.[108] Less than 5% of falls lead to a fracture and only 0.2% to 1.0% of falls result in a hip fracture.[100,106,116-119] In prospective studies, hip fractures occurred in 7 of 507 falls,[119] 4 of 272 falls,[100] and 1 in 490 falls.[106] Thus, exercise may reduce falls but whether it reduces fractures is unclear.[107,120-125]

Not all studies support a reduction in risk for falls.[107,112,126] In some studies, the most inactive and the most active persons have the highest risk for fall.[120-122]

Tinetti and associates and O'Loughlin and associates also found that women who do a variety of different types of physical activity had an increased risk of falls. A Cochrane collaboration review of interventions to prevent falls in elderly people concluded that exercise alone does not reduce the risk for falls.[125-129] One study suggested that the benefits with reduced fall frequency achieved by intervention disappear 2 years after the completion of the intervention.[130] Thus, the literature is inconsistent in the reported benefits of exercise against falls, and whether exercise reduces the incidence of fractures in elderly men and women remains uncertain.

REFERENCES

1. Cooper C, Campion G, Melton LJD: Hip fractures in the elderly: a world-wide projection. Osteoporos Int 1992;2:285-89.
2. Gregg EW, Cauley JA, Seeley DG, et al: Physical activity and osteoporotic fracture risk in older women. Study of Osteoporotic Fractures Research Group. Ann Intern Med 1998;129:81-8.
3. Wickham CA, Walsh K, Cooper C, et al: Dietary calcium, physical activity, and risk of hip fracture: a prospective study. BMJ 1989;299:889-92.
4. Cooper C, Barker DJ, Wickham C: Physical activity, muscle strength, and calcium intake in fracture of the proximal femur in Britain. BMJ 1988;297:1443-46.
5. Coupland C, Wood D, Cooper C: Physical inactivity is an independent risk factor for hip fracture in the elderly. J Epidemiol Community Health 1993;47:441-43.
6. Cummings SR, Nevitt MC, Browner WS, et al: Risk factors for hip fracture in white women. Study of Osteoporotic Fractures Research Group. N Engl J Med 1995;332:767-73.
7. Paganini-Hill A, Chao A, Ross RK, Henderson BE: Exercise and other factors in the prevention of hip fracture: the Leisure World Study. Epidemiology 1991;2:16-25.
8. Farmer ME, Harris T, Madans JH, et al: Anthropometric indicators and hip fracture. The NHANES I epidemiologic follow-up study. J Am Geriatr Soc 1989;37:9-16.
9. Joakimsen RM, Fonnebo V, Magnus JH, et al: The Tromso Study: physical activity and the incidence of fractures in a middle-aged population. J Bone Miner Res 1998;13:1149-57.
10. Meyer HE, Tverdal A, Falch JA: Risk factors for hip fracture in middle-aged Norwegian women and men. Am J Epidemiol 1993;137:1203-11.
11. Johnell O, Gullberg B, Kanis JA, et al: Risk factors for hip fracture in European women: the MEDOS Study. Mediterranean Osteoporosis Study. J Bone Miner Res 1995;10:1802-15.
12. Silman AJ, O'Neill TW, Cooper C, et al: Influence of physical activity on vertebral deformity in men and women: results from the European Vertebral Osteoporosis Study. J Bone Miner Res 1997;12:813-19.
13. O'Neill TW, Marsden D, Adams JE, Silman AJ: Risk factors, falls, and fracture of the distal forearm in Manchester, UK. J Epidemiol Community Health 1996;50:288-92.
14. Mallmin H, Ljunghall S, Persson I, Bergstrom R: Risk factors for fractures of the distal forearm: a population-based case-control study. Osteoporos Int 1994;4:298-304.
15. Kelsey JL, Browner WS, Seeley DG, et al: Risk factors for fractures of the distal forearm and proximal humerus. The Study of Osteoporotic Fractures Research Group [published erratum appears in Am J Epidemiol 1992 May 15;135(10):1183]. Am J Epidemiol 1992;135:477-89.
16. Kujala UM, Kaprio J, Kannus P, et al: Physical activity and osteoporotic hip fracture risk in men. Arch Intern Med 2000;160:705-8.
17. Gregg EW, Pereira MA, Caspersen CJ: Physical activity, falls, and fractures among older adults: a review of the epidemiologic evidence. J Am Geriatr Soc 2000;48:883-93.
18. Grisso JA, Kelsey JL, O'Brien LA, et al: Risk factors for hip fracture in men. Hip Fracture Study Group. Am J Epidemiol 1997;145:786-93.
19. Chan HH, Lau EM, Woo J, et al: Dietary calcium intake, physical activity and the risk of vertebral fracture in Chinese. Osteoporos Int 1996;6:228-32.
20. Greendale GA, Barrett-Connor E, Edelstein S, et al: Lifetime leisure exercise and osteoporosis. The Rancho Bernardo study. Am J Epidemiol 1995;141:951-59.
21. Nguyen TV, Eisman JA, Kelly PJ, Sambrook PN: Risk factors for osteoporotic fractures in elderly men. Am J Epidemiol 1996;144:255-63.
22. Karlsson MK, Linden C, Karlsson C, et al: Exercise during growth and bone mineral density and fractures in old age [letter]. Lancet 2000;355:469-70.
23. Wyshak G, Frisch RE, Albright TE, et al: Bone fractures among former college athletes compared with nonathletes in the menopausal and postmenopausal years. Obstet Gynecol 1987;69:121-26.
24. Jones HH, Priest JD, Hayes WC, et al: Humeral hypertrophy in response to exercise. J Bone Joint Surg Am 1977;59:204-8.
25. Huddleston AL, Rockwell D, Kulund DN, Harrison RB: Bone mass in lifetime tennis athletes. JAMA 1980;244:1107-9.
26. Kannus P, Haapasalo H, Sievanen H, et al: The site-specific effects of long-term unilateral activity on bone mineral density and content. Bone 1994;15:279-84.
27. Haapasalo H, Sievanen H, Kannus P, et al: Dimensions and estimated mechanical characteristics of the humerus after long-term tennis loading. J Bone Miner Res 1996;11:864-72.
28. Kannus P, Haapasalo H, Sankelo M, et al: Effect of starting age of physical activity on bone mass in the dominant arm of tennis and squash players. Ann Intern Med 1995;123:27-31.
29. Dyson K, Blimkie CJ, Davison KS, et al: Gymnastic training and bone density in pre-adolescent females. Med Sci Sports Exerc 1997;29:443-50.
30. Bass S, Pearce G, Bradney M, et al: Exercise before puberty may confer residual benefits in bone density in adulthood: studies in active prepubertal and retired female gymnasts. J Bone Miner Res 1998;13:500-7.
31. Slemenda CW, Reister TK, Hui SL, et al: Influences on skeletal mineralization in children and adolescents: evidence for varying effects of sexual maturation and physical activity. J Pediatr 1994;125:201-7.
32. Cooper C, Cawley M, Bhalla A, et al: Childhood growth, physical activity, and peak bone mass in women. J Bone Miner Res 1995;10:940-47.
33. Bailey DA, McKay HA, Mirwald RL, et al: A six-year longitudinal study of the relationship of physical activity to bone mineral accrual in growing children: the University of Saskatchewan Bone Mineral Accrual Study. J Bone Miner Res 1999;14:1672-79.
34. Morris FL, Naughton GA, Gibbs JL, et al: Prospective ten-month exercise intervention in premenarcheal girls: positive effects on bone and lean mass. J Bone Miner Res 1997;12:1453-62.
35. Bradney M, Pearce G, Naughton G, et al: Moderate exercise during growth in prepubertal boys: changes in bone mass, size, volumetric density, and bone strength: a controlled prospective study. J Bone Miner Res 1998;13:1814-21.
36. McKay HA, Petit MA, Schutz RW, et al: Augmented trochanteric bone mineral density after modified physical education classes: a randomized school-based exercise intervention study in prepubescent and early pubescent children . J Pediatr 2000;136:156-62.
37. Heinonen A, Kannus P, Sievanen H, et al: Good maintenance of high-impact activity-induced bone gain by voluntary, unsupervised exercises: An 8-month follow-up of a randomized controlled trial. J Bone Miner Res 1999;14:125-28.

38. Bradney M, Karlsson MK, Duan Y, et al: Heterogeneity in the growth of the axial and appendicular skeleton in boys: implications for the pathogenesis of bone fragility in men. J Bone Miner Res 2000;15:1871-78.

39. Bass S, Saxon L, Daly R: Heterogeneity in the osteotrophic response to physical loading during different stages of puberty. J Bone Miner Res 1999;15(Suppl 1):558.

40. Turner RT, Hannon KS, Demers LM, et al: Differential effects of gonadal function on bone histomorphometry in male and female rats. J Bone Miner Res 1989;4:557-63.

41. Garn S: The earlier gain and later loss of cortical bone: nutritional perspectives. Springfield, Ill: Charles C. Thomas, 1970: 3-120.

42. Woo SL, Kuei SC, Amiel D, et al: The effect of prolonged physical training on the properties of long bone: a study of Wolff's Law. J Bone Joint Surg Am 1981;63:780-87.

43. Ruff CB, Walker A, Trinkaus E: Postcranial robusticity in Homo. III: Ontogeny. Am J Phys Anthropol 1994;93:35-54.

44. Wronski TJ, Smith JM, Jee WS: Variations in mineral apposition rate of trabecular bone within the beagle skeleton. Calcif Tissue Int 1981;33:583-86.

45. Ashizawa N, Nonaka K, Michikami S, et al: Tomographical description of tennis-loaded radius: reciprocal relation between bone size and volumetric BMD. J Appl Physiol 1999;86:1347-51.

46. Margulies JY, Simkin A, Leichter I, et al: Effect of intense physical activity on the bone-mineral content in the lower limbs of young adults. J Bone Joint Surg Am 1986;68:1090-93.

47. Haapasalo H, Kontulainen S, Sievanen H, et al: Exercise-induced bone gain is due to enlargement in bone size without a change in volumetric bone density: a peripheral quantitative computed tomography study of the upper arms of male tennis players. Bone 2000;27:351-57.

48. Damien E, Price JS, Lanyon LE: Mechanical strain stimulates osteoblast proliferation through the estrogen receptor in males as well as females. J Bone Miner Res 2000;15:2169-77.

49. Jessop HL, Suswillo RFL, Rawlinson SCF, et al: Osteoblast-like cells from estrogen receptor alpha knockout mice have deficient responses to mechanical strain. J Bone Miner Res 2004;19:938-46.

50. Bouxsein ML, Marcus R: Overview of exercise and bone mass. Rheum Dis Clin North Am 1994;20:787-802.

51. Drinkwater BL: Exercise in the prevention of osteoporosis. Osteoporos Int 1993;3(Suppl 1):169-71.

52. Forwood MR, Burr DB: Physical activity and bone mass: exercises in futility? Bone Miner 1993;21:89-112.

53. Friedlander AL, Genant HK, Sadowsky S, et al: A two-year program of aerobics and weight training enhances bone mineral density of young women. J Bone Miner Res 1995;10:574-85.

54. Gleeson PB, Protas EJ, LeBlanc AD, et al: Effects of weight lifting on bone mineral density in premenopausal women. J Bone Miner Res 1990;5:153-58.

55. Lohman T, Going S, Pamenter R, et al: Effects of resistance training on regional and total bone mineral density in premenopausal women: a randomized prospective study. J Bone Miner Res 1995;10:1015-24.

56. Rockwell JC, Sorensen AM, Baker S, et al: Weight training decreases vertebral bone density in premenopausal women: a prospective study. J Clin Endocrinol Metab 1990;71:988-93.

57. Snow-Harter C, Bouxsein ML, Lewis BT, et al: Effects of resistance and endurance exercise on bone mineral status of young women: a randomized exercise intervention trial. J Bone Miner Res 1992;7:761-9.

58. Kerr D, Morton A, Dick I, Prince R: Exercise effects on bone mass in postmenopausal women are site-specific and load-dependent. J Bone Miner Res 1996;11:218-25.

59. Bassey EJ, Ramsdale SJ: Weight-bearing exercise and ground reaction forces: a 12-month randomized controlled trial of effects on bone mineral density in healthy postmenopausal women. Bone 1995;16:469-76.

60. Heinonen A, Sievanen H, Kannus P, et al: Effects of unilateral strength training and detraining on bone mineral mass and estimated mechanical characteristics of the upper limb bones in young women. J Bone Miner Res 1996;11:490-501.

61. Vuori I, Heinonen A, Sievanen H, et al: Effects of unilateral strength training and detraining on bone mineral density and content in young women: A study of mechanical loading and deloading on human bones. Calcif Tissue Int 1994;55:59-67.

62. Cann CE, Martin MC, Genant HK, Jaffe RB: Decreased spinal mineral content in amenorrheic women. JAMA 1984;251:626-29.

63. Drinkwater BL, Nilson K, Chesnut CH, et al: Bone mineral content of amenorrheic and eumenorrheic athletes. N Engl J Med 1984;311:277-81.

64. Pearce G, Bass S, Young N, et al: Does weight-bearing exercise protect against the effects of exercise-induced oligomenorrhea on bone density? Osteoporos Int 1996;6:448-52.

65. Drinkwater BL, Nilson K, Ott S, Chesnut CH: Bone mineral density after resumption of menses in amenorrheic athletes. JAMA 1986;256:380-82.

66. Keen AD, Drinkwater BL: Irreversible bone loss in former amenorrheic athletes [editorial]. Osteoporos Int 1997;7:311-15.

67. Micklesfield LK, Reyneke L, Fataar A, Myburgh KH: Long-term restoration of deficits in bone mineral density is inadequate in premenopausal women with prior menstrual irregularity. Clin J Sport Med 1998;8:155-63.

68. Otis CL: Exercise-associated amenorrhea. Clin Sports Med 1992;11:351-62.

69. Dalsky GP, Stocke KS, Ehsani AA, et al: Weight-bearing exercise training and lumbar bone mineral content in postmenopausal women. Ann Intern Med 1988;108:824-28.

70. Nelson ME, Fiatarone MA, Morganti CM, et al: Effects of high-intensity strength training on multiple risk factors for osteoporotic fractures: a randomized controlled trial. JAMA 1994;272:1909-14.

71. Ebrahim S, Thompson PW, Baskaran V, Evans K: Randomized placebo-controlled trial of brisk walking in the prevention of postmenopausal osteoporosis. Age Ageing 1997;26:253-60.

72. Lau EM, Woo J, Leung PC, et al: The effects of calcium supplementation and exercise on bone density in elderly Chinese women. Osteoporos Int 1992;2:168-73.

73. McMurdo ME, Mole PA, Paterson CR: Controlled trial of weight bearing exercise in older women in relation to bone density and falls. BMJ 1997;314:569.

74. Prince R, Devine A, Dick I, et al: The effects of calcium supplementation (milk powder or tablets) and exercise on bone density in postmenopausal women. J Bone Miner Res 1995;10:1068-75.

75. Pruitt LA, Taaffe DR, Marcus R: Effects of a one-year high-intensity versus low-intensity resistance training program on bone mineral density in older women. J Bone Miner Res 1995;10:1788-95.

76. Hartard M, Haber P, Ilieva D, et al: Systematic strength training as a model of therapeutic intervention: a controlled trial in postmenopausal women with osteopenia. Am J Phys Med Rehabil 1996;75:21-8.

77. Kelley GA: Aerobic exercise and bone density at the hip in postmenopausal women: a meta-analysis. Prev Med 1998;27:798-807.

78. Karlsson MK, Johnell O, Obrant KJ: Bone mineral density in professional ballet dancers. Bone Miner 1993;21:163-69.

79. Karlsson MK, Johnell O, Obrant KJ: Is bone mineral density advantage maintained long-term in previous weight lifters? Calcif Tissue Int 1995;57:325-28.

80. Karlsson MK, Hasserius R, Obrant KJ: Bone mineral density in athletes during and after career: A comparison between loaded and unloaded skeletal regions. Calcif Tissue Int 1996;59:245-48.

81. Karlsson MK, Johnell O, Obrant KJ: Bone mineral density in weight lifters. Calcif Tissue Int 1993;52:212-15.

82. Khan KM, Green RM, Saul A, et al: Retired elite female ballet dancers and nonathletic controls have similar bone mineral density at weightbearing sites. J Bone Miner Res 1996;11:1566-74.

83. Duppe H, Johnell O, Lundborg G, et al: Long-term results of fracture of the scaphoid: a follow-up study of more than thirty years. J Bone Joint Surg Am 1994;76:249-52.

84. Etherington J, Harris PA, Nandra D, et al: The effect of weight-bearing exercise on bone mineral density: a study of female ex-elite athletes and the general population. J Bone Miner Res 1996;11:1333-38.

85. Kontulainen S, Kannus P, Haapasalo H, et al: Changes in bone mineral content with decreased training in competitive young adult tennis players and controls: a prospective 4-yr follow-up. Med Sci Sports Exerc 1999;31:646-52.

86. Michel BA, Lane NE, Bjorkengren A, et al: Impact of running on lumbar bone density: a 5-year longitudinal study. J Rheumatol 1992;19:1759-63.

87. Lipsitz LA, Nakajima I, Gagnon M, et al: Muscle strength and fall rates among residents of Japanese and American nursing homes: an International Cross-Cultural Study. J Am Geriatr Soc 1994;42:953-59.

88. Lord SR, Ward JA: Age-associated differences in sensori-motor function and balance in community dwelling women. Age Ageing 1994;23:452-60.

89. Hakkinen K, Hakkinen A: Neuromuscular adaptations during intensive strength training in middle-aged and elderly males and females. Electromyogr Clin Neurophysiol 1995;35:137-47.

90. Tracy BL, Ivey FM, Hurlbut D, et al: Muscle quality. II. Effects of strength training in 65- to 75-yr-old men and women. J Appl Physiol 1999;86:195-201.

91. Roman WJ, Fleckenstein J, Stray-Gundersen J, et al: Adaptations in the elbow flexors of elderly males after heavy-resistance training. J Appl Physiol 1993;74:750-54.

92. Hyakutake S, Goto S, Yamagata M, Moriya H: Relationship between bone mineral density of the proximal femur and lumbar spine and quadriceps and hamstrings torque in healthy Japanese subjects. Calcif Tissue Int 1994;55:223-29.

93. Snow-Harter C, Bouxsein M, Lewis B, et al: Muscle strength as a predictor of bone mineral density in young women. J Bone Miner Res 1990;5:589-95.

94. Pocock N, Eisman J, Gwinn T, et al: Muscle strength, physical fitness, and weight but not age predict femoral neck bone mass. J Bone Miner Res 1989;4:441-48.

95. Seeman E, Hopper JL, Young NR, et al: Do genetic factors explain associations between muscle strength, lean mass, and bone density? A twin study. Am J Physiol 1996;270:E320-7.

96. Kritz-Silverstein D, Barrett-Connor E: Grip strength and bone mineral density in older women. J Bone Miner Res 1994;9:45-51.

97. Tinetti ME, Williams TF, Mayewski R: Fall risk index for elderly patients based on number of chronic disabilities. Am J Med 1986;80:429-34.

98. Wolfson LI, Whipple R, Amerman P, Kleinberg A: Stressing the postural response: a quantitative method for testing balance. J Am Geriatr Soc 1986;34:845-50.

99. Overstall PW, Johnson AL, Exton-Smith AN: Instability and falls in the elderly. Age Ageing 1978;Suppl:92-6.

100. Tinetti ME, Speechley M, Ginter SF: Risk factors for falls among elderly persons living in the community. N Engl J Med 1988;319:1701-7.

101. Myers AH, Young Y, Langlois JA: Prevention of falls in the elderly. Bone 1996;18(1 Suppl):87S-101S.

102. Fiatarone MA, O'Neill EF, Ryan ND, et al: Exercise training and nutritional supplementation for physical frailty in very elderly people. N Engl J Med 1994;330:1769-75.

103. Daley MJ, Spinks WL: Exercise, mobility and aging. Sports Med 2000;29:1-12.

104. Nevitt MC, Cummings SR, Hudes ES: Risk factors for injurious falls: a prospective study. J Gerontol 1991;46:M164-70.

105. Hu MH, Woollacott MH: Multisensory training of standing balance in older adults: II. Kinematic and electromyographic postural responses. J Gerontol 1994;49:M62-71.

106. Nevitt MC, Cummings SR, Kidd S, Black D: Risk factors for recurrent nonsyncopal falls: a prospective study. JAMA 1989;261:2663-68.

107. Province MA, Hadley EC, Hornbrook MC, et al: The effects of exercise on falls in elderly patients. A preplanned meta-analysis of the FICSIT Trials. Frailty and Injuries: Cooperative Studies of Intervention Techniques. JAMA 1995;273:1341-47.

108. Fiatarone MA, Marks EC, Ryan ND, et al: High-intensity strength training in nonagenarians: effects on skeletal muscle. JAMA 1990;263:3029-34.

109. Hakkinen K, Komi PV: Alterations of mechanical characteristics of human skeletal muscle during strength training. Eur J Appl Physiol 1983;50:161-72.

110. Narici MV, Roi GS, Landoni L, et al: Changes in force, cross-sectional area and neural activation during strength training and detraining of the human quadriceps. Eur J Appl Physiol 1989;59:310-19.

111. Pyka G, Lindenberger E, Charette S, Marcus R: Muscle strength and fiber adaptations to a year-long resistance training program in elderly men and women. J Gerontol 1994;49:M22-7.

112. Lord SR, Ward JA, Williams P, Strudwick M: The effect of a 12-month exercise trial on balance, strength, and falls in older women: a randomized controlled trial. J Am Geriatr Soc 1995;43:1198-206.

113. Heislein DM, Harris BA, Jette AM: A strength training program for postmenopausal women: a pilot study. Arch Phys Med Rehabil 1994;75:198-204.

114. Ryan AS, Treuth MS, Rubin MA, et al: Effects of strength training on bone mineral density: hormonal and bone turnover relationships. J Appl Physiol 1994;77:1678-84.

115. Campbell AJ, Borrie MJ, Spears GF: Risk factors for falls in a community-based prospective study of people 70 years and older. J Gerontol 1989;44:M112-7.

116. Grisso JA, Kelsey JL, Strom BL, et al: Risk factors for falls as a cause of hip fracture in women. The Northeast Hip Fracture Study Group. N Engl J Med 1991;324:1326-31.

117. Greenspan SL, Myers ER, Maitland LA, et al: Fall severity and bone mineral density as risk factors for hip fracture in ambulatory elderly. JAMA 1994;271:128-33.

118. Hayes WC, Myers ER, Morris JN, et al: Impact near the hip dominates fracture risk in elderly nursing home residents who fall. Calcif Tissue Int 1993;52:192-98.

119. Campbell AJ, Borrie MJ, Spears GF, et al: Circumstances and consequences of falls experienced by a community population 70 years and over during a prospective study [published erratum appears in Age Ageing 1990 Sep;19(5):345-6]. Age Ageing 1990;19:136-41.

120. Tinetti ME, Inouye SK, Gill TM, Doucette JT: Shared risk factors for falls, incontinence, and functional dependence: unifying the approach to geriatric syndromes. JAMA 1995;273:1348-53.

121. O'Loughlin JL, Robitaille Y, Boivin JF, Suissa S: Incidence of and risk factors for falls and injurious falls among the community-dwelling elderly. Am J Epidemiol 1993;137:342-54.

122. Graafmans WC, Ooms ME, Hofstee HM, et al: Falls in the elderly: a prospective study of risk factors and risk profiles. Am J Epidemiol 1996;143:1129-36.

123. Wolf SL, Barnhart HX, Kutner NG, et al: Reducing frailty and falls in older persons: an investigation of Tai Chi and comput-erized balance training. Atlanta FICSIT Group. Frailty and Injuries: Cooperative Studies of Intervention Techniques. J Am Geriatr Soc 1996;44:489-97.

124. Tinetti ME, Baker DI, McAvay G, et al: A multifactorial intervention to reduce the risk of falling among elderly people living in the community. N Engl J Med 1994;331:821-27.

125. Campbell AJ, Robertson MC, Gardner MM, et al: Falls prevention over 2 years: a randomized controlled trial in women 80 years and older. Age Ageing 1999;28:513-8.

126. Hornbrook MC, Stevens VJ, Wingfield DJ, et al: Preventing falls among community-dwelling older persons: results from a randomized trial. Gerontologist 1994;34:16-23.

127. Mulrow CD, Gerety MB, Kanten D, et al: A randomized trial of physical rehabilitation for very frail nursing home residents. JAMA 1994;271:519-24.

128. Gillespie LD, Gillespie WJ, Cumming R, et al: Interventions for preventing falls in the elderly. Cochrane Database Syst Rev 2000;(2):CD000340.

129. Rubenstein LZ, Josephson KR, Robbins AS: Falls in the nursing home. Ann Intern Med 1994;121:442-51.

130. Wagner EH, LaCroix AZ, Grothaus L, et al: Preventing disability and falls in older adults: a population-based randomized trial. Am J Public Health 1994;84:1800-6.

13

The Use of Calcium Supplementation in the Management and Prevention of Osteoporosis

Dina Kulik and Rick Adachi

OSTEOPOROSIS: A DEBILITATING DISEASE THAT CAN BE PREVENTED AND TREATED

Osteoporosis is a progressive skeletal disease in which bones become fragile and more likely to break. Bone fragility is due to the low bone mass and microarchitectural deterioration of bone tissue in osteoporotic patients.[1] If not prevented or if left untreated, osteoporosis can progress painlessly until a bone breaks. These broken bones, or fractures, occur typically in the hip, spine, and wrist.[1] Osteoporosis can occur as a result of poor bone growth in childhood and adolescence, or as a result of bone loss.[2] Although women are more likely than men to develop the disease, men also suffer from osteoporosis and fractures.[3] Both men and women have a decline in bone mineral density (BMD) beginning in the fourth decade of life, and women experience an accelerated decline after menopause.[4] Because women have a longer lifespan than men, have smaller bones, and suffer an accelerated loss of bone mass after menopause, their lifetime risk of osteoporotic fracture is higher than that of men. The lifetime risk of osteoporotic fracture at the age of 50 years for white people, taking into account future mortality trends, has been estimated at 47% for women and 22% for men.[5]

Any bone can be affected, but of special concern are fractures of the hip and spine. A hip fracture almost always requires hospitalization and major surgery. It can impair a person's ability to walk unassisted and may cause prolonged or permanent disability or even death. The risk of sustaining a hip fracture throughout life is 23% for women and 11% for men at 50 years of age.[5] Spinal or vertebral fractures also have serious consequences, including loss of height, severe back pain, and deformity. The risk of sustaining vertebral fractures is approximately 15% for women and 8% for men.[5] More recent data suggest that there may be an even greater prevalence of vertebral fractures in men.[3] The prevalence of all types of fractures rises with increasing age, and the risk of hip and vertebral fracture rises exponentially.[6] Farmer and colleagues[6] found that in white women, the incidence of hip fracture rises from 50 per 100,000 at 50 years of age to 237 per 100,000 at 65 years of age. It is projected that as the global population ages, there will be dramatic increases in the incidence of osteoporosis and the risk of fracture. In addition, the rise of osteoporotic fracture is independent of demographic changes, owing to factors such as less active lifestyles, increased use of alcohol and psychotropic drugs, and increased body height.[7,8] Therefore, osteoporosis has become a growing health care problem across Europe and North America.

CONSEQUENCES OF OSTEOPOROSIS

Osteoporotic fractures not only have physical consequences for the patient but can have psychological and social consequences as well. Fractures in the vertebrae can cause loss of height, back pain, immobility, and deformity and can lead to decreased pulmonary function,[9-13] whereas hip fractures can cause chronic pain, disability, and dependence on others.[14] Depression and poor body image can result, as can a loss of self-esteem.[9,12,15-19] As a result of these fractures, the rate of nursing home admissions rises with age, and 10% to 20% of patients living in the community require long-term care after sustaining a hip fracture.[20]

Excess mortality is a result of osteoporotic fractures.[21,22] A 50-year-old woman's risk of dying as a result of sustaining a hip fracture is equivalent to the risk of death from breast cancer and four times higher than the risk of death from endometrial cancer.[23] Patients younger than 70 years also contribute to the excess mortality associated with osteoporosis.[24]

Osteoporosis has a major financial consequence as well, owing to the disease's high prevalence and morbidity rate. Lippunner and associates found that the cost of hospitalization for people sustaining osteoporotic fractures in Switzerland was higher than the cost for those admitted with myocardial infarction, breast cancer, and stroke.[25] Nearly 500,000 Europeans sustain hip fracture each year, costing approximately € 4.8 billion.[26] Costs associated with patients after hospital release, including nursing care, are substantial.[27] Although techniques used to diagnose and treat osteoporosis have been developed, men and women are still underdiagnosed and undertreated; therefore, health care costs associated with osteoporosis are expected to rise dramatically.[28,29]

CALCIUM SUPPLEMENTATION AND ITS EFFECTS

Although the focus of this chapter is on calcium, it is very difficult to discuss calcium in isolation from vitamin D. Hence, where appropriate, we have included vitamin D in our discussion; however, it is discussed in greater depth in Chapter 14. The medical and nutritional communities have known of the importance of calcium and vitamin D in bone health since the early 1990s,[30-33] as women with low milk intake during childhood and adolescence have been shown to have less bone mass in adulthood and greater risk of fracture.[34] For example, Matkovic and coworkers[35] found that nutrition, particularly calcium intake, is an important determinant of bone mass in young adults. However, it was found that nutritional intake had little effect on age-related bone loss in males and females. Other nutrients have been shown to be critical to BMD as well, such as energy, protein, calcium, magnesium, zinc, and vitamin C.[36] Peak bone mass is determined in part by calcium intake, which helps develop strong bones in adolescence and slows bone loss later in life.[30-33] Vitamin D deficiency impairs calcium absorption and causes an increase in parathyroid hormone, leading to bone resorption and increased bone loss.[4,37-41] Therefore, calcium and vitamin D are important elements that protect against osteoporosis by preventing increased bone resorption caused by secondary hyperparathyroidism. Because elderly people are particularly susceptible to vitamin D deficiency owing to lack of sunlight exposure and the decreased capacity of the skin to produce vitamin D_3 with age, vitamin D deficiency is an important risk factor for osteoporosis, especially in elderly populations.

Although there is no universal consensus on the optimal daily calcium intake, the Food and Nutrition Board of the Institute of Medicine, National Academy of Sciences in the United States, predicts that 1200 mg/day of calcium for people older than 50 years is adequate and 1000 mg/day for younger adults is appropriate.[42] In Europe, the recommended intake for all ages is 700 to 800 mg/day.[43] The amount of vitamin D that is required depends on the presence of ultra-violet light exposure and race, age, social condition, and geographic location. Europeans are advised to have an intake of up to 400 IU of vitamin D daily up to the age of 65 and 400 IU daily after 65 years of age.[43] Unfortunately, many do not reach the ideal intake of calcium and vitamin D.[41,44] Elderly individuals are least likely to reach adequate daily intakes because of low dietary intakes and inadequate sun exposure.[45] As the elderly are often deficient in both calcium and vitamin D, both calcium and vitamin D should be supplemented to improve bone health.

Organization	Recommended Calcium Intake	Recommended Vitamin D Intake
The Food and Nutrition Board of the Institute of Medicine	1200 mg/day for those >50 yr 1000 mg/day for those <50 yr	
Europe	700-800 mg/day	400IU/day

The World Health Organization (WHO) Collaborating Centre for Public Health Aspects of Rheumatic Diseases (Liege, Belgium) and the WHO Collaborating Centre for Osteoporosis Prevention (Geneva, Switzerland) along with an international expert panel met in Barcelona in 2002 to discuss the implications for the use of calcium and vitamin D in the prevention and treatment of osteoporosis. As a result of this meeting, the European Union (EU) Directive 2002/46/EC on vitamins and minerals used as ingredients of food supplements with physiological of nutritional effect was enforced in 2003. The panel concluded that osteoporosis requires continuing medical attention to ensure the best therapeutic effects and that calcium and vitamin D supplementation have been shown to be safe and effective agents in the prevention and treatment of osteoporosis and osteoporotic fractures. It was determined that calcium and vitamin D are first-line medications in the management of osteoporosis and are cost-efficient options in the prevention and treatment of this disease. However, the panel found that many patients with osteoporosis would also require antiresorptive therapy in addition to this vitamin and mineral supplementation. The panel concluded that the public does not know the efficacy of this form of osteoporosis treatment, and that awareness among physicians and patients, particularly women, is low. It was suggested that calcium and vitamin D continue to be produced to Good Manufacturing Practice standards and that they be prescribed in optimal amounts so that they can continue to be classified as medicinal products.[46]

CALCIUM SUPPLEMENTATION IN CHILDREN

Johnston and colleagues[47] found that prepubertal twins given calcium supplements had significantly greater increases in bone mineral density at radial sites and in the lumbar spine after 3 years than twins who did not receive supplementation. It was concluded that even in prepubertal children whose dietary intake of calcium approached that of the recommended dietary allowance, calcium supplementation increased the rate of increase in BMD. If this gain persisted, a high peak bone density and a reduced risk of fracture were deemed possible. Rozen and colleagues[48] demonstrated in 2003 that calcium supplementation of postmenarcheal girls with low calcium intakes enhances bone mineral acquisition, especially in girls more than 2 years past the onset of menarche. Similarly, calcium supplementation and exercise enhance bone mineral status in adolescent girls.[49]

DIETARY CALCIUM IN POSTMENOPAUSAL WOMEN

Providing women with high-calcium skimmed milk has also been shown to reduce the rate of bone loss at clinically important lumbar spine and hip sites in postmenopausal Chinese women in Malaysia.[50] Similarly, dietary improvements in elderly women with low bone mass index is associated with a reduction in bone resorption with a small but "net" positive effect on bone formation.[51]

CALCIUM SUPPLEMENTATION IN POSTMENOPAUSAL WOMEN

As many individuals have been found to be deficient in calcium or vitamin D, or both, researchers have begun to study the effects of supplementation (Figure 13-1). Some researchers, such as Ulrich and associates,[52] found that there is no significant short-term effect of calcium supplementation on biochemical markers of either bone resorption or formation. Michaelson and associates[53] and Lamke and associates[54] have found no evidence to indicate that a high dietary calcium or vitamin D intake is of value in the primary prevention of osteoporotic fractures in women. Other studies, however, have shown the benefits of supplementation. For example, Dawson-Hughes and colleagues[55] concluded that healthy older postmenopausal women with a daily calcium intake of 400 mg or less can significantly reduce bone loss by increasing calcium intake to 800 mg per day and that calcium citrate malate supplementation was a more effective supplement than calcium carbonate. Similarly, Recker and colleagues[56] found that in elderly postmenopausal women with spinal fractures and calcium intakes of less than 1 g/day, calcium supplementation of 1.2 g/day reduces the incidence of spinal fractures and prevents bone loss. Prince and colleagues[57] found that calcium supplementation in postmenopausal women (at least 10 years after menopausal onset) by either calcium tablets or milk powder resulted in the prevention of bone loss and fracture at the intertrochanteric hip site, the

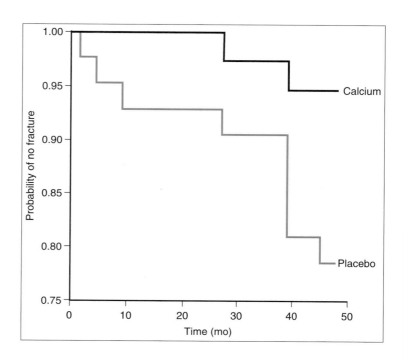

Figure 13-1. Probability of no fracture in postmenopausal women treated with calcium supplementation or placebo for 4 years. The difference in fracture rates between the two groups was significant ($P = .037$). (From Nieves JW, Komar L, Cosman F, Lindsay R: Calcium potentiates the effect of estrogen and calcitonin on bone mass: review and analysis. Am J Clin Nutr 1998:67:18-24.)

trochanteric hip site, the femoral neck site and at the tibia. Reid and coworkers[58] found that calcium supplementation in postmenopausal women (at least 3 years after menopausal onset) reduced the rate of loss of BMD of the total body. Much of the difference in trial results would appear to be related to differences in age. Young postmenopausal women do not have any apparent benefit whereas elderly postmenopausal women do benefit. This may be explained by the dominant effects of menopause over calcium on bone metabolism. In addition, it may be that many younger postmenopausal women are more likely to have adequate vitamin D stores compared with older women, who may be less efficient in synthesizing vitamin D and metabolizing it to its active metabolites.

Cooper and colleagues[59] found that in younger postmenopausal women whose average baseline serum 25-hydroxyvitamin D concentration was well within the normal range, the addition of 10,000 IU vitamin D_2 per week to calcium supplementation at 1000 mg per day did not confer benefits on BMD beyond those achieved with calcium supplementation alone. Therefore, individuals may only benefit from calcium and vitamin D supplementation if they have insufficient calcium and vitamin D intakes. Similarly, it has been shown that calcium and vitamin D_3 supplements only had minor influences of uncertain significance on the calcium balance in healthy, calcium- and vitamin D–sufficient early postmenopausal women.[60] In addition, Riis and associates[61] found that calcium supplementation has only a minor effect on the loss of cortical bone and no effect on the loss of trabecular bone in early postmenopausal women.

In older individuals, however, Grados and colleagues[62] confirmed that there is a high prevalence of calcium and vitamin D deficiencies in elderly female outpatients in France. In this population, calcium and vitamin D supplementation was effective in correcting these deficiencies and in returning 25-hydroxyvitamin D values to normal. Simultaneously, bone remodeling slowed and BMD increased. Grados[63] also demonstrated that short-term changes in bone resorption markers can predict long-term variations in BMD in elderly women with vitamin D insufficiency receiving calcium and vitamin D supplementation. A study by Larsen and associates[64] supported the idea that vitamin D and calcium supplementation may prevent osteoporotic fractures in community-dwelling elderly people in the northern European region known to be deficient in vitamin D, especially during winter periods. Dawson-Hughes and associates[65] found that healthy postmenopausal women with vitamin D intakes of 100 IU daily can significantly reduce spinal bone loss in the winter by increasing the intake of vitamin D to 500 IU each day. They observed that changes

in bone, lean tissue, and fat were related to season. Furthermore, Dawson-Hughes[66] has concluded that adequate calcium intake may help promote the favorable effect of dietary protein (which promotes osteoblast-mediated bone formation) on the skeleton in older individuals.

The combined supplementation of calcium and vitamin D reduces the risk of fractures. Chapuy and coworkers showed in a randomized, double-blind, multicenter, placebo-controlled trial that providing elderly people in institutions with both calcium and vitamin D reduces the risk of nonvertebral fractures.[67-69] A total of 3270 women with inadequate dietary calcium intakes at baseline were included in this study, and 44% of these subjects were vitamin D deficient as well. At 36 months, the supplementation was shown to reduce the incidence of hip fractures by 23% and of all nonvertebral fractures by 17.2%.[68] Of those who received vitamin D therapy, there was a 29% reduction in hip fractures and a 24% reduction in all nonvertebral fractures. The benefits of this calcium and vitamin D supplementation were seen after 1 year,[67,69] and 46 hip fractures and 21 nonvertebral fractures were prevented. BMD changes were seen at 18 months, with the BMD of the proximal femur increasing by 2.7%, with a 4.6% decrease in the placebo group. The researchers also noticed improvements in secondary hyperparathyroidism. Average parathyroid hormone levels decreased by 35% and vitamin D levels increased by 150%. Most benefits from the supplementation were seen at 6 months, and several of the patients with elevated parathyroid hormone and low vitamin D levels at the beginning of the study had normal values by the end of the study.[68] Harwood and colleagues[70] found similar results in their 2003 study. They found that vitamin D supplementation, either orally or injected, suppressed parathyroid hormone, increased bone mineral density, and reduced the incidence of falls. They concluded that these effects might be more marked with calcium co-supplementation, highlighting the benefits of supplementation with both calcium and vitamin D. Riggs and colleagues[71] found that long-term administration of calcium to elderly women partially reversed age-related increases in parathyroid hormone and decreased bone loss. They concluded that calcium supplementation could be effectively used to prevent bone loss in elderly postmenopausal women with normal bone mineral density values for their age.

Daily supplementation with 500 mg of calcium and 700 IU of vitamin D more than halved the incidence of nonvertebral fractures in a study of 389 subjects 65 years of age and older. During the course of the study, members of the placebo group sustained 26 fractures, whereas members of the supplemented group sustained only 11 fractures.[72] Trivedi and coworkers[73] studied the benefits of high doses of vitamin D over long periods. Researchers provided 100,000 IU of vitamin D_3 to patients every 4 months and saw a decrease in the incidence of fractures caused by osteoporosis.

Recently Shea and associates[74] concluded that calcium and vitamin D supplementation has some benefit in preventing the onset of osteoporosis. The addition of calcium alone, although not significant, was found to have some beneficial effects on its own.[74] The addition of vitamin D supplementation, however, provided a further significant reduction on osteoporotic fractures.[75] Although no specified type of calcium has been proven to prevent fractures better than any other type, Kenney and colleagues[76] have shown that calcium citrate supplementation decreases the collagen cross-link resorption markers, urinary N-telopeptide, C-telopeptide, free deoxypyridinoline, and serum N-telopeptide, compared with no significant change after calcium carbonate supplementation. Further studies of various calcium treatments can help elucidate the most effective form of calcium supplementation.

CALCIUM AND VITAMIN D SUPPLEMENTATION: A COST-EFFECTIVE MEASURE

It has been determined that calcium and vitamin D supplementation has proved efficacy in preventing osteoporotic fractures. This form of prevention and treatment is a cost-effective one, owing to the high economic cost of treating osteoporotic patients and the low cost of providing patients and those at risk of developing osteoporosis with this supplementation. Lilliu and colleagues[77] studied the cost-effectiveness of supplying institutionalized women with 1200 mg/day of calcium and 800 IU/day of vitamin D. Using the seven European countries involved in the Chapuy trial, they found that the total costs in the placebo groups were higher than in the groups supplemented with calcium and vitamin D. A net benefit of €79,000 to €711,000 per 1000 women was seen. Because treatment is also effective in decreasing the incidence of nonvertebral fractures, this cost analysis may be an underestimate. Therefore, Lilliu and colleagues found that calcium and vitamin D_3 supplementation is cost-effective in hip fracture prevention and concluded that calcium and vitamin D should be a first-line preventative and therapeutic measure of osteoporosis. Rosner and colleagues[78] agree that calcium and vitamin D therapy is in fact cost-saving.

CALCIUM AND VITAMIN D THERAPY IN CLINICAL PRACTICE

Calcium and vitamin D have been shown to be effective in the prevention and management of osteoporosis when prescribed in controlled and appropriate amounts in trials. To ensure optimum efficacy and safety, clinicians should supervise the supplementation of calcium and vitamin D according to the WHO and the panel of osteoporosis experts' guidelines.

According to a survey conducted in 1999 by the International Osteoporosis Foundation,[26] most women are aware of the seriousness of osteoporosis, but only 20% believed they were at risk themselves. Awareness or personal risk of osteoporosis was found to be low among both men and women, and fewer men than women are aware that osteoporosis can affect men.[79] Furthermore, the International Osteoporosis Foundation survey demonstrated that less than one-third of physicians discuss osteoporosis with their patients and their awareness of the disease and its diagnosis is low.

Therefore, although many people know that osteoporosis exists and has serious consequences, most individuals do not think they will be affected by this disease and do not seek preventative and therapeutic care for themselves. Compliance with therapy is likely to be better for individuals who discuss osteoporosis with their physician and follow up with the physician on a regular basis. According to the WHO, if financial reimbursements are provided and calcium and vitamin D are classified as medicinal products, patients are more likely to continue with the long-term supplementation. Dawson-Hughes and colleagues[80] showed that long-term compliance was essential, as the benefits of calcium and vitamin D supplementation fade in the femoral neck 2 years after treatment withdrawal.

CALCIUM AND VITAMIN D SUPPLEMENTATION AS ADJUNCTIVE THERAPY

Hormone replacement therapy (HRT) is commonly used by postmenopausal women to replace lost estrogen and prevent bone loss. However, there is evidence that HRT is less effective in patients with low calcium and vitamin D serum levels, and they cannot reach their full effect.[81-84] For example, a recent Finnish OSTPRE study concluded that low calcium intake might be a risk factor for nonresponse from HRT.[84] Sirola and colleagues found the nutritional calcium intake may protect HRT users from bone loss, and low nutritional calcium intake may be a risk factor for nonresponse to HRT.[84] Similarly, Nieves and coworkers[83] demonstrated that an annual increase in lumbar bone mass of patients given estrogen alone was 1.3%, whereas those receiving calcium and estrogen had an increase of 3.3% (Figure 13-2).

Likewise, Masaud and coworkers[82] found that supplementation with calcium and calcitonin increased lumbar spine bone mass by 2.1%, versus a decrease of 0.2% in those with calcitonin supplementation alone.

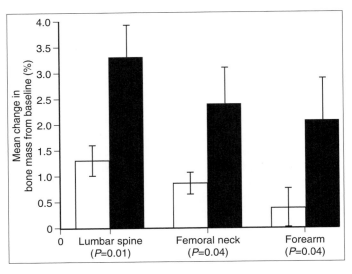

Figure 13-2. Mean (± SEM) annual percentage change in bone mass at the lumbar spine, femoral neck, and forearm in postmenopausal women treated with estrogen alone (white bars; total average calcium intake, 563 mg/d) compared with estrogen and calcium (black bars; total average calcium intake, 1183 mg/d). (From Nieves JW, Komar L, Cosman F, Lindsay R: Calcium potentiates the effect of estrogen and calcitonin on bone mass: review and analysis. Am J Clin Nutr 1998;67:18-24.)

Other studies have shown even greater results with the addition of other hormones.

Prince and associates[85] found that in postmenopausal women with low bone density, bone loss can be slowed or prevented through exercise plus calcium supplementation or hormone replacement therapy. They found that the exercise-hormone regimen was more effective than the exercise-calcium regimen, although it caused more side effects than the other regimen. Ettinger and associates[86] found that with calcium supplementation, the dose of estrogen could be reduced. Similarly, Strause and associates[87] found that bone loss in older postmenopausal women can be prevented with calcium supplementation as well as trace mineral supplementation. Therefore, to achieve maximum benefits, patients with osteoporosis should receive an antiresorptive agent along with calcium and vitamin supplements, and the addition of other agents can further aid in the protection of bone.

THE BENEFITS OF EXERCISE AND CALCIUM IN PREVENTING OSTEOPOROTIC FRACTURES

Patients with osteoporosis can benefit greatly from exercise in addition to calcium and vitamin D supplementation. Results demonstrate that regional BMD can be improved with aerobic, weight-bearing activity combined with weight lifting at clinically relevant sites in postmenopausal women.[88] Overall, in recently postmenopausal women who are in good health and are believed to have a fairly low fracture risk, optimizing the daily calcium intake and faithfully adhering to a program of athletic activities or workouts can help to maintain a satisfactory bone mass.[89] Nelson and coworkers found that trabecular BMD at the lumbar spine increased by 0.5% in exercising postmenopausal women and decreased by 7% in sedentary women. Femoral neck BMD increased by 2% in women consuming high dietary calcium and decreased by 1.1% in those with moderate calcium intake. Therefore, the researchers conclude that a high-calcium diet with exercise can effectively protect against bone loss and fracture.[90] Similarly, calcium supplementation and exercise enhance bone mineral status in adolescent girls.[49] However, whether this is a lasting benefit, leading to the optimization of peak bone mass and a reduction in fracture risk, needs to be determined.

CONCLUSIONS

Osteoporosis is a progressive skeletal disease requiring medical attention and supervision to prevent fracture. Calcium and vitamin D supplementation has been shown to reduce the incidence of osteoporotic fractures if given in appropriate, safe doses. The combined calcium and vitamin D supplementation is a cost-effective measure in preventing and treating osteoporosis. In addition, the combination of calcium, vitamin D, and antiresorptive supplementation will benefit those with osteoporosis. Awareness among physicians, patients, and people at risk is low, and prevention and treatment of osteoporosis can be increased through increased education. If more education and research are conducted regarding osteoporosis and the disease's risks and methods of prevention, the incidence of osteoporotic fracture can be reduced. Specifically, patients and those at risk must be monitored for exercise, calcium, and vitamin D levels to maintain adequate and optimal amounts of this mineral and vitamin both through dietary intake and through supplementation.

REFERENCES

1. Assessment of fracture risk and its application to screening for postmenopausal osteoporosis. Report of a WHO Study Group. World Health Organ Tech Rep Ser 1994;843:1-129.

2. Hui SL, Slemenda CW, Johnston CC Jr: The contribution of bone loss to postmenopausal osteoporosis. Osteoporos Int 1990;1:30-4.

3. Jackson SA, Tenenhouse A, Robertson L: Vertebral fracture definition from population-based data: preliminary results from the Canadian Multicenter Osteoporosis Study (CaMos). Osteoporos Int 2000;11:680-87.

4. Boonen S, Vanderschueren D, Cheng XG, et al: Age-related (type II) femoral neck osteoporosis in men: biochemical evidence for both hypovitaminosis D- and androgen deficiency-induced bone resorption. J Bone Miner Res 1997;12:2119-26.

5. Kanis JA, Johnell O, Oden A, et al: Long-term risk of osteoporotic fracture in Malmo. Osteoporos Int 2000;11:669-74.

6. Farmer ME, White LR, Brody JA, Bailey KR: Race and sex differences in hip fracture incidence. Am J Public Health 1984;74:1374-80.

7. Reginster JY, Gillet P, Gosset C: Secular increase in the incidence of hip fractures in Belgium between 1984 and 1996: need for a concerted public health strategy. Bull World Health Organ 2001;79:942-46.

8. Kannus P, Niemi S, Parkkari J, et al: Hip fractures in Finland between 1970 and 1997 and predictions for the future. Lancet 1999;353:802-5.

9. Gold DT: The clinical impact of vertebral fractures: quality of life in women with osteoporosis. Bone 1996;18(3 Suppl):185S-9S.

10. Schlaich C, Minne HW, Bruckner T, et al: Reduced pulmonary function in patients with spinal osteoporotic fractures. Osteoporos Int 1998;8:261-67.

11. Nevitt MC, Ettinger B, Black DM, et al: The association of radiographically detected vertebral fractures with back pain and function: a prospective study. Ann Intern Med 1998;128:793-800.

12. Lips P, Cooper C, Agnusdei D, et al: Quality of life in patients with vertebral fractures: Validation of the Quality of Life Questionnaire of the European Foundation for Osteoporosis (QUALEFFO). Working Party for Quality of Life of the European Foundation for Osteoporosis. Osteoporos Int 1999;10:150-60.

13. Pluijm SM, Dik MG, Jonker C, et al: Effects of gender and age on the association of apolipoprotein E epsilon4 with bone mineral density, bone turnover and the risk of fractures in older people. Osteoporos Int 2002;13:701-9.

14. Keene GS, Parker MJ, Pryor GA: Mortality and morbidity after hip fractures. BMJ 1993;307:1248-50.

15. Hall SE, Criddle RA, Comito TL, Prince RL: A case-control study of quality of life and functional impairment in women with long-standing vertebral osteoporotic fracture. Osteoporos Int 1999;9:508-15.

16. Gold DT: The nonskeletal consequences of osteoporotic fractures: Psychologic and social outcomes. Rheum Dis Clin North Am 2001;27:255-62.

17. Robbins J, Hirsch C, Whitmer R, et al: The association of bone mineral density and depression in an older population. J Am Geriatr Soc 2001;49:732-36.

18. Lyles KW: Osteoporosis and depression: shedding more light upon a complex relationship. J Am Geriatr Soc 2001;49:827-28.

19. Tosteson AN, Gabriel SE, Grove MR, et al: Impact of hip and vertebral fractures on quality-adjusted life years. Osteoporos Int 2001;12:1042-49.

20. Cree M, Soskolne CL, Belseck E, et al: Mortality and institutionalization following hip fracture. J Am Geriatr Soc 2000;48:283-88.

21. Trombetti A, Herrmann F, Hoffmeyer P, et al: Survival and potential years of life lost after hip fracture in men and age-matched women. Osteoporos Int 2002;13:731-37.

22. Cauley JA, Thompson DE, Ensrud KC, et al: Risk of mortality following clinical fractures. Osteoporos Int 2000;11:556-61.

23. Cummings SR, Black DM, Rubin SM: Lifetime risks of hip, Colles', or vertebral fracture and coronary heart disease among white postmenopausal women. Arch Intern Med 1989;149:2445-48.

24. Center JR, Nguyen TV, Schneider D, et al: Mortality after all major types of osteoporotic fracture in men and women: an observational study. Lancet 1999;353:878-82.

25. Lippuner K, von Overbeck J, Perrelet R, et al: Incidence and direct medical costs of hospitalizations due to osteoporotic fractures in Switzerland. Osteoporos Int 1997;7:414-25.

26. International Osteoporosis Foundation. Survey by Helmut Minne. 2004. Ref Type: Report

27. Autier P, Haentjens P, Bentin J, et al: Costs induced by hip fractures: a prospective controlled study in Belgium. Belgian Hip Fracture Study Group. Osteoporos Int 2000;11:373-80.

28. Kiebzak GM, Beinart GA, Perser K, et al: Undertreatment of osteoporosis in men with hip fracture. Arch Intern Med 2002;162:2217-22.

29. Colditz GA, Manson JE, Hankinson SE: The Nurses' Health Study: 20-year contribution to the understanding of health among women. J Womens Health 1997;6:49-62.

30. Heaney RP: Nutritional factors in osteoporosis. Annu Rev Nutr 1993;13:287-316.

31. Valimaki MJ, Karkkainen M, Lamberg-Allardt C, et al: Exercise, smoking, and calcium intake during adolescence and early adulthood as determinants of peak bone mass. Cardiovascular Risk in Young Finns Study Group. BMJ 1994;309:230-35.

32. Bonjour JP, Carrie AL, Ferrari S, et al: Calcium-enriched foods and bone mass growth in prepubertal girls: a randomized, double-blind, placebo-controlled trial. J Clin Invest 1997;99:1287-94.

33. Lehtonen-Veromaa MK, Mottonen TT, Nuotio IO, et al: Vitamin D and attainment of peak bone mass among peripubertal Finnish girls: a 3-yr prospective study. Am J Clin Nutr 2002;76:1446-53.

34. Kalkwarf HJ, Khoury JC, Lanphear BP: Milk intake during childhood and adolescence, adult bone density, and osteoporotic fractures in US women. Am J Clin Nutr 2003;77:257-65.

35. Matkovic V, Kostial K, Simonovic I, et al: Bone status and fracture rates in two regions of Yugoslavia. Am J Clin Nutr 1979;32:540-49.

36. Ilich JZ, Brownbill RA, Tamborini L: Bone and nutrition in elderly women: protein, energy, and calcium as main determinants of bone mineral density. Eur J Clin Nutr 2003;57:554-65.

37. Boonen S, Aerssens J, Dequeker J: Age-related endocrine deficiencies and fractures of the proximal femur: II. Implications of vitamin D deficiency in the elderly. J Endocrinol 1996;149:13-7.

38. Boonen S, Lesaffre E, Dequeker J, et al: Relationship between baseline insulin-like growth factor-I (IGF-I) and femoral bone density in women aged over 70 years: potential implications for the prevention of age-related bone loss. J Am Geriatr Soc 1996;44:1301-6.

39. Boonen S, Broos P, Verbeke G, et al: Calciotropic hormones and markers of bone remodeling in age-related (type II) femoral neck osteoporosis: alterations consistent with secondary hyperparathyroidism-induced bone resorption. J Gerontol Am Biol Sci Med Sci 1997;52:M286-M293.

40. Reginster JY, Deroisy R, Pirenne H, et al: High prevalence of low femoral bone mineral density in elderly women living in nursing homes or community-dwelling: a plausible role of increased parathyroid hormone secretion. Osteoporos Int 1999;9:121-28.

41. Lips P: Vitamin D deficiency and secondary hyperparathyroidism in the elderly: consequences for bone loss and fractures and therapeutic implications. Endocr Rev 2001;22:477-501.

42. Yates AA, Schlicker SA, Suitor CW: Dietary Reference Intakes: the new basis for recommendations for calcium and related nutrients, B vitamins, and choline. J Am Diet Assoc 1998;98:699-706.

43. European Commission. Directorate V Report on osteoporosis in the European Community: Action for prevention. European Commission, Directorate-General for Employment, Industrial Relations and Social Affairs, Directorate V/F.2.

44. Chapuy MC, Preziosi P, Maamer M, et al: Prevalence of vitamin D insufficiency in an adult normal population. Osteoporos Int 1997;7:439-43.

45. Chapuy MC, Schott AM, Garnero P, et al: Healthy elderly French women living at home have secondary hyperparathyroidism and high bone turnover in winter. EPIDOS Study Group. J Clin Endocrinol Metab 1996;81:1129-33.

46. Boonen S, Rizzoli R, Meunier PJ, et al: The need for clinical guidance in the use of calcium and vitamin D in the management of osteoporosis: a consensus report. Osteoporos Int 2004;15:511-19.

47. Johnston CC Jr, Miller JZ, Slemenda CW, et al: Calcium supplementation and increases in bone mineral density in children. N Engl J Med 1992;327:82-7.

48. Rozen GS, Rennert G, Dodiuk-Gad RP, et al: Calcium supplementation provides an extended window of opportunity for bone mass accretion after menarche. Am J Clin Nutr 2003;78:993-98.

49. Stear SJ, Prentice A, Jones SC, Cole TJ: Effect of a calcium and exercise intervention on the bone mineral status of 16-18-y-old adolescent girls. Am J Clin Nutr 2003;77:985-92.

50. Chee WS, Suriah AR, Chan SP, et al: The effect of milk supplementation on bone mineral density in postmenopausal Chinese women in Malaysia. Osteoporos Int 2003;14:828-34.

51. Hampson G, Martin FC, Moffat K, et al: Effects of dietary improvement on bone metabolism in elderly underweight women with osteoporosis: a randomised controlled trial. Osteoporos Int 2003;14:750-56.

52. Ulrich U, Miller PB, Eyre DR, et al: Short-term calcium supplementation has no effect on biochemical markers of bone remodeling in early postmenopausal women. Arch Gynecol Obstet 2003;268:309-16.

53. Michaelsson K, Melhus H, Bellocco R, Wolk A: Dietary calcium and vitamin D intake in relation to osteoporotic fracture risk. Bone 2003;32:694-703.

54. Lamke B, Sjoberg HE, Sylven M: Bone mineral content in women with Colles' fracture: effect of calcium supplementation. Acta Orthop Scand 1978;49:143-46.

55. Dawson-Hughes B, Dallal GE, Krall EA, et al: A controlled trial of the effect of calcium supplementation on bone density in postmenopausal women. N Engl J Med 1990;323:878-83.

56. Recker RR, Hinders S, Davies KM, et al: Correcting bone nutritional deficiency prevents spine fractures in elderly women. J Bone Miner Res 1996;11:1961-66.

57. Prince R, Devine A, Dick I, et al: The effects of calcium supplementation (milk powder or tablets) and exercise on bone density in postmenopausal women. J Bone Miner Res 1995;10:1068-75.

58. Reid IR, Ames RW, Evans MC, et al: Long-term effects of calcium supplementation on bone loss and fractures in postmenopausal women: a randomized controlled trial. Am J Med 1995;98:331-35.

59. Cooper L, Clifton-Bligh PB, Nery ML, et al: Vitamin D supplementation and bone mineral density in early postmenopausal women. Am J Clin Nutr 2003;77:1324-29.

60. Tfelt-Hansen J, Torring O: Calcium and vitamin D(3) supplements in calcium and vitamin D(3) sufficient early postmenopausal healthy women. Eur J Clin Nutr 2004;58:1420-24.

61. Riis B, Thomsen K, Christiansen C: Does calcium supplementation prevent postmenopausal bone loss? A double-blind, controlled clinical study. N Engl J Med 1987;316:173-77.

62. Grados F, Brazier M, Kamel S, et al: Effects on bone mineral density of calcium and vitamin D supplementation in elderly women with vitamin D deficiency. Joint Bone Spine 2003;70:203-8.

63. Grados F, Brazier M, Kamel S, et al: Prediction of bone mass density variation by bone remodeling markers in postmenopausal women with vitamin D insufficiency treated with calcium and vitamin D supplementation. J Clin Endocrinol Metab 2003;88:5175-79.

64. Larsen ER, Mosekilde L, Foldspang A: Vitamin D and calcium supplementation prevents osteoporotic fractures in elderly community dwelling residents: a pragmatic population-based 3-year intervention study. J Bone Miner Res 2004;19:370-78.

65. Dawson-Hughes B, Dallal GE, Krall EA, et al: Effect of vitamin D supplementation on wintertime and overall bone loss in healthy postmenopausal women. Ann Intern Med 1991;115:505-12.

66. Dawson-Hughes B: Interaction of dietary calcium and protein in bone health in humans. J Nutr 2003;133:852S-54S.

67. Chapuy MC, Arlot ME, Duboeuf F, et al: Vitamin D3 and calcium to prevent hip fractures in the elderly women. N Engl J Med 1992;327:1637-42.

68. Chapuy MC, Arlot ME, Delmas PD, Meunier PJ: Effect of calcium and cholecalciferol treatment for three years on hip fractures in elderly women. BMJ 1994;308:1081-82.

69. Meunier PJ, Chapuy MC, Arlot ME, et al: Can we stop bone loss and prevent hip fractures in the elderly? Osteoporos Int 1994;4(Suppl 1):71-6.

70. Harwood RH, Sahota O, Gaynor K, et al: A randomised, controlled comparison of different calcium and vitamin D supplementation regimens in elderly women after hip fracture: The Nottingham Neck of Femur (NONOF) Study. Age Ageing 2004;33:45-51.

71. Riggs BL, O'Fallon WM, Muhs J, et al: () Long-term effects of calcium supplementation on serum parathyroid hormone level, bone turnover, and bone loss in elderly women. J Bone Miner Res 1998;13:168-74.

72. Dawson-Hughes B, Harris SS, Krall EA, Dallal GE: Effect of calcium and vitamin D supplementation on bone density in men and women 65 years of age or older. N Engl J Med 1997;337:670-76.

73. Trivedi DP, Doll R, Khaw KT: Effect of four monthly oral vitamin D3 (cholecalciferol) supplementation on fractures and mortality in men and women living in the community: randomised double blind controlled trial. BMJ 2003;326:469.

74. Shea B, Wells G, Cranney A, et al: Meta-analyses of therapies for postmenopausal osteoporosis. VII. Meta-analysis of calcium supplementation for the prevention of postmenopausal osteoporosis. Endocr Rev 2002;23:552-59.

75. Papadimitropoulos E, Wells G, Shea B, et al: Meta-analyses of therapies for postmenopausal osteoporosis. VIII: Meta-analysis of the efficacy of vitamin D treatment in preventing osteoporosis in postmenopausal women. Endocr Rev 2002;23:560-69.

76. Kenny AM, Prestwood KM, Biskup B, et al: Comparison of the effects of calcium loading with calcium citrate or calcium carbonate on bone turnover in postmenopausal women. Osteoporos Int 2004;15:290-94.

77. Lilliu H, Pamphile R, Chapuy MC, et al: Calcium-vitamin D3 supplementation is cost-effective in hip fractures prevention. Maturitas 2003;44:299-305.

78. Rosner AJ, Grima DT, Torrance GW, et al: Cost effectiveness of multi-therapy treatment strategies in the prevention of vertebral fractures in postmenopausal women with osteoporosis. Pharmacoeconomics 1998;14:559-73.

79. Juby AG, Davis P: A prospective evaluation of the awareness, knowledge, risk factors and current treatment of osteoporosis in a cohort of elderly subjects. Osteoporos Int 2001;12:617-22.

80. Dawson-Hughes B, Harris SS, Krall EA, Dallal GE: Effect of withdrawal of calcium and vitamin D supplements on bone mass in elderly men and women. Am J Clin Nutr 2000;72:745-50.

81. Koster JC, Hackeng WH, Mulder H: Diminished effect of etidronate in vitamin D deficient osteopenic postmenopausal women. Eur J Clin Pharmacol 1996;51:145-47.

82. Masud T, Mulcahy B, Thompson AV, et al: Effects of cyclical etidronate combined with calcitriol versus cyclical etidronate alone on spine and femoral neck bone mineral density in postmenopausal osteoporotic women. Ann Rheum Dis 1998;57:346-49.

83. Nieves JW, Komar L, Cosman F, Lindsay R: Calcium potentiates the effect of estrogen and calcitonin on bone mass: review and analysis. Am J Clin Nutr 1998;67:18-24.

84. Sirola J, Kroger H, Sandini L, et al: Interaction of nutritional calcium and HRT in prevention of postmenopausal bone loss: a prospective study. Calcif Tissue Int 2003;72:659-65.

85. Prince RL, Smith M, Dick IM, et al: Prevention of post-menopausal osteoporosis: a comparative study of exercise, calcium supplementation, and hormone-replacement therapy. N Engl J Med 1991;325:1189-95.

86. Ettinger B, Genant HK, Cann CE: Postmenopausal bone loss is prevented by treatment with low-dosage estrogen with calcium. Ann Intern Med 1987;106:40-5.

87. Strause L, Saltman P, Smith KT, et al: Spinal bone loss in postmenopausal women supplemented with calcium and trace minerals. J Nutr 1994;124:1060-64.

88. Going S, Lohman T, Houtkooper L, et al: Effects of exercise on bone mineral density in calcium-replete postmenopausal women with and without hormone replacement therapy. Osteoporos Int 2003;14:637-43.

89. Deprez X, Fardellone P: Nonpharmacological prevention of osteoporotic fractures. Joint Bone Spine 2003;70:448-57.

90. Nelson ME, Fisher EC, Dilmanian FA, et al: A 1-y walking program and increased dietary calcium in postmenopausal women: effects on bone. Am J Clin Nutr 1991;53:1304-11.

14 Vitamin D and Its Metabolites in the Prevention and Treatment of Osteoporosis

Philip N. Sambrook

SUMMARY

Numerous studies have demonstrated varying effects of vitamin D and its metabolites to reduce falls risk and prevent or treat postmenopausal osteoporosis. The differences reported on falls risk, bone density, and reduction in fracture rates may be due to differences in pretreatment vitamin D and PTH levels. The main therapeutic effect of vitamin D supplementation appears to be in vitamin D deficient patients, usually considered as a serum 25OHD level less than 50 nmol/L.

The discovery last century that vitamin D plays a role in the regulation of intestinal calcium absorption raised the possibility of using vitamin D and its metabolites as a treatment for osteoporosis. Although a number of steroid compounds are classified as vitamin D, this generic term is usually applied to the following two molecules:

Cholecalciferol (vitamin D_3). This is formed through the action of ultraviolet light on 7-dehydrocholesterol in the skin to form provitamin D_3, which is converted to cholecalciferol.

Ergocalciferol (vitamin D_2). This is a less common form of vitamin D, produced by ultraviolet irradiation of the plant steroid ergosterol.

Vitamin D_3 and vitamin D_2, made in the skin or ingested, are transported to the liver and metabolized to 25-hydroxyvitamin D [25(OH)D], the major circulating form. Further hydroxylation occurs in the kidney to form the biologically active molecule 1,25-dihydroxyvitamin D [1,25(OH)$_2$D], which is transported in the blood bound to albumin and vitamin D binding protein. Only a small fraction of 1,25(OH)$_2$D circulates in its free form to bind to a specific vitamin D receptor. The binding of 1,25(OH)$_2$D to its receptor regulates calcium and phosphate metabolism and induces a wide array of biological responses. The term *calciferol* is often used to refer to both cholecalciferol and ergocalciferol, although recent studies indicate that vitamin D_3 may have substantially greater biological potency and longer duration of action than vitamin D_2.[1] Doses of the calciferols are usually expressed in international units. Metabolites of the calciferols and 1,25(OH)$_2$D are used as therapies in osteoporosis and often referred to as *calcidiol* and *calcitriol*, respectively. However, the distinction between pharmacological and physiological uses of vitamin D is important, because the doses involved and their safety are substantially different. Alfacalcidol is a synthetic vitamin D_3 compound, hydroxylated in position 1. It differs from calcitriol in that it has not been hydroxylated at position 25, but this conversion takes place rapidly in the liver after oral administration. Its biochemical effects are very similar to those of calcitriol, although it may be less likely to cause hypercalcemia.[2]

Calcitriol has several actions, including

1. Increasing absorption of calcium and phosphate from the small intestine. This is possibly the most important function of vitamin D compounds.[3] However, increasing intestinal calcium absorption will not inevitably result in an improvement in bone mineral density (BMD). Its effect on calcium balance is determined by a subject's vitamin D status, and there may be differences between its effect in vitamin D–deficient subjects versus vitamin D–replete subjects.
2. Maintenance of calcium homeostasis in the extracellular fluid directly and in interaction with parathyroid hormone (PTH).
3. Through its feedback mechanisms, regulation of its own renal production and degradation.
4. Facilitating skeletal mineralization largely through enhancing acquisition of environmental minerals from the diet.
5. Stimulation of bone resorption, particularly at high concentrations.

VITAMIN D DEFICIENCY AND BONE

Plasma 25(OH)D and 1,25(OH)$_2$D levels have both been shown to decrease with age. This may occur as a result of age-related factors, such as reduced capacity to produce vitamin D and diminished sunlight exposure,[4] reduced intake, and decline in renal function. Vitamin D insufficiency, usually regarded to occur when serum 25(OH)D concentrations are between 30 and 50 nmol/L, may lead to a progressive increase in PTH secretion, high bone turnover,[5] an increase in age-related bone loss, and an increased risk of developing osteoporosis. Vitamin D insufficiency results in loss of cortical bone predominately, with an increased risk for hip fracture.[6,7] Osteomalacia, on the other hand, is the bone disease seen in cases of true vitamin D deficiency. In severe cases, with serum 25(OH)D levels usually less than 12.5 nmol/L, subjects may present with bone and muscle pains, weakness, and pseudofractures. Low vitamin D status generally has been associated with increased risk of hip fracture in elderly people.[8] Furthermore, low vitamin D status is associated with reduced bone density[9] and high bone turnover.[10]

VITAMIN D DEFICIENCY, MUSCLE FUNCTION, AND FALLS

Falls are a crucial part of the pathogenesis of osteoporotic fractures, and the finding that 1,25(OH)$_2$D may affect skeletal muscle function has gained much attention in recent years. In cases of osteomalacia, a metabolic myopathy has been noted, consisting histologically of atrophied type 2 muscle fibers with fat infiltration, fibrosis, and glycogen granules. Patients typically present with gait disturbances and difficulty in arising from a chair. Abnormal motor performance, increased body sway, and quadriceps weakness have been reported with serum 25(OH)D levels below 20 to 30 nmol/L in elderly men and veiled Arab women.[11,12] One randomized controlled trial in 162 subjects (mean age, 85.3 years) over 12 weeks demonstrated a 49% reduction in falls associated with vitamin D and calcium treatment.[13] Serum 25(OH)D levels rose from 30.8 nmol/L to 65.5 nmol/L with calcium plus vitamin D supplementation, and musculoskeletal function improved significantly. In another 8-week study of 148 women (mean age, 74) with 25(OH)D levels below 50 nmol/L, Pfeifer and associates[14] showed that calcium and supplementation with vitamin D resulted in an increase in serum 25(OH)D levels of 72%, a decrease in serum PTH of 18%, a decrease in body sway of 9%, and a decrease in falls. Over 12 months, the number of falls per subject was 0.45 in the calcium alone group compared with 0.24 in the calcium plus vitamin D group. A number of other studies have shown effects of simple and activated formulations of vitamin D in reducing falls risk,[15-17] and a recent meta-analysis[18] has shown an effect size in reducing falls risk compared with placebo or calcium of 22% (Figure 14-1). Furthermore, polymorphisms in the vitamin D receptor gene have been associated with reduced quadriceps muscle function.[19] These findings suggest a link between vitamin D deficiency, falls, and bone fragility fractures.

SOURCES OF VITAMIN D

The main source of vitamin D is exposure to sunlight. There are seasonal variations in vitamin D status, such that serum 25(OH)D levels are generally lower at the end of winter than at the end of summer. It has been estimated that exposure of the whole body surface to around 10 to 15 minutes of midday sun in summer (i.e., around one minimal erythemal dose) is comparable with taking approximately 15,000 IU (375 µg) of vitamin D orally.[4] Less vitamin D is synthesized at other times of the day, during winter, and in people with dark skin or those who are older.

Vitamin D is added to some foods in some countries, but there may be impaired absorption of dietary vitamin D with aging. Vitamin D$_3$ is generally found in small quantities in foods, but richer sources are fish, especially high-fat fish such as salmon, herring, and mackerel. Other sources of importance are meat and eggs and fortified foods such as margarine. The Food and Nutrition Board of the US Institute of Medicine proposed a Daily Reference Intake (DRI) of 200 IU (5 µg) for people aged 0 to 50 years, 400 IU (10 µg) for those 51 to 70 years, and 600 IU (15 µg) for those older than 70 years.[20] This represents a tripling of the recommended intake for those over the age of 70 years.

DOSAGES REQUIRED TO TREAT VITAMIN D DEFICIENCY

Vitamin D is stored in fat and muscle and is slowly released, particularly during winter.[21] In vitamin D–deficient patients, it is necessary to replenish the vitamin D stores. Although the daily requirement for vitamin D is 400 to 600 IU per day, a much larger dose is used to treat vitamin D–deficient patients. Because vitamin D is fat soluble with a half-life of more than 3 weeks, large doses are needed before changes in serum 25(OH)D are seen. Higher doses (3000-5000 IU daily for 6-12 weeks) may be used to replenish body stores. Even higher doses of 50,000 to 500,000 IU orally or 600,000 IU intramuscularly can effectively treat vitamin D deficiency, but there is the possibility of inducing hypercalcemia/hypercalciuria. The use of active metabolites (calcitriol or alfacalcidol) is not recommended for treating patients with simple vitamin D

Figure 14-1. Meta-analysis of effect size of vitamin D on falls. (From Bischoff-Ferrari HA, Dawson-Hughes B, Willett WC, et al: Effect of vitamin D on falls: a meta-analysis. JAMA, 2004 Apr 28;291(16):1999-2006.)

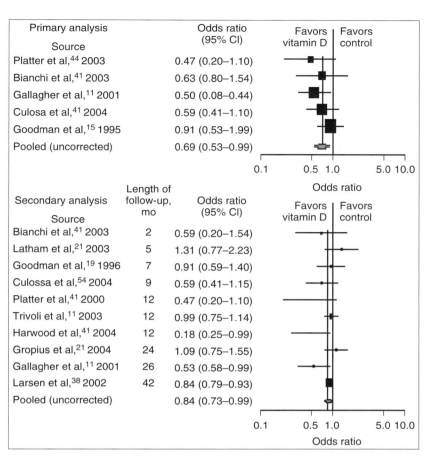

Primary analysis Source	Odds ratio (95% CI)
Platter et al,[44] 2003	0.47 (0.20–1.10)
Bianchi et al,[41] 2003	0.63 (0.80–1.54)
Gallagher et al,[11] 2001	0.50 (0.08–0.44)
Culosa et al,[41] 2004	0.59 (0.41–1.10)
Goodman et al,[15] 1995	0.91 (0.53–1.99)
Pooled (uncorrected)	0.69 (0.53–0.99)

Secondary analysis Source	Length of follow-up, mo	Odds ratio (95% CI)
Bianchi et al,[41] 2003	2	0.59 (0.20–1.54)
Latham et al,[21] 2003	5	1.31 (0.77–2.23)
Goodman et al,[19] 1996	7	0.91 (0.59–1.40)
Culossa et al,[54] 2004	9	0.59 (0.41–1.15)
Platter et al,[41] 2000	12	0.47 (0.20–1.10)
Trivoli et al,[11] 2003	12	0.99 (0.75–1.14)
Harwood et al,[41] 2004	12	0.18 (0.25–0.99)
Gropius et al,[21] 2004	24	1.09 (0.75–1.55)
Gallagher et al,[11] 2001	26	0.53 (0.58–0.99)
Larsen et al,[38] 2002	42	0.84 (0.79–0.93)
Pooled (uncorrected)		0.84 (0.73–0.99)

deficiency, and changes in serum 25(OH)D levels are not a reflection of such therapy.

CALCIUM MALABSORPTION AND OSTEOPOROSIS

As noted, intestinal absorption of calcium declines with age, particularly after the age of 70 years. Several groups have reported calcium absorption in osteoporotic patients and in general have found that calcium absorption is lower in osteoporotic subjects.[22,23] However, most studies of calcium absorption have categorized subjects as either having osteoporosis based on the presence of vertebral fracture or not. The relationship between intestinal calcium absorption and bone density is unknown. In the presence of vitamin D deficiency, low serum calcium concentration stimulates the parathyroid glands to release PTH.[5] High doses of PTH raise serum calcium concentrations through an increase in renal calcium reabsorption, mobilization of calcium from the skeleton, and

intestinal absorption of calcium from the gut. Clinically, the principal index of vitamin D deficiency is the serum 25(OH)D level, but there are arguments about the appropriate threshold to define vitamin D deficiency. Many authors suggest that the vitamin D–replete state is seen when the serum 25(OH)D level approaches 50 nmol/L, but others suggest it is closer to 70 nmol/L.[24,25] Hypovitaminosis D is common in the elderly, and there is some evidence that fluctuations in serum 25(OH)D levels correlate with fluctuations in bone density according to seasonal changes. The principle index of altered vitamin D metabolism is the circulating concentration of $1,25(OH)_2D$. Several groups have reported the latter to be reduced in subjects with vertebral fractures,[26] whereas other investigators have found them to be normal. The effects of advancing old age on renal function and consequently $1,25(OH)_2D$ production and the increasing prevalence of vitamin D deficiency in elderly populations provide a basis for intervention with these compounds in older subjects.

POSTMENOPAUSAL OSTEOPOROSIS: CALCIFEROLS

Considerable interest has focused on the use of physiological doses of the calciferols to correct subclinical vitamin D deficiency. Although the most physiological way to replace vitamin D in the housebound elderly person might seem to be via sunlight exposure, there appears to be impaired synthesis of vitamin D in skin with age. Older subjects may not go outdoors often, and ultraviolet light of the necessary wavelength (285-310 NM) is completely absorbed by glass. Indoor lighting is inadequate for vitamin D synthesis, and so older people are often reliant on dietary sources of vitamin D. There have now been several large studies of the effects of calciferol administration on fractures in the elderly. Most of these studies have been performed in vitamin D–deficient subjects.

Heikenheimo and associates[27] studied approximately 800 elderly subjects living in Finland, of whom approximately two-thirds were living in their own homes and the remainder in municipal accommodation. Subjects were randomized to receive either 150,000 IU vitamin D_2 annually (and in certain years 300,000 IU) or no treatment. The mean age of the subjects was 86 years. Follow-up was from 2 to 5 years, with a mean duration of just over 3 years. Symptomatic fractures, confirmed by radiographs, were the primary endpoint and were reduced by 25% in the vitamin D–treated subjects ($P = 0.03$). Mean serum 25(OH)D levels were 31 and 14 nmol/L in the control groups, either living independently or in municipal homes, respectively.

In contrast, Lips and associates[28] showed no difference in fracture rate in 2578 men and women older than 70 years, living independently in the community, who were randomized to receive either calciferol 400 IU per day or placebo. Over 3.5 years of follow-up, there was no significant difference in fracture rates. Mean serum 25(OH)D levels in the third year were 23 nmol/L in the placebo group and 60 nmol/L in the vitamin D treated group.

In a 3-year study, Chapuy and coworkers[29] reported the effect of treatment with either calcium plus 800 IU of vitamin D_3 or placebo in more than 3000 women in residential care in France. The subjects' mean age was 84 years. There were more than 350 fractures in total, of which 99% resulted from a fall. Among the subjects receiving vitamin D, there were 32% fewer nonvertebral fractures and 43% fewer hip fractures, a difference that is statistically significant. Mean serum 25(OH)D levels were assessed in a subgroup of the patients only. Baseline 25(OH)D levels were 33 and 43 nmol/L in the placebo and vitamin D groups, respectively. Levels were stable in the placebo group but rose to 100 to 105 nmol/L among those receiving active treatment. This was accompanied by a fall in serum PTH concentrations, whereas serum PTH rose in the placebo group.

More recently, Chapuy and coworkers[30] performed a similar study to their initial trial in order to replicate their findings. In a 2-year, multicenter, double-masked trial, 583 patients were randomized to either calcium plus 800 IU of vitamin D or placebo. The relative risk of hip fracture in the placebo group compared with the active treatment group was 1.69, and based on the biochemical changes, the authors concluded that calcium and vitamin D in combination were able to reverse senile secondary hyperparathyoidism and reduce both hip bone loss and the risk of hip fracture in elderly institutionalized women.

Dawson-Hughes and associates[31] randomized 389 men and women older than 65 years to treatment with either calcium plus 700 IU of calciferol per day or placebo. Subjects were living in the community and baseline 25(OH)D levels were 82 nmol/L. The mean changes in BMD with treatment were +0.5% versus −0.7% in the femoral neck, +2.1% versus +1.2% in the spine, and +0.06% versus −1.09% for the total body. At the end of 3 years, these BMD differences were significant only for total body BMD, but there were 26 subjects with nonvertebral fractures in the placebo group versus 11 in the calcium vitamin D group ($P < .02$).

Trivedi and associates[32] reported a randomized, double-blind, controlled trial of 100,000 IU of oral vitamin D_3 given every 4 months versus placebo in 2686 men and women aged 65 to 85 years living in the community. After 5 years, 286 men and women had incident fractures. The relative risk of fracture in the vitamin D group compared with the placebo group were 0.78 ($P < .04$). After treatment, serum 25(OH)D concentrations were 40% higher in a subgroup of the active treatment group than in placebo-treated patients (74.3 versus 53.4 nmol/L).

More recently, the role of vitamin D supplementation in younger subjects has been examined in a randomized, co-twin, placebo-controlled, double-blind trial over 2 years.[33] In this study, 79 monozygotic twin pairs (mean age, 59 years) were randomized to either 800 IU of vitamin D_3 or placebo. At 6 months, the treatment group had an increase in serum 25(OH)D levels, but there were no significant differences in other serum measurements or bone markers at 3 or 6 months. At 24 months, no significant treatment effect was seen on BMD or calcaneal ultrasonogram. It was concluded that vitamin D supplementation on its own cannot be recommended for healthy postmenopausal women with normal vitamin D levels at baseline.

Several recent large studies in which the vitamin D status of the study population has been equivocal also failed to show a benefit of vitamin D therapy. In the RECORD trial, 5292 subjects (85% female) aged 70 years and older and ambulatory prior to a previous low-trauma fracture were randomized to calcium alone (1000 mg daily), vitamin D$_3$ (800 IU daily), the combination of supplements, or placebo.[34] Compliance with medication was only moderate (59% after 2 years) but after follow-up of between 24 and 62 months, there were 698 new low-trauma fractures. However, there were no significant differences in fracture rates between groups. In the Wessex Fracture Prevention Trial, 9440 community-dwelling subjects aged 75 to 100 years were randomized to either an annual injection of 300,000 IU cholecalciferol or placebo.[35] In a subset of patients, mean wintertime serum PTH levels were suppressed by 20% after treatment with vitamin D. After 3 years, 609 subjects had sustained an incident fracture but no protective effect of vitamin D could be shown.

The use of replacement doses of calciferol appears to be a safe intervention. Very few patients in the above trials developed hypercalcemia, and this may be expected in a population in which baseline levels are low and the intention is to restore them to normal values. It is more difficult to assess the safety of pharmacological doses of calciferol, but vitamin D toxicity can result in hypercalcemia due to excessive intestinal calcium absorption.

Recently the Women's Health Initiative (WHI) reported its findings in the calcium plus vitamin D arm of that study in 36,282 postmenopausal women.[36] Compared with placebo, BMD increased significantly at the hip (1.1% over 9 years) but not at other sites in patients treated with 1000 mg of calcium plus 400 IU vitamin D. In the intention to treat analysis, the reduction in hip fracture with calcium plus vitamin D was not significant (HR 0.88, 95% CI 0.72 – 1.10), however the power of the study was reduced from 85% to 48% by a lower than projected hip fracture rate. Moreover the reduction in hip fracture risk was significant in the adherent population (HR 0.71, 95% CI 0.52 – 0.97). The risk of renal calculi was also increased with calcium plus vitamin D (HR 1.17, 95% CI 1.02 – 1.34), however the baseline calcium intake of the study population was high (mean intake 1150mg per day). Taken together all these studies suggest calcium alone or in combination with vitamin D has a modest effect on fracture risk but that they are most effective in those with low dietary calcium intakes or vitamin D deficient individuals.

ACTIVE VITAMIN D METABOLITES

The most consistent biochemical effect of calcitriol or alphacalcidol is stimulation of intestinal calcium absorption. This appears to be dose related and can be seen with doses as small as 0.25 µg per day. The effect of calcitriol on serum calcium concentration is more varied, but in general, serum calcium level is not significantly elevated in patients taking doses of less than 0.5 µg per day. The effect may also be greater with calcitriol than with alphacalcidol.[2] Urine calcium excretion may also be affected by calcitriol and rise significantly with higher doses.

One of the first studies to assess the effects of active metabolites on bone mass was that of Christiansen and associates,[36] who randomized early postmenopausal women to receive calcitriol, hormone replacement therapy (HRT), both, or neither. Bone mass was only assessed in the forearm, however. Subjects taking HRT with or without calcitriol showed increases in forearm bone mineral content of about 1% over 12 months. In contrast, the placebo group and the calcitriol group showed a 2% decline in forearm bone mineral content.

Between 1988 and 1989, three American studies following a similar protocol with calcitriol were published.[37-39] All subjects had at least one vertebral fracture and were randomly allocated to receive therapy with calcitrol or placebo. Subjects on active therapy were started on calcitriol 0.5 µg with dose escalation until hypercalciuria or hypercalcemia occurred. Unfortunately, the dose titration was handled differently in each center, with the result that the patients of Ott[37] received a mean dose of 0.43 µg, those of Gallagher[38] received 0.62 µg, and those of Aloia received 0.8 µg daily.[39] Not surprisingly, the results from the studies were quite different. In the Aloia study, there were significant increases in total body calcium, distal radius bone mineral content, lumbar spine BMD, and metacarpal density with calcitriol but no changes in the placebo group.[39] Fracture rates were slightly but not significantly higher in the placebo group. Hypercalciuria and hypercalcemia were quite common. While concluding that the effect of calcitriol in these subjects was beneficial, the investigators did not advocate this treatment because of the high incidence of side effects. In the Gallagher study,[38] the patients did not have major problems with hypercalcemia, because dietary calcium intake was reduced during dose titration. Total body calcium remained stable over 2 years and fell by approximately 2% in those receiving placebo. The spine subregion of the total body scans demonstrated an increase of 2% in BMD in those on calcitriol and a decrease of greater magnitude in those receiving placebo. However, there was no difference between the groups in the number of new fractures occurring during the study. The study by Ott and Chesnut[37] was the largest of the three studies but, as noted, used the lowest dose of calcitriol. Bone density changes tended to be more positive with calcitriol than in the placebo group at the three sites assessed, although between-group differences were not significant. However, there was a significant decrease in distal radius bone mineral content in the calcitriol group, which did not occur in the placebo group. Fractures seemed to be more common in the placebo group than the calcitriol group, but this difference was not statistically significant. The authors concluded that calcitriol was ineffective in the treatment of established postmenopausal osteoporosis. Ott and Chesnut subsequently published a re-analysis of these data in which the calcitriol group was subdivided according to the average dose of drug taken during the study.[40] The numbers by group in this post hoc analysis were small, but the results were consistent with the data from Aloia and Gallagher and suggested that higher doses of calcitriol produced more beneficial effects on bone density.

The other large study of calcitriol for the treatment of postmenopausal osteoporosis was performed by Tilyard.[41] In this study, 622 women with at least one vertebral fracture were randomly assigned to take calcitriol 0.5 μg a day or calcium and were followed for more than 3 years. Bone density was not measured, the primary endpoint being vertebral fracture. In the 432 subjects who completed the study, there were significantly more fractures in the calcium-treated group than in the calcitriol-treated subjects in both years 2 and 3, but not in year 1. The time trend from this study shows a stable fracture rate in the calcitriol-treated subjects with an increasing incidence of new fractures in those taking calcium. This trend is at variance with other calcium supplementation studies. There are other issues of concern about this study. There were a large number of withdrawals in the first year, and it is also likely that a significant number of subjects were vitamin D deficient.

More recently, Gallagher reported the results of a randomized trial comparing calcitriol (0.25 μg twice daily) with HRT (conjugated estrogens 0.625 mg daily), neither, or both in 480 women aged 65 to 77 years for 3 years.[17] At 3 years, increases in BMD were about twice as great with HRT as those seen in the calcitriol-treated patients. In the intent-to-treat analysis, HRT produced a mean increase in BMD of 3.0% at the femoral neck ($P < .0001$) and 4.4% at the spine ($P < .0001$). Calcitriol increased BMD by 0.10% at the femoral neck ($P = .57$) and 1.7% at the spine ($P < .01$). Combination therapy tended to produce greater increments in BMD (3.8% at the femoral neck [$P < .001$] and 4.9% at the spine [$P < .0001$]) (Figure 14-2). There was a trend for a lower fracture rate to be seen in the calcitriol groups.

Sorenson[42] conducted a study of alphacalcidol in established osteoporosis in Danish women. Substantial increases were found in forearm bone mineral content, but many subjects appeared to have osteomalacia. There was also a substantial reduction in back pain with alfacalcidol but no change in mineralized volume on iliac crest bone biopsy.

Studies in Japan have generally demonstrated benefits of alphacalcidol on bone density and vertebral fractures, but descriptions of these trials are limited.[43] More details are provided in two studies by Orimo and coworkers.[44,45] In one study, 86 Japanese women were randomized to alphacalcidol alone, alphacalcidol plus calcium, or calcium alone and compared with 25 non-treated control subjects.[44] After 2 years, the fracture rates were 960 per 1000 patient-years in the control group, 650 per 1000 patient-years with calcium, and 350 per 1000 patient-years with alphacalcidol. The combination of calcium and alphacalcidol resulted in a fracture rate of 140 per 1000 patient-years. Both groups of alphacalcidol-treated subjects had significantly reduced fracture rates as compared with control subjects. Orimo and associates[45] also reported a prospective, double-blind, placebo-controlled trial of alphacalcidol versus placebo in 80 postmenopausal women. In the lumbar spine, the mean BMD change was 0.65% with alphacalcidol versus −1.14% with placebo ($P=.04$). In the femoral trochanteric area, BMD increased by 4.2% with alphacalcidol compared with a decline of 2.4% with placebo. The vertebral fracture rate with alphacalcidol was 75 per 1000 patient-years compared with 255 per 1000 patient-years with placebo ($P = .03$), although the control group had a higher baseline fracture prevalence.

A number of meta-analyses of the efficacy of vitamin D treatment in preventing osteoporosis in postmenopausal women have been published. In one it was concluded that vitamin D reduced the incidence of vertebral fractures (RR, 0.63; 95% CI, 0.45-0.88; $P < .01$) and showed a trend toward a reduced incidence of nonvertebral fractures (RR, 0.77; 95% CI, 0.57-1.04; $P < .09$).[46] It was noted that most patients in the trials that evaluated vertebral fractures received active vitamin D metabolites and most patients in the trials that evaluated nonvertebral fractures received standard vitamin D. Active vitamin D metabolites had consistently larger effects on bone density than standard vitamin D. It was concluded that vitamin D decreased the risk of vertebral fractures and mainly increased the risk of nonvertebral fracture, but the data were uninformative regarding the relative effects of standard and hydroxylated vitamin D (Figure 14-3).

In the other meta-analysis of simple vitamin D, it was concluded that oral doses between 700 and 800 IU daily were able to reduce the risk of hip and nonvertebral fractures in mainly institutionalized elderly subjects, but a dose of 400 IU daily was insufficient (see Figure 14-3).[47] Meta-analyses of the benefit of active metabolites of vitamin D in corticosteroid osteoporosis have also been published recently[48] but are not reviewed further in this chapter, which primarily deals with postmenopausal osteoporosis.

Figure 14-2. Effect of calcitriol on bone density in comparison with estrogen or placebo. (From Gallagher et al, JCEM, 2001.)

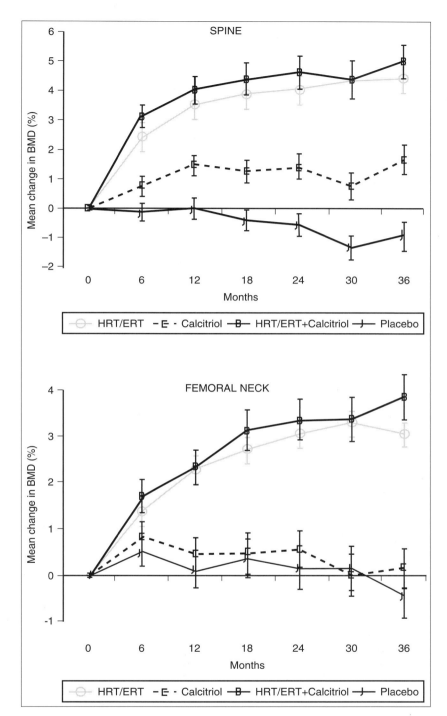

CONCLUSION

Many studies have been undertaken and demonstrate the effects of vitamin D and its metabolites in reducing fall risk and preventing or treating postmenopausal osteoporosis. The varying effects reported on fall risk, bone density, and reduction in fracture rates may be attributed to differences in pretreatment vitamin D and PTH levels. The greatest therapeutic effect of vitamin D supplementation is seen in vitamin D–deficient patients. It is unlikely that vitamin D supplementation has any major role in vitamin D–replete individuals [serum 25(OH)D levels greater than 50 nmol/L].

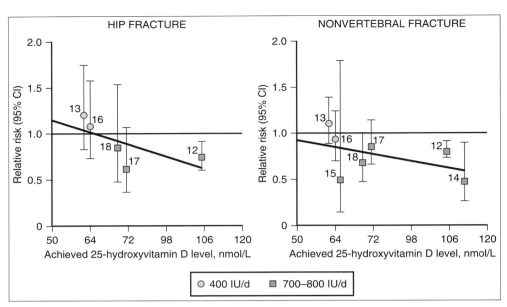

Figure 14-3. Meta-analysis of effect size of vitamin D on fractures. (From Bischoff-Ferrari HA, Dawson-Hughes B, Willett WC, et al: Effect of vitamin D on falls: a meta-analysis. JAMA, 2004 Apr 28;291(16):1999-2006.)

REFERENCES

1. Armas LAG, Hollis B, Heaney RP: Vitamin D2 is much less effective than Vitamin D3 in humans. J Clin Endocrinol Metab 2004;89:5387-91.
2. Gallagher JC, Bishop C, Knutson JC, et al: Effects of increasing doses of 1-alpha-hydroxy vitamin D2 on calcium homeostasis in postmenopausal women. J Bone Miner Res 1994;5:607-14.
3. Malloy PJ, Pike JW, Feldman D: The vitamin D receptor and the syndrome of hereditary 1,25-dihydroxyvitamin D-resistant rickets. Endocr Rev 1999;20:156-88.
4. Holick MF: Vitamin D new horizons for the 21st Century. Am J Clin Nutr 1994;60:619.
5. Holick MF: Vitamin D: photobiology, metabolism, mechanism of action and clinical applications. In: Favus M, editor: Primer on the metabolic bone diseases and disorders of mineral metabolism, 5th ed. American Society for Bone and Mineral Research, 2003:129-37.
6. Parfitt A: Osteomalacia and related disorders. In: Avioli L, Krane S: Metabolic Bone Disease and Clinically Related Disorders, 2nd ed. Philadelphia: WB Saunders, 1999:329-96.
7. Sahota O, Tea M: Vitamin D insufficiency increases bone turnover markers and enhances bone loss at the hip in patients with established vertebral osteoporosis. Clin Endocrinol (Oxf) 1999;51:217-21.
8. Weatherall M: A meta-analysis of 25 hydroxyvitamin D in older people with fracture of the proximal femur. N Z Med J 2000;113:137-40.
9. Outila T, Karkkainen MU, Lamberg-Allandt J: Vitamin D status affects serum parathyroid hormone concentrations during winter in female adolescents: associations with forearm bone mineral density. Am J Clin Nutr 2001;74:206-10.
10. Kipen E, Helme RD, Wark JD, Flicker L: Bone density, vitamin D nutrition, and parathyroid hormone levels in women with dementia. J Am Ger Soc 1995;43:1088-91.
11. Glerup H, Kea M: Commonly recommended daily intake of vitamin D is not sufficient if sunlight exposure is limited. J Intern Med 2000;247:260-68.
12. Dhesi JK, Bearne LM, Moniz C, et al: Neuromuscular and psychomotor function in elderly subjects who fall and the relationship with vitamin D status. J Bone Miner Res 2002;17:891-97.
13. Bischoff H, Stahelin HB, Dick W, et al: Effects of vitamin D and calcium supplementation on falls: a randomized controlled trial. J Bone Miner Res 2003;18:343-51.
14. Pfeifer M, Begerow B, Minne HW, et al: Effects of a short-term vitamin D and calcium supplementation on body sway and secondary hyperparathyroidism in elderly women. J Bone Miner Res 2000;15:1113-18.
15. Dukas L, Bishoff HA, Lindpainter LS, et al: Alfacalcidol reduces the number of fallers in a community dwelling population with a minimal calcium intake. J Am Geriatr Soc 2004;52:230-36.
16. Graafmans WC, Ooms ME, Hofstee HM, et al: Falls in the elderly: a prospective study and risk profiles. Am J Epidemiol 1996;143:1129-36.
17. Gallagher JC, Fowler SE, Detter JR, Sherman SS: Combination treatment with estrogen and calcitriol in the prevention of age-related bone loss. J Clin Endocr Metab 2001;86:3618-28.
18. Bischoff-Ferrari HA, Dawson-Hughes B, Willett WC, et al: Effect of vitamin D on falls: a meta-analysis. JAMA 2004;291:1999-2005.
19. Geusens P, Vandevyver C, Vanhoof J, et al: Quadriceps and grip strength are related to vitamin D receptor genotype in elderly non-obese women. J Bone Miner Res 1997;12:2082-88.
20. US Food and Nutrition Board: Dietary reference intakes for Ca, P, Mg, vitamins D and F. Washington, DC: National Academy Press, 1997.
21. Mawer E, Blackhouse J, Holman CA, et al: The distribution and storage of vitamin D and its metabolites in human tissues. Clin Sci 1972;43:413-31.
22. Lips P: Vitamins D deficiency and secondary hyperparathyroidism in the elderly: consequences for bone loss and fractures and therapeutic implications. Endocr Rev 2001;22:477-501.
23. Gallagher JC, Riggs B, Eisman J, et al: Intestinal calcium absorption and serum vitamin D metabolites in normal subjects

and osteoporotic patients: effect of age and dietary calcium. J Clin Invest 1979;64:729-36.

24. Harris SS, Soteriades E, Coolidge JA, et al: Vitamin D insufficiency and hyperparathyroidism in a low income, multiracial, elderly population. J Clin Endocr Metab 2000;85:4125-30.

25. Chapuy MC, Preziosi P, Maamer M, et al: Prevalence of vitamin D insufficiency in an adult normal population. Osteoporos Int 1997;7:439-43.

26. Ensrud KE, Duong T, Cauley JA, et al: Low fractional calcium absorption increases the risk for hip fracture in women with low calcium intake. Ann Intern Med 2000;132:345-53.

27. Heikinheimo RJ, Inkovaara J, Harju EJ, et al: Annual injection of vitamin D and fractures of aged bones. Calcif Tissue Int 1992;51:105-10.

28. Lips P, Graafmans WC, Ooms ME, et al: Vitamin D supplementation and fracture incidence in elderly persons: a randomized placebo controlled trial. Ann Intern Med 1996;124:400-6.

29. Chapuy MC, Arlot M, Duboeuf F, et al: Vitamin D3 and calcium to prevent hip fractures in the elderly. N Engl J Med 1992;327:1637-42.

30. Chapuy MC, Pamphile R, Paris E, et al: Combined calcium and vitamin D3 supplementation in elderly women: confirmation of reversal of secondary hyperparathyroidism and hip fracture risk. The Decalyos II study. Osteoporos Int 2002;13:257-64.

31. Dawson-Hughes B, Harris SS, Krall EA, Dallal GE: Effect of calcium and vitamin D supplementation on bone, density in men and women 65 years of age or older. N Engl J Med 1997;337:670-76.

32. Trivedi DP, Doll R, Khaw KT: Effect of four monthly oral vitamin D3 (cholecalciferol) supplementation on fractures and mortality in men and women living in the community: randomised double blind controlled trial. BMJ 2003;326:469-75.

33. Hunter D, Major P, Arden N, et al: A randomized controlled trial of vitamin D supplementation on preventing postmenopausal bone loss and modifying bone metabolism using identical twin pairs. J Bone Miner Res 2000:15:2276-83.

34. RECORD Trial Group: Randomised placebo-controlled trial of daily oral vitamin D3 and/or calcium for the secondary prevention of low trauma fractures in the elderly. Lancet 2005;365:1621-28.

35. Anderson FH, Raphael HM, et al: Effect of annual intramuscular vitamin D supplementation on fracture risk in 9440 community

living older people: The Wessex Fracture Prevention Trial. J Bone Miner Res 2004;19:Suppl 1, Abs 1220.

36. Christiansen C, Christensen MS, Rodbro P, et al: Effect of 1,25-dihydroxy-vitamin D3 in itself or combined with hormone treatment in preventing postmenopausal osteoporosis. Eur J Clin Invest 1981;11:305-9.

37. Ott SM, Chesnut CH 3rd: Calcitriol treatment is not effective in postmenopausal osteoporosis. Ann Intern Med 1989;110: 267-74.

38. Gallagher JC, Goldgar D: Treatment of postmenopausal osteoporosis with high doses of synthetic calcitriol: a randomized controlled study. Ann Intern Med 1990;113:649-55.

39. Aloia JF, Vaswani A, Yeh JK, et al: Calcitriol in the treatment of postmenopausal osteoporosis. Am J Med 1988;84:401-8.

40. Ott SM: Tolerance to dose of calcitriol is associated with improved bone density in women with postmenopausal osteoporosis. J Bone Miner Res 1990;5(Suppl):Abs 449.

41. Tilyard MW, Spears GF, Thomson J, Dovey S: Treatment of postmenopausal osteoporosis with calcitriol or calcium. N Engl J Med 1992;326:357-62.

42. Sorenson OH, Christensen MS, et al: Treatment of senile osteoporosis with 1 alpha-hydroxyvitamin D3. Clin Endocrinol 1977;7:169s-175s.

43. Fujita T: Studies of osteoporosis in Japan. Metabolism 1990;39:39-42.

44. Orimo H, Shiraki M, Hayashi T, Nakamura T: Reduced occurrence of vertebral crush fractures in senile osteoporosis treated with 1 alpha (OH)-vitamin D3. Bone Miner 1987;3:47-52.

45. Orimo H, Shiraki M, Hayashi Y, et al: Effects of 1 alpha-hydroxyvitamin D-3 on lumbar bone mineral density and vertebral fractures in patients with postmenopausal osteoporosis. Calcif Tissue Intern 1994;54:370-76.

46. Papadimitropoulos P, Wells G, Shea B, et al: Meta analysis of the effect of vitamin D treatment in preventing osteoporosis in post menopausal women. Endocr Rev 2002;23:560-69.

47. Bischoff-Ferrari HA, Willett WC, Wong JB, et al: Fracture prevention with vitamin D supplementation: a meta-analysis of randomized controlled trials. JAMA 2005;293:2257-64.

48. Richy F, Ethgen O, Bruyere O, Reginster JY: Efficacy of alphacalcidol and calcitriol in primary and corticosteroid induced osteoporosis: a meta-analysis of their effects on bone density and fracture rate. Osteoporosis Int 2004;15:301-10.

15 Selective Estrogen Receptor Modulators (SERMs)

Philip N. Sambrook

SUMMARY

Selective estrogen receptor modulators (SERMS) are a chemically diverse set of compounds that exert selective antagonist or agonist effects in different estrogen target tissues, such as bone, the breast, and the cardiovascular system. The SERM raloxifene can reduce the risk of vertebral fracture, but there remains some uncertainty about its effect on non-vertebral fracture. It is therefore recommended that raloxifene be mainly used in postmenopausal women with milder osteoporosis to prevent bone loss or for treatment in those with predominantly spinal osteoporosis.

Selective estrogen receptor modulators (SERMs) represent a major therapeutic advance in clinical practice for a number of disease states associated with menopause, such as osteoporosis, breast cancer, and cardiovascular disease. Their benefits in these different target tissues and their associated disease states clearly affect clinical decisions about their use as well as cost-benefit considerations when SERMs are considered primarily for osteoporosis.

Unlike estrogens, which are uniformly agonist, the SERMs exert selective antagonist or agonist effects in different estrogen target tissues. They are a chemically diverse set of compounds that lack the steroid structure of estrogen but possess a tertiary structure that allows binding to the estrogen receptor.[1] The first agent to demonstrate a SERM profile was tamoxifen, which was originally developed as an anti-estrogen and produced significant clinical benefit when used as adjuvant therapy in breast cancer patients. Thus, tamoxifen acted as an estrogen antagonist in the breast but as a weak agonist in bone.[2] Gains in bone mineral density (BMD) after 1 to 2 years of tamoxifen therapy in postmenopausal women with or without breast cancer were generally small,[3-5] however, and appeared to diminish over time[6] and resulted in an unclear clinical benefit, at least in terms of hip fracture risk.[7] Toremifene, another SERM, appeared to be an even weaker bone agonist than tamoxifen.[8]

Newer SERMs that have been investigated to treat and prevent osteoporosis, breast cancer, and cardiovascular disease include idoxifene, droloxifene, arzoxifene, and lasofoxifene,[9,10] but the best studied in osteoporosis has been raloxifene. Emphasizing the chemical diversity of SERM compounds, raloxifene has a benzothiophene nucleus, which differs substantially from the triphenylethylene structure of tamoxifen. The effects of raloxifene on markers of bone turnover have generally been modest (e.g., 30-40% reduction) compared with bisphosphonate therapy (typically 50-70%) (Figure 15-1).[11,12] Similarly, the response in BMD has shown modest increases when compared with bisphosphonates,[11,12] averaging between 2% and 3% at different skeletal sites over 3 years.[13] However, there are arguments about the importance of the size of the increase in BMD or suppression of bone turnover in regard to fracture risk reduction,[14-16] and although these surrogate markers provide some insight into mechanisms of action, the effect on fracture risk reduction is most clinically relevant.

The Multiple Outcomes of Raloxifene Evaluation (MORE) study, a large phase III trial of 7705 postmenopausal women, studied the effect of raloxifene on fracture risk. In this pivotal study, raloxifene in doses of 60 to 120 mg per day was compared with placebo. Raloxifene significantly decreased the incidence of vertebral fractures by almost 50% in patients without previous fractures and by 34% in women with previous (prevalent) vertebral fractures.[17,18] The effect on vertebral fractures is comparable with that seen with the bisphosphonates.[19] However, there was no significant decrease in the incidence of nonvertebral fractures or hip fractures. The interpretation of the latter finding is uncertain. It may relate to raloxifene's lesser effects on BMD and remodeling, but may also be related to study design and the population studied. For example, the subjects in the MORE study were on average 3 years younger than those in the alendronate Fracture Intervention Trial (FIT) study and had a vertebral fracture rate in the placebo group about one-third lower than the FIT study.[20] In the MORE study after 3 years, 9.3% of placebo-treated patients sustained nonvertebral

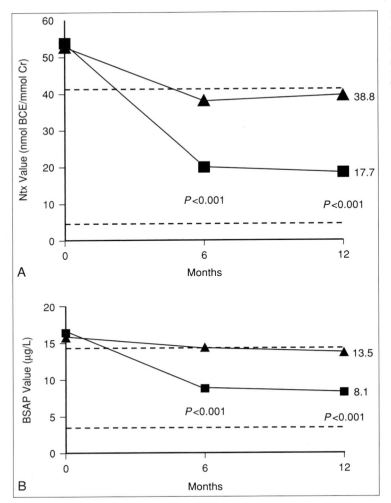

Figure 15-1. Comparison of urinary *N*-telopeptide of type 1 collagen (Ntx) (a) and bone-specific alkaline phosphatase (BSAP) (b) after 12 months of treatment with alendronate 70 mg weekly (square) or raloxifene (triangle). Dotted lines represent the premenopausal normal range.

fractures, with 0.7% sustaining hip fractures. In contrast, in the vertebral fracture arm of the FIT study, the fracture rates were higher, with 14.7% of placebo-treated patients sustaining a nonvertebral fracture and 2.2% a hip fracture.

Recent exploratory analyses in patients with severe-grade vertebral fractures have shown an effect of raloxifene to reduce nonvertebral fracture risk (Figure 15-2),[21] but the interpretation of such post hoc analyses remains unclear.

The MORE study also demonstrated a marked reduction in the risk of breast cancer (62% reduction over 4 years). In the Continuing Outcomes Relevant to Evista (CORE) study, an extension of the MORE study for an additional 4 years in 4011 women to assess the long-term effects of raloxifene on breast cancer, nonvertebral fracture was a secondary endpoint.[22] Again, no significant difference in overall nonvertebral fracture rates was observed between placebo (22.9%) and raloxifene (22.8%) after 8 years, although in post hoc analyses, a decreased risk of nonvertebral fracture was apparent in

subjects with baseline prevalent vertebral fractures (incident rate ratio, 0.78; 95% CI, 0.63-0.96). It is noteworthy that women who enrolled in the CORE study had less severe osteoporosis than those who did not and that use of other bone-active medications was allowed.

Some authors have suggested that one explanation for this apparent lack of effect on nonvertebral fracture incidence is that the more modest antiresorptive effects of raloxifene on cancellous bone are able to "normalize" high bone turnover and prevent further microarchitectural disruption and thus reduce vertebral fracture risk, but to reduce fracture risk at sites of cortical bone such as the hip requires more potent antiresorptive effects.[23]

SELECTIVE ESTROGEN RECEPTOR MODULATORS IN CLINICAL PRACTICE FOR OSTEOPOROSIS

The findings of the Women's Health Initiative that combination hormone therapy can prevent fractures in unselected postmenopausal women but is associated

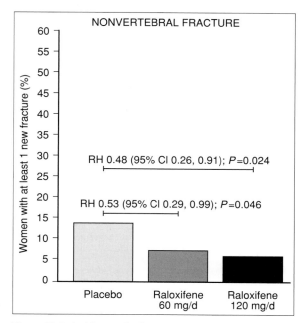

Figure 15-2. Incidence of at least one new nonvertebral fracture at 3 years in women with severe prevalent fractures treated with placebo, raloxifene 60 mg daily, or raloxifene 120 mg daily. (Adapted from Delmas PD, Genant HK, Crans GG, et al: Severity of prevalent vertebral fractures and the risk of subsequent vertebral and nonvertebral fractures: results from the MORE trial. Bone 2003;33:522-32.)

with adverse breast and cardiovascular events[24] provides a strong rationale for an agent that can prevent postmenopausal bone loss while providing benefits in other estrogen-associated target tissues.

An important issue in deciding who will benefit from SERMs in the treatment of osteoporosis is how to compare their efficacy with the bisphosphonates. As noted earlier, there has been increasing recognition that surrogate endpoints of BMD and bone turnover explain only a part of the antifracture efficacy of the antiresorptive agents. Sarkar[25] has reported that the change in BMD with raloxifene treatment accounted for only 4% of the observed reduction in vertebral fracture risk.

Because clinical trials have demonstrated that raloxifene can reduce the risk of vertebral fracture but have not yet definitely demonstrated an effect on nonvertebral fracture, it is recommended that raloxifene be used mainly in postmenopausal women with milder osteoporosis as a preventive measure or for treatment in those with predominantly spinal osteoporosis. It should not be used in women with menopausal hot flashes, because it can exacerbate them and even initiate them in some asymptomatic women.

Data about the optimal duration of therapy with raloxifene are limited. Recently, 7-year data in a subset of 386 women from the CORE study who did not take

other bone-active drugs became available.[22] At the lumbar spine, raloxifene increased BMD by 4.3% compared with baseline, which was 2.2% greater than seen with the calcium plus vitamin D "placebo" group. At the femoral neck, the increase with raloxifene over 7 years was 1.9%, which was 3.0% greater than in the control group.

Similarly, there are only limited data about the effects of withdrawal of raloxifene on BMD and bone turnover. One small study reported the effect of discontinuation of raloxifene versus estrogen therapy on BMD in 38 women after 5 years' prior treatment with either agent.[26] In 10 subjects who had received raloxifene 60 mg daily for 5 years, 1 year after discontinuation lumbar spine BMD had decreased by 2.4% and femoral neck BMD by 3.0%. Also, in the CORE study in the interval in which no study drug was taken, between the 4th and 5th years, the raloxifene group had significant bone loss at both the lumbar spine and the femoral neck.[22] Similarly, a study of 234 women treated with levormeloxifene for 12 months found that BMD approached baseline levels after 12 months without treatment.[27]

Another study examined the effect of raloxifene 60 mg daily on bone markers in 19 elderly women aged 76 to 99 years living in residential care.[28] Serum C-telopeptide of type I collagen decreased by 31% after 12 weeks of raloxifene, but levels returned to normal by 6 weeks after raloxifene was discontinued. Similarly, urinary cross-linked N-telopeptide of type I collagen decreased by 35% with raloxifene, but a more persistent suppressive effect on these levels was seen 6 weeks after cessation. Other data suggesting that bone turnover returns rather rapidly to normal after cessation of raloxifene come from a study of 59 postmenopausal women administered teriparatide for 18 months. Prior treatment with alendronate resulted in baseline bone turnover markers that were about one-half the level of markers in subjects who received prior treatment with raloxifene.[29] Moreover, the bone density response to teriparatide in subjects who received prior raloxifene was no different to the response in treatment-naive patients, whereas those who had received prior treatment with alendronate had an attenuated BMD response. This suggests that if anabolic agents are contemplated, there may be advantages to using a SERM, because they may have quicker off-set effects after withdrawal.

To summarize, because of these more modest effects on BMD and bone turnover that reverse soon after cessation, a conservative approach is to recommend that raloxifene be used as long-term therapy (at least 5 to 10 years) with subsequent decisions based on the bone density level achieved or bone turnover response.

CONCLUSION

Selective estrogen receptor modulators should mainly be used in postmenopausal women with milder osteoporosis or in those with predominantly spinal osteoporosis. The quick offset of SERMs such as raloxifene may offer advantages to more potent antiresorptive agents if use of an anabolic agent is considered in an individual patient. Other SERMs are in phase III clinical trials and the findings concerning their effects on nonvertebral fractures will be of interest.

REFERENCES

1. Riggs BL, Hartmann LC: Selective estrogen-receptor modulators: mechanisms of action and application to clinical practice. N Engl J Med 2003;348:618-29.
2. Turken S, Siris E, Seldin D, et al: Effects of tamoxifen on spinal bone density in women with breast cancer. J Natl Cancer Inst 1989;81:1086-88.
3. Ward RL, Morgan G, Dalley D, Kelly PJ: Tamoxifen reduces bone turnover and prevents lumbar spine and proximal femoral bone loss in early postmenopausal women. Bone Mineral 1993;22:87-94.
4. Love RR, Barden HS, Mazess RB, et al: Effect of tamoxifen on lumbar spine bone mineral density in postmenopausal women after 5 years. Arch Intern Med 1994;154:2585-88.
5. Grey AB, Stapleton JP, Evans MC, et al: The effect of the anti-estrogen tamoxifen on bone mineral density in normal late postmenopausal women. Am J Med 1995;99:636-41.
6. Powles TJ, Hickish T, Kanis JA, et al: Effect of tamoxifen on bone mineral density measured by dual-energy x-ray absorptiometry in healthy premenopausal and postmenopausal women. J Clin Oncol 1996;14:78-84.
7. Kristensen B, Ejlertsen B, Mouridsen HT, et al: Femoral fractures in postmenopausal breast cancer patients treated with adjuvant tamoxifen. Breast Cancer Res 1996;39:321-26.
8. Marttunen MB, Hietanen P, Tiitinen A, Ylikorkala O: Comparison of effects of tamoxifen and toremifene on bone biochemistry and bone mineral density in postmenopausal breast cancer patients. J Clin Endocr Metab 1998;83:1158-62.
9. Sporn MB: Arzoxifene: a promising new selective estrogen receptor modulator for clinical chemoprevention of breast cancer. Clin Cancer Res 2004;10:5403-17.
10. Ke HZ, Foley GL, Simmons HA, et al: Long-term treatment of lasofoxifene preserves bone mass and bone strength and does not adversely affect the uterus in ovariectomized rats. Endocrinol 2004;145:1996-2005.
11. Johnell O, Scheele W, Lu Y, et al: Additive effects of raloxifene and alendronate on bone density and biochemical markers of bone remodeling in postmenopausal women with osteoporosis. J Clin Endocr Metab 2002;87:985-92.
12. Sambrook PN, Geusens P, Ribot C, et al: Alendronate produces greater effects than raloxifene on bone density and bone turnover in postmenopausal women with low bone density: results of EFFECT (Efficacy of FOSAMAX versus EVISTA Comparison Trial) International. J Intern Med 2004;255:503-11.
13. Delmas PD, Bjarnason NH, Mitlak BH, et al: Effects of raloxifene on bone mineral density, serum cholesterol concentrations, and uterine endometrium in postmenopausal women. N Engl J Med 1997;337:1641-47.
14. Eastell R, Barton I, Hannon RA, et al: Relationship of early changes in bone resorption to the reduction in fracture risk with risedronate. J Bone Miner Res 2003;18:1051-56.
15. Delmas PD, Seeman E: Changes in bone mineral density explain little of the reduction in vertebral or nonvertebral fracture risk with anti-resorptive therapy. Bone 2004;34:599-604.
16. Cummings SR, Karpf D, Harris F, et al: Improvement in spine bone density and reduction in risk of vertebral fractures during treatment with antiresorptive drugs. Am J Med 2002;112:281-89.
17. Ettinger B, Black DM, Mitlak BH, et al: Reduction of vertebral fracture risk in postmenopausal women with osteoporosis treated with raloxifene: results from a 3-year randomized clinical trial. Multiple Outcomes of Raloxifene Evaluation (MORE) Investigators. JAMA 1999;282:637-45.
18. Delmas PD, Ensrud KE, Adachi JD, et al: Efficacy of raloxifene on vertebral fracture risk reduction in postmenopausal women with osteoporosis: four-year results from a randomized clinical trial. J Clin Endocr Metab 2002;87:3609-17.
19. Cranney A, Tugwell P, Zytaruk N, et al: Meta-analyses of therapies for postmenopausal osteoporosis. IV. Meta-analysis of raloxifene for the prevention and treatment of postmenopausal osteoporosis. Endocr Rev 2002;23:524-28.
20. Black DM, Cummings SR, Karpf DB, et al: Randomised trial of effect of alendronate on risk of fracture in women with existing vertebral fractures. Fracture Intervention Trial Research Group. Lancet 1996:348:1535-41.
21. Delmas PD, Genant HK, Crans GG, et al: Severity of prevalent vertebral fractures and the risk of subsequent vertebral and nonvertebral fractures: results from the MORE trial. Bone 2003;33:522-32.
22. Siris E, Harris ST, Eastell R, et al: Skeletal effects of raloxifene after 8 years: results from the Continuing Outcomes Relevant to Evista (CORE) Study. J Bone Miner Res 2005;20:1514-24.
23. Riggs B, Melton LJ: Bone turnover matters: the raloxifene treatment paradox of dramatic decreases in vertebral fractures without commensurate increases in bone density. J Bone Miner Res 2002;17:11-14.
24. Rossouw JE, Anderson GL, Prentice RL, et al: Risks and benefits of estrogen plus progestin in healthy postmenopausal women. JAMA 2002;288:321-30.
25. Sarkar S, Mitlak BH, Wong M, et al: Associations between baseline risk factors and vertebral fracture risk in the Multiple Outcomes of Raloxifene Evaluation (MORE) Study. J Bone Miner Res 2002;17:1-10.
26. Neele SJ, Evertz R, De Valk-De Roo G, et al: Effect of 1 year of discontinuation of raloxifene or estrogen therapy on bone mineral density after 5 years of treatment in healthy postmenopausal women. Bone 2002;30:599-603.
27. Warming L, Christoffersen C, Riis BJ, et al: Adverse effects of a SERM (Levormeloxifene): safety parameters and bone mineral density 12 months treatment withdrawal. Maturitas 2003;44:189-99.
28. Hansdottir H, Franzson L, Prestwood K, Sigurdsson G: The effect of raloxifene on markers of bone turnover in older women living in long term care facilities. J Am Geriatr Soc 2004;52:779-83.
29. Ettinger B, San Martin J, Crans G, Pavo I: Differential effects of teriparatide on bone mineral density after treatment with raloxifene or alendronate. J Bone Miner Res 2004;19:745-51.

16 Sex Steroids and Skeletal Health in Men

Christian Meier, Peter Y. Liu, Markus J. Seibel, and David J. Handelsman

SUMMARY

Observational studies of bone development and interventional studies indicate that circulating estradiol is an important factor affecting bone turnover in elderly men. Just how important estradiol is relative to serum testosterone in the maintenance of bone mass in older men remains contentious. Nevertheless, aromatization of testosterone to estradiol plays a significant role in the regulation of bone metabolism and, ultimately, influences age-related bone loss in elderly men.

Osteoporosis is a recognized cause of morbidity and mortality in postmenopausal women. In contrast, osteoporosis in men has only recently received more attention, with studies performed to elucidate the pathogenesis of age-related bone loss in men. It is estimated that about one-third of all osteoporotic fractures occur in men,[1,2] and that the residual lifetime fracture risk in a man aged 60 years may be as high as 30%.[3] These fractures result in significant risks for morbidity and mortality as well as significant health care costs to the community,[4,5] particularly because the mortality and morbidity rates associated with bone fractures in older men exceed those of women.

Accrual of bone mass and age-related bone loss in aging healthy men is multifactorial, with hormonal, environmental, and genetic factors all being important. At puberty, dramatic increases in bone mineral content and bone mass occur, which are associated with sharp increases in blood testosterone, estradiol, and other hormones as well as activation of the nervous system. After peak bone mass has been achieved, bone mineral density (BMD) decreases gradually, but to a much lesser extent than in women. This age-related bone loss in men is accompanied by a slow decrease in blood androgen levels. However, whether a casual relationship exists between the age-associated decreases in androgen levels and bone mass remains unclear. Nevertheless, organic male hypogonadism in younger men with hypothalamic-pituitary or testicular disorders does result in bone loss, and androgen replacement in these men increases bone density.

This chapter summarizes the effects of gonadal steroids on bone turnover and bone mass in men. After a brief introduction on the general aspects of androgen action, observational and interventional data concerning the skeletal effects of gonadal hormones in male hypogonadism and aging men are discussed. In this context, special emphasis is placed on the differential roles of testosterone and estradiol in male skeletal health. Finally, therapeutic effects of testosterone administration in various clinical settings are highlighted.

GENERAL ASPECTS OF SEX HORMONE ACTION

Androgen Metabolism

Androgens are synthesized from cholesterol through several enzymatic pathways in which the side chain of cholesterol is shortened through oxidation from 27 carbons to 19 carbons.[6] In men, androgens are secreted almost exclusively from the testes as testosterone. The adrenal glands also secrete dehydroepiandrosterone, which is a minor androgen that also serves as a substrate for peripheral aromatization to estradiol.

Testosterone is either converted by 5α-reductase to dihydrotestosterone, or metabolized to estradiol by aromatase, a widely distributed microsomal cytochrome P450 enzyme. The former pathway amplifies androgen action locally whereas the latter pathway diversifies androgen action.[6] Hence, enzymatic androgen activation leads to testosterone acting directly or via its more potent metabolite dihydrotestosterone through the androgen receptor (AR) or indirectly via aromatization to estradiol through the estrogen receptors (ERs). The adrenal cortex secretes large amounts of 19-carbon androgens, including dehydroepiandrosterone, dehydroepiandrosterone-sulfate, and androstenedione. These androgens can be metabolized either directly or indirectly to estrone by aromatase or to testosterone by steroid sulfatase, 17β-hydroxysteroid dehydrogenase (17β-HSD) and/or 3β-HSD.[7]

Thus, testosterone, and to a lesser extent dehydroepiandrosterone, function as a precursor for peripheral conversion into biologically highly active hormones. In this respect, it is noteworthy that estradiol, which is believed to play a major role in bone metabolism in men, is largely synthesized by extratesticular aromatization of circulating testosterone with only a small proportion of estradiol (approximately 15-20%) being directly secreted by the testes, although the latter proportion increases with circulating blood luteinizing hormone levels.[8] Nevertheless, only a very small fraction (approximately 0.1%) of testosterone undergoes aromatization, whereas a larger proportion (5-10%) is 5α reduced to dihydrotestosterone and the remainder is inactivated by the liver. Depending on the relative activities of aromatase, 5α-reductase, and dehydrogenases and the relative distribution of AR and ERs in peripheral target tissues, testosterone and its metabolites predominantly activate either the AR or the ER. In bone tissue, the expression of aromatase,[9-15] 5α-reductase,[16-19] 17β-HSD,[10-12, 16, 20] and 3β-HSD[10, 21] has been documented, supporting the concept of tissue-specific peripheral activation of gonadal hormones.

The AR has been identified in most bone cells, including osteoblasts,[22] osteocytes,[23] and osteoclasts.[24, 25] As a result of androgens binding to the AR, the activated ligand-receptor complex acts as a nuclear transcription factor that binds to the androgen response elements located in the promoter region of androgen-responsive genes to regulate their transcription.[26] Estrogen action on bone, in men and women, is mediated via ERs. These nuclear hormone receptors are also expressed in osteoblasts, osteoclasts, and osteocytes.[27, 28] Two ERs have been identified, ERα and ERβ, which are distinct proteins encoded by separate genes.[29, 30] ERα is predominantly expressed in cells resident to cortical bone, whereas ERβ shows higher levels of expression in cells found in cancellous (trabecular) bone.[28] Once activated by their specific ligands, the ERs regulate gene expression by binding to specific response element sequences in the promoter regions of estrogen target genes. Alternate nongenomic pathways have also been described in which ARs and ERs modulate transcription indirectly, via protein-protein interactions.

Age-Related Changes in Gonadal Hormones

Male aging is associated with a gradual, progressive decrease in circulating testosterone.[31, 32] Longitudinal population-based studies show that serum total testosterone concentrations decline by approximately 1% per year in men, but the importance of such a decline remains unclear. A variety of derived testosterone measures ("free," "bioavailable"), which putatively reflect various binding and tissue availabilities of testosterone to carrier proteins, have been postulated to reflect androgen action more closely, but the underlying free hormone hypothesis lacks adequate empirical verification.[33] For example, although "free" testosterone (that is, the fraction of total testosterone that is unbound, particularly to albumin or sex hormone–binding globulin [SHBG]) is reported to fall more rapidly due to a concomitant twofold rise in SHBG binding capacity,[34-36] it is unclear whether this represents more or less net androgen action at a tissue level, because the "free" hormone is more accessible both to sites of hormone action and to degradation.[37] Furthermore, it seems implausible that a single static testosterone measure would adequately reflect androgenic action in all androgen-responsive tissues, including bone, especially given the additional complexity of the local androgen amplification systems involved. Diverse organ-specific factors would seem to be crucial in modulating the net biological action of testosterone within each tissue. Furthermore, declining total, free, or SHBG-bound testosterone levels, although firmly established, are modest in magnitude and may not warrant replacement. Whether the older tissues remain as androgen responsive and whether testosterone replacement is effective or safe remains to be established by appropriate interventional studies.[32, 38]

Although an age-related fall in blood estrone has been observed in men,[36] similar reductions in estradiol have not been well documented. This may be due to increased aromatase activity with age, which in turn is attributed to the age-associated increase in fat mass.[39] Non–SHBG-bound estradiol levels decrease with age (by about 50% over 6 decades) as a consequence of increasing SHBG concentrations.[40] However, the biological validity of this derived estradiol measure remains to be established, because binding to SHBG is competitive with testosterone, which is present in 100-fold higher molar concentrations. Furthermore, nonextraction automated immunoassays are unreliable for the very low serum estradiol concentrations present in men, children, and postmenopausal women. For these reasons, the biological significance of free and SHBG-bound estradiol for bone is even less well-defined than for comparable derived testosterone measurements. Although the available evidence indicates that estradiol has significance for the male skeleton, the circulating blood estradiol concentrations in men are comparable with those of estrogen-deficient postmenopausal women, raising the paradoxical issue of why male bone does not acquire the osteoporotic state of the bone of postmenopausal women. In fact, male bone actually becomes and remains larger, with higher periosteal and endosteal diameters than women, which makes it even stronger than premenopausal female bone. This may be explained, at least in part, by AR-mediated effects and the greater importance of local bone aromatase expression in male bone, so that estrogen action is more dependent on local production than on systemic exposure. However, other factors, some of which relate to larger body and muscle mass, are also likely to be important.

SKELETAL HEALTH WITH VARYING DEGREES OF ANDROGEN DEFICIENCY

Bone mass is the net result of two counteracting metabolic processes, bone formation and bone resorption. This continuous turnover of bone, also referred to as *bone remodeling*, relies on the activity of two major types of cells, namely bone-forming osteoblasts and bone-resorbing osteoclasts.[41] Under normal conditions, bone formation and bone resorption are coupled. To appreciate the effect of gonadal hormones on bone turnover and BMD in men, we now summarize the data from both men with androgen deficiency (male hypogonadism) and healthy men with age-related decreases in androgen levels.

Consequences of Male Hypogonadism and Androgen Resistance in Men

Hypogonadism is present in 15% to 36% of men with documented osteoporosis,[5,42] although this may be an overestimate given the nonspecific effects of acute or chronic illness, particularly fractures, on blood testosterone concentrations. Nevertheless, it is clear that normal gonadal function is crucial for the development and maintenance of male bone integrity. Androgen deprivation therapy (surgical or chemical castration), which is often required in adult men with advanced prostate cancer, for example, results in a profound decline in circulating gonadal hormones. Similar to changes observed in women with surgical ovariectomy or during early menopause, the rapid decline in sex steroids after castration is followed by accelerated and unbalanced bone turnover, which results in net bone resorption. Bone turnover, as assessed by biochemical markers of bone resorption and formation is increased[43-49] and results in rapid and sustained bone loss in hypogonadal men. Bone mineral density is predominately reduced at the lumbar spine, which decreases by about 5% to 10% within the first year of androgen deprivation therapy.[43-48,50] Bone loss is also observed at peripheral skeletal sites, including the hip, although to a lesser extent.[45-47,51-53] Ultimately, bone loss after castration results in an increased risk of osteoporotic fractures.[52,54-59] As reported by Daniell and associates,[52] the cumulative incidence of a first osteoporotic frac-

ture is increased more than fivefold in castrated patients.

Men with overt hypogonadism due to testicular or hypothalamic-pituitary dysfunction present with less dramatic changes in BMD and bone turnover, largely due to less profound and more varying degrees of androgen deficiency. Most men with hypogonadism have significantly lower bone density than age-matched control subjects.[60-64] Luisetto and associates,[65] however, observed that bone mass in 32 men with Klinefelter syndrome was comparable with that of healthy control subjects. This discrepancy is most likely due to the moderate decreases in testicular function and circulating androgen levels present in their specific patient population and reflects the wide phenotypic spectrum of Klinefelter syndrome.[66] In contrast to these mostly uniform alterations in BMD, changes in bone turnover, specifically in bone formation, are less clear. Although bone resorption is accelerated in hypogonadal men as compared with control subjects,[63,67,68] bone formation may be either decreased[63,69,70] or increased[7,67,68] when assessed by biochemical indices of bone formation or histomorphometric studies. Testosterone replacement therapy in hypogonadal men, conversely, decreases bone resorption[68,71-74] and exerts an anabolic effect with increased bone formation,[71,72,75] although some studies failed to show an increase in bone formation.[68,73,74] These inconsistencies may be due to the inadequate androgen replacement and heterogeneity of male hypogonadism.[76]

Recent observations suggest that estradiol may play an important role in the development of male bone. First evidence in support of this concept has emerged from a report of a 28-year-old man with estrogen resistance caused by a homozygous and inactivating mutation in the ERα gene. Despite normal serum testosterone levels, and elevated circulating levels of estradiol, this patient had accelerated bone turnover with increased rates of bone formation and bone resorption and a bone mass in the osteopenic range.[77] Subsequently, clinical findings in adult men with aromatase deficiency caused by inactivating mutations in the aromatase gene and undetectable estradiol confirmed these findings.[78-80] Again, bone turnover and BMD in these men were markedly altered in the presence of undetectable low circulating estradiol levels and normal serum testosterone levels. Furthermore, treatment with estradiol in men with aromatase deficiency suppressed bone resorption[80] and markedly increased bone mass.[79,80] However, these cases reflect developmentally disordered bone formed under conditions of congenital estrogen deficiency, and it is not clear how these findings relate to the maintenance of normal mature bone developed under eugonadal conditions.

Effects of Androgen Replacement in Male Hypogonadism

Most studies of androgen administration in hypogonadal men have reported beneficial effects on BMD, although the gain in bone density is highly variable across studies.[72-74, 81-85] This may be related, at least in part, to differences in the adequacy of testosterone replacement regimens,[76] variable degrees of underlying testosterone deficiencies, and different methods used to quantify bone density (dual x-ray absorptiometry, quantitative computed tomography). In addition, pharmacogenetic characteristics such as the length of the CAG triplet repeat in exon 1 of the AR, which is inversely related to androgen sensitivity, may also contribute to the effectiveness of testosterone treatment on bone (Figure 16-1).[86]

As reported by Behre and colleagues, the most significant increase in BMD is seen during the first year of testosterone treatment and is greatest in patients with the lowest initial BMD. Thereafter, bone density is maintained during long-term testosterone administration (Figure 16-2),[82] so long as adequate testosterone dosage is maintained.[76]

Data from prospective and retrospective studies on the effect of androgen replacement on bone density in hypogonadal men have recently been summarized.[7] From these studies, it is evident that mostly cancellous bone sites (e.g., spine) are more responsive than predominantly cortical sites (e.g., radius, hip), and that measurements based on quantitative computed tomography show much greater responses than studies using

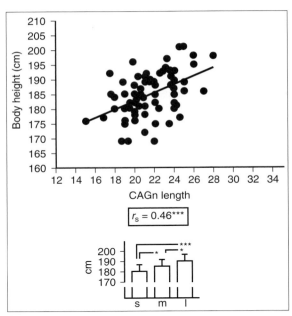

Figure 16-1. Body height in relation to CAGn length of the androgen-receptor genes of patients with Klinefelter syndrome. (Inset) Height distribution according to tertiles of X-weighted biallelic CAGn length. Short (s): CAGn ≤ 20.0; n=27. Medium (m): CAGn 20.0–23.0; n=27. Long (l): CAGn > 23.0; n=23. Significant differences according to Kruskal-Wallis and post hoc tests. Levels of statistical significance are given as asterisks ($^{*}P < .05$; $^{**}P < .01$; $^{***}P < .001$). (Adapted with permission from Zitzmann M, Depenbusch M, Gromoll J, et al: X-chromosome inactivation patterns and androgen receptor functionality influence phenotype and social characteristics as well as pharmacogenetics of testosterone therapy in Klinefelter patients. J Clin Endocrinol Metab 2004;89:6208-17.)

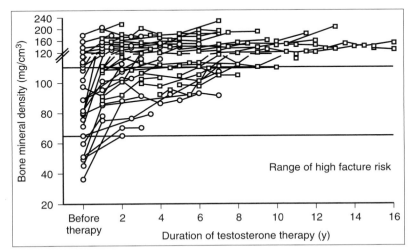

Figure 16-2. Increase in bone mineral density during long-term testosterone substitution therapy up to 16 years in 72 hypogonadal men. Circles indicate hypogonadal patients with first quantitative computed tomography measurement before initiation of testosterone replacement therapy; squares show those patients already receiving testosterone therapy at the first quantitative computed tomography scan. The dark shaded area indicates the range of high fracture risk, the unshaded area shows the range without significant fracture risk, and the light shaded area indicates the intermediate range where fractures may occur. (Adapted with permission from Behre HM, Kliesch S, Leifke E, et al: Long-term effect of testosterone therapy on bone mineral density in hypogonadal men. J Clin Endocrinol Metab 1997;82:2386-90.)

dual x-ray absortiometry or dual- or single-photon absorptiometry. On the other hand, subcortical bone apposition appears to be more important in men and responsible for their larger and stronger bone structure.[87] These differences may be in part due to androgen-induced changes in body composition (i.e., fat mass), which are not corrected for when quantitative computed tomography measures are used to evaluate BMD responses. Furthermore, the adequacy of testosterone administration is an important determinant of its efficacy (Figure 16-3).[76] Intramuscular testosterone

administration may result in supraphysiological circulating testosterone levels and effects on bone may therefore be more prominent. In contrast, transdermal[88,89] or buccal[90] testosterone administration increases serum testosterone levels predominately within the physiological range. However, no prospective studies comparing the effects on skeletal health in accordance with the mode of androgen administration are available. Also, there are no large randomized controlled trials in osteoporotic men using testosterone replacement therapy with fractures as a clinical endpoint.

The effect of androgen replacement on BMD is largely accounted for by its effect on bone turnover. In hypogonadal men, testosterone administration decreases bone resorption[68,71-74] and increases bone formation.[71,72,75] However, beneficial effects on body composition, specifically on muscle mass, are most likely contributing factors to the increase in BMD. Based on several studies, an increase in lean body mass[68,71,74,88] or muscle strength[71,75,91,92] after testosterone administration has been documented.

Consequences of Partial Androgen Deficiency in Elderly Men

Based on observations in men with organic androgen deficiency, sex hormones have been shown to be critical for bone remodeling and maintenance of bone mass during adult life. It is therefore possible that low levels of gonadal hormones would affect skeletal integrity in the elderly male if the deficiency state is sufficiently severe and the skeleton remains sufficiently responsive to steroids. Recently, male reproductive health, specifically androgen-deficiency in aging men, has become an issue of growing interest not only to physicians but also to the wider community. Putative somatic consequences of gradually falling testosterone concentrations, including changes in bone mass, have become the rationale for wider use of testosterone treatment of middle-aged and older men with apparent age-related but no other form of overt androgen deficiency. Such treatment has increased nearly 20-fold worldwide over the last decade, with one-half of this increase occurring in the United States,[38,93] although it has remained largely unchanged in Europe and Australia.[94,95] In this section, we summarize available evidence on age-related changes in bone health, including effects on bone turnover and BMD.

Several cross-sectional and longitudinal studies have investigated the association between sex hormones, biochemical markers of bone turnover, and bone mass in elderly men.[40,96-99] In a cross-sectional study including men between 23 and 90 years of age, Khosla and colleagues[40] reported inverse correlations between urinary cross-linked N-telopeptide levels and both "bioavailable" estradiol and "bioavailable" testosterone.

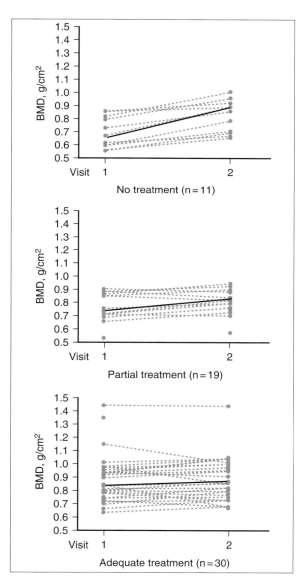

Figure 16-3. Change in bone mineral density (BMD) (g/cm^2) at the lumbar spine (L1-L4) between the first and second visits, depending on treatment at the time of the first BMD ($P < .001$). (Adapted with permission from Aminorroaya A, Kelleher S, Conway AJ, et al: Adequacy of androgen replacement influences bone density response to testosterone in androgen-deficient men. Eur J Endocrinol 2005;152:881-86.)

However, no correlation with total estradiol or testosterone was detected. In contrast, Szulc and colleagues found that in men older than 51 years of age, only bioavailable estradiol levels were negatively correlated with bone turnover, but no associations were observed with total estradiol, or any testosterone measure.[96] The association between estradiol and bone resorption markers has been confirmed in another study in which significant correlations were found only with markers of bone resorption (serum and urinary cross-linked N-telopeptide), but not with biochemical indices of bone formation (osteocalcin [OC], bone specific alkaline phosphatase [BAP]).[98] The available data emphasize that low levels of circulating estradiol are associated with increased bone resorption, and that this increase is only partly compensated for by a concomitant rise in bone formation.

Elderly men, especially those older than 70 years of age, are increasingly at risk of bone loss and osteoporotic fractures. However, the extent to which low levels of testosterone contribute to age-related bone loss in men remains unclear.[7] In analogy to markers of bone turnover, several cross-sectional and longitudinal studies have documented significant correlations between serum levels of "bioavailable" or total estradiol and bone density[100, 101] or change in bone mass during follow-up.[97-99] In contrast, however, studies have failed to show consistent associations between "bioavailable" testosterone and BMD or bone loss.[40,102,103] The failure of studies to show clear relationships with total estradiol casts doubt on the interpretation of these studies. As stated earlier, the relative biological importance of derived estradiol measures such as "free" and "bioavailable" or SHBG-bound estradiol remains to be determined. It is also unclear whether the main mechanism of estrogen action on bone is via local aromatization of testosterone to estradiol within bone or to systemic estradiol exposure. One possible explanation is that there is a threshold for estrogen action, possibly based on some critical level of blood or local estradiol. Alternatively, these observations using derived variables may be computational artifacts due to the strong age dependence of SHBG. When such derived variables are introduced into models, they unintentionally include age, again creating a logical circularity.

All the above-mentioned studies focus on the association between sex hormone levels and bone turnover markers and BMD as surrogate markers of bone integrity. However, data on the relationship between testosterone and estradiol and the risk of osteoporotic fractures are largely unknown. Only recently, Goderie-Plomp and colleagues reported results from a population-based, case-control study investigating the association between endogenous sex hormones and incident vertebral fracture risk in both elderly women and men. In this study, no clear associations were observed between hormonal factors (testosterone, estradiol, SHBG) and the risk for incident vertebral fractures in men, which was probably due to low statistical power.[104]

It is emphasized that bone turnover and BMD only partially contribute to the overall risk for incident fractures in men. Whether, and to what extent, sex hormone levels contribute to fracture risk in men and whether this effect is independent of surrogate markers such as BMD is largely unknown.

Effect of Hormone Replacement in Men with Age-Related Androgen Deficiency

The effects of testosterone treatment on bone in elderly men remain inconclusive and there is no evidence from long-term randomized studies to indicate that androgen treatment reduces bone fractures in men.[32] So far, four randomized placebo-controlled studies in healthy men older than 50 years have examined the impact of androgenic supplementation on bone health, including bone turnover markers[105-108] and bone density.[106-108] All studies treated otherwise healthy, nonosteoporotic men with transdermal testosterone[106,108] or intramuscular testosterone injections.[105,107] Irrespective of baseline blood testosterone concentrations (range, 10.1-13.5 nmol/L), no study showed significant changes in bone turnover markers after 3 to 36 months of treatment. Only in an early small crossover study by Tenover[105] did urinary excretion of hydroxyproline (OHP) decrease in testosterone-treated men while the respective levels remained unchanged in the placebo group. The relevance of this singular finding using a nonspecific marker of collagen turnover remains unclear.

Two placebo-controlled studies investigating the effect on BMD have differed in outcome: the study by Snyder and associates[106] showed no benefit of treatment, but the study by Kenny and associates[108] showed that testosterone is able to prevent ongoing age-related bone loss in one of five bone sites. Post hoc analysis of the larger study by Snyder and associates[106] suggested that bone density gains were inversely related to prestudy baseline levels of blood testosterone, consistent with the idea that the benefits depend on the degree of underlying androgen deficiency (Figure 16-4). In a recent study in which testosterone enanthate was administered at a higher dose, significant increases were found in BMD at the lumbar spine and the hip after 36 months of treatment[107]; however, a reduction in dose for polycythemia was required in 25% of the participating men.[95]

In summary, there appears to be no consistent effect of exogenous testosterone treatment on bone turnover and limited, dose-dependent effect on BMD in older men with low-normal levels of circulating testosterone. Results from placebo-controlled trials including elderly men with consistently lower baseline testosterone levels

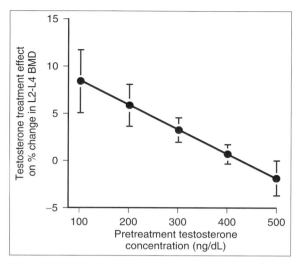

Figure 16-4. The testosterone treatment effect on percentage change in bone mineral density (BMD) during 36 months of testosterone treatment in men older than 65 years of age as a function of the pretreatment serum testosterone concentration. The lower the pretreatment serum testosterone concentration, the greater the effect of testosterone treatment on BMD. The treatment effect was statistically significant ($P < .01$) for pretreatment serum T concentrations of 10 to 300 ng/dL. The values shown are the mean (±SE) changes in BMD during the 36 months of treatment in the testosterone-treated subjects minus those in the placebo-treated subjects. (Adapted with permission from Snyder PJ, Peachey H, Hannoush P, et al: Effect of testosterone treatment on bone mineral density in men over 65 years of age. J Clin Endocrinol Metab 1999;84:1966-72.)

(<8 nmol/L) are needed to unravel the effects of testosterone replacement on bone surrogate markers, such as BMD and bone turnover markers, and ultimately fracture risk, morbidity, and mortality. In the interim, there is no basis for empirical testosterone treatment for men with idiopathic or age-related osteoporosis unless there is concomitant evidence of overt androgen deficiency.

Differential Effects of Testosterone and Estradiol on Bone Metabolism

To understand the physiological roles of sex hormones on skeletal health in men, measurements of biochemical markers of bone turnover have been used as surrogates in many different clinical and research settings. Short-term randomized pharmacological studies have dissected the relative contributions of androgenic and estrogenic actions in the maintenance of bone turnover.[109-112] These studies suggest that bone resorption is largely regulated by local estradiol action, although how much of this effect is due to systemic versus local aromatization of blood testosterone remains unclear. Falahati-Nini and coworkers assessed the relative effects of testosterone and estradiol by either partial (testosterone alone, or estradiol alone) or complete (testosterone and estradiol) sex hormone replacement in 59 elderly men, who prior to the study were rendered acutely androgen- and estrogen-

deficient by combined treatment with a gonadotropin-releasing hormone agonist and an aromatase inhibitor.[109] Bone resorption markers increased significantly in men after acute hormone withdrawal but remained unchanged in subjects with combined testosterone and estradiol replacement therapy. Interestingly, estradiol alone almost completely prevented the increase in bone resorption markers, whereas testosterone alone was much less effective in this respect, although the transdermal patch dosage was probably suboptimal. The authors estimated that, in elderly men, local estradiol accounted for approximately 70% of the total effect of sex hormones on bone resorption, although some of this effect would be mediated by local conversion of systemic testosterone into estradiol[101] (Figure 16-5) and the effect of more adequate testosterone delivery was not determined. The study design does not distinguish between bone effects of estradiol mediated by systemic delivery or local aromatization of testosterone. In another study with pharmacological hormone withdrawal, testosterone replacement alone was partially able to prevent the increase in bone resorption markers (U-DPD, but not S- and U-NTX), whereas in men with combined sex hormone replacement, bone resorption remained unaltered.[112] Although bone resorption seems to be under the predominant control of estradiol in men, an estradiol-independent effect of androgens on bone resorption seems conceivable because androgen receptors were found on human osteoclasts,[25] and in vitro and animal data suggest crucial roles for both estrogens and androgens in male bone metabolism. Owing to limited tolerance for chronic androgen deficiency, both of these studies were short-term, so the effect of longer term hormonal regulation of bone turnover and density remains unclear. Another study showed in chronically glucocorticoid-treated men that even in the presence of adequate androgen exposure, aromatization appears to increase BMD (Figure 16-6).[113] However, 7-alpha-methyl-19-nortestosterone, a novel compound that is minimally reduced by 5α-reductase but is aromatizable to a highly estrogenic compound, did not maintain bone density,[114] although study subjects probably had subtherapeutic T treatment before study entry and these were men with established androgen deficiency. This emphasizes the importance of adequate androgen exposure.

Androgen receptors are found on osteoblasts,[22] suggesting that testosterone per se may have important effects on bone formation. In keeping with this concept, Falahati-Nini and colleagues observed that markers of bone formation (OC, amino terminal propeptide of type 1 collagen [PINP]) decreased significantly in men during acute sex hormone withdrawal. In contrast, these markers remained unchanged in men receiving testosterone and estradiol replacement therapy.[109] Of note, the decrease in serum OC was prevented equally well by

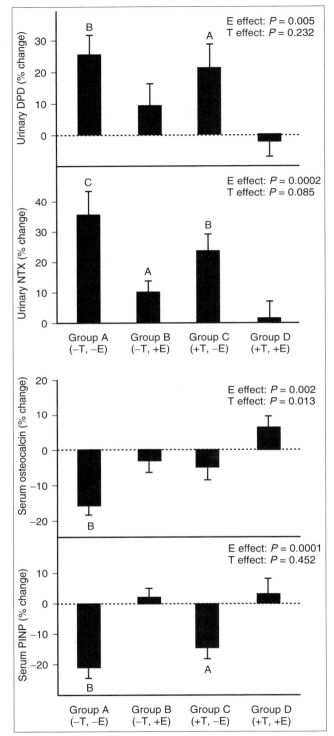

Figure 16-5. Percentage changes in bone resorption markers (urinary DPD and NTX; ^{A} $P < 0.05$, ^{B} $P < 0.005$, and ^{C} $P < 0.001$ for change from baseline) and bone formation markers (serum osteocalcin and PINP; ^{A} $P < 0.005$ and ^{B} $P < 0.001$ for change from baseline) in a group of elderly men (mean age, 68 years) made acutely hypogonadal and treated with an aromatase inhibitor (group A), estradiol (E) alone (group B), testosterone (T) alone (group C), or both estradiol and testosterone (group D). (Adapted with permission from Falahati-Nini A, Riggs BL, Atkinson EJ, et al: Relative contributions of testosterone and estrogen in regulating bone resorption and formation in normal elderly men. J Clin Invest 2000;106:1553-60.)

either testosterone or estradiol, whereas serum PINP levels were affected primarily by estradiol but not by testosterone. In contrast, no such effect on bone formation was observed in a study of sex steroid withdrawal for a period of 12 weeks, which might be due to the longer study duration with an overall increase in bone turnover that had occurred by the time the measurements were made.[112] In addition, the potential effect of estradiol on osteoblastic differentiation was not only observed during selective estradiol replacement in hypogonadal men, but

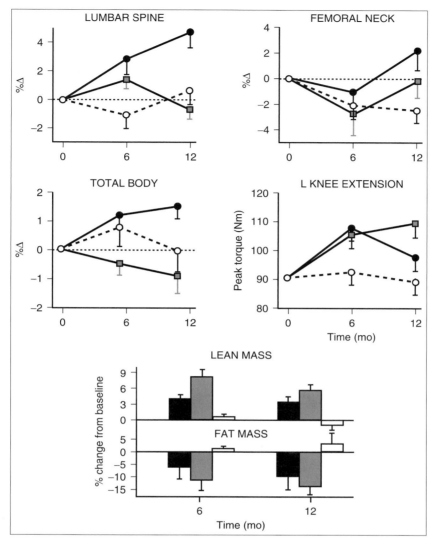

Figure 16-6. Bone mineral density (BMD) changes in the lumbar spine, femoral neck, and total body as well as changes in left knee muscle strength and in lean and fat mass in men treated with testosterone (solid black), minimally aromatizable nandrolone (gray), or placebo (unfilled, with dashed line). The dashed horizontal line through zero represents no change from baseline. Note both androgens increased muscle mass and strength and reduced fat mass, whereas only testosterone has consistent effects on bone density. Between-group difference is significant (*P* < .01). (Modified from Crawford BA, Liu PY, Kean MT, et al: Randomized placebo-controlled trial of androgen effects on muscle and bone in men requiring long-term systemic glucocorticoid treatment. J Clin Endocrinol Metab 2003;88:3167-76.)

also as a result of supraphysiological estradiol treatment (human chorionic gonadotropin treatment) in elderly men with otherwise adequate androgen exposure.[111] Recombinant human chorionic gonadotropin treatment, but not nonaromatizable dihydrotestosterone alone, has been shown to stimulate osteoblastic collagen formation proportionally to increased estradiol concentrations (Figure 16-7).[111] Because S-PINP is generated from newly synthesized collagen, it is considered a measure of newly formed type I collagen and therefore a marker of bone formation (early osteoblastic function).[115] These data would therefore suggest that it is principally estradiol that regulates osteoblastic differenti-

ation, and both testosterone and estradiol may be important in modulating late osteoblastic function.

In summary, results from interventional studies support the findings from observational studies of bone development that estradiol is important for bone turnover in elderly men. These findings suggest that aromatization of testosterone to estradiol plays a significant role in the regulation of bone metabolism and, ultimately, influences age-related bone loss in elderly men.[116] Just how important it is relative to blood testosterone for maintenance of bone in older men and whether the principal effects are due to local aromatization in bone or from circulating estradiol remain contentious points.

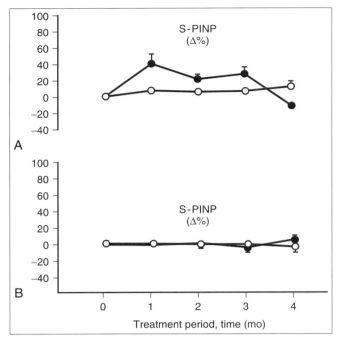

Figure 16-7. ***A,*** Mean percent changes (±SE) in serum PINP levels among 40 men before, during, and after twice-weekly subcutaneous injections of 250 μg (5000 IU) recombinant human chorionic gonadotropin (rhCG) for 3 months. Note the significant increase in S-PINP levels in the treatment (●) compared with the placebo group (○) (*P* = 0.002, repeated-measures general linear model). In contrast, no consistent changes were seen in serum levels of OC and ICTP, or U-DPD. ***B,*** Mean percent changes (±SE) in serum PINP levels among 35 men before, during, and after daily application of 70 mg dihydrotestosterone for 3 months. No significant differences (repeated-measures general linear model) between the treatment (●) and placebo (○) groups were observed during the 3-month treatment period. (Adapted with permission from Meier C, Liu PY, Ly LP, et al: Recombinant human chorionic gonadotropin but not dihydrotestosterone alone stimulates osteoblastic collagen synthesis in older men with partial age-related androgen deficiency. J Clin Endocrinol Metab 2004;89:3033-41.)

REFERENCES

1. Cooper C, Campion G, Melton LJ 3rd: Hip fractures in the elderly: a world-wide projection. Osteoporos Int 1992;2:285-89.
2. Gullberg B, Johnell O, Kanis JA: World-wide projections for hip fracture. Osteoporos Int 1997;7:407-13.
3. Jones G, Nguyen T, Sambrook PN, et al: Symptomatic fracture incidence in elderly men and women: the Dubbo Osteoporosis Epidemiology Study (DOES). Osteoporos Int 1994;4:277-82.
4. Center JR, Nguyen TV, Schneider D, et al: Mortality after all major types of osteoporotic fracture in men and women: an observational study. Lancet 1999;353:878-82,
5. Bilezikian JP: Osteoporosis in men. J Clin Endocrinol Metab 1999;84:3431-34.
6. Handelsman DJ: Androgen action and pharmacologic uses. In: DeGroot L, ed. Endocrinology. Philadelphia: W.B. Saunders, 2001:2232-42.
7. Vanderschueren D, Vandenput L, Boonen S, et al: Androgens and bone. Endocr Rev 2004;25:389-425.
8. de Ronde W, Pols HA, van Leeuwen JP, et al: The importance of oestrogens in males. Clin Endocrinol (Oxf) 2003;58:529-42.
9. Purohit A, Flanagan AM, Reed MJ: Estrogen synthesis by osteoblast cell lines. Endocrinology 1992;131:2027-29.
10. Saito H, Yanaihara T: Steroid formation in osteoblast-like cells. J Int Med Res 1998;26:1-12.
11. Janssen JM, Bland R, Hewison M, et al: Estradiol formation by human osteoblasts via multiple pathways: relation with osteoblast function. J Cell Biochem 1999;75:528-37.
12. Sasano H, Uzuki M, Sawai T, et al: Aromatase in human bone tissue. J Bone Miner Res 1997;12:1416-23.
13. Shozu M, Simpson ER: Aromatase expression of human osteoblast-like cells. Mol Cell Endocrinol 1998;139:117-29.
14. Oz OK, Millsaps R, Welch R, et al: Expression of aromatase in the human growth plate. J Mol Endocrinol 2001;27:249-53.
15. Gennari L, Nuti R, Bilezikian JP: Aromatase activity and bone homeostasis in men. J Clin Endocrinol Metab 2004;89:5898-907.
16. Van Der Eerden BC, Van De Ven J, Lowik CW, et al: Sex steroid metabolism in the tibial growth plate of the rat. Endocrinology 2002;143:4048-55.
17. Shimodaira K, Fujikawa H, Okura F, et al: Osteoblast cells (MG-63 and HOS) have aromatase and 5 alpha-reductase activities. Biochem Mol Biol Int 1996;39:109-16.
18. Schweikert HU, Rulf W, Niederle N, et al: Testosterone metabolism in human bone. Acta Endocrinol (Copenh) 1980;95:258-64.
19. Issa S, Schnabel D, Feix M, et al: Human osteoblast-like cells express predominantly steroid 5alpha-reductase type 1. J Clin Endocrinol Metab 2002;87:5401-7.
20. Feix M, Wolf L, Schweikert HU: Distribution of 17beta-hydroxy-steroid dehydrogenases in human osteoblast-like cells. Mol Cell Endocrinol 2001;171:163-64.
21. Kuwano Y, Fujikawa H, Watanabe A, et al: 3Beta-hydroxysteroid dehydrogenase activity in human osteoblast-like cells. Endocr J 1997;44:847-53.
22. Colvard DS, Eriksen EF, Keeting PE, et al: Identification of androgen receptors in normal human osteoblast-like cells. Proc Natl Acad Sci U S A 1989;86:854-57.
23. Abu EO, Horner A, Kusec V, et al: The localization of androgen receptors in human bone. J Clin Endocrinol Metab 1997;82:3493-97.
24. Mizuno Y, Hosoi T, Inoue S, et al: Immunocytochemical identification of androgen receptor in mouse osteoclast-like multinucleated cells. Calcif Tissue Int 1994;54:325-26.
25. Pederson L, Kremer M, Judd J, et al: Androgens regulate bone resorption activity of isolated osteoclasts in vitro. Proc Natl Acad Sci U S A 1999;96:505-10.
26. Hofbauer LC, Khosla S: Androgen effects on bone metabolism: recent progress and controversies. Eur J Endocrinol 1999;140:271-86.
27. Eriksen EF, Colvard DS, Berg NJ, et al: Evidence of estrogen receptors in normal human osteoblast-like cells. Science 1988;241:84-6.
28. Bord S, Horner A, Beavan S, et al: Estrogen receptors alpha and beta are differentially expressed in developing human bone. J Clin Endocrinol Metab 2001;86:2309-14.
29. Green S, Walter P, Greene G, et al: Cloning of the human oestrogen receptor cDNA. J Steroid Biochem 1986;24:77-83.
30. Kuiper GG, Enmark E, Pelto-Huikko M, et al: Cloning of a novel receptor expressed in rat prostate and ovary. Proc Natl Acad Sci U S A 1996;93:5925-30.
31. Gray A, Berlin JA, McKinlay JB, et al: An examination of research design effects on the association of testosterone and male aging: results of a meta-analysis. J Clin Epidemiol 1991;44:671-84.

32. Liu PY, Swerdloff RS, Veldhuis J: The rationale, efficacy and safety of androgen therapy in older men: future research and current practice recommendations. J Clin Endocrinol Metab 2004;89:4789-96.

33. Ly LP, Handelsman DJ: Empirical estimation of free testosterone from testosterone and sex hormone-binding globulin immunoassays. Eur J Endocrinol 2005;152:471-78.

34. Kaufman JM, Vermeulen A: Declining gonadal function in elderly men. Baillieres Clin Endocrinol Metab 1997;11:289-309.

35. Harman SM, Metter EJ, Tobin JD, et al: Longitudinal effects of aging on serum total and free testosterone levels in healthy men. Baltimore Longitudinal Study of Aging. J Clin Endocrinol Metab 2001;86:724-31.

36. Feldman HA, Longcope C, Derby CA, et al: Age trends in the level of serum testosterone and other hormones in middle-aged men: longitudinal results from the Massachusetts male aging study. J Clin Endocrinol Metab 2002;87:589-98.

37. Liu PY, Death AK, Handelsman DJ: Androgens and cardiovascular disease. Endocr Rev 2003;24:313-40.

38. Liverman CT, Blazer DG, eds: Testosterone and Aging: Clinical Research Directions. Washington, D.C.: National Academic Press, 2003.

39. Vermeulen A, Kaufman JM, Goemaere S, et al: Estradiol in elderly men. Aging Male 2002;5:98-102.

40. Khosla S, Melton LJ 3rd, Atkinson EJ, et al: Relationship of serum sex steroid levels and bone turnover markers with bone mineral density in men and women: a key role for bioavailable estrogen. J Clin Endocrinol Metab 1998;83:2266-74.

41. Seibel MJ, Eastell R, Grundberg CM, et al: Biochemical markers of bone metabolism. In: Bilezikian JP, Raisz LG, Rodan GA, eds: Principles of Bone Biology. San Diego: Academic Press, 2002:1543-71.

42. Leder BZ, Finkelstein JS: Gonadal steroids and the skeleton in men. In: Orwoll ES, Bliziotes M, eds: Contemporary Endocrinology. Osteoporosis: Pathophysiology and Clinical Management. Totowa, NJ: Humana Press, 2003:393-411.

43. Stepan JJ, Lachman M, Zverina J, et al: Castrated men exhibit bone loss: effect of calcitonin treatment on biochemical indices of bone remodeling. J Clin Endocrinol Metab 1989;69:523-27.

44. Goldray D, Weisman Y, Jaccard N, et al: Decreased bone density in elderly men treated with the gonadotropin-releasing hormone agonist decapeptyl (D-Trp6-GnRH). J Clin Endocrinol Metab 1993;76:288-90.

45. Smith MR, McGovern FJ, Zietman AL, et al: Pamidronate to prevent bone loss during androgen-deprivation therapy for prostate cancer. N Engl J Med 2001;345:948-55.

46. Stoch SA, Parker RA, Chen L, et al: Bone loss in men with prostate cancer treated with gonadotropin-releasing hormone agonists. J Clin Endocrinol Metab 2001;86:2787-91.

47. Diamond T, Campbell J, Bryant C, et al: The effect of combined androgen blockade on bone turnover and bone mineral densities in men treated for prostate carcinoma: longitudinal evaluation and response to intermittent cyclic etidronate therapy. Cancer 1998;83:1561-66.

48. Basaria S, Lieb J 2nd, Tang AM, et al: Long-term effects of androgen deprivation therapy in prostate cancer patients. Clin Endocrinol (Oxf) 2002;56:779-86.

49. Mittan D, Lee S, Miller E, et al: Bone loss following hypogonadism in men with prostate cancer treated with GnRH analogs. J Clin Endocrinol Metab 2002;87:3656-61.

50. Wei JT, Gross M, Jaffe CA, et al: Androgen deprivation therapy for prostate cancer results in significant loss of bone density. Urology 1999;54:607-11.

51. Berruti A, Dogliotti L, Gorzegno G, et al: Differential patterns of bone turnover in relation to bone pain and disease extent in bone in cancer patients with skeletal metastases. Clin Chem 1999;45:1240-47.

52. Daniell HW: Osteoporosis after orchiectomy for prostate cancer. J Urol 1997;157:439-44.

53. Kiratli BJ, Srinivas S, Perkash I, et al: Progressive decrease in bone density over 10 years of androgen deprivation therapy in patients with prostate cancer. Urology 2001;57:127-32.

54. Townsend MF, Sanders WH, Northway RO, et al: Bone fractures associated with luteinizing hormone-releasing hormone agonists used in the treatment of prostate carcinoma. Cancer 1997;79:545-50.

55. Hatano T, Oishi Y, Furuta A, et al: Incidence of bone fracture in patients receiving luteinizing hormone-releasing hormone agonists for prostate cancer. BJU Int 2000;86:449-52.

56. Oefelein MG, Ricchuiti V, Conrad W, et al: Skeletal fracture associated with androgen suppression induced osteoporosis: the clinical incidence and risk factors for patients with prostate cancer. J Urol 2001;166:1724-28.

57. Melton LJ 3rd, Alothman KI, Khosla S, et al: Fracture risk following bilateral orchiectomy. J Urol 2003;169:1747-50.

58. Smith MR, Fallon MA, Lee H, et al: Raloxifene to prevent gonadotropin-releasing hormone agonist-induced bone loss in men with prostate cancer: a randomized controlled trial. J Clin Endocrinol Metab 2004;89:3841-46.

59. Lopez AM, Pena MA, Hernandez R, et al: Fracture risk in patients with prostate cancer on androgen deprivation therapy. Osteoporos Int 2005;16:707-11.

60. Francis RM: The effects of testosterone on osteoporosis in men. Clin Endocrinol (Oxf) 1999;50:411-14.

61. Smith DA, Walker MS: Changes in plasma steroids and bone density in Klinefelter's syndrome. Calcif Tissue Res 1977;22(Suppl):225-28.

62. Foresta C, Ruzza G, Mioni R, et al: Testosterone and bone loss in Klinefelter syndrome. Horm Metab Res 1983;15:56-7.

63. Horowitz M, Wishart JM, O'Loughlin PD, et al: Osteoporosis and Klinefelter's syndrome. Clin Endocrinol (Oxf) 1992;36:113-18.

64. Greenspan SL, Neer RM, Ridgway EC, et al: Osteoporosis in men with hyperprolactinemic hypogonadism. Ann Intern Med 1986;104:777-82.

65. Luisetto G, Mastrogiacomo I, Bonanni G, et al: Bone mass and mineral metabolism in Klinefelter's syndrome. Osteoporos Int 1995;5:455-61.

66. Bojesen A, Juul S, Gravholt CH: Prenatal and postnatal prevalence of Klinefelter syndrome: a national registry study. J Clin Endocrinol Metab 2003;88:622-26.

67. Jackson JA, Kleerekoper M, Parfitt AM, et al: Bone histomorphometry in hypogonadal and eugonadal men with spinal osteoporosis. J Clin Endocrinol Metab 1987;65:53-8.

68. Guo CY, Jones TH, Eastell R: Treatment of isolated hypogonadotropic hypogonadism effect on bone mineral density and bone turnover. J Clin Endocrinol Metab 1997;82:658-65.

69. Baran DT, Bergfeld MA, Teitelbaum SL, et al: Effect of testosterone therapy on bone formation in an osteoporotic hypogonadal male. Calcif Tissue Res 1978;26:103-6.

70. Francis RM, Peacock M, Aaron JE, et al: Osteoporosis in hypogonadal men: role of decreased plasma 1,25-dihydroxyvitamin D, calcium malabsorption, and low bone formation. Bone 1986;7:261-68.

71. Wang C, Eyre DR, Clark R, et al: Sublingual testosterone replacement improves muscle mass and strength, decreases bone resorption, and increases bone formation markers in hypogonadal men: a clinical research center study. J Clin Endocrinol Metab 1996;81:3654-62.

72. Wang C, Swerdloff RS, Iranmanesh A, et al: Effects of transdermal testosterone gel on bone turnover markers and bone mineral density in hypogonadal men. Clin Endocrinol (Oxf) 2001;54:739-50.

73. Snyder PJ, Peachey H, Berlin JA, et al: Effects of testosterone replacement in hypogonadal men. J Clin Endocrinol Metab 2000;85:2670-77.

74. Katznelson L, Finkelstein JS, Schoenfeld DA, et al: Increase in bone density and lean body mass during testosterone administration in men with acquired hypogonadism. J Clin Endocrinol Metab 1996;81:4358-65.

75. Morley JE, Perry HM 3rd, Kaiser FE, et al: Effects of testosterone replacement therapy in old hypogonadal males: a preliminary study. J Am Geriatr Soc 1993;41:149-52.

76. Aminorroaya A, Kelleher S, Conway AJ, et al: Adequacy of androgen replacement influences bone density response to testosterone in androgen-deficient men. Eur J Endocrinol 2005;152:881-86.

77. Smith EP, Boyd J, Frank GR, et al: Estrogen resistance caused by a mutation in the estrogen-receptor gene in a man. N Engl J Med 1994;331:1056-61.

78. Morishima A, Grumbach MM, Simpson ER, et al: Aromatase deficiency in male and female siblings caused by a novel mutation

and the physiological role of estrogens. J Clin Endocrinol Metab 1995;80:3689-98.

79. Carani C, Qin K, Simoni M, et al: Effect of testosterone and estradiol in a man with aromatase deficiency. N Engl J Med 1997;337:91-5.

80. Maffei L, Murata Y, Rochira V, et al: Dysmetabolic syndrome in a man with a novel mutation of the aromatase gene: effects of testosterone, alendronate, and estradiol treatment. J Clin Endocrinol Metab 2004;89:61-70.

81. Greenspan SL, Oppenheim DS, Klibanski A: Importance of gonadal steroids to bone mass in men with hyperprolactinemic hypogonadism. Ann Intern Med 1989;110:526-31.

82. Behre HM, Kliesch S, Leifke E, et al: Long-term effect of testosterone therapy on bone mineral density in hypogonadal men. J Clin Endocrinol Metab 1997;82:2386-90.

83. Leifke E, Korner HC, Link TM, et al: Effects of testosterone replacement therapy on cortical and trabecular bone mineral density, vertebral body area and paraspinal muscle area in hypogonadal men. Eur J Endocrinol 1998;138:51-8.

84. Devogelaer JP, De Cooman S, Nagant de Deuxchaisnes C: Low bone mass in hypogonadal males: effect of testosterone substitution therapy, a densitometric study. Maturitas 1992;15:17-23.

85. Isaia G, Mussetta M, Pecchio F, et al: Effect of testosterone on bone in hypogonadal males. Maturitas 1992;15:47-51.

86. Zitzmann M, Depenbusch M, Gromoll J, et al: X-chromosome inactivation patterns and androgen receptor functionality influence phenotype and social characteristics as well as pharmacogenetics of testosterone therapy in Klinefelter patients. J Clin Endocrinol Metab 2004;89:6208-17.

87. Seeman E: The growth and age-related origins of bone fragility in men. Calcif Tissue Int 2004;75:100-9.

88. Wang C, Swerdloff RS, Iranmanesh A, et al: Transdermal testosterone gel improves sexual function, mood, muscle strength, and body composition parameters in hypogonadal men. Testosterone Gel Study Group. J Clin Endocrinol Metab 2000;85:2839-53.

89. Wang C, Cunningham G, Dobs A, et al: Long-term testosterone gel (AndroGel) treatment maintains beneficial effects on sexual function and mood, lean and fat mass, and bone mineral density in hypogonadal men. J Clin Endocrinol Metab 2004;89:2085-98.

90. Wang C, Swerdloff R, Kipnes M, et al: New testosterone buccal system (Striant) delivers physiological testosterone levels: pharmacokinetics study in hypogonadal men. J Clin Endocrinol Metab 2004;89:3821-29.

91. Bhasin S, Storer TW, Berman N, et al: Testosterone replacement increases fat-free mass and muscle size in hypogonadal men. J Clin Endocrinol Metab 1997;82:407-13.

92. Sih R, Morley JE, Kaiser FE, et al: Testosterone replacement in older hypogonadal men: a 12-month randomized controlled trial. J Clin Endocrinol Metab 1997;82:1661-67.

93. Bhasin S, Singh AB, Mac RP, et al: Managing the risks of prostate disease during testosterone replacement therapy in older men: recommendations for a standardized monitoring plan. J Androl 2003;24:299-311.

94. Handelsman DJ: Trends and regional differences in testosterone prescribing in Australia, 1991-2001. Med J Aust 2004;181:419-22.

95. Handelsman DJ, Liu PY: Andropause: invention, prevention, rejuvenation. Trends Endocrinol Metab 2005;16:39-45.

96. Szulc P, Munoz F, Claustrat B, et al: Bioavailable estradiol may be an important determinant of osteoporosis in men: the MINOS study. J Clin Endocrinol Metab 2001;86:192-99.

97. Slemenda CW, Longcope C, Zhou L, et al: Sex steroids and bone mass in older men: positive associations with serum estrogens and negative associations with androgens. J Clin Invest 1997;100:1755-59.

98. Khosla S, Melton LJ 3rd, Atkinson EJ, et al: Relationship of serum sex steroid levels to longitudinal changes in bone density in young versus elderly men. J Clin Endocrinol Metab 2001;86:3555-61.

99. Gennari L, Merlotti D, Martini G, et al: Longitudinal association between sex hormone levels, bone loss, and bone turnover in elderly men. J Clin Endocrinol Metab 2003;88:5327-33.

100. Riggs BL, Khosla S, Melton LJ 3rd: Sex steroids and the construction and conservation of the adult skeleton. Endocr Rev 2002;23:279-302.

101. Khosla S, Melton LJ 3rd, Riggs BL: Clinical review 144: estrogen and the male skeleton. J Clin Endocrinol Metab 2002;87:1443-50.

102. Greendale GA, Edelstein S, Barrett-Connor E: Endogenous sex steroids and bone mineral density in older women and men: the Rancho Bernardo Study. J Bone Miner Res 1997;12:1833-43.

103. Kenny AM, Prestwood KM, Marcello KM, et al: Determinants of bone density in healthy older men with low testosterone levels. J Gerontol A Biol Sci Med Sci 2000;55:M492-M497.

104. Goderie-Plomp HW, van der Klift M, de Ronde W, et al: Endogenous sex hormones, sex hormone-binding globulin, and the risk of incident vertebral fractures in elderly men and women: the Rotterdam Study. J Clin Endocrinol Metab 2004;89:3261-69.

105. Tenover JS: Effects of testosterone supplementation in the aging male. J Clin Endocrinol Metab 1992;75:1092-98.

106. Snyder PJ, Peachey H, Hannoush P, et al: Effect of testosterone treatment on bone mineral density in men over 65 years of age. J Clin Endocrinol Metab 1999;84:1966-72.

107. Amory JK, Watts NB, Easley KA, et al: Exogenous testosterone or testosterone with finasteride increases bone mineral density in older men with low serum testosterone. J Clin Endocrinol Metab 2004;89:503-10.

108. Kenny AM, Prestwood KM, Gruman CA, et al: Effects of transdermal testosterone on bone and muscle in older men with low bioavailable testosterone levels. J Gerontol A Biol Sci Med Sci 2001;56:M266-72.

109. Falahati-Nini A, Riggs BL, Atkinson EJ, et al: Relative contributions of testosterone and estrogen in regulating bone resorption and formation in normal elderly men. J Clin Invest 2000;106:1553-60.

110. Doran PM, Riggs BL, Atkinson EJ, et al: Effects of raloxifene, a selective estrogen receptor modulator, on bone turnover markers and serum sex steroid and lipid levels in elderly men. J Bone Miner Res 2001;16:2118-25.

111. Meier C, Liu PY, Ly LP, et al: Recombinant human chorionic gonadotropin but not dihydrotestosterone alone stimulates osteoblastic collagen synthesis in older men with partial age-related androgen deficiency. J Clin Endocrinol Metab 2004;89:3033-41.

112. Leder BZ, LeBlanc KM, Schoenfeld DA, et al: Differential effects of androgens and estrogens on bone turnover in normal men. J Clin Endocrinol Metab 2003;88:204-10.

113. Crawford BA, Liu PY, Kean MT, et al: Randomized placebo-controlled trial of androgen effects on muscle and bone in men requiring long-term systemic glucocorticoid treatment. J Clin Endocrinol Metab 2003;88:3167-76.

114. Anderson RA, Wallace AM, Sattar N, et al: Evidence for tissue selectivity of the synthetic androgen 7 alpha-methyl-19-nortestosterone in hypogonadal men. J Clin Endocrinol Metab 2003;88:2784-93.

115. Seibel MJ: Biochemical markers of bone remodeling. Endocrinol Metab Clin North Am 2003;32:83-113, vi-vii.

116. Meier C, Liu PY, Handelsman DJ, et al: Endocrine regulation of bone turnover in men. Clin Endocrinol (Oxf) 2005;63:603-16.

17 Calcitonin in the Treatment of Osteoporosis

Stuart L. Silverman

SUMMARY

Calcitonin has a modest effect on bone density of the spine and modestly reduces bone turnover in women with osteoporosis. Calcitonin appears to have a modest effect on vertebral fracture risk in postmenopausal women with osteoporosis. Calcitonin has not been demonstrated to reduce hip fracture risk. Nasal calcitonin is safe and well tolerated. Calcitonin may have analgesic benefit for the patient with acutely painful vertebral fractures. Treatment with calcitonin can be considered for late postmenopausal women with osteoporosis with painful vertebral fractures or for the late postmenopausal woman with mainly spinal osteoporosis, mainly of those unable to take bisphosphonates due to gastrointestinal intolerance or impaired renal function.

The postmenopausal woman with vertebral compression fractures due to osteoporosis presents challenges to the clinician in terms of choosing therapy for her osteoporosis. She may have reduced quality of life due to the pain of her vertebral compression fractures. She may be taking multiple medications. She may be intolerant of oral bisphosphonates. One option may be calcitonin, which provides known efficacy in reducing further vertebral fracture and a possible analgesic effect and is known to be safe and well tolerated in older individuals.

Calcitonin is a 32-amino acid polypeptide hormone of thyroid origin described by Copp in 1961[1] as a regulator of plasma calcium concentration or "tone." Calcitonin is produced by the parafollicular "C" cells of the thyroid,[1] which originate in the neural crest.

Although calcitonin secretion is stimulated by high plasma calcium levels,[1] calcitonin does not appear to play a significant role in the regulation of calcium in normal individuals. Calcitonin knockout mice develop osteopenia by an as yet undefined mechanism. Although calcitonin knockout mice are normal at birth, by 14 months these mice have a significant reduction in cortical thickness and bone mass compared with normal

mice in the appendicular skeleton as well as a significant reduction in trabecular bone in the axial skeleton.[2]

Calcitonin inhibits the activity of osteoclasts by binding to osteoclast receptors. After exposure to calcitonin in vitro, osteoclasts in culture undergo flattening of the ruffled border and withdraw from sites of bone resorption.[3]

Calcitonin is approved by the US Food and Drug Administration (FDA) in the treatment of postmenopausal osteoporosis in women who are more than 5 years postmenopausal.[4] Calcitonin is available as both an injectable and nasal spray formulation.

INJECTABLE CALCITONIN IN POSTMENOPAUSAL OSTEOPOROSIS

Effects on Bone Mineral Density

Injectable calcitonin was approved by the FDA in 1984 using radioactive calcium kinetics and neutron activation analysis data showing positive calcium balance with treatment.[5-8] Injectable calcitonin given daily or every other day at 50 International Units (IU) subcutaneously was found to increase lumbar spine bone mass in late postmenopausal women (mean age, 65 years) in three small randomized, controlled trials.[9-12] The effects of injectable calcitonin on hip bone mineral density (BMD) are not known. The use of injectable calcitonin, however, is limited by side effects of nausea with or without vomiting, local reactions at the injection site, and flushing of the face and hands[13] as well as the inconvenience of injection. Side effects are usually mild and the severity of side effects is dose dependent.

Effects on Fracture

Data on the vertebral fracture efficacy of injectable calcitonin are limited to two studies. In a retrospective cohort study, the Mediterranean Osteoporosis Study, or MEDOS study, Kanis[14] compared the rate of hip fracture in patients taking 50 IU to 100 IU injectable calcitonin with patients taking calcium alone. Patients taking calcitonin had a reduction in rate of hip fracture

(RR, 0.69) that was modestly but not significantly lower than that of patients taking calcium alone (RR, 0.75).

Injectable calcitonin at 100 IU given 10 days/month was shown by Rico[12] to significantly reduce the risk of vertebral fracture in a small randomized single center study of 72 postmenopausal women (mean age, 69 years) with more than one vertebral fracture. The incidence of vertebral fractures was 0.07 per patient year in the group receiving injectable calcitonin and calcium 10 days each month and 0.45 per patient year in the calcium only group ($P < .001$).

NASAL SPRAY SALMON CALCITONIN

Nasal spray calcitonin has been available since 1995 in the United States and is the preferred delivery system. The bioavailability of nasal spray calcitonin is about 25% or less of the administered dose as compared with the intramuscular or subcutaneous preparation, which is 70% bioavailable.[15] An average dose of 200 IU nasal spray calcitonin is thus equivalent to about 50 IU of injectable calcitonin or less.

Efficacy of Nasal Calcitonin in Postmenopausal Osteoporosis

Effect on Bone Mineral Density

There are numerous published randomized clinical trials on the efficacy of nasal calcitonin on BMD,[16-30] of which many are in women older than 55 years.[16,17,26,28,29,30] Limitations of the trials include small sample sizes and single-center trials other than the PROOF trial and the trial by Downs and colleagues.[27]

Overgaard[16] in 1989 randomized 37 late postmenopausal women with a mean age of 55 years and a history of prior forearm fractures to either 200 IU nasal spray calcitonin daily or placebo. All patients received 500 mg calcium carbonate daily. Valid completers who received 200 IU nasal spray calcitonin had a significant increase in lumbar spine BMD of 3.2% compared with the placebo group, who had a decrease of 0.4% ($P = .04$). There was a nonsignificant bone loss at the total body and forearm.

In a second study in 1992, Overgaard[17] studied 208 older females between the ages of 68 and 72 years with low forearm bone density who were randomized to placebo nasal spray or 50 IU, 100 IU, or 200 IU calcitonin nasal spray daily for 2 years. All patients received 500 mg of calcium carbonate daily. Similar to the first study, valid completers (n = 41) who received 200 IU nasal spray calcitonin had a significant increase in lumbar spine BMD of 3.0% (CI, 1.8–4.2) versus completers assigned to calcium only who had a mean increase of 1% (CI, −0.1–1.5).

Ellerington[18] in 1996 compared the efficacy over 2 years of daily and intermittent (3 days weekly) use of 200 IU nasal spray calcitonin in 72 women in early or late postmenopause. No calcium supplementation was given. Lumbar spine BMD did not increase significantly using an intermittent dosing schedule. However, a significant increase in lumbar spine BMD after 2 years was found in late postmenopausal women treated with nasal spray calcitonin daily.

Downs[30] studied 299 women with a mean age of 64 years in a 1-year study of 200 IU nasal calcitonin versus placebo. Compared with baseline, there were significant changes at the lumbar spine (1.18%) but not at the femoral neck (0.6%). There were no significant intergroup differences between calcitonin and placebo at lumbar spine and trochanter using dual x-ray absorptiometry, although a significant difference was seen between the calcitonin and placebo groups at the femoral neck.

Kaskani[19] studied the effects of intermittent administration of 200 IU intranasal salmon calcitonin 1 month on, 1 month off and continuous administration of 0.25 μg of 1-alpha (OH) vitamin D_3 with 500 mg of elemental calcium continuously in a pilot study. Lumbar spine and femoral neck BMD increased significantly compared with baseline and in comparison with the calcium and vitamin D group, with significant effects on bone turnover.

The PROOF study

The PROOF study (Prevent Recurrence of Osteoporotic Fracture)[28] was a large, 5-year, multicenter, double-blind, randomized study, begun in 1991, of the efficacy of nasal spray salmon calcitonin in patients with one to five prior vertebral fractures and low vertebral bone mass (T-score < −2.0). Of the original 1255 postmenopausal women, with a mean age of 68 years, who were randomized by investigators in both the United States and United Kingdom, 817 had one to five prevalent vertebral fractures and had follow-up thoracic and lumbar spine radiographs. Patients were randomized to placebo nasal spray or one of three doses of salmon calcitonin nasal spray daily: 100, 200, or 400 IU. All patients received supplements of 1000 mg elemental calcium carbonate and 400 IU vitamin D daily plus usual dietary calcium for a mean total calcium intake of 1800 mg. Baseline variables were similar across each of the four arms. Although a higher than expected discontinuation rate of 59% was seen in the trial, the discontinuation rate was similar across treatment groups and time. Sixty-two percent of the patients were valid completers of 3 years of the trial.

Lumbar vertebral bone density increased 1.2% in the 200 IU group in the first year, which was significantly different than control at 1 year. There was no further increase in lumbar BMD after 1 year. There was a mean reduction in serum C telopeptide (CTX) from baseline of 25% at 12 months, which was sustained at

20% throughout the 5 years in both the 200 IU group and the 400 IU group.[28] The conditions of individuals who remained in the trial did not differ significantly from those who did not finish the trial.

Effect on fracture

There are two studies of the effect of nasal calcitonin on fracture. Overgaard[17] found that nasal calcitonin significantly reduced the rate of vertebral fractures in 124 women with a mean age of 70 years over 2 years ($P = 0.017$) using pooled data (50, 100, and 200 IU) compared with placebo.

In PROOF, using an intent-to-treat analysis of all randomized patients with one to five prevalent vertebral fractures at baseline who had follow-up thoracic and lumbar spine radiographs resulted in a significant 36% vertebral fracture reduction seen in the 200 IU group with a 36% reduction in relative risk compared with placebo of 0.64 ($P = .03$) with a 45% reduction in the number of patients with multiple new vertebral fractures.[28] These reductions were seen only in the 200 IU group and surprisingly not seen in the 400 IU group. If all patients with follow-up radiographs were included in the analysis (including patients with or without prevalent fracture) then there was a significant 33% reduction ($P = .03$) in the risk of vertebral fracture. Significant vertebral fracture reduction was seen with the 200 IU dose by year 3 and was sustained through year 5.

The PROOF study was not powered to detect nonvertebral fracture reduction.. The number of hip fracture events was small, with only nine hip fracture events in the placebo group. However, there was a nonsignificant 46% reduction in hip/femur fractures in the 200 IU group compared with the placebo group (9/305 in the placebo group and 5/315 in the 200 IU group) and a 28% nonsignificant reduction in humerus/wrist fractures.[28] A post hoc pooled analysis of all doses showed a trend in the reduction of hip fracture risk of 48% ($P = .07$).[31]

Reduction in vertebral fracture risk with calcitonin was independent of baseline variables previously noted to influence fracture risk and response to calcitonin such as age, years since menopause, number of prevalent fractures, baseline bone markers, and baseline spinal BMD.[28]

There are two major limitations of the PROOF Study. The first is that the discontinuation rate of 59% for the 5 years of the study was higher than expected. The second is that a dose response curve of nasal calcitonin with regard to fracture reduction was not seen. Although there was significant reduction in serum CTX and a significant increase in lumbar spine BMD compared with the control group in years 1 and 2 in the 400 IU group, there was no significant fracture reduction in the 400 IU group.[28] However, a valid completer analysis at 3 years has shown similar fracture reduction in the 400 IU group.

Kanis and McCloskey[32] (1999) summarized the fracture efficacy of calcitonin in 1309 women in 14 randomized clinical trials. The relative risk of any fracture for individuals taking calcitonin versus those not taking calcitonin was 0.43 (95% CI, 0.38–0.50). The effect was apparent for both vertebral fractures (RR, 0.45; 95% CI, 0.39–0.53) and nonvertebral fractures (RR, 0.34; 95% CI, 0.17–0.68). When studies identifying the number of patients with fracture were pooled, the magnitude of effect was less (RR, 0.74; 95% CI, 0.60–0.93). The authors concluded that treatment with calcitonin was associated with a significant decrease in the number of vertebral and nonvertebral fractures.

Calcitonin fracture efficacy in older women

A post hoc stratification analysis of PROOF has been done in elderly women by Silverman.[31] In this post hoc analysis, nasal spray calcitonin reduced the risk of new vertebral fracture by 53% in women older than 70 years in PROOF and by 62% in women older than 75 years in PROOF. Nasal calcitonin was well tolerated in these elderly women,[31] with the only major side effect being rhinitis. Data from the PROOF trial suggest therapeutic benefit of nasal calcitonin compared with placebo in postmenopausal osteoporotic older women (age >70 years), with particular and perhaps preferential benefit at the lumbar spine for women older than 70 years. Such findings may be of clinical importance in considering the choice of a therapeutic agent for elderly women with osteoporosis.

Effect on bone markers

Nasal spray calcitonin modestly reduces both urine and serum markers of bone turnover within 4 to 8 weeks,[33–35] with a mean reduction of 26–32%. After cessation of treatment, all biochemical markers of bone turnover return to baseline over a subsequent 12-week period. It has been suggested that patients with a higher bone turnover may have a greater response to injectable calcitonin in terms of BMD.[34] In PROOF, patients with higher levels of bone turnover had the greatest response to treatment in terms of bone marker reduction, although all patients responded to nasal spray calcitonin in terms of fracture efficacy irrespective of tertiles of baseline bone markers (urine N-telopeptide, serum alkaline phosphatase, or osteocalcin).

Mechanism of effect on fracture reduction

The effect of nasal calcitonin on BMD and biochemical markers of bone turnover is modest, yet a significant fracture reduction with 200 IU was observed in PROOF. The degree of vertebral fracture reduction in women with prevalent vertebral fracture was similar to the effect achieved with raloxifene, a selective estrogen receptor modulator whose vertebral fracture reduction has also been found to be associated with modest increases in lumbar BMD. In a post hoc stratification analysis, an even greater reduction in vertebral fractures was seen, comparable with that of bisphosphonates. Recent analyses by Cummings[36] and Sarkar[37] have shown that BMD increases following treatment may explain only 16% and 4% of the fracture reduction seen with alendronate and raloxifene, respectively. Chesnut has hypothesized that nasal spray salmon calcitonin improves bone strength by factors other than BMD. In the QUEST study (QUalitative Effects of Salmon calcitonin), Chesnut[38,39] examined the effects of 200 IU nasal spray salmon calcitonin on bone quality in a 2-year, double-blind, randomized, controlled study of 91 postmenopausal women as measured by a new bone imaging modality, high-resolution magnetic resonance imaging. The QUEST study showed that 2 years of calcitonin nasal spray resulted in no significant increases in lumbar spine BMD but significantly preserved trabecular number at the distal radius at one of four regions (region 3) ($P = .03$) using high-resolution magnetic resonance imaging. This preservation approached significance at regions 1 and 4 ($P = .07$ and .051). Nasal spray calcitonin decreased hip T2* by 0.5% to 3.6% at all measured hip magnetic resonance imaging sites compared with placebo, with significance at the lower trochanter ($P = .008$). This decrease in hip T2* is the equivalent of an increase in trabecular bone density distribution, a composite of bone density and microarchitecture.[40]

Use of Salmon Calcitonin Nasal Spray in Men with Idiopathic Osteoporosis

Up to 20% of symptomatic vertebral fractures and 30% of hip fractures occur in men. Only alendronate has been shown to be effective in male idiopathic osteoporosis. Trovas[41] studied the efficacy of 200 IU nasal salmon calcitonin in a 1-year randomized, double-blind, placebo-controlled study of 28 men with idiopathic osteoporosis ranging in ages from 27 to 74 years (mean, 52.4). All the men received a daily supplement of 500 mg of calcium. There was a significant increase from baseline in lumbar spine BMD of 7.1 ± 1.7% in the group receiving calcitonin compared with an increase of 2.4 ± 1.5% in the placebo group ($P < .05$). There was a nonsignificant increase versus placebo in the femoral neck. Therapy was well tolerated. Nasal salmon calcitonin may be an alternative therapy in men with idiopathic osteoporosis.

Use of Calcitonin in Glucocorticoid-Induced Osteoporosis

Several studies using both injectable and nasal calcitonin have suggested a potential role for salmon calcitonin in the prevention and treatment of lumbar spine bone loss in patients treated with glucocorticoids. However, no data on reduction in fracture risk with calcitonin in glucocorticoid-induced osteoporosis are available. Both Ringe[42] and Luengo[43] found calcitonin to increase or maintain lumbar spine BMD in patients treated with glucocorticoids. Montemurro[44] found calcitonin to prevent lumbar spine bone loss in glucocorticoid-treated patients. In a randomized, controlled trial comparing calcitonin and calcitriol plus calcium, calcitriol plus calcium, and placebo plus calcium over 2 years, Sambrook[45] found that calcitonin and calcitriol in the second year of study prevented lumbar spine bone loss in patients with glucocorticoid-induced osteoporosis whereas calcitriol alone did not.

In summary, although a few small studies demonstrate that nasal salmon calcitonin may maintain lumbar spine BMD in patients who have been treated with glucocorticoids, it is unclear whether calcitonin can prevent bone loss in new patients started on glucocorticoids. More important, no data on fracture reduction with calcitonin are available and no hip BMD data are available. As fracture reduction data are available for the two marketed bisphosphonates, risedronate and alendronate, at this time, nasal spray calcitonin should not be considered a first-line agent agent for treatment of glucocorticoid-induced osteoporosis until fracture reduction data are available.

ORAL CALCITONIN

Oral administration of salmon calcitonin may improve adherence to long-term treatment. Several new oral salmon calcitonins have been developed. Tanko[46] reported the safety and efficacy of an oral formulation using an amino caprylic acid delivery agent in a multicenter trial. Treatment with oral salmon calcitonin resulted in dose-dependent decreases in serum CTX of 60% to 82% from baseline compared with placebo, reaching nadir at 2 to 3 hours after drug intake. The oral formulation was well tolerated. Chin[47] studied single doses of a chemically modified salmon calcitonin orally. The medication was well tolerated and resulted in dose-dependent decreases in total and ionized serum calcium.

ANALGESIC EFFECTS OF CALCITONIN

Calcitonin is unique among osteoporosis therapies in that it may have analgesic efficacy as well as vertebral fracture efficacy. The analgesic effects of salmon calcitonin were recently reviewed by Silverman.[48] Salmon calcitonin binding sites have been found in the human central nervous system using I[125] labeled salmon calcitonin. Intramuscular or nasal salmon calcitonin has been proven to be analgesic for both the acute pain of vertebral fracture[49-51] and the chronic pain after vertebral fracture[48] The analgesic effect of salmon calcitonin was noted at 1 week or less by the visual analog pain scale and by a decrease in analgesic consumption by day 3. Increased mobilization was noted by week 1.[49] A dose of 50 IU of salmon calcitonin intramuscularly is equivalent to 200 IU nasal spray with regard to analgesic efficacy.[52] Salmon calcitonin therefore may have a potential role in reducing the pain of acute vertebral fracture, reducing analgesic dependence, and possibly secondarily decreasing immobilization.

The mechanism of bone pain relief due to calcitonin is not known but appears to be a central effect.[53] The most likely effect is a direct action on central nervous system receptors. The analgesic effect of calcitonin appears to operate through both opioid and nonopioid mechanisms.[54]

ADMINISTRATION AND SIDE EFFECTS OF NASAL CALCITONIN IN OLDER WOMEN WITH OSTEOPOROSIS

The recommended dose of calcitonin nasal spray is 200 IU daily administered intranasally in alternating nostrils. Nasal calcitonin can be taken at any time of day and can be taken without regard to meals. Women should take adequate calcium every day (1000-1500 mg calcium) and 400 to 800 IU vitamin D. Clinical experience has shown the side effects with nasal calcitonin to be minimal in older women.[55] In the PROOF study, the largest study with salmon calcitonin to date, there was a significant increase in rhinitis and a significant decrease in headache[28] compared with placebo nasal spray.

RESISTANCE TO CALCITONIN

Calcitonin is a biological agent for osteoporosis, as opposed to bisphosphonates, which as inorganic agents bind directly to bone. Concerns have been raised about the potential for clinical resistance to calcitonin due to the presence of antibodies or downregulation, based on early reports on calcitonin "escape" with prolonged use in patients with hypercalcemia of malignancy.[56]

Patients may develop antibodies to calcitonin under treatment.[57,58] Binding antibodies with titers of greater than 1:1000 were observed in approximately 20% of patients in the PROOF study.[28] The presence of these antibodies did not appear to affect fracture efficacy as judged by biochemical markers of bone turnover.

One part of the resistance may be downregulation of calcitonin receptors. Downregulation has been reported in mouse calvaria[57] and human carcinoma cell lines. Tissue culture experiments have shown decreased calcitonin receptor mRNA expression for 12 hours after calcitonin treatment of osteoclast-like giant cells.[58] This decreased mRNA expression is reversible, suggesting the need for studies of intermittent use of the medication to avoid clinical resistance and potentially lower costs.

The best way to identify patients who will not respond or become resistant to therapy is not known. Stepan[59] has suggested the use of a loading dose of 400 IU nasal spray followed by serum CTX measurement 90 minutes later. In 24% of the patients, serum CTX suppression did not exceed least significant change. In patients treated over 4 years, this number increased to 34%. If those identified by serum CTX suppression less than least significant are given 10 IU subcutaneous calcitonin, 63% fail to respond.

USE OF CALCITONIN IN COMBINATION THERAPY IN OSTEOPOROSIS

There are few data on the combination of salmon calcitonin and other antiresorptives or anabolic agents for osteoporosis. Meschia[60] combined eel calcitonin and hormonal replacement therapy with a significant 10% gain in lumbar spine bone mass at 1 year. Hodsman[61] found the bone density increased with sequential therapy with calcitonin and parathyroid hormone was no better than cyclic parathyroid hormone alone.

ROLE OF CALCITONIN IN THE THERAPY OF POSTMENOPAUSAL OSTEOPOROSIS

Calcitonin is FDA approved for the treatment but not the prevention of postmenopausal osteoporosis. Nasal spray calcitonin is the most commonly used delivery system. Calcitonin use is very safe. Its efficacy is considered less robust than either estrogen replacement therapy or a bisphosphonate such as alendronate. Calcitonin has been found to reduce the risk of vertebral fracture by 36% in patients with prevalent vertebral fracture, similar to the effect of selective estrogen receptor modulators such as raloxifene. Calcitonin has not been found to significantly reduce risk of hip fracture.

Nasal spray calcitonin should be considered one of the options for the treatment of the late menopausal patient with established osteoporosis who may not be tolerant of alendronate or risedronate. Other options include estrogen and raloxifene.

Nasal spray calcitonin should be considered for patients with established osteoporosis who have a history of estrogen-dependent neoplasia, thromboembolic disease, or active gastrointestinal problems such as gastritis, duodenitis, ulcer, or motility problems. Nasal spray calcitonin should also be considered for patients with renal impairment, multiple medications, or a rigid lifestyle or in the institutionalized older patient who is unable to stay upright for 30 minutes after taking a bisphosphonate.

Nasal spray calcitonin should be considered as one of the options for initial treatment of the symptomatic patient with osteoporotic vertebral fracture because of its potential analgesic effect.

Calcitonin is not recommended for the prevention of osteoporosis in men or in women at the time of menopause because of the absence of efficacy data. In these patient groups, raloxifene and alendronate are available as estrogen alternatives.

CONCLUSION

Calcitonin is FDA approved for the treatment of postmenopausal osteoporosis but not for prevention. The preferred delivery system is nasal. Nasal calcitonin is safe and well tolerated. Calcitonin reduces vertebral fracture risk at a rate similar to that of other antiresorptive agents. Calcitonin has not been demonstrated to reduce hip fracture risk. Calcitonin produces small increments in bone mass of the spine and modestly reduces bone turnover in women with osteoporosis. Calcitonin may have a possible analgesic benefit for the woman with acutely painful vertebral fractures. Treatment with calcitonin should be considered for late postmenopausal women with osteoporosis with painful vertebral fractures or for the late postmenopausal woman with vertebral greater than hip osteoporosis. Calcitonin should be considered for the late postmenopausal woman who is unable to take oral bisphosphonates because of gastrointestinal intolerance or impaired renal function.

REFERENCES

1. Azria M: The calcitonins: physiology and pharmacology. Basel: Karger, 1989.
2. Hoff AO, Thomas M, Cote GJ, et al: Generation of a calcitonin knockout mouse model. Bone 1998;23:abs 1062.
3. Chambers TJ, Moore A: The sensitivity of isolated osteoclasts to morphological transformation by calcitonin. J Clin Endo Metab 1983;57:819-24.
4. Approval letter: Miacalcin NDA. Rockville, MD: Office of Freedom of Information, Department of Health and Human Services, 1995.
5. Cannigia A, Gennari C, Bencini M, et al: Calcium metabolism and 47 Calcium kinetics before and after long term thyrocalcitonin treatment in senile osteoporosis. Clin Sci 1970;38:397-407.
6. Milhaud G, Talbott JN, Coutris G: Calcitonin tratment of postmenopausal osteoporosis: evaluation of efficacy by primary component analysis. Biomedicine 1975;23:223-32.
7. Wallach S, Cohn SH, Atkins HL, et al: Effects of salmon calcitonin on skeletal mass in osteoporosis. Curr Ther Res 1977;22:556-72.
8. Gruber HE, Ivey JL, Baylink DJ, et al: Long-term calcitonin therapy in postmenopausal osteoporosis. Metabolism 1984;33:295-303.
9. Mazzuoli G, Passeri M, Gennari C, et al: Effects of salmon calcitonin in postmenopausal osteoporosis: a controlled double blind clinical study. Calcif Tissue Int 1986;38:3-8.
10. Mazzuoli GF, Tabolli S, Bigi F, et al: Effects of salmon calcitonin on the bone loss induced by ovariectomy. Calcif Tissue Int 1990;47:209-14.
11. Meschia M, Brincat M, Barbaracini P, et al: Effect of hormone replacement therapy and calcitonin on bone mass in post-menopausal women. Eur J Obs Gyn Reprod Biol 1992;47:53-7.
12. Rico H, Revilla M, Hernandez ER, et al: Total and regional bone mineral content and fracture rate in postmenopausal osteoporosis treated with salmon calcitonin: a prospective study. Calcif Tissue Int 1995;56:181-85.
13. Gennari C, Passeri M, Chierichetti SM, Piolini M: Side effects of synthetic salmon and human calcitonin. Lancet 1983;I:594-95.
14. Kanis JA, Johnell O, Gulberg B, et al: Evidence for efficacy of drugs affecting bone metabolism in preventing hip fracture. Br Med J 1992;305:1124-28.
15. Overgaard K, Agnusdei D, Hansen MA, et al: Dose response bioactivity and bioavailability of salmon calcitonin in premenopausal and postmenopausal women. J Clin Endocrinol Metab 1991;72: 344-49.
16. Overgaard K, Riis BJ, Christiansen C, et al: Nasal calcitonin for treatment of established osteoporosis. Clin Endocrinol 1989;30:435-42.
17. Overgaard K, Hansen MA, Jensen SB: Effect of calcitonin given intranasally on bone mass and fracture rates in established osteoporosis: a dose response study. BMJ 1992;305:556-61.
18. Ellerington MC, Whitcroft SJ, Stevenson JC, et al: Intranasal calcitonin for the prevention and treatment of postmenopausal osteoporosis: a double blind placebo controlled study. Calc Tissue Int 1996;59:6-11.
19. Kaskani E, Lyritis GP, Kosmidis C, et al: Effect of intermittent administration of 200 IU intranasal salmon calcitonin and low doses of 1alpha(OH) vitaminD(3) on bone mineral density of the lumbar spine and hip region and biochemical bone markers in women with postmenopausal osteoporosis: a pilot study. Clin Rheumatol 2005 Jan 13 (Epub ahead of print).
20. Reginster JY, Denis D, Albert A, et al: 1 Year controlled randomized trial of prevention of early postmenopausal bone loss by intranasal calcitonin. Lancet 1987;2:1481-83.
21. Reginster JY, Denis D, Deroisy R, et al: Longterm (3 years) prevention of trabecular postmenopausal bone loss with low dose intermittent nasal salmon calcitonin. J Bone Miner Res 1994;9:69-73.
22. Overgaard K, Riis Bj, Christiansen C, et al: Effect of salcatonin given intranasally on early postmenopausal bone loss. BMJ 1989;299:477-79.
23. Overgaard K, Hansen MA, Jensen SB, et al: Effect of salcatonin given intranasally on bone mass and fracture rates in established osteoporosis: a dose response study. BMJ 1992;305:556-61.
24. Agnusdei D, Gonelli S, Camporeale A, et al: Clinical efficacy of treatment with salmon calcitonin, administered intranasally for 1 year, in stablilized postmenopausal osteoporosis. Minerva Endocrinol 1989;14:169-76.
25. Gennari C, Agnuddei D, Monatgnani M, et al: An effective regimen of intranasal salmon calcitonin in early postmenopausal bone loss. Calcif Tissue Int 1992;50:381-83.
26. Reginster JY, Denis D, Deroisy R, et al: Long-term prevention of trabecular postmenopausal bone loss with low dose intermittent nasal salmon calcitonin. J Bone Miner Res 1994;9:69-73.
27. Campodarve I, Drinkwater BL, Insogna KL, et al: Intranasal salmon calcitonin (INSC), 50-200 IU does not prevent bone loss in early postmenopausal women. J Bone Miner Res 1995;S391:abs C264.

28. Chesnut CH, Silverman SL, Andriano K, et al, for the PROOF Study Group: Prospective, randomized trial of nasal spray calcitonin in postmenopausal women with established osteoporosis: the PROOF Study. Am J Med 2000;109:267-76.

29. Flicker L, Hopper JL, Larkins RG, et al: Nandrolone decanoate and intranasal calcitonin as therapy in established osteoporosis. Osteoporosis Int 1997;7:29-35.

30. Downs RW, Bell NH, Ettinger MP, et al: Comparison of alendronate and intranasal calcitonin for treatment of osteoporosis in postmenopausal women. J Clin Endocrinol Metab 2000;85:1783-88.

31. Silverman SL, Chesnut C, Baylink D, et al: Salmon calcitonin nasal spray (SCNS) is effective and safe in older osteoporotic women: results from the PROOF Study. J Bone Miner Res 2001;16(Suppl 1): S530 (abs M414).

32. Kanis JA, McCloskey EV: Effect of calcitonin on vertebral and other fractures. Q J Med 1999;92:143-49.

33. Kraenzlin ME, Seibel MJ, Trechsel U, et al: The effect of intranasal salmon calcitonin on postmenopausal bone turnover as assessed by biochemical markers: evidence of maximal effect after 8 weeks of continuous treatment. Calcif Tissue Int 1996;58:216-20.

34. Ongpghiphadhanakul B, Piaseu N, Chailurkit L, Rajatanavin R: Suppression of bone resorption in early postmenopausal women by intranasal salmon calcitonin in relation to dosage and basal bone turnover. Calcif Tissue Int 1998;62:379-82.

35. Civitelli R, Gonnelli S, Zacchei F, et al: Bone turnover in postmenopausal osteoporosis: effect of calcitonin treatment. J Clin Invest 1988;82:1268-74.

36. Cummings SR, Karpf DB, Harris F, et al: Improvement in spine bone density and reduction in risk of vertebral fractures during treatment with antiresorptive drugs. Am J Med 2002;112:281-89.

37. Sarkar S, Mitlak BH, Wong M, et al: Relationships between bone mineral density and incident vertebral fracture risk with raloxifene treatment. J Bone Miner Res 2002;17:1-10.

38. Chesnut C, Majumdar S, Shields A, et al: Salmon calcitonin nasal spray (CT-NS) may preserve/improve trabecular microarchitecture (TMA) in postmenopausal osteoporotic women (PM-OP); high resolution MRI (HR MRI) results from the QUEST Study. J Bone Miner Res 2003;18(suppl 2):S92 (abs F361).

39. Chesnut C, Shields A, Pitzel P, et al: How do antiresorptive therapies reduced fracture in absence of robust effects on BMD and remodeling? The Qualitative Effects of Salmon Calcitonin Treatment (QUEST) Study. J Bon Miner Res 1999;14:S515 (abs SU335).

40. Majumdar S, Chesnut C, Shields A, et al:. The impact of salmon calcitonin nasal spray (CT-NS) on trabecular bone density distribution as measured by magnetic resonance imaging (MR) T2* times in the proximal femur in a 2 year study. J Bone Miner Res 2003;18(suppl 2):S264 (abs SU353).

41. Trovas GP, Lyritis GP, Galanos A, et al: A randomized trial of nasal spray salmon calcitonin in men with idiopathic osteoporosis: effects on bone mineral density and bone markers. J Bone Miner Res 2002;17:521-27.

42. Ringe JD, Welzel D: Salmon calcitonin in the therapy of corticosteroid induced osteoporosis. Eur J Clin Pharmacol 1987;33:35-9.

43. Luengo M, Pons F, Martinez de Osaba MJ, Picado C: Prevention of further bone mass loss by nasal calcitonin in patients on long

term glucocorticoid therapy for asthma: a two year follow up study. Thorax 1994;49:1099-102.

44. Montemurro L, Schiraldi G, Fraioli P, et al: Prevention of corticosteroid induced osteoporosis with salmon calcitonin in sarcoid patients. Calcif Tissue Int 1991;49:71-6.

45. Sambrook P, Birmingham J, Kelly P, et al: Prevention of corticosteroid osteoporosis: a comparison of calcium, calcitriol and calcitonin. N Engl J Med 1993;328:1747-52.

46. Tanko LB, Bagger YZ, Alexandersen P, et al: Safety and efficacy of a novel salmon calcitonin (sCT) technology based oral formulation in healthy postmenopausal women: acute and three months effects on bonemarkers of bone turnover. J Bone Miner Res 2004;19:1531-38.

47. Chin CM, Gutierrez M, Still JG, Kosutic G: Pharmacokinetics of modified oral calcitonin product in healthy volunteers. Pharmacotherapy 2004;24:994-1001.

48. Silverman SL, Azria M: The analgesic role of calcitonin following osteoporotic fracture. Osteoporos Int 2002;13:858-67.

49. Lyritis GP, Paspati I, Karachalios T, et al: Pain relief from nasal salmon calcitonin in osteoporotic vertebral crush fractures: a double blind placebo controlled study. Acta Orthop Scand 1997;68(Suppl 275):112-14.

50. Lyritis GP, Tsakalakos N, Magiasis B, et al: Analgesic effect of salmon calcitonin in osteoporotic vertebral fractures: a double blind placebo controlled clinical study. Calcif Tissue Int 1991;49:369-72.

51. Pun KK, Chan LW: Analgesic effect of intranasal salmon calcitonin in the treatment of osteoporotic vertebral fractures. Clin Therapeutics 1989;11:205-9.

52. Combe B, Cohen C, Aubin F: Equivalence of nasal spray and subcutaneous formulations of salmon calcitonin. Calcif Tissue Int 1997;61:10-15.

53. Szanto J, Joszef S, Rado J, et al: Pain killing with calcitonin in patients with malignant tumors. Oncology 1986;43:69-72.

54. Gennari C: Clinical aspects of calcitonin in pain. Triangle 1983;2:157-63.

55. Foti R, Martorana U, Broggini M: Long-term tolerability of nasal spray formulation of salmon calcitonin. Curr Ther Res 1995;56:429-35.

56. Mundy GR, Wilkinson R, Heath DA: 1984. A comparative study of medical treatment for hypercalcemia of malignancy. Am J Med 1984;74:421-37.

57. Tashjian AM, Wright DR, Ivey JL, Post A: Calcitonin binding sites in bone and relationships to biological response and escape. Recent Prog Hormone Res 1978;34:285-334.

58. Takahashi S, Goldring S, Katz M, et al: Downregulation of calcitonin receptor m RNA expression by calcitonin during human osteoclast-like cell differentiation. J Clin Invest 1995;95:167-71.

59. Stepan JJ, Virkan V: Calcitonin loading test to assess the sustained efficacy of salmon calcitonin. Osteoporosis International, 2002, 13 Suppl 1, P1685A.

60. Meschia M, Brincat M, Barabcini P, et al: A clinical trial on the effects of a combination of elcatonin (carbocalcitonin) and conjugated estrogens on vertebral bone mass in early postmenopausal women. Calcif Tissue Int 1993;53:17-20.

61. Hodsman AB, Steer BM, Fraher LJ, Drost DJ: Bone densitometric and histomorphometric responses to sequential human parathyroid hormone (1-38) and salmon calcitonin in osteoporotic patients. Bone Miner 1991;14:67-83.

18 Bisphosphonates in the Prevention and Treatment of Postmenopausal Osteoporosis

Ian R. Reid

SUMMARY

Bisphosphonates are first line therapy in the management of osteoporosis with an increasing diversity of agents and regimens. In some countries, generic formulations may be available in the near future, and this is likely to reduce drug costs. Despite their impressive anti-fracture efficacy, a number of issues are arising with regard to bisphosphonates. They remain in the skeleton for decades and their duration of physiological effect is unclear but bone turnover markers can remain suppressed for at least five years after their discontinuation. Morover the benefit of bisphosphonates on fracture endpoints are proven by randomized controlled trials only for the first 4 to 5 years and it remains unclear what is optimal duration of therapy.

HISTORY

The bisphosphonates entered clinical practice in the 1970s with the introduction of etidronate as a therapy for Paget disease of bone. It was not until the end of that decade that their true potential was signaled by two reports from Bijvoet's group, published in *The Lancet*.[1] These papers described the much more potent bisphosphonate pamidronate and demonstrated its efficacy in treating hypercalcemia of malignancy and Paget disease. Although this agent was used increasingly for these indications during the 1980s, it was not until the publication of the first positive randomized controlled trial of a bisphosphonate in the management of osteoporosis[2] that this whole new indication opened up for this class of drugs. The 1990s saw enormous progress in this field. The bisphosphonates went from being experimental agents at the beginning of the decade to becoming the treatments of choice for osteoporosis, Paget disease, hypercalcemia of malignancy, and other skeletal complications of malignancy by the decade's end. The domination of the pharmacological management of osteoporosis by the bisphosphonates has become even more marked since the publication of the adverse safety findings with estrogen/progestin therapy from the Women's Health Initiative in 2002.[3]

STRUCTURE

Drugs in the bisphosphonate class consist of two phosphate groups linked through a central carbon atom (Figure 18-1). The various members of the class are distinguished from one another by the two side chains that bind to the central carbon atom. Two classes of bisphosphonates are distinguished on the basis of their side chains: those that contain a nitrogen atom, and those that do not. The nitrogen atom can be part of a straight carbon chain (as in pamidronate, alendronate, and ibandronate) or part of a ring structure (as in risedronate and zoledronate). The nitrogen-containing bisphosphonates appear to have a different intracellular target from the other drugs in this class and are generally more potent inhibitors of bone resorption.

MECHANISM OF ACTION

The phosphate groups have a strong negative charge, giving them a very high affinity for the positively charged bone surface. Therefore, bisphosphonates are deposited across the surface of bone and remain there for a considerable time, ranging from months to years.[4] They become incorporated into the bone crystal as bone is remodeled and are ingested by osteoclasts when these cells resorb bone.

Within the osteoclast, nitrogen-containing bisphosphonates inhibit the enzyme farnesyl diphosphate synthase. This is a key enzyme in the mevalonate pathway, which leads to the synthesis of cholesterol. Intermediate metabolites of this pathway are necessary for the coupling of key regulatory proteins to the cell membrane. With this loss of protein prenylation, osteoclasts

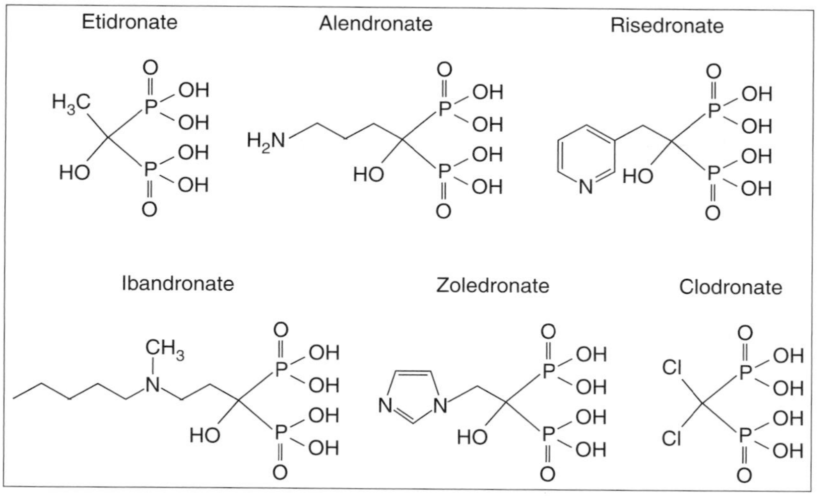

Figure 18-1. Structure of some members of the bisphosphonate class of drugs. The class is defined by the presence of two phosphate groups linked through a central carbon atom. The individual members are distinguished from one another by the other side groups attached to that central carbon.

become unable to resorb bone and ultimately die (apoptosis). In early osteoclast precursors, this results in a blockade of the development of bone-resorbing cells.[5] In contrast, bisphosphonates lacking a nitrogen atom in the side chain (e.g., etidronate, clodronate) are metabolized to form analogues of adenosine triphosphate. These inhibit the adenosine diphosphate/adenosine triphosphate translocase in the mitochondria and again result in osteoclast apoptosis.[6]

Bisphosphonates may also act on osteoblasts, transiently stimulating the proliferation and differentiation of preosteoblast cells,[7] reducing apoptosis in osteoblasts and osteocytes,[8] and increasing osteoblast production of the antiresorptive protein osteoprotegerin.[9]

The reduction in bone turnover caused by bisphosphonates results in an increased lifetime of the bone tissue, providing a longer time in which the secondary mineralization of bone can proceed.[10] This results in an increase in mineral density, which may contribute to the greater strength of bisphosphonate-treated bone,[11] as may the preservation of trabecular thickness and trabecular connectivity.[12,13] Meta-analyses of clinical studies suggest that bisphosphonate-induced changes in bone mineral density (BMD) alone do not account for all the reduction in fracture risk,[14] suggesting that the associated preservation of architecture and possibly other factors are also important.

PHARMACOLOGY

Bisphosphonates have an oral bioavailability of only 1% to 2% and are very poorly absorbed from the gastrointestinal tract. The low oral bioavailability of bisphosphonates is a critical issue in their use. They must be taken in the fasting state with water alone if they are to be absorbed at all. Fasting for 30 minutes after dosing is adequate, but a 60-minute fast may increase the effect on BMD by up to 60%.[15] Amino-bisphosphonates, such as alendronate, can cause upper gastrointestinal irritation, so patients must not lie down for 30 to 60 minutes after oral dosing, to prevent reflux of the tablet into the esophagus. These drugs should not be used in individuals with anatomical or motility disorders of the upper gastrointestinal tract. In others, attention to the dosing regimen prevents difficulties in most patients.[16] Less potent, non-amino-bisphosphonates, such as etidronate, appear to have better upper gastrointestinal tolerability but still need to be taken in the fasting state to optimize bioavailability.

Of the absorbed dose, about one half is deposited on the bone surface, and the balance is excreted unchanged in the urine over the following days. When osteoclasts resorb bone, they ingest the bisphosphonate and are effectively poisoned by it, resulting in a reduction of bone resorption and a redressing of its imbalance with bone formation. Bisphosphonate remains on the bone surface for many years and is gradually incorporated into the structure of bone,[17] so that it can potentially inhibit remodeling cycles that occur years after the time of dosing. This long duration of action opens the possibility of intermittent administration, which is now the most common form of administration. The terminal half-life of bisphosphonates in bone is more than 10 years.[18] The P-C-P bond is very stable, so the bisphosphonates are not metabolized in vivo.

ETIDRONATE

The studies of Storm[19] and Watts[20] using cyclical etidronate (400 mg/day for 2 weeks, repeated every 3 months) indicated that this regimen produced modest increases in BMD and possibly a halving of the number of vertebral fractures. Meta-analysis confirms that etidronate reduces the risk of vertebral fracture (relative risk, 0.63), but there is no evidence for an effect on nonvertebral fracture (relative risk, 0.99), although no adequately powered study has yet been conducted.[21] Etidronate appears to cause fewer gastrointestinal problems than the amino-bisphosphonates, and in some countries is available at low cost. Etidronate use in higher doses in patients with Paget disease was complicated by the development of osteomalacia, indicating that the window of safety is narrow. This, together with the absence of evidence for efficacy against nonvertebral fractures, has led to its being a minor player globally.

ALENDRONATE

The efficacy of alendronate has been assessed in studies of its use in both the prevention of postmenopausal bone loss and the treatment of established osteoporosis.[22] Alendronate in doses of 5 to 10 mg/day reduces bone resorption markers from postmenopausal levels (about twice those in premenopausal women) to values in the lower one-half of the premenopausal range.[23] These changes are maximal within a few months of initiating treatment and are nonprogressive after that time. These declines in bone resorption are mirrored by increases in bone mass. In the spine, BMD increases by about 5% after 3 years on treatment with 5 mg/day, and by about 9% with 10 mg/day.[24] With continuation of therapy, there is a gradual increase in BMD, reaching 14% above baseline after 10 years of 10 mg/day, and 10% above baseline after a similar period of 5 mg/day (Figure 18-2).[25]

In those studies powered to assess fracture rates, alendronate use has been associated with substantial decreases in fracture incidence. Thus, the phase III trial[24] and both arms of the Fracture Intervention Trial[26,27] showed approximately 50% decreases in vertebral fractures, and the pooled estimate from all the alendronate trials is a relative of risk of vertebral fracture of 0.52 (95% CI, 0.43-0.65).[22] Of the two studies carried out in osteopenic populations, one showed a substantial downward trend in vertebral fracture incidence, whereas the other did not. The pooled relative risk of vertebral fracture from these two studies is roughly the same as that in the osteoporotic population, although it is nonsignificant because of the smaller number of fractures.[22]

There is also clear evidence that alendronate decreases the risk of nonvertebral fractures in women with osteoporosis, whether this is defined in terms of prevalent fracture or in terms of BMD.[28] This was first clearly demonstrated by Black[26] (Figure 18-3) and was subsequently independently confirmed by Pols in a 1-year study.[29] The pooled relative risk for osteoporotic women estimated by Cranney is 0.49 (95% CI, 0.36-0.67). The 10-year follow-up of the phase III study suggests that the rate of nonvertebral fractures remains reduced in subjects who continue to take alendronate, but the numbers of subjects were insufficient to be certain of this.[25]

The Fracture Intervention Trial (FIT) has now been extended. A total of 1099 women aged 60 to 86 years who were assigned to active therapy in FIT and had an average duration of alendronate use of 5 years were re-randomized to receive alendronate (30% to 10 mg/day, 30% to 5 mg/day) or to placebo (40% of the cohort) for an additional 5 years. BMD and turnover data for the first 3 years of the extension have been published[30] and show that total hip BMD declined 2.4% in the placebo group (reaching a level still >1% above the FIT baseline), compared with a 0.4% decrease in the alendronate groups (5 and 10 mg/day doses combined). In the spine,

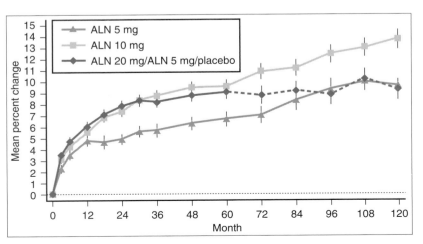

Figure 18-2. Effects of various daily doses of alendronate on lumbar spine bone mineral density, shown as a change from baseline levels. The group shown as diamonds received alendronate 20 mg/day in years 1 and 2, then alendronate 5 mg/day for 3 years, followed by placebo for 5 years (shown as a broken line). (Based on data in Bone et al.[25] Copyright Merck et al, used with permission.)

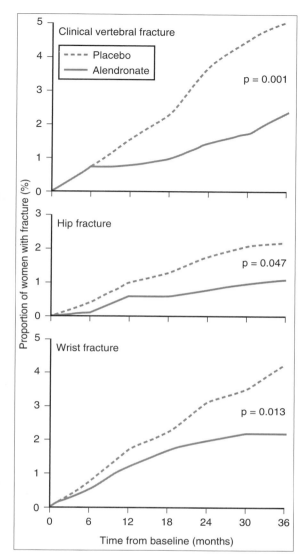

Figure 18-3. Proportions of women in the FIT study[26] with fractures of various types, according to whether they were allocated to treatment with alendronate or placebo. The significances of the between-groups differences are shown. (Redrawn from Black DM, Cummings SR, Karpf DB, et al: Randomised trial of effect of alendronate on risk of fracture in women with existing vertebral fractures. Lancet 1996;3348:1535-41.)

BMD increased 1.0% in placebo subjects, compared with 3.5% in those continuing on active therapy. BMD changes were 0.5% to 1.0% more positive in those taking alendronate 10 mg/day compared with the 5 mg/day group. Bone alkaline phosphatase increased about 15% and urinary N-telopeptide excretion about 20% in those re-randomized to receive placebo (both $P < .001$), but the latter still remained 60% below their levels at the beginning of the FIT study. Preliminary data for the 5-year endpoint of this extension[31] show BMD changes

similar to those at 3 years (hip BMD: placebo −3.4%, alendronate −1.0%; spine BMD: placebo 1.5%, alendronate 5.3%). Most importantly, fracture data are also available, showing a relative risk of clinical spine fracture of 0.45 but for a non-spine fracture of 1.0, when those continuing on either dose of alendronate are compared with those receiving placebo. This indicates that continuation of alendronate for 10 years produces more beneficial fracture outcomes than does its discontinuation after only 5 years.

More recent studies have demonstrated that alendronate administered daily, twice weekly, or once weekly produces the same effects on bone turnover markers and BMD, if the average dose per day is the same.[22] However, there are no fracture data with anything other than daily regimens of administration.

Recently, evidence for efficacy has been extended to other specific groups not studied previously. Greenspan and associates[32] studied osteoporotic women living in a long-term care facility and showed that daily alendronate produced changes in BMD comparable with those demonstrated previously in women living independently. Bell and associates[33] have shown that alendronate produced changes in BMD in African-American women comparable with those observed in the white women. Kushida and associates[34] have shown beneficial effects of alendronate on BMD in a Japanese cohort, which were at least as large as those seen in European and North American studies. Furthermore, they demonstrated that the incidence of vertebral fractures was reduced by 66% in alendronate-treated patients in comparison with those treated with alfacalcidol.

RISEDRONATE

A very similar body of evidence has been assembled for risedronate. In general, the suppression of bone resorption that it produces is slightly less than that for alendronate.[35] This is reflected in slightly smaller increments in BMD, typically about 5% at the lumbar spine after 3 years of therapy, and less than 3% at the hip. Despite this, risedronate reduces vertebral fractures[35,36] with a pooled relative risk across all studies of 0.64 (95% CI, 0.54-0.77).[37] Osteoporotic women without prevalent fractures also have a reduced risk of vertebral facture on risedronate.[38] Risedronate also reduces nonvertebral fractures, with Harris[35] finding a decrease of 39% over 3 years and McClung[39] finding a 30% reduction in hip fracture risk in a population of women over the age of 70 years. When available data on nonvertebral fractures are examined through meta-analysis, relative risk after treatment with risedronate is 0.73 (95% CI, 0.61-0.87).[37] Pooling of data from the risedronate studies indicates that reductions in both vertebral[40] and nonvertebral fractures[41] are apparent within 6 months of starting this drug.

A 2-year extension to one of the risedronate studies has been reported, during which the double-blind design and original randomization were maintained.[42] The risk of new vertebral fractures was reduced by 59% in years 4 and 5 ($P = 0.01$), compared with a 49% reduction in the first 3 years. Continuation of risedronate for a further 2 years is associated with maintenance of low fracture rates.[43] As with the long-term alendronate data, suppression of markers is maintained with long-term treatment, and BMD changes tend to increase, although at a slower rate than in the early years of treatment.

Like alendronate, risedronate is now typically used in a once-a-week dose of 35 mg, rather than the 5 mg/day on which the fracture data are based. As with alendronate, equivalence of efficacy of this dose has been demonstrated only for bone turnover and BMD,[44] although comparison across studies suggests an equivalent fracture reduction.[45]

A key issue in the use of bisphosphonates for treating postmenopausal osteoporosis is determining the appropriate treatment endpoint. The efficacy of these agents has frequently been assessed using measurements of BMD, but it is clear that relatively modest increases in BMD are associated with substantial decreases in fracture risk. Recently, Eastell and colleagues[46] analyzed the relationship between fracture incidence and bone resorption (measured as telopeptides) in the risedronate studies. Pooling placebo and risedronate groups, they found an almost linear relationship between fracture incidence and resorption markers down to a marker value of 1.5 SD below the premenopausal mean (Figure 18-4). At this point, the fracture incidence appears to plateau. The number of individuals reaching this level of bone turnover was relatively small, so this analysis will need to be repeated with other agents to determine whether this truly does represent an optimal turnover rate in patients with postmenopausal osteoporosis.

Although most risedronate data are based on studies in European populations, Shiraki and colleagues[47] have found that risedronate 2.5 mg/day and 5 mg/day produce comparable changes in BMD and markers in Japanese patients, and they conclude that the smaller dose is likely to be adequate for management of osteoporosis in Japan.

IBANDRONATE

Ibandronate is another potent nitrogen-containing bisphosphonate that has been studied using a variety of regimens. Ibandronate was first studied in patients

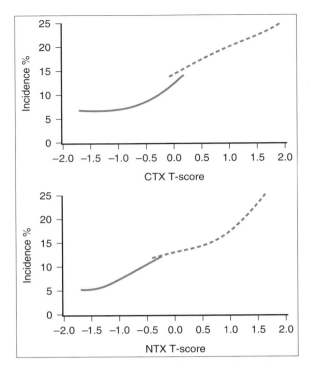

Figure 18-4. Relationship between bone resorption markers expressed as a T-score and the 0- to 3-year incidence of new vertebral fractures. The placebo group is represented by the broken line and the risedronate 5 mg/day group by the solid line. All patients received calcium supplementation (1000 mg/day) and vitamin D (if levels were low). (From Eastell R, Barton I, Hannon RA, et al: Relationship of early changes in bone resorption to the reduction in fracture risk with risedronate. J Bone Mineral Res 2003;18:1051-56, with permission of the American Society for Bone and Mineral Research.)

with osteoporosis as an intravenous injection[48] and showed beneficial effects on BMD. However, ibandronate 1 mg intravenously every 3 months did not result in a reduction in fracture numbers,[49] possibly because this regimen does not stably suppress bone resorption markers over the inter-dose interval[50] and does not increase BMD as much as the potent oral bisphosphonates. Oral ibandronate, either continuously (2.5 mg/day) or intermittently (20 mg every other day for the first 24 days, followed by 9 weeks without active drug) produces changes in BMD comparable with those found with oral alendronate or risedronate,[51] and a monthly dose of 150 mg appears to be comparably effective.[52, 53] Both daily and cyclic regimens have now been shown to reduce vertebral fractures by about one-half, and nonvertebral fractures were reduced in subjects with femoral neck T-scores less than −3.[53] Intravenous ibandronate 2 mg, every three months, produces similar changes in BMD[54, 55] but its anti-facture efficacy is not yet known.

ZOLEDRONATE

The advent of the extremely potent intravenous bisphosphonate zoledronate (also referred to as zoledronic acid) provided the opportunity to test more thoroughly the potential of intermittent intravenous bisphosphonate administration.[56] In a phase II trial involving 350 women with low BMD, participants were randomized to receive placebo or one of five zoledronate regimens. Three of these regimens involved the use of a 3-month dose interval, one a 6-month dose interval, and one a single dose at the beginning of the 1-year study. While BMD and markers of bone turnover were stable in the placebo group, these indices changed almost identically in the five zoledronate groups, indicating that the regimens were therapeutically equivalent (Figure 18-5). The changes in both markers and BMD were comparable with those seen with standard daily regimens of oral bisphosphonates, which are of proven antifracture efficacy. This suggests that annual administration of zole-

dronate is likely to prevent fractures, although the results of phase III studies currently underway will need to be awaited for confirmation of this.

It should be noted that this study does not establish a maximum effective dose interval, because there is no evidence of loss of efficacy even 12 months after a single dose. Thus, it is possible that a greater spacing between doses could be effective, and the maximum interval is likely to be dependent on both the dose and the bisphosphonate used. If the antifracture efficacy of zoledronate is confirmed, then it is likely that many individuals at risk for osteoporosis will opt for the convenience of infrequent intravenous dosing in preference to daily or even weekly use of tablet preparations.

OTHER BISPHOSPHONATES

There are also data indicating that a number of other bisphosphonates are effective. Pamidronate has been

Figure 18-5. Effect of five regimens of administration of zoledronate or placebo on (a) lumbar spine bone density and on (b) bone resorption (measured as serum *C*-telopeptide of type I collagen). The regimens are shown in the inset as the (number of infusions) × (dose in mg) during the 1-year study. All findings in the groups undergoing zoledronate regimens were significantly different from those in the placebo group but none was different from the others. (From Reid IR, Brown JP, Burckhardt P, et al: Intravenous zoledronic acid in postmenopausal women with low bone mineral density. N Engl J Med 2002;346:653-61. Copyright 2002 Massachusetts Medical Society.)

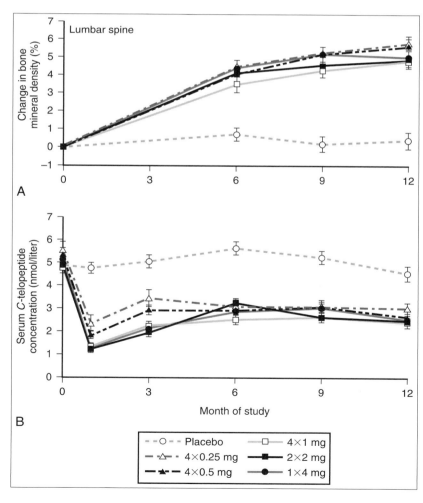

used orally[57,58] and as intermittent infusions.[59,60] Several studies have been reported with clodronate, most recently as a daily oral formulation.[61] In this study of 593 osteoporotic women, the incidence of vertebral fractures was significantly reduced by 46% in subjects assigned to clodronate.

BISPHOSPHONATES IN THE PREVENTION OF OSTEOPOROSIS

Bisphosphonates have positive effects on BMD in women who do not have osteoporosis. For example, in a study of recently menopausal women, alendronate treatment for 7 years increased spine and trochanter BMD by 3% to 4%, whereas femoral neck BMD was maintained.[62] A 2-year study with risedronate produced similar results.[63] An important unresolved issue with regard to the use of both bisphosphonates and other anti-osteoporotic medications, however, is whether they prevent fractures in individuals who do not already have osteoporosis. Studies with both alendronate[27] and risedronate[39] have suggested that they do not, although neither of these studies was powered to specifically address this issue. The findings of the Women's Health Initiative suggest that estrogen/progestin prevents fractures in unselected older women, and a recent study comparing clodronate 800 mg/day with placebo in 5592 women aged 75 years or older also found fewer clinical fractures (reduced by 20%) over 3 years.[64] Antifracture efficacy was independent of age, body mass index, baseline BMD, or prior fracture history. This represents a potential significant expansion to the indications for the use of bisphosphonates, particularly as they become more affordable in the coming years.

COMBINATION THERAPY

Recently, much interest has focused on the use of combinations of a bisphosphonate with another agent, particularly parathyroid hormone (PTH). The PaTH Study randomized 238 postmenopausal women with BMD T-scores of less than −2 to PTH, alendronate, or the combination.[65] Bone turnover markers were almost doubled with PTH, and more than halved with alendronate. With combination therapy, formation markers rose at 1 month, but subsequently both formation and resorption markers paralleled the changes seen with alendronate alone. PTH produced larger changes in spine BMD than did alendronate, whereas the reverse tended to be the case at the hip. Combination therapy resulted in changes that were intermediate between those found with the respective monotherapies. Similar results have been found in a study in male osteoporosis.[66] However, adding PTH on top of a bisphosphonate does appear to produce more positive changes in BMD than does continuation of the bisphosphonate alone.[67] Thus, it is unclear what role combinations of PTH and bisphosphonates have in osteoporosis management.

TREATMENT OFFSET

After discontinuation of alendronate, bone turnover rises to some extent, but even several years after the end of long-term use, bone resorption rates have not returned to baseline.[68,69] Preliminary data have been presented suggesting that the offset of risedronate's effect is more rapid, but the degree of suppression was less than in the alendronate studies, so these data are not directly comparable.[70] Greenspan and coworkers[71] found that there was a significant loss of BMD after the termination of 2 years of treatment with estrogen/progestin, whereas there was no loss of BMD after termination of alendronate after a similar period of treatment. McClung and coworkers[69] found that there was some loss of BMD after 2 or 4 years of therapy with alendronate, but that this was again much less than that after a similar period of treatment with estrogen/progestin. Bagger and coworkers assessed women 7 years after treatment withdrawal and found that those who received alendronate (2.5-10 mg per day) for 2 years had a 3.8% higher BMD than those who received placebo.[68] The residual effect was proportionally larger in women who had received treatment for longer periods (4 years, 5.9%, $P = 0.02$; 6 years, 8.6%, $P = 0.002$). The slow offset of the bisphosphonate effect is not surprising in light of their long residence time in bone. This prolonged duration of action raises important, unanswered questions about the optimal duration of continuous therapy.

LONG-TERM EFFECTS

There is substantial uncertainty regarding the optimal use of bisphosphonates for long-term therapy. The continuing rise in spine BMD with long-term use implies that bisphosphonates have progressive effects on bone, and it appears that they are progressively accumulated in bone mineral. Therefore, it is possible that at some point this accumulation will become deleterious. On the basis of these findings, several courses are open. One is to conclude that treatment up to 10 years is safe and effective, and to continue treating most patients for this period of time. This course is supported by both of the extended studies of alendronate. A second course is to reduce alendronate doses from 10 mg/day to 5 mg/day (or its equivalent) in patients who have been taking alendronate for periods greater than 5 years. This is consistent with the FIT extension, which does not appear to show a fracture advantage of alendronate 10 mg/day over 5 mg/day during the second quinquennium of treatment, although a detailed breakdown of the data by dose is not yet available. Whether such a dose reduction is appropriate for risedronate cannot be determined. A third course is suggested by the recent analysis of the relationship between fracture incidence and bone resorption in the risedronate studies.[46] This suggests that the intermittent use of bisphosphonates to maintain resorption markers 1.5 SD below the premenopausal mean might produce maintenance of fracture prevention. However, there are no data to address this in the context of use for 5 to 10 years, nor in direct comparison with other treatment strategies.

In recent years, there has been a general acceptance that the surrogate endpoints of BMD and bone turnover do not guarantee antifracture efficacy. Therefore, it is not possible to determine which of the above approaches is optimal in terms of the one endpoint that really matters: fracture. The least speculative course is to continue bisphosphonates until year 10 and then consider dose reduction along with monitoring of BMD and turnover. Unfortunately, there is no prospect of authoritative data beyond 10 years becoming available in the foreseeable future.

SAFETY

A number of different safety issues have arisen with bisphosphonate use in osteoporosis. There was initial concern that these potent antiresorptives would decrease bone turnover to a level at which microdamage would not be repaired, resulting in decreased biomechanical strength. Although such effects have been demonstrated in animal models treated with high doses of bisphosphonates,[72] this phenomenon has not been found in human studies, where, in contrast, fracture rates are found to decrease. Isolated reports of stress fracture occurrence in patients treated with bisphosphonates have appeared,[73] but in the absence of persuasive control data, the consensus is that this is not a major issue.

A second concern was that bisphosphonates would interfere with the normal mineralization process. This is clearly true of etidronate when used in high doses for the treatment of Paget disease but has not been found to be a widespread problem with the lower dose cyclic regimen used in osteoporosis. Again, isolated case reports have appeared,[74] but long-term follow-up of the original trial groups[75] and large-scale observational studies[76] (albeit without bone biopsies) indicate that this is an uncommon problem.

Gastrointestinal side effects are now the principal concern with the use of oral bisphosphonates. Patients with preexisting inflammatory bowel disease some-

times suffer exacerbations when taking etidronate, but upper gastrointestinal inflammatory effects are not increased by the use of this drug.[77] The same is true when these agents are used in association with nonsteroidal anti-inflammatory drugs or corticosteroids.

Randomized controlled trials of alendronate produced similarly reassuring results, demonstrating that gastrointestinal adverse effects are no more common in the active therapy group than in the placebo group.[78] However, case reports of upper gastrointestinal problems have appeared, including descriptions of esophageal and gastric erosions and ulcers.[79] The latter probably result either from reflux of bisphosphonate tablets from the stomach or from abnormalities in the esophagus, which interfere with tablet transit. These anecdotes are supported by observational post-marketing data, indicating that alendronate users are 60% more likely to visit doctors or hospitals complaining of dyspeptic symptoms.[80] The discrepancy between trial and post-marketing data may have arisen because patients with significant upper gastrointestinal disease did not enter the trial program, or because dosing regimens were more strictly adhered to in the disciplined environment of a clinical trial.

A number of short-term randomized controlled trials have now been carried out to use endoscopy to assess the gastrointestinal effects of these agents. Graham and colleagues[81] have shown a significantly increased risk of endoscopic abnormalities after only several weeks of alendronate therapy, whereas other investigators have not.[82,83] The propensity of aminobisphosphonates to damage mucosal surfaces has resulted in oral ulceration in a case report of a patient who sucked alendronate tablets.[84]

Like alendronate, risedronate was not associated with an increased risk of gastrointestinal adverse events in the phase 3 study program, even in those with predisposing medical histories and medications.[85] Endoscopic studies are also generally reassuring with this agent.[86-88]

When adverse gastrointestinal experiences occur with the aminobisphosphonates, these agents do not necessarily need to be abandoned. Miller and coworkers[89] found that, of patients intolerant of alendronate, only 15% were still intolerant of the agent when rechallenged, in comparison with 17% of those rechallenged with placebo. Similar data have been published for subjects intolerant of alendronate being rechallenged with risedronate or placebo; discontinuation rates are 16.1% and 11.4%, respectively.[90] To minimize the likelihood of gastrointestinal problems with oral aminobisphosphonates, these medicines should be taken with a full glass of water and the patient should remain upright over the following hour to minimize the likelihood of tablet reflux into the esophagus. Weekly alendronate or risedronate are at least as safe as daily therapy in terms of gastrointestinal side effects.[44,91-93]

One way of circumventing the possible problem of gastrointestinal intolerance of potent bisphosphonates is to administer these drugs intravenously.[57] This route of administration is well tolerated, although some patients develop a mild influenza-like illness after the first injection of these drugs. This has been attributed to an acute phase reaction and, in the doses of zoledronate used in treating osteoporosis, occurs in about 10% of individuals. It leads to withdrawal from treatment in less than 2% of patients. This problem has occasionally been reported with the use of oral aminobisphosphonates.[94]

Other bisphosphonate side effects are rare. Intravenous dosing with pamidronate has been associated with iritis[95] and, less commonly, with impaired hearing,[96] but these problems have not been reported with the doses used in osteoporosis. There is one report of disordered liver function test findings with the use of clodronate.[97] Recently, a syndrome of either a non-healing tooth extraction socket or an exposed jawbone after dental procedures in patients receiving high-dose bisphosphonate for malignancy has been described.[98] These lesions are refractory to débridement and antibiotic therapy. Although a few patients receiving osteoporotic doses of bisphosphonates have been described with this problem, the great majority of those affected have malignancy.

CONCLUSIONS

The bisphosphonates now hold center stage in the management of osteoporosis. An increasing diversity of agents and regimens are available, and evidence for their safety and efficacy continues to grow. In some countries, generic formulations may be available in the near future, and this is likely to reduce drug costs. As this trend progresses and the bisphosphonates become even more cost-effective, there will be a need to continually review the indications for the use of these powerful agents to optimize their effects on bone health.

REFERENCES

1. Frijlink WB, te Velde J, Bijvoet OLM, et al: Treatment of Paget's disease with (3-amino-1-hydoxypropylidene)-1,1-bisphosphonate (APD). Lancet 1979;i:799-803.
2. Reid IR, King AR, Alexander CJ, et al: Prevention of steroid-induced osteoporosis with (3-amino-1-hydroxypropylidene)-1,1-bisphosphonate (APD). Lancet 1988;i:143-46.
3. Rossouw JE, Anderson GL, Prentice RL, et al: Risks and benefits of estrogen plus progestin in healthy postmenopausal women: principal results from the Women's Health Initiative randomized controlled trial. JAMA 2002;288:321-33.
4. Masarachia P, Weinreb M, Balena R, et al: Comparison of the distribution of 3H-alendronate and 3H-etidronate in rat and mouse bones. Bone 1996;19:281-90.
5. Van Beek ER, Lowik CWGM, Papapoulos SE: Bisphosphonates suppress bone resorption by a direct effect on early osteoclast precursors without affecting the osteoclastogenic capacity of osteogenic cells: the role of protein geranylgeranylation in the action of nitrogen-containing bisphosphonates on osteoclast precursors. Bone 2002;30:64-70.
6. Lehenkari PP, Kellinsalmi M, Napankangas JP, et al: Further insight into mechanism of action of clodronate: inhibition of mitochondrial ADP/ATP translocase by a nonhydrolyzable, adenine-containing metabolite. Mol Pharmacol 2002;61:1255-62.
7. Fromigue O, Body JJ: Bisphosphonates influence the proliferation and the maturation of normal human osteloblasts. J Endocr Invest 2002;25:539-46.
8. Plotkin LI, Weinstein RS, Parfitt AM, et al: Prevention of osteocyte and osteoblast apoptosis by bisphosphonates and calcitonin. J Clin Invest 1999;104:1363-74.
9. Viereck V, Emons G, Lauck V, et al: Bisphosphonates pamidronate and zoledronic acid stimulate osteoprotegerin production by primary human osteoblasts. Biochem Biophys Res Commun 2002;291:680-86.
10. Boivin G, Meunier PJ: Changes in bone remodeling rate influence the degree of mineralization of bone. Conn Tissue Res 2002;43:535-37.
11. Borah B, Dufresne TE, Chmielewski PA, et al: Risedronate preserves trabecular architecture and increases bone strength in vertebra of ovariectomized minipigs as measured by three-dimensional microcomputed tomography. J Bone Mineral Res 2002;17:1139-47.
12. Ding M, Day JS, Burr DB, et al: Canine cancellous bone microarchitecture after one year of high-dose bisphosphonates. Calcif Tissue Int 2003;72:737-44.
13. Dufresne TE, Chmielewski PA, Manhart MD, et al: Risedronate preserves bone architecture in early postmenopausal women in 1 year as measured by three-dimensional microcomputed tomography. Calcif Tissue Int 2003;73:423-32.
14. Cummings SR, Karpf DB, Harris F, et al: Improvement in spine bone density and reduction in risk of vertebral fractures during treatment with antiresorptive drugs. Am J Med 2002;112:281-9.
15. Tanko LB, McClung MR, Schimmer RC, et al: The efficacy of 48-week oral ibandronate treatment in postmenopausal osteoporosis when taken 30 versus 60 minutes before breakfast. Bone 2003;32:421-6.
16. Lanza F: Bisphosphonate mucosal injury: the end of the story? Dig Liver Dis 2003;35:67-70.
17. Masarachia P, Weinreb M, Balena R, et al: Comparison of the distribution of h-3-alendronate and h-3-etidronate in rat and mouse bones. Bone 1996;19:281-90.
18. Khan SA, Kanis JA, Vasikaran S, et al: Elimination and biochemical responses to intravenous alendronate in postmenopausal osteoporosis. J Bone Mineral Res 1997;12:1700-7.
19. Storm T, Thamsborg G, Steiniche T, et al: Effect of intermittent cyclical etidronate therapy on bone mass and fracture rate in women with postmenopausal osteoporosis. N Engl J Med 1990;322:1265-71.
20. Watts NB, Harris ST, Genant HK, et al: Intermittent cyclical etidronate treatment of postmenopausal osteoporosis. N Engl J Med 1990;323:73-9.
21. Cranney A, Guyatt G, Krolicki N, et al: A meta-analysis of etidronate for the treatment of postmenopausal osteoporosis. Osteoporos Int 2001;12:140-51.

22. Cranney A, Wells G, Willan A, et al: Meta-analysis of alendronate for the treatment of postmenopausal women. Endocrine Reviews 2002;23:508-16.

23. Greenspan SL, Bone G, Schnitzer TJ, et al: Two-year results of once-weekly administration of alendronate 70 mg for the treatment of postmenopausal osteoporosis. J Bone Mineral Res 2002;17:1988-96.

24. Liberman UA, Weiss SR, Broll J, et al: Effect of oral alendronate on bone mineral density and the incidence of fractures in postmenopausal osteoporosis. N Engl J Med 1995;333:1437-43.

25. Bone HG, Hosking D, Devogelaer J, et al: Ten years' experience with alendronate for osteoporosis in postmenopausal women. N Engl J Med 2004;350:1189-99.

26. Black DM, Cummings SR, Karpf DB, et al: Randomised trial of effect of alendronate on risk of fracture in women with existing vertebral fractures. Lancet 1996;348:1535-41.

27. Cummings SR, Black DM, Thompson DE, et al: Effect of alendronate on risk of fracture in women with low bone density but without vertebral fractures: results from the fracture intervention trial. JAMA 1998;280:2077-82.

28. Black DM, Thompson DE, Bauer DC, et al: Fracture risk reduction with alendronate in women with osteoporosis: the Fracture Intervention Trial. J Clin Endocrinol Metab 2000;85:4118-24.

29. Pols HAP, Felsenberg D, Hanley DA, et al: Multinational, placebo-controlled, randomized trial of the effects of alendronate on bone density and fracture risk in postmenopausal women with low bone mass: results of the FOSIT study. Osteoporos Int 1999;9:461-68.

30. Ensrud KE, Barrett-Connor EL, Schwartz A, et al: Randomized trial of effect of alendronate continuation versus discontinuation in women with low BMD: results from the Fracture Intervention Trial long-term extension. J Bone Mineral Res 2004;19:1259-69.

31. Black D, Schwartz A, Ensrud K, et al: A 5 year randomized trial of the long-term efficacy and safety of alendronate: the FIT Long-term EXtension (FLEX). J Bone Miner Res 2004;19 (suppl 1): S45.

32. Greenspan SL, Schneider DL, McClung MR, et al: Alendronate improves bone mineral density in elderly women with osteoporosis residing in long-term care facilities: a randomized, double-blind, placebo-controlled trial. Ann Intern Med 2002;136:742-46.

33. Bell NH, Bilezikian JP, Bone HG, et al: Alendronate increases bone mass and reduces bone markers in postmenopausal African-American women. J Clin Endocrinol Metab 2002;87:2792-97.

34. Kushida K, Shiraki M, Nakamura T, et al: The efficacy of alendronate in reducing the risk for vertebral fracture in Japanese patients with osteoporosis: a randomized, double-blind, active-controlled, double-dummy trial. Curr Therapeut Res Clin Exp 2002;63:606-20.

35. Harris ST, Watts NB, Genant HK, et al: Effects of risedronate treatment on vertebral and nonvertebral fractures in women with postmenopausal osteoporosis: a randomized controlled trial. JAMA 1999;282:1344-52.

36. Reginster JY, Minne HW, Sorensen OH, et al: Randomized trial of the effects of risedronate on vertebral fractures in women with established postmenopausal osteoporosis. Osteoporos Int 2000;11:83-91.

37. Cranney A, Tugwell P, Adachi J, et al: Meta-analysis of risedronate for the treatment of postmenopausal osteoporosis. Endocrine Rev 2002;23:517-23.

38. Heaney RP, Zizic TM, Fogelman I, et al: Risedronate reduces the risk of first vertebral fracture in osteoporotic women. Osteoporos Int 2002;13:501-5.

39. McClung MR, Geusens P, Miller PD, et al: Effect of risedronate on the risk of hip fracture in elderly women. N Engl J Med 2001;344:333-40.

40. Roux C, Seeman E, Eastell R, et al: Efficacy of risedronate on clinical vertebral fractures within six months. Curr Med Res Opinion 2004;20:433-39.

41. Harrington JT, Ste-Marie LG, Brandi ML, et al: Risedronate rapidly reduces the risk for nonvertebral fractures in women with postmenopausal osteoporosis. Calcif Tissue Int 2004;74:129-35.

42. Sorensen OH, Crawford GM, Mulder H, et al: Long-term efficacy of risedronate: a 5-year placebo-controlled clinical experience. Bone 2003;32:120-26.

43. Goemaere S, Sorensen OH, Johnson TD, et al: Sustained anti-fracture efficacy of risedronate treatment over 7 years in postmenopausal women. J Bone Miner Res 2003;18(suppl 2): S90.

44. Harris ST, Watts NB, Li Z, et al: Two-year efficacy and tolerability of risedronate once a week for the treatment of women with postmenopausal osteoporosis. Curr Med Res Opin 2004;20:757-64.

45. Watts NB, Lindsay R, Li ZQ, et al: Use of matched historical controls to evaluate the anti-fracture efficacy of once-a-week risedronate. Osteoporos Int 2003;14:437-41.

46. Eastell R, Barton I, Hannon RA, et al: Relationship of early changes in bone resorption to the reduction in fracture risk with risedronate. J Bone Mineral Res 2003;18:1051-56.

47. Shiraki M, Fukunaga M, Kushida K, et al: A double-blind dose-ranging study of risedronate in Japanese patients with osteoporosis (a study by the Risedronate Late Phase II Research Group). Osteoporos Int 2003;14:225-34.

48. Thiebaud D, Burckhardt P, Kriegbaum H, et al: Three monthly intravenous injections of ibandronate in the treatment of postmenopausal osteoporosis. Am J Med 1997;103:298-307.

49. Recker R, Stakkestad JA, Chesnut CH, et al: Insufficiently dosed intravenous ibandronate injections are associated with suboptimal antifracture efficacy in postmenopausal osteoporosis. Bone 2004;34:890-99.

50. Christiansen C, Tanko LB, Warming L, et al: Dose dependent effects on bone resorption and formation of intermittently administered intravenous ibandronate. Osteoporos Int 2003;14:609-13.

51. Riis BJ, Ise J, Von Stein T, et al: Ibandronate: a comparison of oral daily dosing versus intermittent dosing in postmenopausal osteoporosis. J Bone Mineral Res 2001;16:1871-78.

52. Miller PD, McClung MR, Macovei L, et al: Monthly oral ibandronate therapy in postmenopausal osteoporosis: one year results from the MOBILE study. J Bone Miner Res 2005;20:1315-1322.

53. Chesnut CH, Skag A, Christiansen C: Effects of oral ibandronate administered daily or intermittently on fracture risk in postmenopausal osteoporosis. J Bone Miner Res 2004;19:1241-49.

54. Schimmer RC, Bauss F: Effect of daily and intermittent use of ibandronate on bone mass and bone turnover in postmenopausal osteoporosis: a review of three phase II studies. Clin Therapeut 2003;25:19-34.

55. Adami S, Felsenberg D, Christiansen C, et al: Efficacy and safety of ibandronate given by intravenous injection once every 3 months. Bone 2004;34:881-9.

56. Reid IR, Brown JP, Burckhardt P, et al: Intravenous zoledronic acid in postmenopausal women with low bone mineral density. N Engl J Med 2002;346:653-61.

57. Reid IR, Wattie DJ, Evans MC, et al: Continuous therapy with pamidronate, a potent bisphosphonate, in postmenopausal osteoporosis. J Clin Endocrinol Metab 1994;79:1595-99.

58. Orr-Walker B, Wattie DJ, Evans MC, et al: Effects of prolonged bisphosphonate therapy and its discontinuation on bone mineral density in post-menopausal osteoporosis. Clin Endocrinol 1997;46:87-92.

59. Gallacher SJ, Fenner JAK, Anderson K, et al: Intravenous pamidronate in the treatment of osteoporosis associated with corticosteroid dependent lung disease: an open pilot study. Thorax 1992;47:932-36.

60. Thiebaud D, Burckhardt P, Melchior J, et al: Two years' effectiveness of intravenous pamidronate (APD) versus oral fluoride for osteoporosis occurring in the postmenopause. Osteoporos Int 1994;4:76-83.

61. McCloskey E, Selby P, Davies M, et al: Clodronate reduces vertebral fracture risk in women with postmenopausal or secondary osteoporosis: results of a double-blind, placebo-controlled 3-year study. J Bone Mineral Res 2004;19:728-36.

62. Sambrook PN, Rodriguez JP, Wasnich RD, et al: Alendronate in the prevention of osteoporosis: 7-year follow-up. Osteoporos Int 2004;15:483-88.

63. Mortensen L, Charles P, Bekker PJ, et al: Risedronate increases bone mass in an early postmenopausal population: two years of treatment plus one year of follow-up. J Clin Endocrinol Metab 1998;83:396-402.

64. McCloskey E, Jalava T, Oden A, et al: The efficacy of clodronate (Bonefos) to reduce the incidence of osteoporotic fractures in

elderly women is independent of the underlying BMD. J Bone Mineral Res 2003;18(suppl 2):S92.

65. Black DM, Greenspan SL, Ensrud KE, et al: The effects of parathyroid hormone and alendronate alone or in combination in postmenopausal osteoporosis. N Engl J Med 2003;349:1207-15.

66. Finkelstein JS, Hayes A, Hunzelman JL, et al: The effects of parathyroid hormone, alendronate, or both in men with osteoporosis. N Engl J Med 2003;349:1216-26.

67. Cosman F, Nieves JW, Luckey MM, et al: Daily versus cyclic PTH combined with alendronate versus alendronate alone for treatment of osteoporosis. J Bone Min Metab 2003;18(suppl 2):S32.

68. Bagger YZ, Tanko LB, Alexandersen P, et al: Alendronate has a residual effect on bone mass in postmenopausal Danish women up to 7 years after treatment withdrawal. Bone 2003;33:301-7.

69. McClung M: Resolution of effect following alendronate: six-year results from the Early Postmenopausal Interventional Cohort (EPIC) Study. J Bone Miner Res 2002;17(suppl 1):s134.

70. Watts NB, Olszynski W, McKeever C: Effect of risedronate treatment discontinuation on bone turnover and BMD. Calcif Tissue Int 2004;74(suppl 1):S79.

71. Greenspan SL, Emkey RD, Bone HG, et al: Significant differential effects of alendronate, estrogen, or combination therapy on the rate of bone loss after discontinuation of treatment of postmenopausal osteoporosis: a randomized, double-blind, placebo-controlled trial. Ann Intern Med 2002;137:875-83.

72. Mashiba T, Hirano T, Turner CH, et al: Suppressed bone turnover by bisphosphonates increases microdamage accumulation and reduces some biomechanical properties in dog rib. J Bone Mineral Res 2000;15:613-20.

73. Guanabens N, Peris P, Monegal A, et al: Lower extremity stress fractures during intermittent cyclical etidronate treatment for osteoporosis. Calcif Tissue Int 1994;54:431-34.

74. Thomas T, Lafage MH, Alexandre C: Atypical osteomalacia after 2 year etidronate intermittent cyclic administration in osteoporosis. J Rheumatol 1995;22:2183-85.

75. Miller PD, Watts NB, Licata AA, et al: Cyclical etidronate in the treatment of postmenopausal osteoporosis: efficacy and safety after seven years of treatment. Am J Med 1997;103:468-76.

76. Vanstaa TP, Leufkens H, Abenhaim L, et al: Postmarketing surveillance of the safety of cyclic etidronate. Pharmacotherapy 1998;18:1121-28.

77. Vanstaa T, Abenhaim L, Cooper C: Upper gastrointestinal adverse events and cyclical etidronate. Am J Med 1997;103:462-67.

78. Bauer DC, Black D, Ensrud K, et al: Upper gastrointestinal tract safety profile of alendronate: the fracture intervention trial. Arch Int Med 2000;160:517-25.

79. de Groen PC, Lubbe DF, Hirsch LJ, et al: Esophagitis associated with the use of alendronate. N Engl J Med 1996;335:1016-21.

80. Ettinger B, Pressman A, Schein J: Clinic visits and hospital admissions for care of acid-related upper gastrointestinal disorders in women using alendronate for osteoporosis. Am J Manag Care 1998;4:1377-82.

81. Graham DY, Malaty HM: Alendronate gastric ulcers. Aliment Pharmacol Therapeut 1999;13:515-19.

82. Lanza F, Rack MF, Simon TJ, et al: Effects of alendronate on gastric and duodenal mucosa. Amer J Gastroenterol 1998;93:753-57.

83. Lowe CE, Depew WT, Vanner SJ, et al: Upper gastrointestinal toxicity of alendronate. Am J Gastroenterol 2000;95:634-40.

84. Demerjian N, Bolla G, Spreux A: Severe oral ulcerations induced by alendronate. Clin Rheumatol 1999;18:349-50.

85. Hosking D, Keller M, Hooper M, et al: Risedronate is well tolerated in postmenopausal osteoporotic women using NSAIDs or with underlying gastrointestinal disorder. Calcif Tissue Int 2000;66(suppl 1):s120.

86. Lanza FL, Rack MF, Li Z, et al: Placebo-controlled, randomized, evaluator-blinded endoscopy study of risedronate vs. aspirin in healthy postmenopausal women. Aliment Pharmacol Therapeut 2000;14:1663-70.

87. Lanza FL, Hunt RH, Thomson ABR, et al: Endoscopic comparison of esophageal and gastroduodenal effects of risedronate and alendronate in postmenopausal women. Gastroenterology 2000;119:631-38.

88. Lanza F, Schwartz H, Sahba B, et al: An endoscopic comparison of the effects of alendronate and risedronate on upper gastrointestinal mucosae. Am J Gastroenterol 2000;95:3112-7.

89. Miller PD, Woodson G, Licata AA, et al: Rechallenge of patients who had discontinued alendronate therapy because of upper gastrointestinal symptoms. Clin Therapeut 2000;22:1433-42.

90. Adachi JD, Adami S, Miller PD, et al: Tolerability of risedronate in postmenopausal women intolerant of alendronate. Aging Clin Exp Res 2001;13:347-54.

91. Lanza F, Sahba B, Schwartz H, et al: The upper GI safety and tolerability of oral alendronate at a dose of 70 milligrams once weekly: a placebo-controlled endoscopy study. Am J Gastroenterol 2002;97:58-64.

92. Greenspan S, Field-Munves E, Tonino R, et al: Tolerability of once-weekly alendronate in patients with osteoporosis: a randomized, double-blind, placebo-controlled study. Mayo Clin Proc 2002;77:1044-52.

93. Eisman JA, Rizzoli R, Roman-Ivorra J, et al: Upper gastrointestinal and overall tolerability of alendronate once weekly in patients with osteoporosis : results of a randomized, double-blind, placebo-controlled study. Curr Med Res Opin 2004;20:699-705.

94. Schweitzer DH, Vanderuit MO, Vanderpluijm G, et al: Interleukin-6 and the acute phase response during treatment of patients with Paget's disease with the nitrogen-containing bisphosphonate dimethylaminohydroxypropylidene bisphosphonate. J Bone Mineral Res 1995;10:956-62.

95. Macarol V, Fraunfelder FT: Pamidronate disodium and possible ocular adverse drug reactions. Am J Ophthalmol 1994;118:220-24.

96. Reid IR, Mills DA, Wattie DJ: Ototoxicity associated with intravenous bisphosphonate administration. Calcif Tissue Int 1995;56:584-85.

97. Laitinen K, Taube T: Clodronate as a cause of aminotransferase elevation. Osteoporos Int 1999;10:120-2s2.

98. Ruggiero SL, Mehrotra B, Rosenberg TJ, et al: Osteonecrosis of the jaws associated with the use of bisphosphonates: a review of 63 cases. J Oral Maxillofacial Surg 2004;62:527-34.

19 Parathyroid Hormone for the Treatment of Osteoporosis: The Science and the Therapy

Nancy E. Lane

Osteoporosis is a disease that is characterized by both a deterioration of the bone structure and a reduction in bone mass such that the bone fractures with very little impact. Therefore, the ideal treatment for osteoporosis would be with agents that would improve the bone strength and reduce bone fracture rates.[1] Over the past 10 years, a number of new medications have been approved for the prevention and treatment of osteoporosis, including selective estrogen receptor modulators (raloxifene),[1,2] bisphosphonates,[3-5] and calcitonin,[6] just to name a few. All of these agents' main effect is to reduce bone turnover, as they are referred to as antiresorptive agents. However, by reducing bone turnover, they effectively prolong the secondary mineralization phase of the bone remodeling cycle and improve bone strength.[7] Sodium fluoride was also tried as an agent to treat osteoporosis. Although sodium fluoride is referred to as an anabolic agent because it stimulates osteoblasts to form new osteoid, it was not found to have antifracture efficacy initially due to its incorporation into the hydroxyapatite crystal as fluoroapatite, which turned out not to be as strong as the hydroxyapatite. Subjects treated with this agent sustained more fractures than those treated with placebo.[8] However, when a lower dose of a slow-release sodium fluoride preparation was used (75 mg twice a day), a reduction in vertebral fracture risk was observed in only one study, but because fracture reduction was not found in another study, the agent has not been approved for the treatment of osteoporosis.[9,10]

Despite the availability and the efficacy in fracture reduction with approved antiresorptive agents, a significant argument can still be made for expecting only modestly good results from an antiresorptive agent that is targeted to osteoclasts. Once adult peak bone mass is achieved, the skeleton has limited capacity to form new bone from soft tissue sites. Adult bone is strengthened in response to different forms of mechanical loading by thickening of the bone that is already present.[11,12] On the endosteal surfaces of the cortical bone and on the trabecular bone surfaces, packets of new bone form at these sites where there has previously been bone resorption. Also, bone can slowly accumulate by continuous slow accretion only on periosteal surfaces, but this occurs at very low levels in adults. Therefore, if bone resorption is reduced with antiresorptive agents, even fewer sites will be available for formation of thickened packets of new bone. Although the balance of bone formation over bone resorption is positive with antiresorptive agent treatment, as evidenced by a significant increase in bone mineral density (BMD) within the first 2 to 4 years of therapy, the effect does plateau.[4] Also, although antiresorptive agents, especially the bisphosphonates, do reduce fracture risk by 50% or more in osteoporotic subjects, because these agents only modestly alter trabecular and cortical bone structure, subjects still are at a relatively high risk of fracture despite compliance with these therapies.[4,5]

HISTORICAL BACKGROUND ON PARATHYROID HORMONE

Parathyroid hormone (PTH) (1-84) is the principal regulator of calcium homeostasis in mammals. PTH is released when serum calcium levels are low and it is suppressed when calcium levels increase. PTH also regulates bone metabolism as it stimulates 1-α-hydroxylase activity in the kidney, thereby increasing 1,25-dihydroxyvitamin D levels, which promote intestinal calcium absorption.[12]

It has been know since the 1930s that parathyroid hormone has anabolic properties on bone.[13] Importantly, these data were somewhat ignored due to manufacturing issues that were resolved in the 1970s when synthetic PTH could be manufactured. Biosynthetic intact PTH (1-84), many synthetic or biosynthetic PTH fragments, and PTH-peptide have been developed and studied in both preclinical and clinical trials during recent years.[12]

PATHOPHYSIOLOGY OF THE ACTION OF PARATHYROID PEPTIDES

Parathyroid hormone exerts most of its biological functions on bone through the PTH1 receptor it shares with the PTH-related peptide (PTHrP) (Figure 19-1). The effects of the PTH2 receptor on bone have not yet been clearly delineated.[12,14,15] Interestingly, the PTH1 receptors are generally not found on osteoclasts but are found in high numbers on stromal cells that generate osteoblasts, and on growth plate chondrocytes in growing animals. When PTH activates its receptor, it results in intracellular activation of cyclic adenosine monophosphate (cAMP) and cAMP-dependent protein kinase-A. At high concentrations, the phospholipase-c system can also be activated.[12,15] The osteoclastic bone resorption that accompanies prolonged daily PTH administration or continuous PTH administration most likely occurs from the osteoblast/stromal cells release of RANKL, interleukin-6, and other osteoclast-activating proteins that activate RANK on the osteoclast surface and result in maturation and activation of osteoclast activity.[16,17] Also, PTH treatment may inhibit osteoprotogerin (OPG), which is a decoy receptor of RANKL and an inhibitor of osteoclast maturation and activation. Small clinical studies appear to support these findings.[17]

In preclinical and clinical studies, it has been observed that a daily injection of PTH fragments leads to stimulation of bone formation followed by some bone resorption. However, with continuous high levels of PTH fragments, as are seen in the clinical disease of hyperparathyroidism, there is bone formation but greater bone resorption, usually resulting in a new loss of bone. Because of observations that bone cells react differently to exposure to intermittent and continuous levels of PTH, attention has focused on why this phenomenon occurs. The anabolic actions of the daily PTH administration has been a topic of great interest. How PTH increases bone mass is not completely clear. However, Dobnig and Turner found that a single subcutaneous administration of hPTH (1-34) or a 1-hour infusion resulted in a significant increase in the number of osteoblasts in previous nonremodeling bone surface.[18] However, if the infusion of hPTH (1-34) was continued for 12 to 24 hours, there was a significant increase in osteoclasts on the trabecular bone surface. The authors concluded that the one subcutaneous administration or the 1-hour infusion of hPTH (1-34) may have activated previously inactive lining cells to redifferentiate into an osteoblast phenotype and form bone.[18] Leaffer and colleagues[19] performed a more detailed ultrastructural study and made similar conclusions. Also, a short-term, 28-day treatment with hPTH (1-34) resulted in an increase in osteoblast number on the trabecular bone surface, as compared with results in control subjects.[20] Another research group has devoted more effort to defining the anabolic

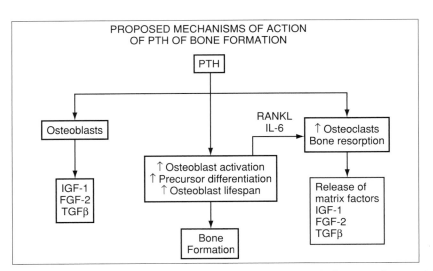

Figure 19-1. Parathyroid hormone (PTH) promotes bone formation through a number of different mechanisms. PTH promotes the osteoblast proliferation via several mechanisms. PTH stimulates preosteoblasts and osteoblasts to make growth factors (IGF-1, FGF-2, TGFβ) that promote proliferation of mesenchymal stem cells to differentiate into preosteoblasts. PTH stimulates the conversion of bone lining cells to osteoblasts and it prevents osteoblast and osteocyte apoptosis.[18] Also, with continued PTH treatment, osteoblasts are stimulated to produce RANKL and interleukin-6 which stimulates osteoclast maturation and activity. Osteoclastic bone resorption, releases more bone growth factors (IGF-1, FGF-2, TGFβ) from the bone matrix that further stimulate the maturation and activity of osteoblasts. FGF-2 = fibroblast growth factor-2; IGF-1 = insulin-growth factor-1; TGFβ = transforming growth factor β. (Adapted from Whitfield[85] and Lane and Kelman.[86])

action of PTH and has in vitro evidence that PTH increases bone formation by preventing osteoblast apoptosis, thereby prolonging the bone-forming time.[21] All of these data support a role of PTH given by a method that exposes the bone-forming cells to the protein for only a short period of time in initially causing a very rapid increase in bone formation. Most likely, this rapid anabolic action is the result of a combination of factors that includes increasing osteoblast lifespan and activity.

It is well known, however, that PTH has different effects on the skeleton depending on the time of exposure of the bone cells to the protein. Collagen synthesis was inhibited in cavarial cultures when continuous PTH exposure was provided, but increased with intermittent exposure of PTH. The stimulatory effect of PTH on collagen synthesis was found to be through the stimulation of insulin-like growth factor (IGF)-1 production by bone cells or released from the calvarial bone matrix.[22,23] Additional molecular biological examination was done to further elucidate this finding of increased mRNA transcripts for IGF-1 when cancellous osteoblasts from ovariectomized rats were exposed to PTH.[24] Although it is still not fully understood how IGFs act to increase the formation of new bone with PTH treatment, it is believed that the IGFs probably act locally and are either produced by osteoblast-like cells or are released from the nearby bone matrix and prolong the osteoblast phenotype to increase new bone formation packets. In addition, the IGFs may inhibit osteoblast apoptosis, prolonging osteoblast survival and thereby increasing bone mass. Recent data from an IGF-1 knockout mouse experiment found that treatment with hPTH (1-34) did not increase bone formation, suggesting that IGF-1 was again clearly involved in the mechanism for PTH-activated bone formation.[25]

Insulin-like growth factors are not the only bone growth factors that may be influenced by PTH treatment. Basic fibroblast growth factor (FGF) is also released from the bone matrix and can influence stromal cell differentiation into osteoblasts. Basic FGF is known also to stimulate the production of new trabeculae and improve trabecular thickness in mouse and rat models of osteoporosis.[26, 27] Also, an FGF-2 (bFGF) knockout mouse, when treated with hPTH (1-34), did not have an increase in bone formation, suggesting that bFGF is an important factor in the bone formation action of PTH.[28] Lastly, a clinical study in which daily hPTH (1-34) treatment was given to osteoporotic postmenopausal women taking glucocorticoids found that bFGF levels increased nearly 150% over the baseline after 3 months of treatment and remained elevated at nearly this level until the PTH therapy was discontinued after 1 year. At the time of discontinuation, the levels fell toward the baseline levels very quickly.[29] Importantly, there was no change in serum bFGF levels in the control group who were just treated with calcium and vitamin D supplementation.[29]

There are probably a number of other bone growth factors that are stimulated with PTH treatment within the local bone environment. Data are available showing that PTH affects transforming growth factor-1 activity and prostaglandin production.[12,30]

The Wnt Signaling Pathway and Parathyroid Hormone

Recently, a very important biological pathway was delineated, the canonical Wnt signaling pathway, which is composed of secreted glycoproteins that participate in morphogenesis, determination of cell polarity, and regulation of cell proliferation and differentiation during embryogenesis.[31] In addition, this pathway plays a major role in postnatal bone accrual. Major advances in our understanding of skeletal biology that could lead to therapeutic advances and understanding of diseases of altered bone have and will continue to emerge as this pathway is further elucidated. A subgroup of Wnts induces a cascade of intracellular events that stabilize B-catenin, facilitating its transport to nuclei where it binds to Lef1/Tcf transcription factors and alters gene expression to promote osteoblast expansion and function. Natural extracellular Wnt antagonists, Dickkopfs and secreted frizzled-related proteins, impair osteoblast function and block bone formation. In a number of genetic disorders of skeletal mass, mutations of Wnt signaling proteins, including LRP5, create gain-of-function or loss-of-function receptors that tend to be resistant to the normal regulatory mechanisms and cause higher or lower bone density. Recently, families have been identified in whom a gain-of-function mutation of the LRP5 cell surface receptor results in extremely high bone mass.[31, 32] In addition, small rodent models in which the genes for the Wnt proteins are either knocked out or overexpressed reveal that the mice with the LRP5 mutation have a greater increase in bone mass in response to loading than control mice.[32] This information synthesizes the long-held belief that a mechanism or "mechanostat" exists in which the skeleton responds to loading by forming bone and that the Wnt pathway most likely is the link to the skeleton responding to load by increasing bone mass. The Wnt signaling pathway is also important in the sequence of events on how PTH increases bone formation. Because the canonical Wnt signaling pathway promotes the proliferation, expansion, and survival of premature and immature osteoblasts, Dickoff-1, secreted frizzled related proteins, and Wif-1 antagonize Wnt signaling in osteoblasts to promote the death of immature cells.

However, they can also downregulate the pathway in mature cells to induce terminal differentiation.[31] Recent data demonstrate that treatment of osteoblast cells with PTH results in a decrease in Dickoff-1 production and an increase in canonical signaling that stimulates osteoblasts to mature and form bone.[31,33] Additional research on this pathway will surely expand our knowledge of how skeletal tissues are both formed and maintained.

Preclinical Studies of Parathyroid Hormone

In the clinical development of any agent for osteoporosis, the US Food and Drug Administration (FDA) requires that an agent demonstrate significant efficacy in a small animal model and a larger animal model with known intracortical bone remodeling. In addition, the FDA requires study endpoints of bone mass and biomechanical tests of bone strength. Interestingly, quite a large number of animal studies were done with PTH both for the process of clinical approval by the FDA and also by curious scientists interested in its novel mechanism of action on the skeleton. Because the number of animal studies performed with PTH is in the hundreds, this chapter will review just a few of them.

Numerous studies in animal models have demonstrated that intermittent PTH injections have an anabolic effect on cancellous bone at multiple skeletal sites. As early as the late 1920s and 1930s, daily injections of a peptide extract of human PTH into rats were found to increase bone density.[34,35] Initial observations included proliferation of both osteoclasts and osteoblasts after a single injection of 20 units of parathyroid extract. When the injections were continued, bone tissue increased and the number of osteoclasts (but not osteoblasts) declined.[35,36]

The anabolic effect of hPTH has been documented in healthy adult female rats. Rats injected with varying doses of hPTH (1-38) 5 days per week for 2 to 8 weeks demonstrated anabolic responses in both femoral cortical and trabecular bone. Observed microarchitectural changes included increased cancellous bone mass due to trabecular thickening, small increases in the quantity of woven bone in marrow cavities, and the presence of lamellar bone formation on all surfaces.[35,37] Interestingly, rats treated for 8 weeks with hPTH (1-38) had increased bone mass compared with animals treated with hPTH (1-38) for 4 weeks followed by 4 weeks of placebo, and both groups had significantly greater bone mass compared with placebo. This anabolic action of hPTH (1-38) occurs relatively rapidly after initiation of therapy. In a study of the action of different durations of 50 μg/kg hPTH (1-38) in 48 10-week-old healthy female rats, animals treated for only 10 days demonstrated statistically significant increases in bone mass, bone mineral content (as measured by ash weight), and BMD measured by dual x-ray absorptiometry (DXA).[35,38] Animals treated for 15 days had additional improvements, including improved biomechanical properties of the hip and increased width of the femoral neck.

The effect of intermittent PTH injections was also assessed in the ovariectomized rat, the primary animal model of postmenopausal osteoporosis. The adult female rat, when rendered estrogen deficient by bilateral ovariectomy, loses trabecular bone mass very rapidly from sites with red marrow (high turnover trabecular bone), which includes both the proximal tibial and distal femoral metaphyses, very similar to the postmenopausal female human. However, the loss of trabecular bone mass in the adult female rat is much more rapid than in the postmenopausal female human in that the rat loses nearly 30% in 6 to 8 weeks whereas the postmenopausal women loses 30% over a 20- to 30-year period.[39] A study of immature female Sprague-Dawley rats treated immediately after ovariectomy for 25 weeks with multiple weekly injections of hPTH (1-34) revealed that hPTH (1-34) prevented the reduction in bone weight and mineral content observed in the ovariectomized controls.[35,40] In other words, three-times-weekly injections of hPTH (1-34) prevented the development of low bone mass in ovariectomized rats.

Intermittent PTH is also effective in reversing osteoporosis due to estrogen deficiency. In a 6-month course of daily injections of 8 or 40 μg/kg of hPTH (1-34) in 9-month-old ovariectomized rats, both doses substantially increased bone mass in the proximal tibia and femur compared with ovariectomized controls.[35,41] Significant dose-dependent anabolic actions on femoral bone at the metaphysis, diaphysis, and, to a lesser extent the epiphysis were observed. Mechanical resistance to fracture and compression, particularly in the lumbar spine, was also significantly increased. In this instance, hPTH (1-34) therapy reversed bone loss associated with estrogen deficiency and markedly improved many biomechanical properties of bone.

Similarly, a 1995 study of daily treatment with 62.5 μg/kg/d hPTH (1-34) for 56 days in 2-year-old male rats demonstrated a statistically significant increase in cancellous bone volume and trabecular thickness of the L1-6 vertebral bodies.[35,42] In addition, hPTH (1-34) induced accelerated bone formation (as evidenced by the increased mineral apposition rate), increased mineralizing surface, and increased volume-related and surface-related bone formation rates. An analysis of the strength of the L4 vertebra after completion of hPTH (1-34) therapy revealed increases of 66% in total load, 47% in total stiffness, and 98% in total energy absorption, which remained even after correction for increased bone mass. Also, a measurement of total bone calcium found that hPTH (1-34) dramatically improved this in addition to the total bone dry weight after 12 days of therapy.[35,43]

A more recent study documented that treatment with hPTH (1-34) in 2-year-old male rats with age-related osteoporosis in the distal femur led to a statistically significant increase in trabecular bone volume and trabecular thickness, as measured by micro-computed tomography (micro-CT), and compressive strength.[35,44] Thus, hPTH (1-34) led to the formation of new cancellous bone and substantially improved bone strength in sites where osteoporosis had developed in older male rats. Studies in other animal models, including cynomolgus monkeys, greyhounds, beagles, and rabbits, have demonstrated similar effects of intermittent hPTH fragments on bone.

In summary, intermittent PTH therapy augments bone mass in healthy rats, prevents bone loss in newly estrogen-deficient rats, and increases bone mass in rats with low bone mass or established osteoporosis. The majority of the beneficial activity is observed in areas rich in trabecular bone, which include the lumbar spine, distal femur, and proximal tibia. Continued work in our laboratory evaluating the effects of hPTH (1-34) versus bFGF in the treatment of estrogen-deficiency osteoporosis find that the major effect of PTH in reversing osteoporosis in the rat is to thicken existing trabecular plates, thereby improving bone strength. Interestingly, bFGF treatment of osteoporotic rats also improves bone mass and bone strength like hPTH (1-34), but it increases trabecular number by stimulating osteoblast progenitors to differentiate into osteoblasts and form new trabeculae. The new trabeculae formed by bFGF appear to connect to existing trabeculae and again, like hPTH (1-34), improve bone strength, albeit by different mechanisms.[26]

The effect of hPTH fragments on cortical BMD and strength appears to differ across species. Initial fears that hPTH therapy may lead to increased cancellous bone mass at the expense of cortical bone, the "cortical steal" phenomenon, have not been conclusively confirmed in animal models, in clinical trials of hPTH in men and women with osteoporosis, or in histomorphometric analyses of men and women with osteoporosis.

Because the FDA requires that studies for osteoporosis agents be done in an animal species that is larger than the rat, studies with hPTH-related fragments were performed. It was also critical for the preclinical development of PTH to perform studies in an animal model that had intracortical bone remodeling similar to the human, as the ovariectomized rat does not remodel its cortical bone. Adult cynomolgus ovariectomized monkeys or sham-operated controls were given hPTH (1-34) subcutaneously at 10 µg/kg for 3 days a week for 6 months. The investigators reported that PTH treatment resulted in a 6.7%

increase in spinal BMD, but no increase in total body bone mass was found. Mechanical testing revealed that PTH treatment significantly increased bone strength at the axial skeleton in a large estrogen-deficient animal model and that hPTH (1-34) improved bone mass and bone strength both at trabecular and cortical bone enriched sites.[45]

One interesting aspect of the animal studies was the effect of PTH on the response of bone to mechanical loading. As stated earlier in this chapter, PTH appears to link the mechanical loading of bone to the bone-forming genes and proteins (Wnt signaling pathway) in the osteoblast. A study by Chow and associates found that PTH increased the bone formation from mechanical stimulation in the caudal vertebrae in rats. Interestingly, the increase in bone formation in response to mechanical loading could be further augmented with the injection of PTH about 60 minutes before the loading.[46] Again, this was additional evidence that PTH augments bone cells to respond to mechanical load and form bone, most likely increasing Wnt signaling pathway in osteogenic cells.

Several additional preclinical studies were performed with PTH in combination with antiresorptive agents, including estrogen, calcitonin, and bisphosphonates, to determine whether the combination of an antiresorptive agent that would prevent cortical bone remodeling would be superior to PTH alone. The majority of these studies were performed in mature ovariectomized rats, and outcome variables included histomorphometry at high-turnover trabecular bone skeletal sites with mechanical testing of bone strength. Nearly all of the studies found that PTH was as effective alone as in combination.[47-49] One study by Shen and colleagues[50] reported that PTH and estrogen increased trabecular connectivity and bone mass more than either alone, but other investigators could not reproduce this findings.[51]

Another important aspect of interest from the preclinical animal studies for the development of PTH was that PTH increased bone mass during the therapy, but immediately after PTH was discontinued the bone mass accrued during the therapy rapidly disappeared. However, if treatment of the osteoporotic rats was sequential with the course of PTH therapy being followed by a bisphosphonate, the newly formed bone from the PTH treatment was maintained.[52]

CLINICAL STUDIES

Pharmacokinetic Properties of Parathyroid Hormone

Recombinant human PTH (1-34) or teriparatide is the only PTH fragment currently approved for the treatment of osteoporosis in women and prevention of bone loss in men. Teriparatide reaches serum peak concentrations about 30 minutes after a subcutaneous administration for the approved 20 µg dose, and its serum concentration rapidly decreases within 3 hours. The systemic clearance of teriparatide is about 62 L/hour in women and 94 L/hour in men. This clearance rate exceeds the rate of normal hepatic plasma flow, which is consistent with both extrahepatic and hepatic clearance. The serum distribution half-life is about 1 hour when administered by subcutaneous injection.[53] Peripheral metabolism of PTH most likely occurs by nonspecific enzymatic mechanisms in the liver with excretion in the kidney.

Clinical Efficacy Studies

A number of small randomized clinical trials were performed with PTH. Many of these studies were in postmenopausal women with severe osteoporosis. The outcome measures in these studies were not standard, as the DXA and quantitative computed tomography (QCT) instruments we now have to assess bone mass and bone volume were still under development. In general, most of these studies found that PTH [most of the studies were done with hPTH (1-34)] was anabolic to the skeleton, with large increases in bone mass of the lumbar spine assessed by QCT and by iliac crest histomorphometry. Early studies, while confirming the preclinical animal study findings that PTH dramatically increased trabecular bone mass, also revealed evidence for increased cortical bone remodeling both within the cortex and on the endocortical surface. An increase in the cross-sectional area of the cortical bone was also observed as additional evidence that PTH increased bone mass on both the periosteal surface and the endocortical surface. Many of these early studies were innovative and clearly confirmed the hypotheses that PTH, when given as a daily injection with bone cell exposure only limited to a short period, was anabolic to bone. This was in contrast to the catabolic effects of PTH on the skeleton when exposed to continuous high levels, as in hyperparathyroidism.

Clinical Studies with Antifracture Efficacy

Small investigator-initiated or phase I and phase II trials of either hPTH (1-34) or PTH (1-84) have been performed and their findings reported in a number of review articles.[35, 54] In this chapter we comprehensively review the two large phase III studies with rhPTH (1-34) and rhPTH (1-84), because both studies demonstrate fracture efficacy and rhPTH (1-34) is currently approved in a number of countries for the treatment of osteoporosis.

To date, the most comprehensive randomized, placebo-controlled, double-blinded clinical trial of rhPTH (1-34) in postmenopausal osteoporosis was conducted in 1637 postmenopausal women with prior vertebral fractures and low BMD, who were randomized to receive rhPTH (1-34) 20 or 40 µg daily.[35,55] The planned duration of the study was 24 months, but the trial was discontinued after a median follow-up of 21 months because of a report that osteosarcomas had developed in Fischer 344 rats exposed to lifelong rhPTH (1-34). In the active drug-treatment groups, lumbar spine BMD increased by 9% and 13%, respectively, femoral neck BMD increased by 3% and 6%, respectively, and total body BMD increased by 2% to 4% in both groups. In the shaft of the radius, BMD decreased from baseline in all three study groups, and the percentage change compared with the placebo group (approximately a 2% decrease) reached statistical significance in those receiving 40 µg rhPTH. The risk of one or more new vertebral fractures was decreased by 69% in the 20 µg group and by 65% in the 40 µg group, as compared with the placebo group. The risk of new vertebral fragility fractures was also decreased, by 53% and 54% versus placebo, respectively. Additionally, in women who experienced a new vertebral fracture, the mean loss of height was significantly less in both rhPTH (1-34) groups than in subjects receiving placebo, and there was a marked decrease in symptoms of back pain in both active-treatment groups. Adverse events were generally mild and infrequent, with nausea, headache, dizziness, and leg cramps most commonly reported. Mild hypercalcemia occurred in 2% of the placebo group, 11% in the 20 µg group, and 28% in those receiving 40 µg. Nine patients were withdrawn from the 40 µg group due to persistent hypercalcemia, as compared with one patient in the 20 µg group.[35,55]

The investigators concluded that treatment of postmenopausal osteoporosis with rhPTH (1-34) not only improved BMD at the lumbar spine, femoral neck, and total body, but also decreased the risk of vertebral and nonvertebral fractures. Although the effect on trabecular bone was well defined, the action on cortical bone (as evidenced by a decrease in BMD of the radial shaft) was less clear. Mid-radius and distal radius BMD decreased in this phase III study of rhPTH (1-34) for the treatment of postmenopausal osteoporosis. This anatomic region of the forearm is composed primarily of cortical bone. The effect of rhPTH (1-34) on cortical bone is best described from iliac crest biopsy samples taken from a small subset of subjects in the phase III study. After approximately 21 months of rhPTH (1-34) treatment, two-dimensional histomorphometry of iliac crest biopsy samples revealed a 14% increase in trabecular bone mass in the rhPTH (1-34) group and a decrease of 24% in the placebo group. However, three-dimensional micro-CT assessment of the same specimens found that compared with the placebo group, rhPTH (1-34) treatment increased trabecular connectivity (+19% with rhPTH versus −15% with placebo), changed the structure model index to reflect a more platelike structure, and increased cortical thickness (rhPTH (1-34), +22%; placebo, +3%).[54,56] However, consistent with the knowledge that rhPTH (1-34) does increase bone resorption, an increase in cortical porosity was observed both by bone histomorphometry and by micro-CT evaluations in the rhPTh (1-34) group compared with the placebo-treated group.[54,56] Interestingly, at the same time, an increase in cortical thickness with rhPTH (1-34) was observed; in fact, the cross-sectional area of the bone actually increased significantly compared with the placebo-treated groups. Because the BMD is a ratio of bone mineral content to the cross-sectional area of the scan measurement, an increase in cortical thickness that was greater than the increase in bone mineral content in the scanned region, this resulted in a modest reduction in BMD in the forearm of patients treated with rhPTH (1-34). Because bone strength is a function of both bone mass and cross-sectional area, calculations of bone strength demonstrated an increase in the forearm of patients treated with rhPTH (1-34).[54] In addition, other data to support the finding that subjects treated with rhPTH (1-34) have increased cortical bone thickness by stimulating new bone apposition on both the periosteal and endosteal surfaces were found in a subset of study subjects from this trial that underwent pQCT of the distal tibia during the study. Zanchetta and coworkers reported significant changes in bone size and cortical thickness in rhPTH (1-34)–treated subjects compared with the placebo-treated group.[54,55,57]

Treatment with rhPTH (1-34) was associated with a rapid increase within a month of initiation of therapy of bone formation markers (>100% above baseline) and a slower but equally large increase in bone resorption markers (>100% above baseline levels). The increase in the biochemical markers of bone turnover started to decline after 12 months of the therapy, although they remained elevated above the baseline levels until the treatment was stopped.[55] A post hoc analysis of the biochemical markers of bone turnover with rhPTH (1-34) treatment found that study subjects in the highest group for bone turnover markers at the baseline evaluation had a more rapid increase in lumbar spine BMD and a greater increase in BMD compared with study subjects who had lower baseline bone turnover markers (R. Marcus, personal communication, January 10, 2005.)

The finding of an increased risk of osteogenic sarcoma in 344 6-week-old Fisher rats exposed to high-dose lifelong rhPTH (1-34) is worthy of discussion. Two experiments were performed,[35,58] the first of which exposed rats to rhPTH (1-34) beginning at 2 months of age, at doses that were 3, 20, and 60 times higher than the recommended human dose. All doses resulted in the development of osteosarcomas, in a dose-dependent manner. The second study demonstrated that tumor development was a function of both dose and duration of therapy. At the time of this writing, no primate studies have demonstrated any increased risk of osteosarcoma with hPTH fragment therapy. Analyses of more than 2500 humans with primary, secondary, or tertiary hyperparathyroidism have failed to document a single case of osteogenic sarcoma. Studies in humans with osteoporosis who were treated with rhPTH to date have found no increased incidence of osteosarcomas. Finally, early standard safety studies of hPTH (1-34) failed to show a mutagenic or genotoxic potential; hPTH fragment therapy is considered safe in humans for up to 24 months. However, osteosarcomas are tumors that usually develop in late adolescence and early adulthood. Therefore, rhPTH (1-34) is not to be prescribed to subjects with open epiphyses, subjects with Paget disease, or subjects who have had radiation to the skeleton or an unexplained elevation of alkaline phosphatase level.[58] Additional laboratory research is still need to determine whether there are surrogate markers that can identify individuals who might be at risk for this complication. Until that time, it is critical that physicians follow the warning in the FDA label in the United States.

Recombinant human PTH (1-84), or Preos, has also been evaluated in a phase III study for antifracture efficacy. The TOP study randomized 2532 postmenopausal women who were older than 55 years of age, with lumbar spine, femoral neck, and total BMD T-score of less than −2.5 (or ≤ −2.0 with a prevalent vertebral fracture) or postmenopausal women between the ages of 45 and 54 years with a T-score of less than or equal to −3.0 or less than or equal to −2.5 with a prevalent fracture. Throughout the trial, all subjects received 700 mg calcium and 400 IU vitamin D supplements daily and were randomized to either placebo or PTH 100 µg daily. Characteristics of the study subjects included an average age of 64 years (range, 45-94 years) and mean spine, total hip, and femoral neck BMD T-scores of −3.0, −1.9, and −2.2, respectively. Prevalent vertebral fractures were present in 19% of the 1737 subjects. About 70% of the placebo group and 65% of the PTH group completed the trial. In subjects who were 75% or more compliant with the study medication and the study protocol, the new vertebral fracture incidence was 3.33% and 1.14% in the placebo and PTH groups, respectively ($P = .002$), a relative fracture risk reduction of 66%. In study subjects who were compliant with the study protocol and without a prevalent vertebral fracture, PTH decreased new vertebral fracture from 2.22% to 0.83% ($P = .028$), resulting in a relative fracture risk reduction of 63%. PTH decreased new vertebral fracture incidence from 8.38% to 2.63% ($P = .025$) in subjects with a prevalent vertebral fracture, a relative fracture risk reduction of 69%. At month 18, mean spine, total hip, and femoral neck BMD scores increased by 7.2%, 2.2%, and 2.5%, respectively, in the PTH group relative to the placebo group ($P < .001$ for each). Overall, the percentage of subjects experiencing adverse events, including serious adverse events was comparable in both groups. Some study subjects in the PTH group withdrew from the study (9%), and reasons given included headache, dizziness, nausea or vomiting, and elevated serum or urine calcium levels. Two percent of placebo subjects discontinued due to one or more similar adverse events. Interestingly, in this study, 16% of PTH subjects and 12% of placebo subjects discontinued due to any adverse events.

The results of this pivotal phase III study of PTH (1-84) found significant protection against first vertebral fractures in a high-risk population of postmenopausal osteoporotic women and provided significant protection against additional fractures in women who had already experienced an osteoporotic fracture. At this time, a new drug application is under review at the US Food and Drug Administration for rhPTH (1-84) for the treatment of osteoporosis.[59]

In summary, the results of these two phase III studies of recombinant PTH peptides (1-34) and (1-84) show that both are effective in reducing vertebral fracture risk in osteoporotic and osteopenic postmenopausal women. At this time, the nonvertebral fracture risk reduction has only been reported for rhPTH (1-34) and is still under analysis for rhPTH (1-84). The study populations evaluated in these two large clinical trials of antifracture efficacy were not exactly similar. All of the rhPTH (1-34) subjects had osteoporotic fractures, so the therapy was secondary prevention of an additional bone fracture, and those in the rhPTH (1-84) study group had only 19% prevalent vertebral fractures at the baseline evaluation, so that about 80% in this study were evaluated with this compound for primary prevention of vertebral osteoporotic fractures. We believe the over-riding conclusion is that both agents are effective as both primary prevention and secondary prevention of osteoporotic fractures. Additional studies will need to be performed if rhPTH (1-84) is approved for the treatment of osteoporosis to identify other similarities and differences between these two anabolic bone agents. In addition, these study results suggest that intermittent or daily PTH injections in postmenopausal women and men is safe and effective treatment for osteoporosis. Initially, there is a great increase in BMD at skeletal sites rich in trabecular bone. Next, bone remodeling dramatically increases with PTH, with markers of bone formation rising early, followed by equally increased levels of bone resorption by 6 months of the therapy. These clinical studies demonstrate that bone strength is significantly enhanced at several skeletal sites with greater trabecular and cortical bone thickness and a marked increase in bone volume if measured by QCT. These changes in bone mass, bone structure, and bone strength result in rapid and significant fracture risk reduction after 12 to 18 months of daily PTH injections.

Combination Therapy with rhPTH (1-34) and rhPTH (1-84)

Because PTH is known to cause increased cortical bone remodeling with continued use, bone investigators were at one time concerned that the increase in trabecular bone mass might be occurring at the expense of the cortical bone. These observations also emerged from the review of iliac crest biopsies in patients with hyperparathyroidism in which it was observed that these patients had sufficient trabecular bone mass and evidence of high bone formation on the trabecular and endocortical surfaces, but they also had cortical remodeling or porosity. To try to minimize the cortical remodeling that occurs with PTH treatment and to evaluate whether the addition of an antiresorptive agent might prevent bone resorption and shorten the duration of PTH therapy, a number of combination studies with PTH were undertaken. None of these studies has fracture endpoints, but they are important to review to provide history and insight into the actions and use of PTH as an osteoporosis agent.

Combined Human Parathyroid Hormone and Hormone Replacement Therapy or Selective Estrogen Receptor Modulator Therapy in Postmenopausal Women

Several clinical trials have addressed the efficacy of hPTH amino-terminal fragments in combination with postmenopausal hormone replacement therapy (HRT). HRT is a recognized and often used antiresorptive therapy that helps prevent bone loss in states of estrogen deficiency. In 2003, however, the Women's Health Initiative (WHI)[60] found the risks of HRT including myocardial infarctions, cerebrovascular accident, and thromboembolism were greater than expected. Since then, the use of HRTs for the prevention and treatment of osteoporosis has virtually stopped in the United States. The studies presented in this section were all performed before the WHI study results were known. Although HRT is effective in protecting the skeleton from ongoing bone loss, its function as an anabolic agent is limited. Because hPTH (1-34) clearly has anabolic actions on cancellous bone but may cause cortical bone remodeling, it was hypothesized that the addition of an antiresorptive agent such as HRT might prevent cortical bone loss and thus result in an even greater gain in BMD than with hPTH (1-34) monotherapy. In addition, it was believed that HRT could help to maintain the improved BMD after a relatively short course of hPTH (1-34).

This issue was assessed in a 3-year randomized controlled trial in women with postmenopausal osteoporosis receiving HRT.[35,61] A total of 34 women with T-scores of less than −2.5 or atraumatic fractures were first treated with standard HRT for at least 24 months. Then, the patients were randomized to receive either hPTH (1-34) 25 μg subcutaneously and HRT daily or HRT alone for 3 years. No placebo injections were used. In the hPTH (1-34) group, lumbar spine bone mass increased continuously throughout the study period, improving by 13% over baseline values after 3 years, compared with a nonsignificant decrease in lumbar spine mass in the HRT-only group at the same timepoint. Total hip and total body bone mass increased significantly, by 2.7% and 7.8%, respectively, in the hPTH (1-34) group, versus no significant change in the control group. Vertebral fractures (as measured by either a 15% or 20% reduction in vertebral height) declined significantly in the combined treatment group. Osteocalcin, a marker of bone formation, increased significantly during the first month of therapy, peaked at 6 months, and then gradually returned to baseline levels at 3 years. Urinary N-telopeptide, a marker of bone resorption, increased more slowly to a peak at 6 months, followed by a gradual decline to baseline levels. These changes in the levels of biochemical markers suggest an uncoupling of bone formation and resorption, allowing for a rapid increase in bone formation, with a more gradual but ultimately equal increase in bone resorption. Importantly, bone mass was at least conserved at all skeletal sites in the hPTH (1-34) HRT group, and no significant decline in cortical bone was observed. The authors concluded that the combination of hPTH (1-34) and HRT significantly increased bone mass in the spine, decreased vertebral fracture rates, and was not detrimental to cortical bone.[35,61]

Iliac crest bone biopsies in HRT-treated women with osteoporosis before and after 3 years of hPTH (1-34) therapy showed significant improvements in bone histomorphometric indices.[35,62] Cancellous bone area was maintained in all subjects. Cortical width and thickness significantly increased in women on HRT and hPTH (1-34), and there was no increase in cortical porosity. Micro-CT analysis revealed an increase in trabecular connectivity density. These findings in part help explain the unique improvements in both quantity and quality of bone after hPTH (1-34) therapy.[34,35]

An additional analysis of the longer term data on the combination of HRT and hPTH (1-34) was done.[35,63] After 3 years of hPTH (1-34) 40 μg/d and HRT, bone mass increased by about 13% in the lumbar spine, 4% in the total hip, and about 4% in the total body, compared with nonsignificant increases in the HRT-only group at each skeletal site. The number of women experiencing a vertebral fracture decreased from 37.5% to 8.3% (based on 15% vertebral height reduction criteria; 12 fractures versus 2) and from 25% to 0% (using 20% height reduction; 7 versus 0). Notably, all patients were continued on HRT and followed for an additional 12 months after hPTH therapy was stopped. After this observation period, bone mass decreased very slightly in a nonsignificant manner at all body sites, but still remained significantly greater than baseline levels. Again, there was no evidence of a catabolic effect on cortical bone, and an important new finding suggesting that HRT could preserve the increased bone mass caused by short-term hPTH therapy. Changes in bone turnover markers were similar to those previously described.[35,61,63]

Also, a 2-year randomized, double-blinded, placebo-controlled trial of the efficacy of daily subcutaneous hPTH (1-34) plus HRT was performed.[64] Postmenopausal women with osteoporosis diagnosed by DXA (T-score at the lumbar spine or femoral neck of < −2.5) who were receiving 1500 mg of calcium and 800 IU of vitamin D daily were treated for 2 years with hPTH (1-34) and HRT, or placebo and HRT. BMD as measured by DXA increased steadily in the lumbar spine and peaked at 29.2% above baseline levels at 24 months in the hPTH group. Significant, but less striking, improvements were observed in the femoral neck. Lumbar spine trabecular density measured by QCT demonstrated a dramatic 74% increase above baseline, compared with a 2.1% decrease in the placebo group.[35,64]

Recently, a 12-month randomized, double-blinded, placebo-controlled trial evaluated the efficacy of daily subcutaneous rhPTH (1-34) plus raloxifene versus placebo PTH plus raloxifene.[65] Postmenopausal women with osteoporosis diagnosed by DXA (T-score of either the lumbar spine or femoral neck of < −2.5) who also received calcium (1000 mg/d) and vitamin D (800 IU/d) were treated for 1 year with either rhPTH (1-34) and raloxifene (60 mg/d) or placebo and raloxifene (60 mg/d). BMD as measured by DXA increased in the lumbar spine by 5.2% in the PTH plus raloxifene group compared with 6.2% in the placebo plus raloxfene group. Total hip BMD increased 2.3% in the PTH plus raloxifene group compared with 0.7% in the PTH plus placebo group ($P < .04$). Interestingly, CTX, a marker of bone resorption, was 50% lower in the

PTH plus raloxifene group compared with the PTH plus placebo group ($P < .01$).[65]

Combined hPTH/Bisphosphonate Therapy in Postmenopausal Osteoporosis

A number of studies have now been performed to evaluate whether PTH in combination with a bisphosphonate could improve bone mass and bone strength.

A recent study, the parathyroid hormone and alendronate (PATH) study illustrated the effectiveness of rhPTH (1-84) at 100 µg/d alone or in combination with bisphosphonate alendronate (10 mg/d) for treatment of osteoporosis/osteopenia. Women with a lumbar spine or femoral neck BMD T-score of less than −2 were randomized into three groups receiving 10 mg/d alendronate and placebo injections, 10 mg/d of alendronate and rhPTH (1-84) 100 µg/d injections, or placebo alendronate and rhPTH (1-84) 100 µg/d injections for 1 year.[54,66] After 12 months of these treatments, BMD at the lumbar spine increased in all treatment groups, and there was no significant difference between the PTH alone and the combination groups. However, the volumetric bone density of the trabecular bone of the lumbar spine measured by QCT was increased in all treatment groups, but the PTH alone group had nearly twice as high a value as the other groups, and this difference was statistically significant. Compared with the other study groups, those receiving rhPTH and alendronate showed significantly greater improvements in BMD of the vertebrae (+6% both PTH groups versus +4% alendronate alone) but all hip BMD measurements and the distal one-third radius BMD measurements found that alendronate alone either increased BMD more at the hip or prevented BMD loss at the radius more than either rhPTH (1-34) treatment group by DXA measurements. In addition, hip QCT increases were lessened with rhPTH (1-84) with alendronate or alendronate alone.[54,66] The changes in the biochemical markers of bone turnover were highly correlated with the BMD findings. Study subjects treated with rhPTH (1-84) alone had rapid and sustained increases in PINP and bone alkaline phosphatase and urine CTX, and the increases in these markers were less in both the rhPTH (1-84) group with alendronate and the alendronate-only group. The significance of these findings related to antifracture efficacy is not known. Recently, a post hoc analysis was performed on the PATH data and found significant heterogeneity of the BMD and biochemical bone turnover marker response to rhPTH (1-34) therapy, greater than in alendronate-treated subjects. Seventeen percent of the PTH-treated patients had no increase in cancellous bone BMD measured by QCT, whereas 39% had a greater than 30% increase in the measurement.

Importantly, all subjects evaluated were very compliant with the study medications.[67] Of note, 21% of the subjects treated with alendronate only had no increase in cancellous BMD. These data suggest that there is heterogeneity in the response to bone-active agents. Additional investigation is needed to determine what factors identify patients who will maximally respond to PTH. It may be that additional work in baseline bone turnover markers will answer this question from the PATH data.[66,67]

SEQUENTIAL THERAPY: PARATHYROID HORMONE FOLLOWED BY AN ANTIRESORPTIVE AGENT

Probably the first study evaluating the sequential therapy of PTH followed by a bisphosponate was reported by Rittmaster and associates.[35,54,68] In a sequential combination study, 66 postmenopausal women with osteoporosis were treated with daily subcutaneous injections of 50, 75, or 100 µg rhPTH (1-84) or placebo for 1 year, followed by 1 year of 10 mg alendronate a day.[68,69] After 1 year of therapy, lumbar spine BMD increased by 1.3% ($P > .05$) with placebo, compared with 4.3% ($P > .05$), 6.9% ($P < .001$), and 9.3% ($P < .001$) in the three rhPTH (1-84) dosage groups, respectively. After 12 months of alendronate therapy, lumbar spine BMD compared with baseline increased by 7.1 ± 5.3%, 11.3 ± 5.7%, 13.4 ± 5.0% ($P < .01$), and 14.6 ± 7.9% ($P < .001$) in the placebo and 50, 75, and 100 µg rhPTH (1-84) groups, respectively. Femoral neck BMD did not change significantly after rhPTH (1-84) therapy but did increase after the course of alendronate. Compared with placebo, whole-body BMD decreased significantly in each rhPTH (1-84) group, but after 12 months of alendronate, there was no significant difference between the placebo group and any rhPTH (1-84) group. These results suggested that 75 and 100 µg of rhPTH (1-84) significantly increased lumbar spine BMD, and that the addition of alendronate protected and further augmented lumbar spine BMD as well as reversing the mild negative impact of rhPTH (1-84) on cortical bone.[35,68]

Another study of sequential therapy was performed by Lindsay and colleagues.[70] These investigators evaluated study subjects who had been enrolled in the phase III rhPTH (1-34) trial that was discontinued approximately 21 months after it was initiated. This follow-up study of 18 months found the absolute risk reduction with PTH treatment was about 13% for both doses of PTH. Although other osteoporosis medications were used in 47% of the study subjects during the follow-up period, the persistent fracture protection observed during this 18-month follow-up study was attributed only to the previous PTH treatment. In fact, a post hoc analysis found that previous PTH treatment was a significant predictor of continued fracture reduction in the follow-up period.[70]

In another sequential therapy study with a study design similar to that of the study by Rittmaster and associates, treatment with rhPTH (1-84) was given for 1 year followed by alendronate for 1 year.[71] The original PATH study protocol required study subjects to be randomized for 1 year to rhPTH (1-84), rhPTH (1-84) with alendronate (10 mg/dL) or placebo plus alendronate (10 mg/dL) in a 2:1:1 randomization. After 1 year of therapy, subjects in the PTH only group were then rerandomized to treatment with alendronate (10 mg/d) or placebo; the other study groups continued alendronate. As was reported by Rittmaster and associates, subjects treated initially with rhPTH (1-34) who were then treated with alendronate had a total increase over 2 years of 12%, as compared with 4% in subjects treated with PTH followed by placebo (a difference of 8% over 2 years) in lumbar spine BMD.[71] Subjects who were treated with placebo after the rhPTH (1-84) lost about 2% bone mass and the two other study groups maintained the BMD values from the first year of therapy.[71] These data again support the concept that PTH increases bone mass but also bone remodeling space and that a potent bisphosphonate, alendronate, prevents additional remodeling space from opening up while allowing the open space to fill in and fully mineralize. This sequential therapy with an anabolic agent followed by a potent antiresorptive agent appears to allow for optimization of the bone-forming effects of rhPTH (1-84) after only 1 year of therapy.

Another sequential study reported only in abstract form raises the question of what might be the optimal duration of PTH therapy to maximize new bone formation. Cosman and colleagues performed a study that treated all postmenopausal women with osteoporosis (T-score of lumbar spine or femoral neck of < −2.5) with alendronate (10 mg/d or 70 mg/wk) for 1 to 3 years and then randomized the study subjects to hPTH (1-34) to receive placebo injection, hPTH (1-34) daily for months 0 through 3, then months 6 through 9, and then months 12 through 15 or hPTH (1-34) daily for 15 months. At the 15-month timepoint, the increase in lumbar spine BMD was similar in the daily and sequential PTH groups (6.5% vs. 5.4%) and no change was observed in the alendronate-only group. Total hip BMD increased about 2% in all treatment groups and the difference between the groups was not significant. Interestingly, vertebral fracture numbers were assessed and subjects treated either daily or sequentially appeared to have a significantly reduced incidence of fractures; however, the numbers in each group were small.[54,72]

Another study evaluated sequential therapy in postmenopausal women who had been treated for 3 years with either raloxifene (60 mg/d) or alendronate (10 mg/d) with continued osteopenia were all discontinued from their antiresorptive agents and started on rhPTH (1-34) for 18 to 36 months.[73] At 1 month after rhPTH (1-34) started, both groups had significant increases in most biochemical markers of bone turnover, but those previously treated with raloxifene had significantly greater increases that remained more than 30% greater for 18 months. In addition, the BMD increases in the lumbar spine in patients treated previously with raloxifene (10.2%) compared with those treated previously with alendronate (4.1%) as well as in the hip (1.8% vs. 0%). Although both groups of patients responded to the rhPTH (1-34), the rate of increase was greater in the prior raloxifene group compared with the prior alendronate group. These results suggest that some bone remodeling is important to a rapid PTH anabolic response. Because this was a small study, additional studies will be needed to confirm or refute these findings. Overall, it appears that the bone surface needs to be able to remodel or, as mentioned earlier, release bone matrix proteins that stimulate osteoblast maturation to obtain a maximal and/or rapid response to PTH.

hPTH as Monotherapy for Men with Osteopenia/Osteoporosis

The significant public health problem of osteoporosis is not simply confined to estrogen-deficient women. Elderly men frequently have decreased BMD, and it is estimated that approximately 20% of all osteoporotic fractures in the United States occur in men.[35,74,75] As the elderly population continues to increase, this percentage will increase. Worldwide figures suggest that 27% of all hip fractures occur in men.[35,74,75] Similarly, vertebral fractures are also found with greater frequency in older men, with a 1996 European Osteoporosis Study reporting that the prevalence of vertebral deformity in elderly European white men was approximately 30%.[35,76] The association of both hip and vertebral fractures with pain, decreased mobility, and loss of independence in both men and women is well recognized and represents a massive and costly public health challenge.[35]

Osteoporosis in men is most often due to such conditions as alcohol abuse, glucocorticoid excess, hypogonadism, malabsorption, and hyperthyroidism. Although treatment of any underlying disorder is the most appropriate medical intervention, in many cases no distinct cause can be identified. Antiresorptive therapy with a bisphosphonate has proved beneficial in men with idiopathic osteoporosis,[35,76] but few studies have evaluated the efficacy of hPTH in male osteoporosis (Table 19-1).

TABLE 19-1 A REPRESENTATIVE SAMPLE OF CLINICAL TRIALS OF PARATHYROID HORMONE FRAGMENTS, CHANGE IN BONE MINERAL DENSITY, AND FRACTURE RISK REDUCTION, IF AVAILABLE[*]

Study	Patients	Treatment Regimen	Lumbar Spine BMD	Total Hip BMD	Femoral Neck BMD	Radial BMD	Fracture Risk
Monotherapy							
Neer RM et al, 2001	PMOP	rhPTH (1-34) 20 or 40 μg/d for median of 18-21 months	+9.7% and 13.7% in 20 and 40 μg PTH groups ($p<0.001$) from placebo	+2.6% and 3.6% in 20 and 40 μg PTH groups ($p<0.001$) from placebo	+2.8% and 5.1% in 20 and 40 μg PTH groups ($p<0.001$) from placebo		Reductions of 65-69% in 20 and 40 μg PTH ($p<0.001$) from placebo in both groups
Ettinger et al, 2004	PMOP	rhPTH (1-84) 100 μg/d	+7.2% from placebo ($p<0.001$)	+2.2% from placebo ($p<0.001$)	+2.5% from placebo ($p<0.001$)		Reduction in relative risk of 66% from placebo ($p<0.001$)
Monotherapy in Men							
Orwoll et al,[*] 2003	Men with osteoporosis	rhPTH (1-34) 20 μg or 40 μg/d or placebo for 11 months	+ about 6% in 20 μg and 9% in 40 μg groups vs. placebo ($p < 0.001$) for both		+1.5% and 2.9% in 20 μg % 40 μg from placebo ($p<0.05$) [AU4]	No significant differences	Not available
Kurland ES et al, 2000	Men with osteoporosis	HPTH (1-34) at 25 μg/d for 18 months	+13.5% PTH vs. placebo ($p < 0.001$)	No significant change in either group	+2.9% in hPTH vs. placebo ($p<0.05$)	−1% in hPTH vs. placebo ($p<0.05$)	Not available
Combination							
Lindsay et al, 1997	PMOP	HRT alone, HRT + hPTH (1-34) 25 μg/d × 3 years	+13% PTH + HRT from baseline vs. HRT no decline ($p < 0.01$)	+17% PTH + HRT vs. HRT alone ($p<0.01$)			Using 15% vertebral height reduction, n=3 PTH + HRT, 10 HRT only, 70% reduction
Black et al, 2003	PMOP	RhPTH (1-84) alone, rhPTH (1-84) + alendronate, alendronate	+6 PTH alone and PTH+A vs. 4% A alone ($p = 0.15$)	+0.2% PTH alone, +2% PTH+A vs. +2.5% A alone ($p<0.02$ PTH alone vs PTH+A)	+1 PTH alone, +2% PTH+A vs. 2.5% A alone ($p=0.5$)	−2.5% PTH, −1% PTH+A vs. −0.5% A alone ($p<0.001$ PTH alone vs. PTH+A ($p<0.01$)	Not done

Study	Population	Regimen				
Finkelstein 2003	Men with osteoporosis	Alendronate for 6 months, then PTH alone, PTH+alendronate, or alendronate alone	+12% PTH alone, +12% PTH+A, +5% A alone, p<0.0 both PTH groups vs. A alone	+8% PTH alone. +6% PTH+A vs. 3%, p<0.01	+6% PTH alone, +6% PTH+A vs. +4% A alone	
Sequential						
Rittmaster et al, 2000	PMOP	rhPTH (1-84) 50-, 75-, 100 µg/d or placebo for 1 year followed by alendronate for 1 year	+15% 1 yr PTH (100 µg/d dose) +1 yr A, +11% 75 µg, +9% PTH 50 µg + A, vs. 6% placebo	+4% all PTH followed by A, vs. 3% A alone	Not done	Not available
Black, 2005		PTH for 1 year followed by alendronate for 1 year, or placebo for 1 year.	+12% A vs. 4% placebo, difference of 8% over 2 years (p < 0.01) between and within groups	+4.5% vs. −0.1%. (p<0.01) within PTH+A from baseline		None available
Cosman, 2005	PMOP	Alendronate for 1-3 years, then 15-month study PTH+A daily, PTH 3 months. Off, 3 cycles, and A alone	+5-6 % increase in both PTH+A daily and PTH in 3 months on and 3 months off cycles, no change in A alone	All 3 treatment groups had about a 2% increase		PTH+A and PTH+A cyclically significantly reduced vertebral fractures compared with alendronate
Kurland, 2004	Men with osteoporosis	HPTH (1-34) for 2 years then alendronate for 1 and 2 years	+24% for 4 years (PTH+A). PTH+ 1 year. A=+5.1%, PTH+ no Rx=+5.5% after PTH			

*Adapted from Buxton and Primer***.

Two early uncontrolled studies in idiopathic male osteoporosis demonstrated an increase in BMD after low-dose intermittent injections of hPTH (1-34).[35,76,77] In the first study, 21 osteoporotic men were treated with hPTH (1-34) for 6 to 24 months, resulting in a mean increase in iliac trabecular bone volume of 70% above baseline values. The second study, which assessed the impact of 12 months of daily hPTH (1-34) and $1,25(OH)_2$-vitamin D therapy in middle-aged men with osteoporosis, found that trabecular BMD assessed by QCT in the spine was significantly increased.[35,77]

The findings of these small initial studies have been confirmed by more recent randomized, double-blind, placebo-controlled clinical trials. One such study assessed the impact of 18 months of daily injections of 400 IU of hPTH (1-34) in young and middle-aged men (mean age: 50 ± 1.9 years) with idiopathic osteoporosis.[35,79] Seventy-eight percent of the patients had a fracture at baseline, and all had a Z-score of less than −2.0 or a T-score of less than −2.5 at the lumbar spine or femoral neck. After 12 to 15 months of initial observation, during which all patients were encouraged to take 1500 mg of calcium and 400 IU of vitamin D daily, patients were randomized into either the placebo or hPTH (1-34) group. The active treatment resulted in a linear increase in lumbar spine BMD as measured by DXA of about 5% compared with controls at 6 months; about 9.5% at 12 months; and about 13.5% at 18 months. There was a smaller but significant increase in BMD at the femoral neck (about 3% at 18 months compared with controls), and no change in total hip density. Cortical bone density at the distal radius declined slightly in the treatment group (about 1%), but this difference from baseline values within this group was not statistically significant. However, the difference between the groups at 18 months was significant (< +0.5% control group vs. −1% decrease in PTH group, respectively). Adverse events associated with hPTH (1-34) were few and mild, with minimal hypercalcemia in two patients that responded to hPTH (1-34) dose reduction, and slightly higher rates of injection-site irritation.[78] Interestingly, in the PTH-treated group of subjects, after the PTH treatment ended they were then started on bisphosphonate therapy and after a 24-month follow-up period increases in lumbar spine BMD increased to more than 20% above the baseline value.[79]

Very recently, a large multicenter, international, randomized, double-blind, placebo-controlled study of the effects of daily rhPTH (1-34) injections in men with a Z-score of less than −2.0 randomized 437 patients (mean age, 59 years) to placebo, rhPTH (1-34) 20 μg daily, or rhPTH (1-34) 40 μg daily.[35,80] Nearly all patients were white, all received supplemental calcium and vitamin D, and all had similar baseline BMD values. The median treatment duration was 11 months.

The study was terminated early following the previously discussed study finding of osteosarcoma in 344 Fischer rats exposed to chronic rhPTH (1-34) injections. rhPTH (1-34) treatment resulted in a dose-dependent increase in BMD at the lumbar spine and femoral neck. Whole-body BMD increased significantly in both treatment groups, and there was no change in BMD in the radius. The improvement in BMD occurred regardless of gonadal status. Dose-dependent increases in markers of bone formation and resorption were also observed. Both dosages of the active drug were well tolerated, with similar incidences of mild side effects in the placebo and 20 μg rhPTH (1-34) groups, and slightly higher rates of nausea in those receiving 40 μg.[35,54,80]

The possibility that combining the anabolic agent hPTH with an antiresorptive bisphosphonate may lead to even greater improvements in BMD was addressed in a 30-month study. Men aged 46 to 85 with idiopathic osteoporosis were all initially treated with alendronate for a period of time then randomized to either randomly assigned to receive alendronate 10 mg daily, hPTH 40 μg daily, or both in combination.[35,82] Results at 30 months were a mean increase of lumbar spine BMD of approximately 7%, 13%, and 14% in the alendronate, hPTH, and combination groups, respectively. Total hip BMD increased by 4%, 5%, and 6% in all three treatment groups, respectively. Total body BMD was significantly greater in the combination group compared with either the hPTH- or alendronate-alone groups, and there was a trend toward improved BMD in the radial shaft and total hip in the combined-treatment group compared with either monotherapy. These data suggest that the combination of hPTH with a bisphosphonate is superior to hPTH alone in improving total body, and to a lesser extent total hip and radial shaft, BMD. However, these data suggest that combining the antiresorptive alendronate and hPTH therapy may lead to a blunting of the maximum anabolic effect of hPTH on the lumbar spine. Larger studies of longer duration with fracture incidence rates will be needed to further elucidate these initial observations.[35,54,81]

hPTH in Glucocorticoid-Induced Osteoporosis

Lane and associates reported that hPTH reversed glucocorticoid-induced osteoporosis in a year-long, randomized, controlled study.[35,83] Postmenopausal women with osteoporosis receiving HRT and at least 5 mg of prednisone daily for the past 12 months were randomized to 1 year of combined therapy with hPTH (1-34) and HRT, or HRT alone. Lumbar spine BMD compared with baseline increased by 35.2 ± 5.5% as measured by QCT, and 11.1 ± 1.4% as measured by DXA in the combination treatment group. No significant change was observed in the HRT-only group. BMD of the hip and forearm did not significantly change in any group. Concentrations of serum osteocalcin and bone-specific alkaline phosphatase increased more rapidly than urinary excretion of deoxypyridinoline cross-links, suggesting an uncoupling between bone formation and resorption that favored bone formation.[35,82]

Questions that Arise about Parathyroid Hormone for the Treatment of Osteoporosis

In the past 5 years, it has been convincingly found that monotherapy with rhPTH (1-34) and rhPTH (1-84) increases bone mass, especially in the lumbar spine, increases bone size by increasing cortical thickness, and improves bone strength as evidenced by significant antifracture efficacy. In addition, rhPTH (1-34) also has been found to reduce nonvertebral fracture risk. There appears to be no added advantage to using PTH in combination with other antiresorptive agents, and sequential therapy with a potent bisphosphonate prior to PTH therapy may lessen or slow the bone mass gain from PTH. However, PTH followed by potent antiresorptive therapy appears to optimize the increase in bone mass from PTH and maintain the bone mass gained from PTH. A number of questions still remain regarding PTH therapy for osteoporosis including the optimal duration of PTH therapy to maximize antifracture efficacy, the number of treatment cycles that an individual patient can safety undergo, and if an optimal bone turnover state is required to maximize the PTH effect. Lastly, additional studies must be done to be define how PTH increases bone mass through a combination of increasing bone formation and bone remodeling. Indeed, there are clearly some aspects of bone remodeling and releasing bone growth factors stored in the bone matrix that potentiate the PTH effect. This is an exciting time in which we can grow bone and improve bone size and bone strength.[83]

REFERENCES

1. Eastell R: Treatment of postmenopausal osteoporosis. N Engl J Med 1998;338:736-46.
2. Ettinger B, Black DM, Mitlak BH, et al, for the Multiple Outcomes of Raloxifene Evaluation (MORE) Investigators: Reduction of vertebral fracture risk in postmenopausal women with osteoporosis treated with raloxifene: results from a 3-year randomized clinical trial. JAMA 1999;282:637-45.
3. Harris ST, Watts NB, Genant HK, et al: Effects of risedronate treatment on vertebral and nonvertebral fractures in women with postmenopausal osteoporosis: a randomized controlled trial. Vertebral Efficacy with Risedronate Therapy (VERT) Study Group. JAMA 1999;282:1344-52.
4. Black DM, Cummings SR, Karpf DB, et al, for the Fracture Intervention Trial Research Group: randomised trial of effect of alendronate on risk of fracture in women with existing vertebral fractures. Lancet 1996;348:1535-41.
5. Cummings SR, Black DM, Thompson DE, et al: Effect of alendronate on risk of fracture in women with low bone density but without vertebral fractures: results from the Fracture Intervention Trial. JAMA 1998;280:2077-82.
6. Chesnut CH III, Silverman S, Andriano K, et al, for the PROOF Study Group: a randomized trial of nasal spray salmon calcitonin in postmenopausal women with established osteoporosis: The Prevent Recurrence of Osteoporotic Fractures Study. Am J Med 2000;109:267-76.
7. Boivin G, Meunier PJ: Changes in bone remodeling rate influence the degree of mineralization of bone. Connect Tissue Res 2002;43:535-37.
8. Riggs BL, O'Fallon WM, Lane A, et al: Clinical trial of fluoride therapy in postmenopausal osteoporotic women: extended observations and additional analysis. J Bone Miner Res 1994;9:265-75.
9. Pak CY, Zerwekh JE, Antich P: Anabolic effects of fluoride on bone. Trends Endocrinol Metab 1995;6:229-34.
10. Pak CY, Sakhaee K, Rubin CD, Zerwekh JE: Sustained-release sodium fluoride in the management of established postmenopausal osteoporosis. Am J Med Sci 1997;313:23-32.
11. Hillam RA, Skerry TM: Inhibition of bone resorption and stimulation of formation by mechanical loading of the modeling rat ulna in vitro. J Bone Miner Res 1995;10:683-89.
12. Mosekilde L, Reeve J: Treatment with PTH peptides. In: Marcus RS, Feldman D, Kelsey J, eds: Osteoporosis, 2nd ed. San Diego, CA: Academic Press, 2001:725-46.
13. Selye H: On the stimulation of new bone formation with parathyroid hormone extract and irradiated ergosterol. J Endocrinol 1932:16:547-58.
14. Usdin TB, Gruber C, Bonner TI: Identification and functional expression of a receptor selectively recognizing parathyroid hormone, PTH2 receptor. J Biol Chem 1995;270:15455-58.
15. Schneider H, Feyen JHM, Seuwen K, Movva NR: Cloning and functional expression of a human parathyroid hormone receptor. Eur J Pharmacol 1993;246:149-55.
16. Khosla S: Minireview: The OPG/RANKL/RANK system. Endocrinology 2001;142:5050-55.
17. Buxton EC, Yao W, Lane NE: Changes in serum RANKL: OPG and IL-6 levels in glucocorticoid-induced osteoporosis patients treated with hPTH (1-34). JCEM 2004;89:3332-36.
18. Dobnig H, Turner RT: Evidence of intermittent treatment with parathyroid hormone increases bone formation in adult rats by activation of bone lining cells. Endocrinology 1995;136:3632-38.
19. Leaffer D, Sweeney M, Kellerman LA, et al: Modulation of osteogenic cell ultrastructure by RS-23581, an analog of human parathyroid hormone (PTH)-related peptide (1-34) and bovine PTH (1-34). Endocrinology 1995;136:3624-31.
20. Hodsman AB, Steer BM: Early histomorphometric changes in response to PTH therapy in osteoporosis: evidence for de novo bone formation on quiescent cancellous surfaces. Bone 1993;14:523-27.
21. Jilka RL, Weinstein RS, Bellido T, et al: Increased bone formation by prevention of osteoblast apoptosis with parathyroid hormone. J Clin Invest 1999;104:439-46.
22. Canalis E, Centrella M, Burch W, McCarty TL: Insulin-like growth factor-1 mediates selective anabolic effects of parathyroid hormone in bone cultures. J Clin Invest 1989;83:60-5.
23. McCarthy TL, Centrella M, Canalis E: Parathyroid hormone enhances the transcription and polypeptide levels of insulin-like growth factor I in osteoblast-enriched cultures from fetal rat bone. Endocrinology 1989;124:1247-53.
24. Watson P, Lazowski D, Han V, et al: Parathyroid hormone restores bone mass and enhances osteoblast insulin-like growth factor I gene expression in ovariectomized rats. Bone 1995;16:357-65.
25. Bikle DD, Sakata T, Leary C, et al: Insulin-like growth factor I is required for the anabolic actions of parathyroid hormone on mouse bone. J Bone Miner Res 2002;17:1570-78.

26. Lane NE, Yao W, Kinney JH, et al: Both hPTH(1-34) and bFGF increase trabecular bone mass in osteopenic rats but they have different effects on trabecular bone architecture. J Bone Miner Res 2003;18:2105-15.

27. Iwaniec UT, Mosekilde L, Mitova-Caneva NG, et al: Sequential treatment with FGF and PTH is more efficacious than treatment with PTH alone for increased bone mass and strength in ostepenic ovariectomized rats. Endocrinology 2002;143:2515-26.

28. Okada Y, Montero A, Zhang X, et al: Impaired osteoclast formation in bone marrow cultures of Fgf2 null mice in response to parathyroid hormone. J Biol Chem 2003;278:21258-66.

29. Hurley MM, Yao W, Lane NE: Changes in serum fibroblast growth factor-2, (FGF or bFGF) in patients with glucocorticoid induced osteoporosis treated with hPTH (1-34). JBMR 2004;19(suppl 1):S458.

30. Oursler MH, Cortese C, Keeting P, et al: Modulation of transforming growth factor-B production in normal human osteoblast-like cells by 17 B estradiol and parathyroid hormone. Endocrinology 1991;129:3313-20.

31. Westendorf JJ, Kahler RA, Schroeder TM: Wnt signaling in osteoblasts and bone diseases. Gene 2004;341:19-39.

32. Little RD, Carulli JP, Del Mastro RG, et al: A mutation in the LDL receptor-related protein 5 gene results in the autosomal dominant high-bone mass trait. Am J Hum Genet 2002;70:11-19.

33. Kulkarni NH, Halladay DH, Miles RR, et al: Wnt signaling pathway: a target for PTH action in bone and bone cells. J Bone Miner Res 2004;95(6):1178-90.

34. Pugsley LI, Selye H: The histological changes in the bone responsible for the action of parathyroid hormone on the calcium metabolism of the rat. J Physiol (Lond) 1933;79:113-17.

35. Buxton EC, Fitzgerald IK, Lane NE: Parathyroid hormone as a treatment for osteoporosis. Today's Therapeutic Trends 2004;21:345-72.

36. MacDonald BR, Gallagher JA, Russell RG, et al: Parathyroid hormone stimulates the proliferation of cells derived from human bone. Endocrinology 1986;118:2445-49.

37. Jerome CP: Anabolic effect of high doses of human parathyroid hormone (1-38) in mature intact female rats. J Bone Miner Res 1994;9:933-42.

38. Toromanoff A, Ammann P, Riond JL: Early effects of short-term parathyroid hormone administration on bone mass, mineral content, and strength in female rats. Bone 1998;22:217-23.

39. Wronski TJ, Walsh CC, Ingaszewski LJ: Histologic evidence for osteopenia and increased bone turnover in ovariectomized rats. Bone 1990;7:119-23.

40. Hori M, Uzawa T, Morita K, et al: Effect of human parathyroid hormone (PTH (1-34)) on experimental osteopenia of rats induced by ovariectomy. J Bone Miner Res 1988;3:193-99.

41. Sato M, Zeng GQ, Turner CH: Biosynthetic human parathyroid hormone (1-34): effects on bone quality in aged ovariectomized rats. Endocrinology 1997;138:4330-37.

42. Ejersted C, Andreassen TT, Oxlund H, et al: Human parathyroid hormones (1-34) and (1-84) increase the mechanical strength and thickness of cortical bone in rats. J Bone Miner Res 1993;8:1097-101.

43. Hock J, Gera I, Fonseca J, Raisz LG: Human PTH (1-34) increases bone mass in ovariectomized and orchidectomized rats. Endocrinology 1988;122:2899-904.

44. Oxlund H, Dalstra M, Ejersted C, Andreassen TT: Parathyroid hormone induces formation of new cancellous bone with substantial mechanical strength at a site where it had disappeared in old rats. Eur J Endocrinol 2002;146:431-38.

45. Jerome CP, Johnson CS, Vafai HT, et al: Effect of treatment for 6 months with human parathyroid hormone (1-34) peptide in ovariectomized cynomolgus monkeys. Bone 1999;25:302-9.

46. Chow JWM, Fox S, Jagger CJ, Chambers TJ: Role for parathyroid hormone in mechanical responsiveness of rat bone. Am J Physiol Endocrinol Metab 1998;37:E146-54.

47. Wronski TJ, Yen C-F, Qi H, Dann LM: Parathyroid hormone is more effective than estrogen or bisphosphonates for restoration of lost bone mass in ovariectomized rats. Endocrinology 1993;132:823-33.

48. Mosekilde L, Danielsen CC, Gasser JSA: The effect on vertebral bone mass and strength of long term treatment with anti-resorptive agents (estrogen and calcitonin), human PTH (1-38), and combination therapy, assessed in aged ovariectomized rats. Endocrinology 1994;135:2126-34.

49. Mosekilde L, Danielsen CC, Sogaard CHS, et al: The anabolic effects of parathyroid hormone on cortical bone mass, dimensions and strength-assessed in a sexually mature ovariectomized rat model. Bone 1995;16:223-30.

50. Shen V, Dempster DW, Birchman R, et al: Loss of cancellous bone mass and connectivity in ovariectomized rats can be restored by combined treatment with PTH and estradiol. J Clin Invest 1999;91:2479-87.

51. Lane NE, Haupt D, Kimmel D, et al: Estrogen increases trabecular bone mass in estrogen deficiency: results from three dimensional XTM longitudinal study in rats. J Bone Miner Res 1999;14:206-14.

52. Ejersted C, Oxlund H, Andreassen TT: Bisphosphonate maintains PTH (1-34) induced cortical bone mass and mechanical strength in old rats. Calcif Tissue Int 1998;62:316-22.

53. Forteo (teriparatide [rDNA origin] injection) [package insert]. Product information. Indianapolis, Ind: Eli Lily, 2002

54. Lane NE: Parathyroid hormone: evolving and therapeutic concepts. Curr Opin Rheumatol 2004;16:457-63.

55. Neer RM, Armand CD, Zanchetta JR, et al: Effect of parathyroid hormone (1-34) on fractures and bone mineral density in postmenopausal women with osteoporosis. N Engl J Med 2001;344:1434-41.

56. Jiang Y, Zhao J, Mitlak B, et al: Recombinant human PTH (1-34) teriparatide improves both cortical and trabecular bone structure. J Bone Miner Res 2003;18:1932-41.

57. Zanchetta JR, Bogado C, Ferrretti JL, et al: Effects of rhPTH (1-34) on cortical bone strength indices as assessed by peripheral quantitative computed tomography. Bone 2002;28:S86.

58. Forteo prescribing information. Indianapolis, IN: Eli Lily, 2005. Available at www.LillyMedical.com.

59. Ettinger MP, Greenspan SL, Barriott TB, et al: PTH (1-84) prevents first vertebral fracture in postmenopausal women with osteoporosis. Results from the TOP study. Arthritis and Rheumatism , American College of Rheumatology, San Antonio Texas, L16, October 21, 2004.

60. Lemay A: The relevance of the WHI results on combined HRT in clinical practice. WHI-J Obstet Gynaecol Can 2002;24:711-15.

61. Lindsay R, Nieves J, Formica C, et al: Randomised controlled study of effect of parathyroid hormone on vertebral-bone mass and fracture incidence among postmenopausal women on oestrogen with osteoporosis. Lancet 1997;350:550-55.

62. Dempster DW, Cosman F, Kurland ES, et al: Effects of daily treatment with parathyroid hormone on bone microarchitecture and turnover in patients with osteoporosis: a paired biopsy study. J Bone Miner Res 2001;16:1846-53.

63. Cosman F, Nieves J, Woelfert L, et al: Parathyroid hormone added to established hormone therapy: effects on vertebral fracture and maintenance of bone mass after parathyroid hormone withdrawal. J Bone Miner Res 2001;16:925-31.

64. Roe EB, Sanchez SD, del Puerto GA, et al: Parathyroid hormone 1-34 (hPTH 1-34) and estrogen produce dramatic bone density increases in postmenopausal osteoporosis: results from a placebo-controlled randomized trial. J Bone Miner Res 1999;14(Suppl 1):S137.

65. Deal C, Omizo M, Schwatz EN, et al: Raloxifene in combination with teriparatide reduced teriparatide induced stimulation of bone resorption but not formation in postmenopausal women with osteoporosis. J Bone Mineral Res 2004;19(Suppl 1):S44, 1169.

66. Black DM, Greenspan LS, Ensrud EK, et al: The effects of PTH and alendronate alone or in combination in post-menopausal osteoporosis. N Engl J Med 2003;349:1207-15.

67. Sellmeyer DE, Palermo L, Bouxsein ML, et al: Heterogeneity in skeletal response to full-length parathyroid hormone (PTH). J Bone Miner Res 2004;9(Suppl 1):S96.

68. Rittmaster RS, Bolognese M, Ettinger MP, et al: Enhancement of bone mass in osteoporotic women with parathyroid hormone followed by alendronate. J Clin Endocrinol Metab 2000;85:2129-34.

69. Lindsay R, Hodsman AB, Genant HK, et al: A randomized controlled multi-center study of 1-84 hPTH for treatment of postmenopausal osteoporosis. Bone 1998;23(suppl 1):S175.

70. Lindsay R, Scheele WH, Neer R, et al: Sustained vertebral fracture risk reduction after withdrawal of teriparatide in postmenopausal women with osteoporosis. Arch Intern Med 2004;164:2024-30.

71. Black DM, Rosen CJ, Palermo L, et al: The effect of one year of alendronate following 1 year of PTH (1-84): second year results from PTH and Alendronate (PaTH) Trial. J Bone Miner Res. 1998;19(suppl 10):S26.

72. Cosman F, Nieves JW, Luckey MM, et al: Daily versus cyclic PTH combined with alendronate versus alendronate alone for treatment of osteoporosis. J Bone Miner Res 2003;X:S32,

73. Ettingern B, San Martin JA, Crans G, Pavo I: Differential effects of teriparatide on BMD after treatment with raloxifene or alendronate. J Bone Miner Res 2004;19:745-51.

74. Gullberg B, Ohnell O, Kanis JA: World-wide projections for hip fracture. Osteoporos Int 1997;7:407-13.

75. O'Neill TW, Felsenberg D, Varlow J, et al: The prevalence of vertebral deformity in European men and women: the European Vertebral Osteoporosis Study. J Bone Miner Res 1996;11:1010-18.

76. Orwoll E, Ettinger M, Weiss S, et al: Alendronate for the treatment of osteoporosis in men. N Engl J Med 2000;343:604-10.

77. Slovik DM, Rosenthal DI, Doppelt SH, et al: Restoration of spinal bone in osteoporotic men by treatment with human parathyroid hormone (1-34) and 1,25-dihydroxyvitamin D. J Bone Miner Res 1986;1:377-81.

78. Kurland ES, Cosman F, McMahon DJ, et al: Parathyroid hormone as a therapy for idiopathic osteoporosis in men: effects on bone mineral density and bone markers. J Clin Endocrinol Metab 2000;85:3069-76.

79. Kurland ES, Heller SL, Diamond B, et al: The importance of bisphosphonate therapy in maintaining bone mass in men after therapy with teriparatide [human parathyroid hormone (1-34). Osteoporos Int 2004;15:992-97.

80. Orwoll ES, Scheele WH, Paul S, et al: The effect of teriparatide [human parathyroid hormone (1-34)] therapy on bone density in men with osteoporosis. J Bone Miner Res 2003;18:9-17.

81. Finkelstein JS, Hayes A, Hunzelman JL, et al: The effects of parathyroid hormone, alendronate or both in men with osteoporosis. N Engl J Med 2003;349:1216-26.

82. Lane NE, Sanchez S, Modin GW, et al: Parathyroid hormone treatment can reverse corticosteroid-induced osteoporosis: results of a randomized controlled clinical trial. J Clin Invest 1998;102:1627-33.

83. Rosen CJ: What's new with PTH in osteoporosis: where are we and where are we headed? Trends Endocrinol Metab 2004;15:229-35.

84. Whitfield JF, Morley P, Willick GE: The parathyroid hormone: an unexpected bone builder for treating osteoporosis. Austin, TX: Landes Bioscience, 1998.

85. Lane NE, Kelman A: A review of anabolic therapies for osteoporosis. Arthritis Res Ther 2003;5:214-21.

20 Combination Therapy for Osteoporosis: What Do the Data Show Us?

Paul D. Miller

SUMMARY

Combination therapies, in which two osteoporosis-specific agents are used at the same time, are based on the observation that small increments in endpoints such as bone density, additional to that seen with either agent alone, are often observed with the combination. However, the rationale for combining agents with similar actions on bone remodelling (e.g., inhibition of resorption), are unclear and the effects of such combinations on fracture endpoints are generally unproven. For this reason combination therapies are generally not advised. However sequential therapies, where one agent follows another, especially after anabolic therapy, have a stronger rationale.

Combination therapy for postmenopausal or glucocorticoid-induced osteoporosis incorporates the concepts of two distinctly different pharmacotherapeutic principles: (1) concomitant therapy, in which two osteoporosis-specific agents are used at the same time, and (2) sequential therapy, in which one osteoporosis pharmacological agent follows after the use and discontinuation of a different osteoporosis-specific pharmacological agent.

Although the concept of sequential therapy was most recently enhanced by the availability of the anabolic agent 1-34 parathyroid hormone (PTH) (teriparatide), in which antiresorptive therapy is generally advised after discontinuation of PTH,[1,2] it is also important to consider the data on sequential therapy situations involving switching from one antiresorptive agent to another antiresorptive agent. A frequent example is the situation in which hormone replacement therapy (HRT) is discontinued because of the US Food and Drug Administration recommendations not to use HRT to benefit skeletal health, after the publication of the Women's Health Initiative (WHI) findings.[3] Hence, there is the potential of switching from HRT to a different antiresorptive agent. This potential sequence is important to examine, because anti-resorptive agents differ in their effects on bone mineral density (BMD), biochemical markers of bone turnover (BTM), or the types of fracture risk reduction (vertebral versus nonvertebral).[4-8]

CONCOMITANT THERAPY

This chapter assumes that all patients on osteoporosis-specific pharmacological therapies will also be provided with adequate calcium and vitamin D. The adequacy of vitamin D replacement has recently changed, with the increasing published data showing the higher than expected prevalence of vitamin D insufficiency in the world's population.[9-12] Although most osteoporosis-specific pharmacological clinical trials added calcium and vitamin D to their "placebo" as well as their treatment groups, the supplementation of these important skeletal-strengthening elements is inconsistent in dosages between different clinical trials. This latter point will not be discussed as a potential factor influencing outcomes of combination or sequential therapies in this chapter. The reader is directed to separate issues on the doses of calcium and vitamin D administered among the different clinical trials to study the potential impact that variable doses of vitamin D and/or calcium supplementation may have on any of the differences in outcomes among the clinical trial results.[13,14]

Finally, it is of utmost importance that readers realize that in the following datasets of combination or sequential therapy, no fracture data are given. All results of combination or sequential therapy are based on changes in BMD or BTM, or both. These two surrogate markers may provide indirect evidence of pharmacologically induced improvements in bone strength, although there is a great deal of debate and uncertainty surrounding the exact relationship between changes in BMD or BTM that are induced by pharmacological intervention and changes in bone strength.[5,15-24] Certainly, the relationship between pharmacologically induced changes in BMD and risk reduction is not linear, but some contribution to improvements in bone strength as bone mineral is added

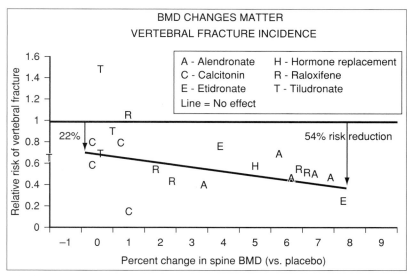

Figure 20-1. The relationship between changes in axial bone mineral density mediated by antiresorptive agents and incident vertebral fracture risk reduction.

is universally accepted (Figure 20-1).[18] The recent US Surgeon General's report on the status of America's bone health has stated that "although the most important study outcome is fracture risk reduction, changes in BMD or markers of bone turnover can be used (in the context of clinical studies) as supportive evidence of the effectiveness of treatment."[15] Although it is generally agreed that increasing BMD and/or reducing bone turnover explain some of the changes in fracture risk,[25,26] the relationship is neither linear nor proportional. Hence, it must rest on the opinion of the individual reader to interpret whether the pharmacologically induced changes in BMD or BTM in the following studies of combination or sequential therapy are reflective of changes in bone strength.

ANTIRESORPTIVE TO ANTIRESORPTIVE THERAPY

Why would one even consider such a combination for skeletal health benefits alone? If a physician is using HRT or a selective estrogen receptor modulator (SERM) for an indication other than bone strength (e.g., menopausal symptoms or reduction of breast cancer risk) and decides that there is a need for additional skeletal benefit, then adding an agent for bone benefit may be reasonable. The basis of such a decision could be (1) no change or even loss of BMD with monotherapy, (2) continual fracture development with monotherapy, or (3) a persistently very low T-score in a high-risk patient. Defining "non-response" to justify such a consideration is difficult, because a stable BMD on monotherapy may be an acceptable endpoint,[27] and

no treatment can abolish fracture risk. Nevertheless, it is often intuitive in patient management that if a fracture occurs while the patient is on monotherapy with no secondary cause discovered, a combination therapeutic approach might provide additional benefit.

Early observations of the effects of adding a bisphosphonate to HRT were made in patients previously receiving HRT and suggested that the addition of alendronate provided a greater gain in BMD than continuation of HRT alone.[28] Subsequent clinical trials examined the effect of HRT alone versus HRT plus a bisphosphonate on surrogate endpoints in treatment-naive patients. In these clinical trials, both alendronate and risedronate combined with HRT induced greater increases in BMD and reduction of BTM than either agent alone (Figures 20-2 and 20-3).[29-31] Likewise, in previously treatment-naive patients, the combination of raloxifene and alendronate increased BMD and reduced BTM to a greater extent than either agent alone (Figure 20-4).[32] As previously stated, without fracture data it is impossible to know whether these greater improvements in BMD and reduction in BTM with combination therapy translate into any greater differences in bone strength. Of equal theoretical concern is whether combining two antiresorptive agents simultaneously could lead to a reduction in bone strength. This hypothesis is based on the observations that a certain amount of bone turnover is necessary to repair the daily microdamage in bone that occurs with normal activity[33,34] and on the observations in nonhuman subjects that high doses of bisphosphonates[35,36] may mitigate this repair process. Additional experimental data suggest that excessive suppression of bone turnover may result in

193

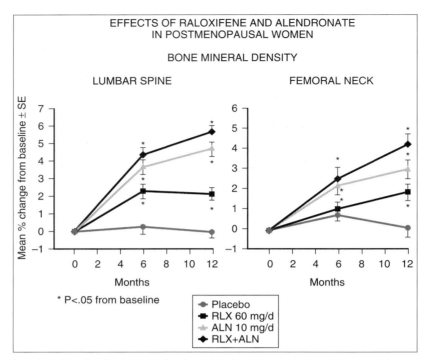

Figure 20-2. The effect of combination therapy with alendronate and estrogen versus monotherapy and subsequent effect of discontinuation.

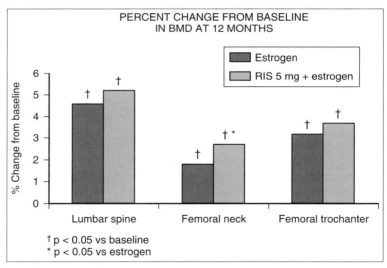

Figure 20-3. The effect of combination therapy with risedronate and hormonal therapy as opposed to risedronate or hormonal therapy alone on axial bone mineral density in postmenopausal women.

"hypermineralization" of bone, which may lead to bone brittleness.[37-42] Yet, none of these hypothetical concerns has any good scientific evidence supporting any safety issue in human beings.[43-45] The recent anecdotal case reports of increased bone fragility and histomorphometric evidence of very low bone turnover reported in nine patients taking alendronate (three of whom were also receiving HRT and two of whom were also taking glucocorticoids) is a small observational study with no control group.[46] More recent careful histomorphometric data in patients in the FLEX trial (Fosamax Long-Term Extension) show double tetracycline labels in all biopsy samples; that is, no "frozen-bone."[47] Nevertheless, we must have a level of watchfulness and seek better long-term scientific data to see if there is any potential for bisphosphonates to induce bone fragility.[48,49]

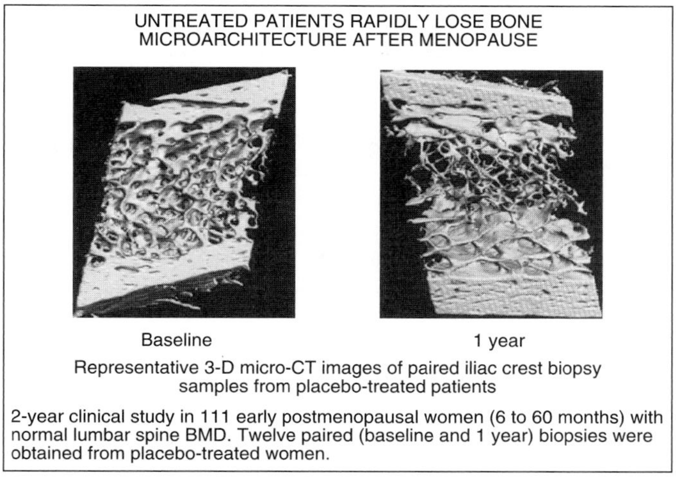

UNTREATED PATIENTS RAPIDLY LOSE BONE
MICROARCHITECTURE AFTER MENOPAUSE

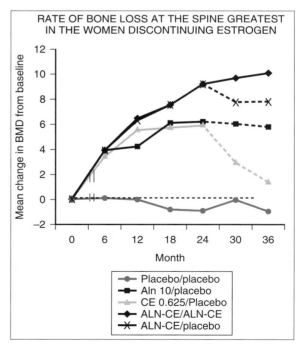

Baseline | 1 year

Representative 3-D micro-CT images of paired iliac crest biopsy
samples from placebo-treated patients

2-year clinical study in 111 early postmenopausal women (6 to 60 months) with
normal lumbar spine BMD. Twelve paired (baseline and 1 year) biopsies were
obtained from placebo-treated women.

Figure 20-4. Early micoarchitectural deterioration after discontinuing hormonal therapy in postmenopausal women: paired three-dimensional quantitative computed tomography bone biopsy study.

The ultimate decision about adding a second agent to an existing osteoporotic-specific pharmacological agent is a purely clinical one. It is often based on a situation in which one agent (such as HRT or raloxifene) is being used for nonskeletal benefits and the patient is discovered to have a low hip BMD, where the bisphosphonates or teriparatide [recombinant human PTH (1-34)] have the best evidence of nonvertebral and hip fracture reduction benefits.[50-54] When the physician adds a second agent for its skeletal benefit, it is usually done to achieve a greater increase in BMD or reduction in BTM than had been achieved with the single agent alone, and the physician should do it with the knowledge that there is no evidence of a greater benefit in fracture risk reduction. Nevertheless, in the real world of clinical practice, individual patient management, including patient compliance and trust issues, might be facilitated by feedback to the patient that a "better" effect has been achieved with combination therapy.

What about the issue of the many women worldwide who discontinue HRT as a result of the WHI findings and now have concerns about their skeletal health? This is a very common scenario since the July 9, 2002 publication of the WHI findings.[3] One approach to this issue, assuming that the patient has a skeletal risk, either defined by low BMD (T-score −2.0 or lower or −1.5 or lower with other significant skeletal risk factors) or prior fracture is to begin administering raloxifene if the patient is at increased risk for vertebral fracture and a bisphosphonate if the patient has an increased risk for nonvertebral or hip fracture. There is evidence that women who discontinue HRT may have a greater risk for either fracture or microarchitectural deterioration of bone early after discontinuation (Figure 20-5).[55-58] Therefore, substituting, in sequence, an alternate osteoporosis-specific pharmacological agent makes clinical sense.

ANABOLICS AND ANTIRESORPTIVES

Because of the fundamental coupling of bone remodeling in normal human bone biology, it has been conceived that if one could "uncouple" bone resorption of bone formation (or vice versa), one could achieve even greater increases in BMD, and, by inference, bone strength, than if coupling continues as it does in either normal bone biology or whenever we try to modulate

RATE OF BONE LOSS AT THE SPINE GREATEST
IN THE WOMEN DISCONTINUING ESTROGEN

- Placebo/placebo
- Aln 10/placebo
- CE 0.625/Placebo
- ALN-CE/ALN-CE
- ALN-CE/placebo

Figure 20-5. The effect of combination therapy with raloxifene and alendronate versus monotherapy with raloxifene or alendronate alone on axial bone mineral density in postmenopausal women.

a bone cell line. For example, whenever osteoclast activity is increased, ultimately osteoblastic activity will also increase. Likewise, whenever we inhibit osteoclastic activity (as we do with antiresorptive agents), we ultimately reduce osteoblastic activity. Hence, with antiresorptive agent administration, we see a reduction in BTM of bone resorption first, then a later, delayed reduction in BTM of bone formation, until a new steady-state of lower bone turnover is achieved. If one could "uncouple" this normal process, the goal of increasing bone formation without a concomitant increase in bone resorption might be achievable. Even when one stimulates bone formation (e.g., with intermittent parathyroid hormone) and one initially sees an increase in BTM of bone formation, there will be a delayed, albeit predictable, increase in the BTM of bone resorption. Hence, intuitively, it would be possible to "uncouple" this bone biological process if one could give an anabolic agent in some combination or sequence with an inhibitor of bone resorption.

A few earlier studies examined the effect of administering the anabolic agent PTH to women previously receiving HRT for either postmenopausal osteoporosis or glucocorticoid-induced osteoporosis.[59,60] In these studies, PTH was added to HRT. The slope of the gain in BMD seen with combination therapy was greater than in the group who continued only monotherapy with HRT, and this BMD rise was similar to the rise in BMD induced by PTH alone in PTH-only clinical trials, suggesting that there may be no mitigation of the PTH effect by prior exposure to HRT. However, there was no PTH-only arm in these early combination studies, so it cannot be known for certain if there may have been some mitigation of the PTH response. The only valid conclusion that can be made is that the addition of PTH to patients previously receiving HRT for postmenopausal osteoporosis or glucocorticoid-induced osteoporosis induces an additional gain in BMD as compared with the maintenance of BMD in the groups that only continued HRT alone.

In an observational-type clinical study design, Ettinger and associates examined the effect of sequential therapy with PTH in a small group of self-selected postmenopausal women who had been taking either alendronate or raloxifene for 18 to 36 months.[61] Those patients who agreed to be taken off their antiresorptive agent and given PTH were then followed for 2 additional years. The patients who had previously been taking raloxifene increased their BMD and bone formation markers to a greater extent than those patients who had previously been taking alendronate. The implication is that prior raloxifene exposure has a less "blunting of PTH effect" than prior alendronate exposure. During the second year of this study, however, the slope of the rise in axial BMD induced by PTH in

previously treated raloxifene as well as alendronate patients was the same. Thus, any potential mitigation of the PTH response with alendronate seemed to wane over time. However, just as in the previously mentioned HRT/PTH studies, there was no PTH-only arm in the Ettinger study either, so it can only be speculated that there may have been potential mitigation of PTH effect by prior exposure to antiresorptive agents.

Two recently published companion papers in *The New England Journal of Medicine* examined the effect of PTH monotherapy compared with alendronate monotherapy versus combination therapy using PTH plus alendronate.[62,63] The PaTH (parathyroid hormone alendronate treatment) clinical trial examined these combinations in treatment-naive postmenopausal women. The bone formation marker (or to be more correct, the marker of osteoblast activity) PINP increased significantly more with PTH alone and was mitigated in its response with combination therapy (Figure 20-6). In the same manner, axial BMD as measured by dual x-ray absorptiometry (DXA) increased equally with combination therapy as with monotherapy, whereas axial BMD measured by quantitative computed tomography (QCT) increased more with PTH monotherapy than with combination therapy or with alendronate monotherapy (Figure 20-7). The real clinical meaning of the QCT changes are unknown, because there are no fracture risk reduction data as a function of QCT changes. On the other hand, in the PaTH trial, the total hip BMD by DXA increased significantly more with combination therapy than with monotherapy with PTH or alendronate (Figure 20-8). In the male study,[63] patients previously treated for 6 months with alendronate had PTH added and this combination group of previously short-term alendronate therapy group was compared with two monotherapy groups of PTH or alendronate alone. As in the PaTH study, the axial BMD measured by DXA and QCT increased significantly more in the PTH monotherapy group than in the combination group and the total serum alkaline phosphatase (an index of osteoblast activity) also increased significantly more in the combination group. However, just as in the PaTH trial, there were also some results that seemed to favor combination therapy: the total body BMD by DXA increased significantly more in the combination group than in either monotherapy group. The general opinion from the results of these two clinical trials is that combination therapy has no advantages over PTH monotherapy and it is possible that alendronate exposure (short-term or concurrent) may mitigate the anabolic effect of PTH (vis-a-vis the formation marker data). Neither study provided any fracture data or quantitative bone histomorphometry data.

What is the basis of the hypothesis that combination therapy with PTH-bisphosphonates may not be desir-

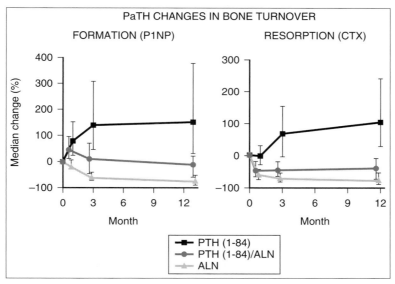

Figure 20-6. Changes in the bone formation marker (PINP) and the bone resorption marker (CTX) in postmenopausal women treated with parathyroid hormone or alendronate alone versus combination therapy with parathyroid hormone and alendronate.

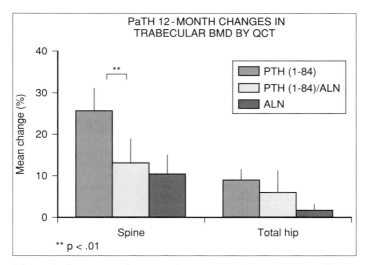

Figure 20-7. Changes in axial quantitative computed tomography parameters in postmenopausal women treated with parathyroid hormone or alendronate alone versus combination therapy with parathyroid hormone and alendronate.

able?[64] The prevailing opinion is that antiresorptive agents, especially bisphosphonates, reduce the remodeling space and in turn the measurable osteoblast pool, making fewer osteoblasts available for PTH to activate. Thus, in the presence of bisphosphonates, the anabolic effect of PTH will be mitigated to the extent that the available osteoblast pool is reduced. However, PTH also activates resting preosteoblasts just outside the bone remodeling unit as well as bone marrow–derived and circulating preosteoblasts, cells that are not known to be affected by prior bisphosphonate exposure.[66,67] Hence, it is a theoretical possibility that PTH could activate these preosteoblasts that are unaffected by

prior bisphosphonate exposure to become plump bone-forming osteoblasts and be followed by a potentiation of the PTH response, because osteoclast activity would be inhibited by the bisphosphonate presence. This hypothesis needs scientific validation but is plausible from a bone biological point of view. There could be differences in the PTH response as a function of the prior duration of bisphosphonate exposure or the type of bisphosphonate used. Potentiation of the PTH response in the presence of an antiresorptive agent has, in fact, been shown. In a very recent study examining the effect of PTH alone or PTH combined with raloxifene in treatment-naive postmenopausal women,

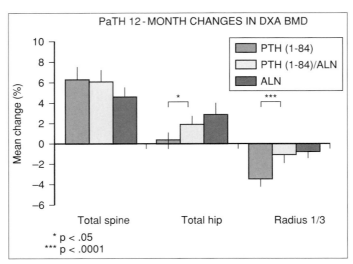

Figure 20-8. The effect on axial BMD of parathyroid hormone or alendronate versus combination therapy with parathyroid hormone and alendronate on axial and total hip BMD in postmenopausal women.

there was a significantly greater increase in total hip BMD by DXA in the combination group as compared with monotherapy with PTH alone.[67] In addition, in rats given the anti-osteoclastic agent osteoprotogerin (OPG) alone or PTH alone or combination OPG-PTH, a much larger increase in axial BMD was found with combination therapy than with either mono-therapy.[68] Hence, it may be premature to conclude that antiresorptive therapy and PTH combined are an unfavorable combination, and there certainly is a need for far more data surrounding these interactions before we have more definitive answers. Although the prevailing opinion currently is that combination therapy with an antiresorptive agent and PTH may not have any advantages for improving skeletal strength as opposed to monotherapy, this conclusion is based on very limited clinical trial data. Nevertheless, until we have better data examining these PTH-combination issues, the standard of care would suggest not using combination PTH-antiresorptive therapies.

There are two scenarios that do have far more consensus than the concomitant use issue just discussed: one is that in high-risk patients it may be favorable to use PTH first, followed by an antiresorptive; the other is that, after discontinuing PTH, it is important to add an antiresorptive agent to maintain the improvements in BMD (especially axial) that have been attained with PTH use.[1,2] The first scenario is based on the concept that if prior exposure to bone of an antiresorptive agent might mitigate a PTH effect, it might be more favorable to stimulate new bone formation with PTH without any potential encumbrance by an antiresorptive agent and then follow with an antiresorptive agent. In addition, with the "black-box" warning that

limits the use of PTH to 18 to 24 months, clinicians have a limited window of opportunity to use PTH and would want to maximize the effect within this window of use. The second scenario has better data to support it: in all follow-up studies examining BMD after PTH discontinuation, axial BMD declines unless an anti-resorptive agent is utilized,[69,70] and in the post-PTH studies, the BMD actually increased with the addition of a bisphosphonate following PTH.[71,72] Thus, at the current time, there is general agreement that an antiresorptive agent should be started after discontinuation of PTH.[1,2]

STRONTIUM RANELATE: A COMBINATION ALL IN ONE?

Strontium ranelate (Protelos) was recently registered in Europe for the treatment of postmenopausal osteoporosis and indicated to reduce incident vertebral, nonvertebral, and hip fractures.[73,74] The mechanism or mechanisms of action whereby strontium ranelate improves bone strength are putative at the current time but may be due to a dual effect, one that is both anabolic and anti-catabolic. In mouse and rat models, strontium ranelate stimulates preosteoblast replication as well as collagen synthesis and decreases osteoclastic activity and bone resorption.[75,76] In the pivotal phase III clinical trial of 2 g/day of strontium ranelate, postmenopausal women with either prevalent vertebral or nonvertebral fractures experienced a significant reduction in incident vertebral, nonvertebral, and hip fractures, the latter analysis being post hoc (Figures 20-9 and 20-10). There was an impressive increase in axial BMD (mean, +14%) as well as femoral neck BMD

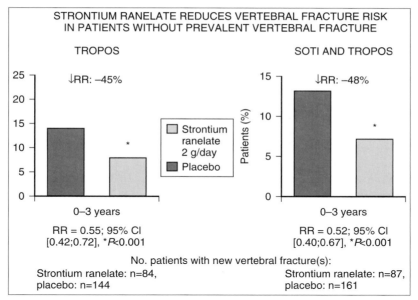

Figure 20-9. The effect of strontium ranelate on incident vertebral fractures in postmenopausal women.

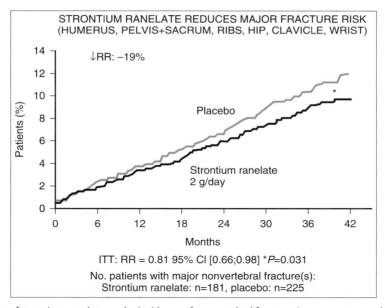

Figure 20-10. The effect of strontium ranelate on the incidence of nonvertebral fractures in postmenopausal women.

(mean, +8%) in the studied population, although approximately 50% of the BMD changes are due to the effect of the heavy metal, strontium, to block the photons.[77] There was a simultaneous increase in bone formation markers (BSAP) and decrease in resorption markers (CTX) with this dose of strontium ranelate. Hence, this very interesting compound may be a "combination" all in one and one that seems to uncouple bone coupling in the correct direction, anabolic as well as anti-catabolic.

CONCLUSIONS

Combination therapy for a single clinical benefit—improving skeletal strength—may have appeal from the greater BMD gains consistently seen with the combination of two antiresorptive agents, and, in a few measured studies, with combinations of PTH and antiresorptive agents; however, there are no fracture data to show whether bone strength is better with combination therapy than with monotherapy. In addition, there are some hypothetical concerns that the simultaneous administration of two antiresorptive agents could lead to excessive suppression of bone turnover and could impair microdamage repair to the point of leading to more skeletal fragility. Although this latter possibility remains unproven by good scientific data in human beings given approved doses of antiresorptives for the treatment of osteoporosis, there seems to be no sound reason to take any potential risk without proved benefit (better fracture risk reduction).

It seems far more reasonable to use sequential therapies, going from one antiresorptive to another. Obviously, the most common scenario for this is starting a SERM, bisphosphonates, or calcitonin in women who are discontinuing HRT but are still at increased fracture risk. In addition, going from a SERM to a bisphosphonate or calcitonin is also not an uncommon sequence when women have SERM-induced side-effects or have a newly discovered risk for nonvertebral fractures, in which situation the bisphosphonates or teriparatide have the only evidence for reducing the risk of nonvertebral fracture.

With the introduction of the anabolic agent teriparatide [rhPTH (1-34)] came the general agreement that an antiresorptive agent should be provided after 18 to 24 months of teriparatide to prevent the loss in axial BMD that is seen after teriparatide discontinuation. Based on very preliminary data, most physicians would also discontinue the antiresorptive agent when initiating teriparatide. As previously discussed, much of this opinion is based on the blunting of the bone formation markers in patients pretreated with alendronate for a short time or simultaneous administration of alendronate and PTH, remembering that for some skeletal sites, combination therapy was significantly better than monotherapy. The area of combination therapy with PTH and an antiresorptive agent is one where we need far more data before we have a level of evidence that is strong enough to declare whether there is a blunting or potentiating of the PTH effect, whether there may be differences between the types of bisphosphonates used with PTH, the prior duration of exposure, and the potential for intermittent sequential therapy (PTH-antiresorptive-PTH).

Combination therapies for osteoporosis are generally not advised.[78-80] Until we have evidence for a greater degree of fracture risk reduction with combination therapy as opposed to monotherapy, the potential risks and increased costs of using two drugs as opposed to one drug make combination therapy not advisable as a general recommendation. Certainly, however, there may be special individual circumstances based on individual clinical judgment in which combination therapy might be utilized.

REFERENCES

1. Miller PD, Bilezikian JP, Deal C, et al: Clinical use of teriparatide in the real world: initial insights. Endo Prac 2004;10:139-48.
2. Hodsman AB, Bauer DC, Dempster D, et al: Parathyroid hormone and teriparatide for the treatment of osteoporosis: a review of the evidence and suggested guidelines for it use. Endocr Rev 2005;10:2004-6.
3. Writing Group for The Women's Health Initiative Investigators: Risks and benefits of estrogen plus progestin in healthy postmenopausal women: principal results from the women's health initiative randomized control trial. JAMA 2002;288:321-23.
4. Miller PD: Optimizing the management of postmenopausal osteoporosis with bisphosphonates: the emerging role of intermittent therapy. Clin Ther 2005;27:1-16.
5. Miller PD, Hockberg MC, Wehren LE, et al: How useful are measures of BMD and bone turnover? Curr Med Res Opin 2005;21:545-54.
6. Miller PD: The treatment of osteoporosis: antiresorptive therapy. Clin Lab Med 2000;20:603-22.
7. Miller PD: Osteoporosis treatment outcomes: the factors that lead to the ultimate end point of osteoporosis therapies—fracture risk reduction. Endocrinologist 2003;13:S4-S9.
8. Guyatt GH, Cranney A, Griffith L, et al: Summary of meta-analyses of therapies for postmenopausal osteoporosis and the relationship between bone density and fractures. Endocrinol Metab Clin North Am 2002;31:659.
9. Leboff MS, Karkkainen MU, Lamberg-Allardt CJ: Occult vitamin D deficiency in postmenopausal US women with acute hip fracture. JAMA 1999;281:1505-11.
10. Heaney RP, Davies KM, Chen TC, et al: Human serum 25-hydroxycholecalciferol response to extended oral dosing with cholecalciferol. Am J Clin Nutr 2003;74:206-10.
11. Reid IR: Vitamin D and its metabolites in the management of osteoporosis. Osteoporosis 2001;2:553-75.
12. Lips P: Vitamin D deficiency and secondary hyperparathyroidism in the elderly: consequences for bone loss and fractures and therapeutic implications. Endocr Rev 2001;22:477-501.
13. Dawson-Hughes B, Dallai GE, Krall EA, et al: A controlled trial of the effects of calcium supplementation on bone density in postmenopausal women. N Engl J Med 1990;323:878-83.
14. US Department of Health and Human Services: Bone health and osteoporosis: a report of the Surgeon General. Rockville MD: US Department of Health and Human Services, Office of the Surgeon General, 2004. Available at http://www.hhs.gov/surgeongeneral/ library/bonehealth/content.html. Accessed May 3, 2005.
15. Kleerekoper M: Use of biomarkers in the management of women with low bone density. Menopausal Med 2002;10:4-7.
16. Miller PD, Baran DT, Bilezikian JP, et al: Practical clinical application of biochemical markers of bone turnover. J Clin Densitom 1999;2:323-42.
17. Watts NB, Miller PD: Changing perceptions in osteoporosis: markers should be used as adjunct to bone densitometry. BMJ 1999;319:1371-72.
18. Wasnich RD, Miller PD: Antifracture efficacy of antiresportive agents are related to changes in bone density. J Clin Endocr Metab 2000;85:1-6.
19. Delmas PD, Eastell R, Garnero P, et al, for the Committee of Scientific Advisors of the International Osteoporosis Foundation: a position paper on the use of biochemical markers of bone turnover in osteoporosis. Osteoporosis Int 2000;11:S2-S17.
20. Hochberg M, Greenspan S, Wasnich R, et al: Changes in bone density and turnover explain the reductions in incidence of nonvertebral fractures that occur during treatment with antiresorptive agents. J Clin Endocrinol Metab 2002;87:1586-92.

21. Watts NB, Cooper C, Lindsay R, et al: Relationship between changes in bone mineral density and vertebral fracture risk associated with risedronate. J Clin Densit 2004;7:255-61.

22. Eastell R, Barton I, Hannon RA, et al: Relationship of early changes in bone resorption to the reduction in fracture risk with risedronate. J Bone Miner Res 2003;18:1051-56.

23. Bauer DC, Black DM, Ganero P, et al: Change in bone turnover and hip, non-spine and vertebral fractures in alendronate treated women: Fracture Intervention Trial. J Bone Miner Res 2004;19:1250-8.

24. Delmas PD, Seeman E: Changes in bone mineral density explain little of the reduction in vertebral or non-vertebral fracture risk with anti-resorptive therapy. Bone 2004;34:599-604.

25. Leib ES, Lewiecki EM, Binkley N, Hamdy RC: Official positions of the International Society for Clinical Densitometry. J Clin Densit 2004;7:1-6.

26. Cummings SR, Karpf DB, Harris F, et al: Improvements in spine bone density and reduction in risk of vertebral fractures during treatment with antiresorptive drugs. Am J Med 2002;112:281-89.

27. Chapurlat RD, Palermo L, Ramsay P, Cummings SR: Risk of fracture among women who lose bone density during treatment with alendronate. The Fracture Intervention Trial. Osteoporos Int 2005;16:842-48.

28. Lindsay R, Cosman F, Lobo RA, et al: Addition of alendronate to ongoing hormonal therapy in the treatment of postmenopausal osteoporosis: a randomized controlled clinical trial. J Clin Endocrinol Metab 1999;84:3076-81.

29. Bone HG, Greenspan SL, McKeever C, et al: Alendronate and estrogen effects in postmenopausal women with low bone mineral density. J Clin Endocrinol Metab 2000;85:720-26.

30. Greenspan SL, Emkey RD, Bone H III, et al: Significant differential effects of alendronate, estrogen or combination therapy on the rate of bone loss after discontinuation of treatment of postmenopausal osteoporosis. Ann Intern Med 2002;137:875-83.

31. Harris ST, Eriksen EF, Davidson M, et al: Effect of combined risedronate and hormone replacement therapies on bone mineral density in postmenopausal women. J Clin Endocrinol Metab 2001;86:1890-7.

32. Johnell O, Scheele WH, Regisnter JY, et al: Additive effects of raloxifene and alendronate on bone mineral density and biochemical markers of bone remodeling in postmenopausal women with osteoporosis. J Clin Endocrinol Metab 2002;87:985-92.

33. Heaney R: Remodeling and skeletal fragility. Osteoporos Int 2003;14(suppl 5):S12-S15.

34. Burr DB, Turner CH: Biomechanics of bone. In: Favus M, ed: Primer on the Metabolic Bone Diseases and Disorders of Mineral Metabolism. Washington, D.C.: American Society for Bone and Mineral Research, 2003:58-64.

35. Mashiba T, Hirano T, Turner CH, et al: Suppressed bone turnover by bisphosphonates increases microdamage accumulation and reduces some biomechanical properties in dog rib. J Bone Miner Res 2000;15:613-20.

36. Mashiba T, Turner CH, Hirano T, et al: Effects of suppressed bone turnover by bisphosphonates on microdamage accumulation and biomechanical properties in clinically relevant skeletal sites in beagles. Bone 2001;28:524-31.

37. Weinstein RS: True strength [editorial]. J Bone Miner Res 2000;15:613-20.

38. Renshow CE, Schulson EM: Universal behavior in compressive failure of brittle materials. Nature 2001;412:897-900.

39. Bouxsein ML: Bone quality: where do we go from here? Osteoporos Int 2003;14(suppl 5):S118-S27.

40. Boivin G, Meunier PJ: The mineralization of bone tissue: a forgotten dimension in osteoporosis research. Osteoporos Int 2003;14:S19-S24.

41. Roschger P, Rinnerthaler S, Yates J, et al: Alendronate increases degree and uniformity of mineralization in cancellous bone and decreases the porosity in cortical bone of osteoporotic women. Bone 2001;29:185-91.

42. Roschger P, Gupta HS, Berzlanovich A, et al: Constant mineralization density distribution in cancellous human bone. Bone 2003;32:316-23.

43. Chavassieux PM, Arlot ME, Reda C, et al: Histomorphometric assessment of the long-term effects of alendronate on bone quality and remodeling in patients with osteoporosis. J Clin Invest 1997;100:1475-80.

44. Bone HG, Hosking D, Devogelaaer JP, et al: Alendronate phase III osteoporosis treatment study group: ten Years' experience with alendronate for osteoporosis in postmenopausal women. N Engl J Med 2004;350:1189-99.

45. Miller PD, Watts NB, Licata AA, et al: Cyclical etidronate in the treatment of postmenopausal osteoporosis: efficacy and safety after seven years of treatment. Am J Med 1997;103:468-76.

46. Odvina CV, Zerwekh JE, Rao DS, et al: Severely suppressed bone turnover: a potential complication of alendronate therapy. J Clin Endocrinol Metab 2005;90:1294-301.

47. Recker R, Masarachia P, Santora A, et al: Trabecular bone microarchitecture after alendronate treatment of osteoporotic women. Curr Med Res Opin 2005;21:185-94.

48. Miller PD: Efficacy and safety of long-term bisphosphonates in postmenopausal osteoporosis. Exp Opin Pharmacother 2003;4:1-6.

49. Ott S.: Long-term safety of bisphosphonates [editorial]. J Clin Endocrinol Metab 2005;90:1897-99.

50. Black DM, Cummings SR, Karpf DB, et al: Randomized trial of the effect of alendronate on risk of fracture in women with existing vertebral fractures. Fracture Intervention Trial Research Group. Lancet 1996;348:1535-41.

51. Harris S, Watts NB, Genant HK, et al: Effects of risedronate on vertebral and non-vertebral fractures in women with postmenopausal osteoporosis: a randomized controlled trial. JAMA 1999;282:1344-52.

52. McClung M, Geusens P, Miller PD, et al: Effect of risedronate on the risk of hip fracture in the elderly. N Engl J Med 2001;344:333-40.

53. Harrington JT, Ste-Marie LG, Brandi ML, et al: Risedronate rapidly reduces the risk for nonvertebral fractures in women with postmenopausal osteoporosis. Calcif Tissue Int 2004;74:129-35.

54. Neer RM, Arnaud CD, Zanchetta JR, et al: Effect of parathyroid hormone (1-34) on fractures and bone mineral density in postmenopausal women with osteoporosis. N Engl J Med 2001;344:1434-41.

55. Barrett-Connor E, Wehren L, Siris E, et al: Recency and duration of postmenopausal hormone therapy: effects on bone mineral density and fracture risk in the National Osteoporosis Risk Assessment (NORA) study. Menopause 2003;10:412-19.

56. Yates J, Barrett-Connor E, Barlas S, et al: Rapid loss of hip fracture protection after estrogen cessation: evidence from the National Osteoporosis Risk Assessment. Obstet Gynecol 2004;103:440-46.

57. Dufresne TE, Chmielewski PA, Manhart MD, et al: Risedronate preserves bone architecture in early postmenopausal women in 1 year as measured by three-dimensional microcomputed tomography. Calcif Tissue Int 2003;73:423-32.

58. Mosekilde L, Beck-Nielsen H,Sorenson OH, et al: Hormonal replacement therapy reduces forearm fracture incidence in recent postmenopausal women: results of the Danish Osteoporosis Prevention Study. Maturitas 2000;36:181-93.

59. Lindsay R, Nieves J, Formica C, et al: Effects of adding parathyroid hormone to ongoing estrogen replacement therapy vs. continuation of estrogen on BMD in postmenopausal women. Lancet 1997;350:550-55.

60. Lane NE, Sanchez, Modin GW, et al: Parathyroid hormone treatment can reverse corticosteroid-induced osteoporosis: results of a randomized controlled clinical trial. J Clin Invest 1998;102:1627-33.

61. Ettinger B, San Martin J, Crans G, Pavo I: Differential effects of teriparatide on BMD after treatment with raloxifene or alendronate. J Bone Miner Res 2004;19:745-51.

62. Black DM, Greenspan SL, Ensrud KE, et al, PaTH Study Investigators: the effects of parathyroid hormone and alendronate alone or in combination in postmenopausal osteoporosis. N Engl J Med 2003;349:1207-15.

63. Finkelstein JS, Hayes A, Hunzelman JL, et al: The effects of parathyroid hormone, alendronate, or both in men with osteoporosis. N Engl J Med 2003;349:1216-26.

64. Khosla S: Parathyroid hormone plus alendronate: a combination that does not add up. N Engl J Med 2003;349:1277-79.

65. Russell RGG, Rogers MJ: Bisphosphonates: from the laboratory to the patient and back again. Bone 1999;25:97-106.

66. Russell RGG, Rogers MJ, Frith J, et al: The pharmacology of bisphosphonates and new insights into their mechanisims of action. J Bone Miner Res 1999;14:53-65.

67. Deal C, Omizo M, Schwartz EN, et al: Raloxifene in combination with teriparatide reduces teriparatide-induced stimulation of bone resorption but not formation in postmenopausal women with osteoporosis J Bone Miner Res 2004;19(Suppl 1):S44.

68. Kostenulk et al: OPG and PTH have additive effects on BMD in aged osteopenic OVX rats. Endocrinology 2001;142:4295-304.

69. Kurland ES, Heller SL, Diamond B, et al: The importance of bisphosphonate therapy in maintaining bone mass in men after therapy with teriparatide [human parathyroid hormone(1-34)]. Osteoporos Int 2004;15:992-97.

70. Lindsay R, Scheele WH, Neer R, et al: Sustained vertebral fracture risk reduction after withdrawal of teriparatide in postmenopausal women with osteoporosis. Arch Intern Med 2004;164:2024-30.

71. Rittmaster RS, Bolognese M, Ettinger MP, et al: Enhancement of bone mass in osteoporotic women with parathyroid hormone followed by alendronate. J Clin Endocrinol Metab 2000;85:2129-34.

72. Black DM, Bilezikian JP, Ensrud KE, et al: PaTH Study Investigators: One year of alendronate after one year of parathyroid hormone (1-84) for osteoporosis. N Engl J Med. 2005;353(6):555-65.

73. Meunier PJ, Roux C, Seeman E, et al: The effects of strontium ranelate on the risk of vertebral fracture in women with postmenopausal osteoporosis. N Engl J Med 2004;350:459-68.

74. Reginster JY, Seeman E, De Vernejoul MC, et al: Strontium ranelate reduces the risk of nonvertebral fractures in postmenopausal women with osteoporosis: Treatment of Peripheral Osteoporosis (TROPOS) Study. J Clin Endocrinol Metab 2005;90:2816-22.

75. Marie P, Hott M, Modrowski D, et al: Strontium ranelate decreases bone resorption in oophorectomized rats. J Bone Miner Res 1993;8:607-15.

76. Canalis E, Hott M, Deloffre P, et al: The divalent strontium salt S12911 enhances bone cell replication and bone formation in vitro. Bone1996;18:517-23.

77. Meunier PJ, Slosman DO, Delmas PD, et al: Strontium ranelate: dose-dependent effects in established postmenopausal vertebral osteoporosis—a 2-year randomized placebo controlled trial. J Clin Endocrinol Metab. 2002 May;87(5):2060-66.

78. Lecart MP, Bruyere O, Reginster JY: Combination/sequential therapy in osteoporosis. Curr Osteoporos Rep 2004;2:123-30.

79. Binkley N, Krueger D: Combination therapy for osteoporosis: considerations and controversy. Curr Rheumatol Rep 2005;7:61-5.

80. McDermott MT, Zapalowski C, Miller PD: Treatment of osteoporosis. In: Hot Topics-Osteoporosis. Philadelphia: Elsevier, 2004:71-110.

21

The Pathogenesis of Glucocorticoid-Induced Bone Loss

Jean Pierre Devogelaer, Yves Boutsen, and Daniel Henri Manicourt

SUMMARY

Glucocorticoids induce a rapid dose dependent bone loss and it is unclear whether any dose can be considered safe. Glucocorticoid-induced bone loss is faster and more marked in the first 6 to 12 months of therapy, and trabecular bone is more affected than cortical bone. Numerous mechanisms are involved in the development of glucocorticoid-induced osteoporosis, especially effects on bone formation. However synergistic actions of glucocorticoids may explain more why some patients seem to be relatively protected and why others lose bone rapidly leading to bone fragility and fracture.

Because of their potent anti-inflammatory and immuno-suppressive actions, glucocorticoids are commonly used to treat a large variety of debilitating and potentially life-threatening conditions such as arthritides, vasculitides, allergic disorders, diseases of the liver and intestinal tract, multiple myeloma, and graft rejection. This list is not restrictive. However, the side effects of glucocorticoids are as protean as their therapeutic indications (e.g., truncal obesity, posterior subcapsular cataract, disturbances of glucose and lipid metabolism, myopathy, cutaneous atrophy, salt and fluid retention) and they usually prevent the unconsidered usage of these drugs. This notwithstanding, the most frequent and devastating complication of glucocorticoid therapy is the occurrence of a brittle and osteoporotic bone, and many authors believe that glucocorticoid-induced osteoporosis (GCIOP) is the most common cause of "secondary" osteoporosis.

Prior and current exposure to glucocorticoids confers an increased risk of fracture that is of substantial importance beyond that explained by the measurement of bone mineral density (BMD). In a meta-analysis of data from seven cohort studies of approximately 42,000 men and women,[1] the relative risk of any fracture ranged from 1.98 at the age of 50 years to 1.66 at the age of 85 years. For osteoporotic fracture, the range of relative risk was 2.63 to 1.71, and for hip fracture it was 4.42 to 2.48. Further, the fracture risk was independent of prior fracture and was similar in both men and women. It is also worth noting that, in patients who were on current glucocorticoid treatment, BMD was significantly reduced at the femoral neck, but fracture risk was still only partly explained by BMD.

An increased fracture risk during oral glucocorticoid therapy, with greater effects on the hip and spine than on the forearm, has also been observed in another retrospective cohort study that comprised 244,235 oral glucocorticoid users and 244,235 control subjects who were matched for age and gender.[2] The relative rate of nonvertebral fracture during oral glucocorticoid treatment was 1.33 (95% CI, 1.29-1.38), that of hip fracture 1.61 (95% CI, 1.47-1.76), that of forearm fracture 1.09 (95% CI, 1.01-1.17), and that of vertebral fracture 2.60 (95% CI, 2.31-2.92). Importantly, the study pointed out that the fracture risk was dose dependent. With a standardized daily dose of less than 2.5 mg prednisolone, hip fracture risk was 0.99 (95% CI, 0.82-1.20) relative to control, rising to 1.77 (95% CI, 1.55-2.02) at daily doses of 2.5 to 7.5 mg, and 2.27 (95% CI, 1.94-2.66) at doses of 7.5 mg or greater. For vertebral fracture, the relative rates were 1.55, (95% CI, 1.20-2.01), 2.59 (95% CI, 2.16-3.10), and 5.18 (95% CI, 4.25-6.31), respectively. Further, all fracture risks declined toward baseline rapidly after cessation of oral glucocorticoid treatment, a point worth stressing and apparently peculiar to GCIOP.

Glucocorticoid-induced osteoporosis is not restricted to adults. When compared with children taking nonsystemic corticosteroids (n = 345,748), children taking oral corticosteroids (n = 37,562; age range, 4-17 y) exhibit an adjusted odds ratio for fracture of 1.32 (95% CI, 1.03-1.69).[3] Further, and as observed in adults, stopping oral glucocorticoid therapy is associated with a rapid decrease in the risk of fracture, which then becomes similar to the risk observed in the control group.

The fact that, for a similar BMD, the bone is more brittle in people with GCIOP than in people with postmenopausal osteoporosis is worth stressing. The exact mechanisms accounting for this important observation are probably multifactorial. The role played by the nature and severity of the underlying disease is not clear.

On the other hand, it is clear that the faster rate of bone loss induced by glucocorticoids is more marked at the highly metabolically active trabecular sites of the skeleton, and the fragility fractures affect mostly ribs and vertebral bodies, than in the less metabolically active cortical bone compartment such as at the upper extremity of the femur and in long bones, which are, nonetheless, not devoid of bone loss. It is also clear that the severity of osteoporosis is related to the dose and duration of glucocorticoid therapy and that weaning from glucocorticoids rapidly resets the fracture risk toward that of normal control subjects, an observation that might be related, at least in part, to the observation that, in GCIOP, the decline in osteoblast activity is associated with a gradual thinning of the trabecular plates, in contrast to the case of postmenopausal osteoporosis in which overenthusiastic osteoclastic activity leads to perforation and, ultimately, resorption of the trabecula.

A schematic view of the clinical mechanisms potentially involved in the development of GCIOP is shown in Figure 21-1. The large variety of these mechanisms might account for the rapid onset of bone complications. Although not exhaustive and maybe oversimplistic, this approach has the merit of delineating therapeutic avenues to control one of the most devastating effects of glucocorticoid therapy.

GLUCOCORTICOID FORMS AND ROUTES OF ADMINISTRATION

Cortisol is the principal naturally occurring plasma corticosteroid in humans. Modification of various sites on the cortisol molecule has resulted in the development of synthetic corticosteroids to enhance anti-inflammatory activity, prolong half-life, and reduce sodium-retaining potency (Table 21-1). Values of equivalent doses given in the table are average values rather than fixed face values, the individual responses being potentially at small variance with these mean values.

The introduction of a 1,2 double bond in ring A (prednisone and prednisolone) increases the anti-inflammatory potency by an order of magnitude of 4 and yields compounds that are metabolized more slowly than cortisol. 6-α-Methylation (methylprednisolone) of the B ring also increases the anti-inflammatory potency but reduces the electrolyte-retaining properties. While 9-α-fluorination enhances all biological activities, 16-α-hydroxylation, 16-α-methylation, and 16-β-methylation all eliminate the sodium-retaining effect. Substitution at the 17-α-ester position produces a group of extremely potent steroids, beclomethasone dipropionate and budesonide, which are effective when applied topically to skin or administered by inhalation. Deflazacort, an oxazoline derivative of prednisone, has been developed with the hope of reducing the catabolic effects of glucocorticoids while maintaining anti-inflammatory effects. Whether the anti-inflammatory potency of 6 mg of this compound corresponds to that of 5 mg of prednisone remains a matter of debate.

With the notable exception of the high-dose methylprednisolone pulse therapy,[4] unfortunately, most of these synthetic analogues still exhibit a significant effect on BMD and on biochemical markers of bone metabolism, whether they are administered orally, by

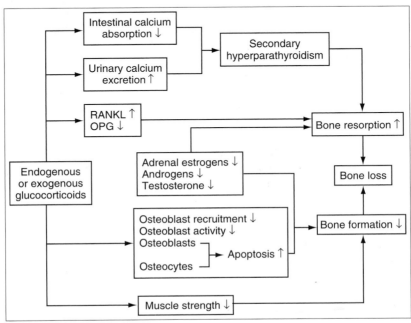

Figure 21-1. Schematic representation of various mechanisms leading individually or synergistically to glucocorticoid-induced bone loss and osteoporosis.

TABLE 21-1 AVAILABLE GLUCOCORTICOID PREPARATIONS		
	Respective Potencies	
Preparation	Anti-inflammatory	Equivalence (mg)
With a biological half-life <12 hours		
Hydrocortisone	1	20
Cortisone	0.8	25
With a biological half-life 12-36 hours		
Prednisone (Δ-1-cortisone)	4	5
Prednisolone (Δ-1-cortisol)	4	5
6-α-Methylprednisolone	5	4
Triamcinolone (9- α-fluoro-16-α-hydroxyprednisolone)	5	4
Deflazacort	4	6
With a biological half-life >48 hours		
Paramethasone (6-α-fluoro-16-α-methylprednisolone)	10	2
Betamethasone (9-α-fluoro-16-β-methylprednisolone)	25	0.60
Dexamethasone (9-α-fluoro-16-α-methylprednisolone)	30	0.75

inhalation,[5] or by topical application to the skin. It has been hypothesized that the side effects of glucocorticoids are due to the transactivation of genes through the binding of glucocorticoid receptor (GR) dimers to DNA, whereas their anti-inflammatory effects result from the binding of a single GR to transcription factors or coactivators, resulting in transrepression of genes.[6] However, although they exert strong transrepression but little or no transactivation, the newly developed glucocorticoids still induce osteoporosis.[7]

PATHOPHYSIOLOGY OF GLUCOCORTICOID-INDUCED OSTEOPOROSIS

The pathophysiology of GCIOP is not yet fully understood. The rate at which GCIOP develops is influenced by a number of factors, namely the glucocorticoid dose (the daily dose, the treatment duration, or the cumulative dose).[8] The age, gender, and menopausal status of the patient, as well as the BMD prior to initiation of glucocorticoid therapy, may also have roles to play. The indication for glucocorticoid therapy may consist of various systemic conditions, such as rheumatoid arthritis, that might by themselves predispose patients to lose BMD.[9] The complexity of the interaction of these various factors may explain why the pathophysiology of GCIOP has not yet been definitely apprehended. The isolated and/or synergistic action of the more or less involved factors might also be central to the rapidity of bone loss that is observed in glucocorticoid-treated patients. The aim of the paper is to review the various mechanisms leading to bone loss and bone fragility.

Age: Children and Adolescents

Glucocorticoid action on the skeleton of children is also particularly complex. In children, glucocorticoids reduce bone turnover, impair linear growth, and lower BMD.[10-12] They are toxic for the growth plate: they inhibit the elongation of the skeleton and the creation of trabeculae by complex mechanisms.[13] Besides hampering the intestinal absorption of calcium, glucocorticoids interfere with the growth hormone (GH)–insulin growth factor-1 (IGF-1) axis at the hypothalamic, pituitary, and target organ levels, affecting hormone release, receptor abundance, and gene transcription. Glucocorticoids also exert deleterious effects on the growth plate by inhibiting chondrocyte proliferation, proteoglycan synthesis, and mineralization. Further, these drugs increase the apoptosis of hypertrophic chondrocytes, enhance the activity of osteoclasts, suppress the recruitment and function of osteoblasts, and disrupt the normal control of vascular invasion at the cartilage-bone interface. Fortunately, preliminary studies indicate that the growth-suppressing effect of glucocorticoids can be counterbalanced by daily administration of recombinant GH at doses comparable with those prescribed for treatment of GH deficiency (0.3 mg/kg week).[14] Further, responsiveness to GH seems to be inversely related to the glucocorticoid dose but does not depend on the type of glucocorticoid-dependent disease. However, the effects of GH therapy on body composition and metabolism in children receiving long-term glucocorticoid therapy remain to be explored.

Several mechanisms may account for the decrease in BMD observed in children treated with glucocorticoids. First, as growth is impaired, the decrease in height might account, at least in part, for the reduction in BMD.[12] Second, glucocorticoids inhibit remodeling and modeling, which both accelerate again rapidly after tapering of the glucocorticoid dose.[15,16] Whereas remodeling—bone resorption by osteoclasts followed by bone formation by osteoblasts—does not lead to changes in bone shape but maintains bone strength, modeling modifies the shape of bone,[11] promotes bone formation independently of the sites of bone resorption, and leads to an increase in BMD. On the other hand, the underlying condition might have a significant impact,[9,11] and one cannot exclude the possibility that low-dose glucocorticoids have little effect on bone modeling in prepubertal children but exert a strong effect in adolescents.[17] Further, in glucocorticoid-treated young patients, the link between the final outcomes of growth and peak bone mass could be dependent on the pubertal stage at which therapy intervenes, just as for the relation between growth spurt and BMD accrual in healthy adolescents.[11,18]

Orally administered glucocorticoids are likely to be more harmful both to growth and to BMD than inhaled glucocorticoids because the systemic doses are higher.[10,19] The skeleton undergoing growth and modeling seems to be more vulnerable than the mature skeleton to the osteoblast-inhibiting effects of long-term exposure to glucocorticoids, with consequent long-term deficits in cortical and trabecular bone masses.[20,21] Moreover, the effects of glucocorticoids might differ in cortical and in trabecular compartments in children just as in adults, cortical bone being much less affected.[20] The risk of permanent stunting of the height and BMD could be reduced when glucocorticoid-treatment is withdrawn before the pubertal growth spurt has started. Serum bone formation markers are lowered in glucocorticoid-treated children, which is due to a direct suppressive effect of glucocorticoids on osteoblasts.

Although the production of IGF-1 is not impaired, the increased concentrations of IGF binding protein 3 might inhibit IGF-1 bioactivity.[22] The lack of specificity of biochemical markers of bone remodeling does not permit a distinction between modeling, remodeling, and disturbances due to the disease itself.[23] Changes in the levels of biochemical markers might also be dependent on the manner (oral or inhaled) and period (prepubertal or postpubertal) of administration of glucocorticoids.[23] It is therefore difficult to assess the net result of glucocorticoids on BMD, because, owing to the scarcity of normative data on BMD in children, we lack values standardized for bone age, skeleton height and skeletal area, lean body mass, and body mass index.[11,20,24]

Age: Adults

Saville and Kharmash had already found in 1967, before more precise BMD measurements were available, a significantly increased incidence of osteoporosis only in patients over the age of 50 years. With more modern methods of evaluation, a greater loss of bone has been observed in individuals older than 50 years of age (males or postmenopausal females).[25]

Gender

At doses lower than or equivalent to 7.5 mg/day of prednisolone, glucocorticoids do not induce significant changes in the BMD of the forearm, lumbar spine, and hip in premenopausal women, in contrast to men and postmenopausal women who both are more sensitive to GCIOP.[26,27] At higher doses, however, glucocorticoids have a devastating effect on BMD, irrespective of menopausal status or gender.[27] These differences in sensitivity to glucocorticoid side effects might be, at least in part, related to differences in the relative levels of both androgens and glucocorticoids that these patients exhibit during glucocorticoid therapy. Indeed, androgen receptors and GRs not only mediate opposite effects on cellular metabolism and proliferation, but their signaling pathways are mutually inhibitory.[28] Androgen receptors and GRs, which display a high degree of sequence homology and bind to a common DNA site, inhibit each other's transcriptional activities by forming heterodimers.[29] Therefore, when glucocorticoid levels rise to predominate over androgen levels, heterodimer formation will ensure that the anabolic effects mediated by androgen receptor homodimers are curtailed at the same time that glucocorticoid homodimers begin to activate transcription of genes involved in catabolism.

Although glucocorticoids can inhibit the production of testosterone by the testes both directly and indirectly via the reduced secretion of gonadotropin-releasing hormone, which also contributes to lower the serum levels of estradiol,[30] the serum levels of testosterone in patients treated with glucocorticoids are reported to be decreased in some study groups[23] and unchanged in others.[31] Nevertheless, all studies point out that decreased serum levels of estradiol, an observation in close agreement with several reports suggesting that estradiol rather than testosterone might be the gonadal hormone active in bone that maintains a positive formation/resorption balance.[32] This hypothesis is supported by the observation that, in elderly men[33] and in men also treated with glucocorticoids,[31] estradiol rather than free or total testosterone is most correlated with bone mass. Further, deficiency in aromatase, an enzyme expressed in bone tissue and known to play a key role in the conversion of both testosterone and adrenal androgens into estradiol,[34] has been associated with severe osteoporosis that responds to estradiol treatment.[35] On the other hand, thus far, it is not known to what extent glucocorticoids might regulate the aromatase activity in bone as it has been reported in adipose tissue.[36]

In postmenopausal women, glucocorticoid-induced depression of the hypothalamic-pituitary-gonadal axis leads to a decrease in the serum levels of estradiol, androstenedione, dehydroepiandrosterone sulfate, and progesterone,[37] which all are known to play a crucial role in the maintenance of BMD.[38,39]

Doses of Glucocorticoids and Timing

As pointed out by in vitro studies, the time period during which osteoblasts are exposed to physiological doses of glucocorticoids may lead to marked changes in the overall metabolism of these bone-forming cells. Thus, after short time periods, the differentiated function of osteoblasts is maintained, whereas after long periods, the very same glucocorticoid concentrations inhibit the synthesis of both collagens (types I and III) and noncollagenous proteins.[40,41] This biphasic effect might explain, at least in part, why low doses of glucocorticoids are not completely devoid of adverse effect on BMD and bone mechanical resistance, as stressed by longitudinal studies demonstrating that even at so-called physiological glucocorticoid doses (i.e., <10 mg of predniso(lo)ne equivalent per day), a significant bone loss and even an increase in fracture risk both can be observed, chiefly in the trabecular compartment of the skeleton,[26,42,43] which exhibits a marked depression of the mineral apposition rate[44] as well as a marked thinning of trabecular width when compared with the same site in gender- and age-matched control subjects.[44-47]

These findings notwithstanding, the rationale for using the lowest possible glucocorticoid doses stems from histomorphometric data of transilial bone biopsies showing that low glucocorticoid doses modestly increase the trabecular resorption surface and preserve the trabecular architecture.[48,49] This is in sharp contrast to the findings in specimens from postmenopausal osteoporosis patients, which, for a similar loss of trabecular bone volume, show a rapid decline in trabecular number with an increased resorption leading to plate perforations and to deterioration of trabecular architecture.[46] At higher glucocorticoid doses, however—that is, greater than 10 g prednisolone cumulative dose—trabecular connectivity is no longer preserved.[49]

These histomorphometric findings strongly suggest that the mechanism or mechanisms responsible for the maintenance of bone microarchitecture might be quite different in GCIOP than in postmenopausal osteoporosis, at least after exposure to low glucocorticoid dose.[49] The maintenance of a critical amount of trabecular bone volume might be central to the persistence of the trabecular network along different glucocorticoid doses during the course of therapy.[48] Alternatively, the persistence of the integrity of the trabecular architecture could help to explain why bone biopsies performed in patients with Cushing syndrome revealed, after adrenalectomy, a rapidly resumed osteoblastic activity with extended osteoid surfaces and normalized appositional rate resulting in a positive bone tissue balance,[44,50] leading macroscopically to a dramatic increase in BMD after adrenalectomy or hypophysectomy (Figure 21-2).[50] The same resumption of increase in BMD has been observed after weaning from oral glucocorticoid therapy.[42] GCIOP is to a certain extent reversible when exposure to excessive exogenous or endogenous glucocorticoids stops, thus accounting for a rapid reset to normal of the fracture risk.[3] When and under which conditions irreversibility sets in remain to be determined.

Alternate-day therapy has been added to the armamentarium of glucocorticoid therapy to reduce the side effects of glucocorticoids without impairing too much their therapeutic efficacy. However, if growth was preserved in children, BMD was in fact not protected in children or in adults.[51,52] The explanation for the persistent bone loss could lie in the prolonged depression of adrenal androgen secretion not only during the day on but also during the day off glucocorticoids.[53] The crucial role of adrenal androgens in BMD maintenance has already been formerly underlined.[38]

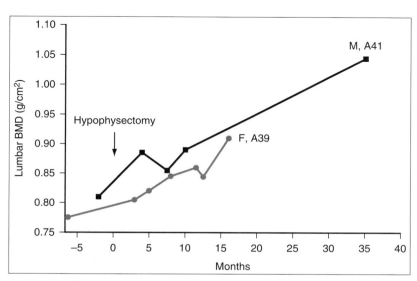

Figure 21-2. Rapid increase of lumbar BMD after surgical hypophysectomy in a male and a female patient suffering from Cushing syndrome.

Pulsed intravenous high-dose glucocorticoids (up to 1 g methylprednisolone) do not seem to be deleterious to BMD,[2] probably because their metabolic action is short lived. An alternative explanation for their beneficial action with lack of BMD changes could be that supersaturation or even downregulation of cytosolic GRs could occur with this kind of rapid administration, with an imbalance between nongenomic and genomic glucocorticoid effects.[54,55] A fast reduction in the intense activity of the inflammatory processes could also be protective for BMD.

Bone loss is more marked during the first 6 months after initiation of glucocorticoid therapy[56] and from then on tends to have a slower pace. This could be partly due to the fact that higher doses are frequently used to start therapy, with progressive tapering later on when the patient's state improves. However, this is far from being the only explanation. Several authors have observed a faster bone loss early in therapy with a subsequent slowing down, even despite maintenance of high steroid dosage,[27] an observation that could be consistent with the hypothesis that histochemical changes and catabolic effects of glucocorticoids on bone are more pronounced early in the course of treatment.[56] The dosage constitutes an important determinant of bone loss. However, there is largely no real scientific basis for the use of various doses of glucocorticoids in the various indications. Therefore, the prescribed glucocorticoid dosage in a given patient suffering from a given disease should be empirically maintained as low as possible, even if the exact threshold dose necessary and sufficient to avoid detrimental effects in a given individual has not yet been established. This lack of rules of prescription could also be due to the numerous factors unevenly involved in that process, interfering with the expected positive effect of GCs. Moreover, the variability in the clearance rates of predniso(lo)ne and in the circulating half-lives of steroids,[57] the specificity in glucocorticoid receptor haplotype,[58] and the potential amplifier role of 11β-hydroxysteroid dehydrogenase isoenzyme[59] could explain the paradoxic difference in individual severity of glucocorticoid side effects, some patients developing almost no after effects on large glucocorticoid doses, whereas others have obvious side effects on much smaller doses.

Osteoblast and Osteocyte Function

The histomorphometric features of GCIOP have been well characterized.[44-47] Although the prevalence of resorption lacunae and osteoclasts is frequently enhanced, an observation that might be related to the promotion of osteoclast survival by glucocorticoids,[60] the most impressive findings point to a major impairment in bone formation: the number and longevity of active osteoblasts as well as the mean wall thickness of completed trabecular plates are markedly decreased. Relevant to this decrease in bone formation are a decrease in the bioactivity of skeletal growth factors such as IGF-1 as well as the effects of glucocorticoids on osteoblastogenesis. Indeed, glucocorticoids are likely to inhibit the proliferation and/or the differentiation of the stromal cell-osteoblast family at an early stage and thereby to reduce not only the number of matrix-secreting osteoblasts but also the number of osteoblastic cells that support osteoclast development.[61] Further, glucocorticoids not only decrease the formation of osteoblasts but also promote the apoptosis of osteoblasts. The decreases in the number and activity of bone-forming cells are reflected by an early and dramatic reduction in the serum levels of osteocalcin (OC) in human subjects taking glucocorticoids.[62]

Glucocorticoids also increase the prevalence of apoptosis of osteocytes, the most abundant bone cells.[61,63,64] Because the network of osteocytes is believed to participate in the detection of microdamage and in the transmission of signals that lead to its repair by remodeling, disruption of this network by apoptosis might lead to accumulation of microdamage and increased bone fragility.[65] On the other hand, as it is a cumulative and unrepairable defect, glucocorticoid-induced osteocyte apoptosis might contribute to the pathophysiology of avascular necrosis of bone, a dramatic event that may occur late after glucocorticoid administration has ceased.[66]

Role of Secondary Hyperparathyroidism

It is often believed that glucocorticoids act initially to depress intestinal calcium absorption[67] and increase urinary calcium excretion,[68] leading to compensatory hypersecretion of parathyroid hormone (PTH).[44,67-69] By activating the formation of new remodeling units, PTH then increases bone turnover, but at the same time the depressive effect of glucocorticoids on osteoblasts directly uncouples remodeling so that bone loss accelerates. Although this PTH-based model of glucocorticoid-induced osteoporosis is attractive, sufficient ambiguity remains that it is premature to consider it validated at the present time. Indeed, although it is clear that glucocorticoids depress intestinal calcium absorption, the mechanisms remain controversial: the induction of a resistance of intestinal cells to 1,25-dihydroxyvitamin D_3 has been advocated,[67] whereas other evidence indicates that glucocorticoids directly inhibit calcium transport by mechanisms that are independent of the vitamin D system.[70] On the other hand, studies exploring the effects of glucocorticoids on renal calcium handling are scarce and their results conflicting.[71] Further, and importantly, studies conducted with recent PTH assays[72] do not support the concept that the serum PTH levels are enhanced in patients taking high doses of glucocorticoids.

Thus, it may prove useful to consider alternative models. It is indeed possible that glucocorticoids amplify the response of bone to normal levels of PTH,[73] a contention strengthened by the observation that glucocorticoids enhance the PTH-dependent cyclic adenosine monophosphate production in bone cells.[74] Another but not exclusive possibility is that the calcium-sensing receptor of parathyroid cells is altered by glucocorticoids.

Biological Parameters of Bone Remodeling

The discovery and characterization of essential cytokines for osteoclast biology, that is, the receptor activator of nuclear factor NF-κB ligand (RANK-L), its receptor RANK, and its decoy receptor osteoprotegerin (OPG) have improved our understanding of bone metabolism in both healthy and disease states (Figure 21-3).[75] Stromal cells, osteoblasts, and activated T lymphocytes all express RANK-L, also termed OPG-L, that exists in a cell membrane–associated form and in a soluble form, both of which stimulate osteoclastogenesis and osteoclast action after binding to and activating RANK, a high-affinity receptor located on osteoclast precursors. The soluble cytokine receptor OPG, which lacks a transmembrane-spanning domain, counteracts the biological effects of RANK-L by competing for both forms of RANK-L and preventing them from binding to the RANK receptor on osteoclast precursors. Although the production of OPG is stimulated by various hormones (1,25-dihydroxyvitamin D, bone morphogenic protein-2, estrogen) and cytokines (tumor necrosis factor-α and -β, interleukin-1α and -β), glucocorticoids concurrently decrease OPG and increase RANK-L production by human osteoblastic lineage cells.[76] These findings might provide a potential major mechanism for glucocorticoid effects on bone resorption,[61] a hypothesis strengthened by the observation that glucocorticoid administration results in a rapid (within 2 weeks) and marked decrease in the circulating levels of OPG.[77-79] In contrast, in patients with Cushing syndrome, serum levels of OPG are enhanced and correlate significantly with the increased circulating levels of cortisol.[80] The reasons for these apparently conflicting results are not known. It is possible that endogenous and exogenous glucocorticoids differ by some inherent properties. On the other hand, unknown mechanisms might shift the low OPG levels and the rapid rate of bone loss that are observed in early glucocorticoid treatment[27,80,81] to an increase in OPG levels and to a reduction in the rate of bone loss, which both are seen in long-standing cortisol excess. Further studies pertaining to the OPG/RANKL/RANK system in postmenopausal osteoporosis compared with GCIOP are urgently needed.

Examples of changes in biochemical parameters of bone remodeling in patients receiving glucocorticoids are given in Table 21-2 and illustrated in Figure 21-4.[82] No increase in serum C-telopeptide cross-links of type I collagen, a parameter of bone resorption, was observed immediately after the start of therapy or later on in a

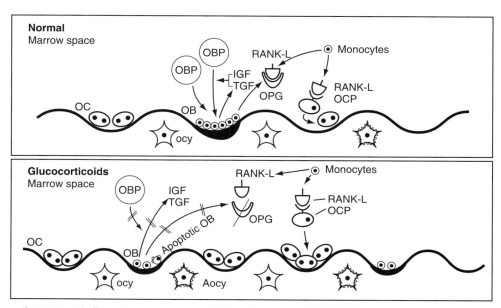

Figure 21-3. Glucocorticoid effects. Decreased release of OPG with increased RANKL/OPG ratio causes an increase in osteoclasts and an increased number of sites undergoing remodeling. Decreased differentiation, function, and lifespan of osteoblasts result in decreased bone formation. An increased number of apoptotic osteocytes causes decreased bone strength. Aocy = apoptotic osteocyte; OB = osteoblast; OBP = osteoblast precursor; OC = osteoclast; OCP = osteoclast precursor; ocy = osteocyte; OPG = osteoprotegerin. (From Lukert BP: Glucocorticoid-induced osteoporosis. In: Favus MJ, ed: Primer on the Metabolic Bone Diseases and Disorders of Mineral Metabolism, 5th ed., Washington, D.C.: ASBMR, 2003. With permission.)

TABLE 21-2 CHANGES IN BIOCHEMICAL PARAMETERS OF BONE REMODELING IN PATIENTS RECEIVING GLUCOCORTICOIDS*

Time	Prednisolone Doses (mg), mean ± SD (median)	Total ALP (NV: 90-265 IU/L)	B-ALP (NV: 13.2 ± 4.7 µg/L)	OC (NV: 28.9 ± 9.7 ng/mL)	CTx (NV: 3634 ± 833 pM)	Femoral Neck L1-L4 BMD (g/cm²)	Total Hip BMD (g/cm²)	Trochanter BMD (g/cm²)	BMD (g/cm²)
Start	22.5 ± 19.9 (15.0)	269 ± 200	9.4 ± 8.1	9.3 ± 3.3	2648 ± 1115	0.963 ± 0.173	0.723 ± 0.110	0.803 ± 0.134	0.641 ± 0.132
3 mo	11.4 ± 2.1 (11.3)	174 ± 58	6.0 ± 3.5	7.2 ± 3.9	1973 ± 1134				
6 mo	8.6 ± 5.0 (7.5)	161 ± 59	5.0 ± 1.0	6.2 ± 4.6	1457 ± 1420	0.941 ± 0.155	0.708 ± 0.093	0.812 ± 0.124	0.646 ± 0.090
9 mo	7.2 ± 5.2 (7.5)	169 ± 32	5.6 ± 1.2	6.2 ± 3.4	1004 ± 491				
12 mo	5.3 ± 3.5 (6.8)	184 ± 42	5.5 ± 1.6	9.1 ± 8.5	1569 ± 1517	0.916 ± 0.144	0.695 ± 0.082	0.783 ± 0.121	0.622 ± 0.092

*Daily glucocorticoid doses expressed as milligrams of prednisolone.

ALP = alkaline phosphatase; B-= bone specific; CTx = C-telopeptide cross-link of type I collagen; NV = normal values; OC = osteocalcin; SD = standard deviation.

Modified from Boutsen et al.[82]

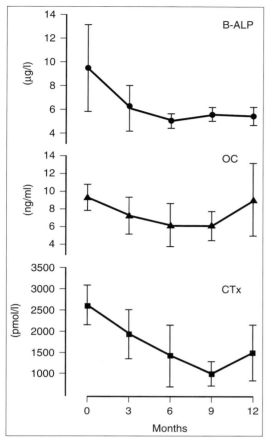

Figure 21-4. Evolution of serum levels of bone-specific alkaline phosphatase (B-ALP), osteocalcin (OC), and C-telopeptide cross-links of type I collagen (CTx) in patients treated with glucocorticoids and put on calcium supplements.

group of patients treated with high-dose prednisolone (>10 mg/day).[82] There was, however, a dramatic decrease in the parameters of bone formation (total alkaline phosphatase, bone-specific alkaline phosphatase, and OC) during the first 6 months, but leveling off was observed later on. The increase in the levels of C-telopeptide cross-links observed after 9 months might be explained by an improvement in the underlying

rheumatic conditions.[82] BMD decreased significantly in the calcium group during the year of follow-up, without any evident leveling off. The changes in biochemical parameters of bone remodeling could be partly explained by a progressive tapering of glucocorticoid daily doses (on average 15 mg/day at the start, 11 mg/day between 3 and 6 months, and 7.5 mg/day thereafter). Another explanation could be the protective intrinsic mechanism alluded to earlier.[80,81]

Glucocorticoid-Induced Myopathy

Glucocorticoid may provoke a decrease in muscle strength.[34] The myopathy could constitute in itself a cause of bone loss. This mechanism cannot explain the bone loss observed with low glucocorticoid doses, a clinically significant myopathy being observed only after administration of high glucocorticoid doses.

CONCLUSIONS

Although glucocorticoids induce a rapid bone loss that is more marked with high doses than with low doses, the bone loss occurs at all doses and hence no glucocorticoid dose can be considered safe. Further, the bone loss is faster and more marked in the first 6 months of therapy than later on, and the trabecular bone compartment is more exposed than the cortical bone. Numerous mechanisms are involved in the development of GCIOP. They act either separately or synergistically. This synergy, more or less marked, could help to explain why some patients seem to be protected and why in others, the velocity of bone loss leads rapidly to an enhanced bone fragility. The large variety of presumed or demonstrated mechanisms could also explain why so many various therapies have been proposed to try to circumvent the most crippling complication of glucocorticoids.

ACKNOWLEDGMENTS

We thank Marie-Christine Hallot for her invaluable assistance in typing the manuscript.

REFERENCES

1. Kanis JA, Johansson H, Oden A, et al: A meta-analysis of prior corticosteroid use and fracture risk. J Bone Miner Res 2004;19:893-99.
2. Van Staa TP, Leufkens HGM, Abenhaim L, et al: Use of oral corticosteroids and risk of fractures. J Bone Miner Res 2000;15:993-1000.
3. Van Staa TP, Cooper C, Leufkens HGM, et al: Children and the risk of fractures caused by oral corticosteroids. J Bone Miner Res 2003;18:913-18.
4. Frediani B, Falsetti P, Bisogno S, et al: Effects of high dose methylprednisolone pulse therapy on bone mass and biochemical markers of bone metabolism in patients with active rheumatoid arthritis: a 12-month randomized prospective controlled study. J Rheumatol 2004;31:1083-87.
5. Richy F, Bousquet J, Ehrlich GE, et al: Inhaled corticosteroids effects on bone in asthmatic and COPD patients: a quantitative systematic review. Osteoporos Int 2003;14:179-90.
6. Resche-Rigon M, Gronemeyer H: Therapeutic potential of selective modulators of nuclear receptor action. Curr Opin Chem Biol 1998;2:501-7.
7. Belvisi MG, Wicks SL, Battram CH, et al: Therapeutic benefit of a dissociated glucocorticoid and the relevance of in vitro

separation of transrepression from transactivation activity. J Immunol 2001;166:1975-82.

8. van Staa TP, Leufkens HGM, Abenhaim L, et al: Oral corticosteroids and fracture risk: relationship to daily and cumulative doses. Rheumatology 2000;39:1383-89.

9. Peel NFA, Moore DJ, Barrington NA, et al: Risk of vertebral fracture and relationship to bone mineral density in steroid treated rheumatoid arthritis. Ann Rheum Dis 1995;54:801-6.

10. Wolthers OD, Pedersen S: Short term linear growth in asthmatic children during treatment with prednisolone. Br Med J 1990;301:145-48.

11. Leonard MB, Zemel BS: Pediatric gastroenterology and nutrition: current concepts in pediatric bone disease. Pediatr Clin North Am 2002;49:143-73.

12. Boot AM, de Jongste JC, Verberne AAPH, et al: Bone mineral density and bone metabolism of prepubertal children with asthma after long-term treatment with inhaled corticosteroids. Pediatr Pulmonol 1997;24:379-84.

13. Hochberg Z: Mechanisms of steroid impairment of growth. Horm Res 2002;58(Suppl 1):33-8.

14. Allen DB, Julius JR, Breen TJ, et al: Treatment of glucocorticoid-induced growth suppression with growth hormone. National Cooperative Growth Study. J Clin Endocrinol Metab 1998;83:2824-29.

15. Crofton PM, Ahmed SF, Wade JC, et al: Effects of intensive chemotherapy on bone and collagen turnover and the growth hormone axis in children with acute lymphoblastic leukemia. J Clin Endocrinol Metab 1998;83:3121-29.

16. Atkinson SA, Halton JM, Bradley C, et al: Bone and mineral abnormalities in childhood acute lymphoblastic leukemia: influence of disease, drugs and nutrition. Int J Cancer 1998;11(suppl):35-9.

17. Wolthers OD, Heuck C: Differential effects of inhaled budesonide on serum osteocalcin in children and adolescents with asthma. Pediatr Allergy Immunol 1998;9:150-55.

18. Bonjour JP, Theintz G, Buchs B, et al: Critical years and stages of puberty for spinal and femoral bone mass accumulation during adolescence. J Clin Endocrinol Metab 1991;73:555-63.

19. Wolthers OD, Riis BJ, Pedersen S: Bone turnover in asthmatic children treated with oral prednisolone or inhaled budesonide. Pediatr Pulmonol 1993;16:341-46.

20. Leonard MB, Feldman HI, Shults J, et al: Long-term, high-dose glucocorticoids and bone mineral content in childhood glucocorticoid-sensitive nephrotic syndrome. N Engl J Med 2004;351:868-75.

21. Freundlich M, Jofe M, Goodman WG, et al: Bone histology in steroid-treated children with non-azotemic nephrotic syndrome. Pediatr Nephrol 2004;19:400-7.

22. Wolthers OD, Juul A, Hansen M, et al: The insulin-like growth factor axis and collagen turnover during prednisolone treatment. Arch Dis Child 1994;71:409-13.

23. Szulc P, Seeman E, Delmas PD: Biochemical measurements of bone turnover in children and adolescents. Osteoporos Int 2000;11:281-94.

24. Crabtree NJ, Kibirige MS, Fordham JN, et al: The relationship between lean body mass and bone mineral content in paediatric health and disease. Bone 2004;35:965-72.

25. Dykman TR, Gluck OS, Murphy WA, et al: Evaluation of factors associated with glucocorticoid-induced osteopenia in patients with rheumatic diseases. Arthritis Rheum 1985;28:361-68.

26. Nagant de Deuxchaisnes C, Devogelaer JP, Esselinckx W, et al: The effect of low dosage glucocorticoids on bone mass in rheumatoid arthritis: a cross-sectional and a longitudinal study using single photon absorptiometry. Adv Exp Med Biol 1984;171:209-39.

27. Jardinet D, Lefèbvre C, Depresseux G, et al: Longitudinal analysis of bone mineral density in pre-menopausal female systemic lupus erythematosus patients: deleterious role of glucocorticoid therapy at the lumbar spine. Rheumatology 2000;39:389-92.

28. Monder C, Sakai RR, Miroff Y, et al: Reciprocal changes in plasma corticosterone and testosterone in stressed male rats maintained in a visible burrow system: evidence for a mediating role of testicular 11 beta-hydroxysteroid dehydrogenase. Endocrinology 1994;134:1193-98.

29. Chen S-Y, Wang J, Yu G-Q, et al: Androgen and glucocorticoid receptor heterodimer formation: a possible mechanism for

30. mutual inhibition of transcriptional activity. J Biol Chem 1997;272:14087-92.

31. Hampson G, Bhargava N, Cheung J, et al: Low circulating estradiol and adrenal androgens concentrations in men on glucocorticoids: a potential contributory factor in steroid-induced osteoporosis. Metabolism 2002;51:1458-62.

31. Iqbal F, Michaelson J, Thaler L, et al: Declining bone mass in men with chronic pulmonary disease: contribution of glucocorticoid treatment, body mass index, and gonadal function. Chest 1999;116:1616-24.

32. Riggs BL, Khosla S, Melton LJ 3rd: A unitary model for involutional osteoporosis: estrogen deficiency causes both type I and type II osteoporosis in postmenopausal women and contributes to bone loss in aging men. J Bone Miner Res 1998;13:763-73.

33. Slemenda CW, Christian JC, Reed T, et al: Long-term bone loss in men: effects of genetic and environmental factors. Ann Intern Med 1992;117:286-91.

34. Crawford BAL, Liu PY, Kean MT, et al: Randomized placebo-controlled trial of androgen effects on muscle and bone in men requiring long-term systemic glucocorticoid treatment. J Clin Endocrinol Metab 2003;88:3167-76.

35. Bilezikian JP, Morishima A, Bell J, et al: Increased bone mass as a result of estrogen therapy in a man with aromatase deficiency. N Engl J Med 1998;339:599-603.

36. McTernan PG, Anderson LA, Anwar AJ, et al: Glucocorticoid regulation of p450 aromatase activity in human adipose tissue: gender and site differences. J Clin Endocrinol Metab 2002;87:1327-36.

37. Montecucco C, Caporali R, Caprotti P, et al: Sex hormones and bone metabolism in postmenopausal rheumatoid arthritis treated with two different glucocorticoids. J Rheumatol 1992;19:1895-1900.

38. Devogelaer JP, Crabbé J, Nagant de Deuxchaisnes C: Bone mineral density in Addison's disease: evidence for an effect of adrenal androgens on bone mass. Br Med J 1987;294:798-800.

39. Cauley JA, Robbins J, Chen Z, et al: Effects of estrogen plus progestin on risk of fracture and bone mineral density: the Women's Health Initiative randomized trial. JAMA 2003;290:1729-38.

40. Bellows CG, Aubin JE, Heersche JNM: Physiological concentrations of glucocorticoids stimulate formation of bone nodules from isolated rat calvaria cells in vitro. Endocrinology 1987;121:1985-92.

41. Oikarinen A, Autio P, Vuori J, et al: Systemic glucocorticoid treatment decreases serum concentrations of carboxyterminal propeptide of type I procollagen and aminoterminal propeptide of type III procollagen. Br J Dermatol 1992;126:172-78.

42. Laan RFJM, van Riel PLCM, van de Putte LBA, et al: Low-dose prednisolone induces rapid reversible axial bone loss in patients with rheumatoid arthritis. Ann Intern Med 1993;119:963-68.

43. Eastell R, Devogelaer JP, Peel NFA, et al: Prevention of bone loss with risedronate in glucocorticoid-treated rheumatoid arthritis patients. Osteoporos Int 2000;11:331-37.

44. Bressot C, Meunier PJ, Chapuy MC, et al: Histomorphometric profile, pathophysiology and reversibility of corticosteroid-induced osteoporosis. Metab Bone Dis Relat Res 1979;1:303-11.

45. Stellon AJ, Webb A, Compston JE: Bone histomorphometry and structure in corticosteroid treated chronic active hepatitis. Gut 1988;29:378-84.

46. Aaron JE, Francis RM, Peacock M, et al: Contrasting microanatomy of idiopathic and corticosteroid-induced osteoporosis. Clin Orthop 1989;243:294-305.

47. Dempster DW: Perspectives: bone histomorphometry in glucocorticoid-induced osteoporosis. J Bone Miner Res 1989;4:137-41.

48. Chappard D, Legrand E, Basle MF: Altered trabecular architecture induced by corticosteroids: a bone histomorphometric study. J Bone Miner Res 1996;11:676-85.

49. Dalle Carbonare L, Arlot ME, Chavassieux PM, et al: Comparison of trabecular bone microarchitecture and remodeling in glucocorticoid-induced and postmenopausal osteoporosis. J Bone Miner Res 2001;16:97-103.

50. Pocock NA, Eisman JA, Dunstan C, et al: Recovery from steroid-induced osteoporosis. Ann Intern Med 1987;107:319-23.

51. Gluck OS, Murphy WA, Hahn TJ, et al: Bone loss in adults receiving alternate day glucocorticoid therapy: a comparison with daily therapy. Arthritis Rheum 1981;24:892-98.

52. Rüegsegger P, Medici TC, Anliker M: Corticosteroid-induced bone loss: a longitudinal study of alternate day therapy in patients with bronchial asthma using quantitative computed tomography. Eur J Clin Pharmacol 1983;25:615-20.

53. Avgerinos PC, Cutler GB, Tsokos GC, et al: Dissociation between cortisol and adrenal androgen secretion in patients receiving alternate day prednisone therapy. J Clin Endocrinol Metab 1987;65:24-9.

54. Lipworth BJ: Therapeutic implications of non-genomic glucocorticoid activity. Lancet 2000;356:87-9.

55. Buttgereit F, Straub RH, Wehling M, et al: Glucocorticoids in the treatment of rheumatic diseases: an update of the mechanisms of action. Arthritis Rheum 2004;50:3408-17.

56. LoCascio V, Bonucci E, Imbimbo B, et al: Bone loss in response to long-term glucocorticoid therapy. Bone Miner 1990;8:39-51.

57. Kozower M, Veatch L, Kaplan MM: Decreased clearance of prednisolone, a factor in the development of corticosteroid side effects. J Clin Endocrinol Metab 1974;38:407-12.

58. Stevens A, Ray DW, Zeggini E, et al: Glucocorticoid sensitivity is determined by a specific glucocorticoid receptor haplotype. J Clin Endocrinol Metab 2004;89:892-97.

59. Tomlinson JN, Walker EA, Bujalska IJ, et al: 11 β-hydroxysteroid dehydrogenase type 1: a tissue-specific regulator of glucocorticoid response. Endocr Rev 2004;25:831-66.

60. Weinstein RS, Chen JR, Powers CC, et al: Promotion of osteoclast survival and antagonism of bisphosphonate-induced osteoclast apoptosis by glucocorticoids. J Clin Invest 2002;109:1041-48.

61. Weinstein RS, Jilka RL, Parfitt AM, et al: Inhibition of osteoblastogenesis and promotion of apoptosis of osteoblasts and osteocytes by glucocorticoids: potential mechanisms of their deleterious effects on bone. J Clin Invest 1998;102:274-82.

62. Godschalk MF, Downs RW: Effect of short-term glucocorticoids on serum osteocalcin in healthy young men. J Bone Miner Res 1988;3:113-15.

63. Noble BS, Stevens H, Loveridge N, et al: Identification of apoptotic changes in osteocytes in normal and pathological human bone. Bone 1997;20:273-82.

64. Qiu S, Rao DS, Palnitkar S, et al: Reduced iliac cancellous osteocyte density in patients with osteoporotic fracture. J Bone Miner Res 2003;18:1657-63.

65. Noble BS, Reeve J: At the cutting edge: osteocyte function, osteocyte death and bone fracture resistance. Mol Cell Endocrinol 2000;159:7-13.

66. Felson DT, Anderson JJ: Across-study evaluation of association between steroid dose and bolus steroids and avascular necrosis of bone. Lancet 1987;1:902-6.

67. Morris HA, Need AG, O'Loughlin PD, et al: Malabsorption of calcium in corticosteroid-induced osteoporosis. Calcif Tissue Int 1990;46:305-8.

68. Suzuki Y, Ichikawa Y, Saito E, et al: Importance of increased urinary calcium excretion in the development of secondary hyperparathyroidism of patients under glucocorticoid therapy. Metabolism 1983;32:151-56.

69. Prummel MF, Wiersinga WM, Lips P, et al: The course of biochemical parameters of bone turnover during treatment with corticosteroids. J Clin Endocrinol Metab 1991;72:382-86.

70. Yeh JK, Aloia JF: Influence of glucocorticoids on calcium absorption in different segments of the rat intestine. Calcif Tissue Int 1986;38:282-88.

71. Marcus R: Secondary forms of osteoporosis. In: Coe FC, Favus MJ, eds: Disorders of Bone and Mineral Metabolism. New York: Raven Press, 1992:889-904.

72. Paz-Pacheco E, El-Hajj Fuleihan G, Leboff MS: Intact parathyroid hormone levels are not elevated in glucocorticoid-treated subjects. J Bone Miner Res 1995;10:1713-18.

73. Silve C, Fritsch J, Grosse B, et al: Corticosteroid-induced changes in the responsiveness of human osteoblast-like cells to parathyroid hormone. Bone Miner 1989;6:65-75.

74. Rodan SB, Fischer MK, Egan JJ, et al: The effect of dexamethasone on parathyroid hormone stimulation of adenylate cyclase in ROS 17/2.8 cells. Endocrinology 1984;115:951-58.

75. Manolagas SC: Birth and death of bone cells: basic regulatory mechanisms and implications for the pathogenesis and treatment of osteoporosis. Endocr Rev 2000;21:115-37.

76. Hofbauer LC, Gori F, Riggs BL, et al: Stimulation of osteoprotegerin ligand and inhibition of osteoprotegerin production by glucocorticoids in human osteoblastic lineage cells: potential paracrine mechanisms of glucocorticoid-induced osteoporosis. Endocrinology 1999;140:4382-89.

77. Sasaki N, Kusano E, Ando Y, et al: Glucocorticoid decreases circulating osteoprotegerin (OPG): possible mechanism for glucocorticoid induced osteoporosis. Nephrol Dial Transplant 2001;16:479-82.

78. Sasaki N, Kusano E, Ando Y, et al: Changes in osteoprotegerin and markers of bone metabolism during glucocorticoid treatment in patients with chronic glomerulonephritis. Bone 2002;30:853-58.

79. von Tirpitz C, Epp S, Klaus J, et al: Effect of systemic glucocorticoid therapy on bone metabolism and the osteoprotegerin system in patients with active Crohn's disease. Eur J Gastroenterol Hepatol 2003;15:1165-70.

80. Ueland T, Bollerslev J, Godang K, et al: Increased serum osteoprotegerin in disorders characterized by persistent immune activation or glucocorticoid excess: possible role in bone homeostasis. Eur J Endocrinol 2001;145:685-90.

81. Hofbauer LC, Kühne CA, Viereck V: The OPG/RANKL/RANK system in metabolic bone diseases. J Musculoskel Neuron Interact 2004;4:268-75.

82. Boutsen Y, Jamart J, Esselinckx W, et al: Primary prevention of glucocorticoid-induced osteoporosis with intravenous pamidronate and calcium: a prospective controlled 1-year study comparing a single infusion, an infusion given once every 3 months, and calcium alone. J Bone Miner Res 2001;16:104-12.

22

Corticosteroid-Induced Osteoporosis

Philip N. Sambrook and Nancy E. Lane

SUMMARY

Corticosteroids affect bone through multiple effects but especially inhibitory actions on bone formation. Bone loss with corticosteroids is most rapid in the first year after starting, but is also dose dependent and influenced by the underlying disease. Postmenopausal women receiving corticosteroids are at the highest risk of rapid bone loss and should be actively considered for intervention. The first choice for prevention would be a potent oral bisphosphonate such as alendronate or risedronate. In patients intolerant of oral bisphosphonates, intravenous bisphosphonates should be considered or a vitamin D metabolite. Calcium and vitamin D should always be considered as adjunctive therapy.

Corticosteroids are widely used and effective for control of many inflammatory diseases, but corticosteroid-induced osteoporosis is a common problem associated with long-term high-dose use. Prevention of corticosteroid-induced bone loss is preferable to treatment of established corticosteroid-induced osteoporosis.

Cushing first described patients chronically treated with corticosteroids as having truncal obesity, proximal muscle wasting, thinning of the skin, increased skin fragility with ecchymoses, proximal muscle weakness, fluid retention, hyperglycemia, and vertebral compression fractures.[1] The most disabling side effect is osteoporotic fracture.[2,3]

PATHOPHYSIOLOGY OF CORTICOSTEROID-INDUCED BONE LOSS

Corticosteroids are known to affect bone through multiple pathways, influencing both bone formation and bone resorption.[2,4,5]

Corticosteroids have inhibitory effects on the osteoblast and osteoblast precursors, with studies also showing that corticosteroids can decrease messenger RNA levels encoding for osteoblast products such as osteocalcin.[6] At the organ level, direct inhibitory effects of corticosteroids on bone formation have also been observed in histomorphometric studies.[7,8]

Corticosteroids also decrease intestinal absorption of calcium[9-11] and increase urinary phosphate and calcium loss by direct effects on the kidney,[12] which, together with impaired calcium absorption, lead to secondary hyperparathyroidism[12] and hence enhanced bone resorption. The combination of enhanced activation frequency of bone remodeling units due to secondary hyperparathyroidism, together with an inadequate amount of new bone synthesis due to suppression of osteoblastic function, result in net bone loss with corticosteroid use. Enhanced osteoctye apoptosis has also recently been implicated as an important mechanism.[13,14]

The complex effects of corticosteroids on bone metabolism are reflected in marked changes in biochemical markers of bone turnover. Markers of bone formation such as serum osteocalcin fall rapidly after treatment with corticosteroids.[15] The degree of suppression of osteocalcin levels is related to corticosteroid dose.[15] Increased bone resorption has been demonstrated in histomorphometric studies,[7] and markers of bone resorption have been shown to rise after acute corticosteroid administration.[12] The histomorphometric picture that is characteristic of corticosteroid-treated patients is initially trabecular plate thinning, which may be followed by perforation and removal of entire trabecular plates.[16]

FRACTURES AND CORTICOSTEROID-INDUCED OSTEOPOROSIS

Osteoporosis has been reported to occur in up to 50% of persons who require long-term corticosteroid therapy. Some studies have reported a four- to fivefold increase in vertebral fracture prevalence in patients treated with corticosteroids, when compared with non-corticosteroid–treated patients.[10,17,18] In a large retrospective cohort study conducted in the United Kingdom,[3] subjects taking corticosteroids (n = 244, 235) were matched with control patients (n = 244, 235). The relative risk during oral corticosteroid therapy for vertebral fractures was 2.6, for hip fracture 1.6, and for nonvertebral fracture 1.3. Fracture risk increased with increasing daily doses of corticosteroids,[3] and when corticosteroids were discontinued, the fracture risk appeared to return to baseline. A study by Naganathan and coworkers[19] has shown the greatest risk of vertebral fracture is in older postmenopausal women and age was a risk factor independent of bone mineral density (BMD).

Fracture risk with corticosteroids is determined by several factors, including

- BMD, both its starting value before corticosteroid therapy and the amount of subsequent corticosteroid associated loss; thus, bone loss from an initially normal T-score in a premenopausal woman creates a different fracture risk to bone loss from a low T-score, for example, in a postmenopausal woman (Figure 22-1)[20,21]
- corticosteroid dose, as bone loss is dependent on cumulative and daily dosage
- duration of exposure, that is, a relatively short course of corticosteroids will cause bone loss that is largely reversible after stopping corticosteroids, but a sustained reduction in BMD from chronic steroid therapy increases the likelihood that a fracture will occur eventually
- the underlying disease for which corticosteroids are prescribed, which may be independently associated with increased fracture risk

Some studies have suggested that vertebral fractures due to corticosteroids occur at higher BMD values than observed in other types of osteoporosis. Van Staa and associates[22] reported higher fracture risks in postmenopausal women taking corticosteroids at similar BMD levels to postmenopausal women not taking corticosteroids. In contrast, Selby and associates[23] observed no increased risk of vertebral fracture in glucocorticoid-treated patients compared with other causes of osteoporosis when cumulative fracture prevalence was compared with BMD.

PATTERN OF BONE LOSS WITH CORTICOSTEROID TREATMENT

Bone loss with corticosteroid treatment appears most rapid in the first 12 months after starting therapy, followed by a slower decline in patients on chronic therapy. When high-dose corticosteroids are used, rates of loss in the spine range between 5% and 15% per annum.[24] In a longitudinal histomorphometric study, treatment with prednisone (10-25 mg/day) resulted in a 27.1% decrease in iliac crest cancellous bone volume by 6 months.[8] In patients on chronic low-dose therapy, continuing slower bone loss or no loss occurs.[25] Corticosteroid-induced bone loss may be reversible on cessation, as illustrated by recovery in bone density after successful treatment of Cushing syndrome.[26]

Corticosteroid bone loss appears dose dependent, although a longitudinal study observed loss averaging 9.5% over 20 weeks from spinal trabecular bone in patients receiving a mean dose of 7.5 mg prednisone per day,[27] suggesting that even lower doses of corticosteroids can cause bone loss in some patients.

Although inhaled steroids are less likely to have systemic effects than oral corticosteroids, in higher doses they result in adrenal suppression, growth impairment, and reduced bone density.[28-30] Wong and colleagues[31] reported a large cross-sectional study of patients receiving long-term inhaled corticosteroids for asthma and found a significant inverse relationship between corticosteroid dose (or duration of corticosteroid therapy) and bone density at the spine and hip.

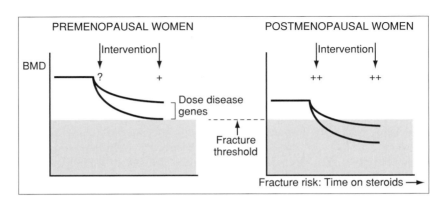

Figure 22-1. The degree of bone loss from corticosteroids varies according to dose, underlying disease, and possibly genetic factors. The case for intervention is strong early (primary prevention) in postmenopausal women but is less clear in premenopausal women. Because fracture risk is a function of the duration of corticosteroid use, secondary prevention is appropriate to consider in pre- and postmenopausal women on long-term corticosteroid treatment with low BMD. (From Sambrook PN: Corticosteroid osteoporosis: practical implications of recent trials. J Bone Miner Res 2000;15:1645-49.) (See Color Plates.)

INVESTIGATION OF PATIENTS TREATED WITH CORTICOSTEROIDS

Bone Mineral Density

The effects of corticosteroids on BMD can be measured precisely and accurately using dual-energy x-ray absorptiometry (DXA) of the lumbar spine, hip, and distal forearm or quantitative computed tomography for the lumbar spine. The earliest changes of glucocorticoid-induced bone loss are seen in the lumbar spine because of its high content of trabecular bone. It is recommended that physicians obtain a DXA measurement of the lumbar spine (anteroposterior scan) and femoral neck when subjects are initiating corticosteroid treatment or soon after. Lateral DXA measurement is not recommended due to positioning issues and its poorer precision and accuracy. Repeat DXA scans are recommended to monitor for bone loss. The role of biochemical markers of bone turnover in diagnosis and management remains unclear.

TREATMENT

Because the most rapid bone loss occurs in the first 12 to 24 months in patients commencing high-dose corticosteroids, it is important to consider two therapeutic situations: (a) primary prevention in patients starting corticosteroids and (b) treatment (or secondary prevention) in patients on chronic corticosteroids who will almost certainly have some significant degree of existing corticosteroid-related bone loss.[32] Although the terms *secondary prevention* and *treatment* can be used interchangeably, from a clinical point of view, primary prevention of bone loss in patients starting high-dose corticosteroids for the first time is preferred.[32,33]

Current therapeutic approaches include

- use of the lowest corticosteroid dose possible
- use of agents that prevent or reverse bone loss.

Agents that have been investigated for potential benefit include antiresorptive agents (such as calcium, vitamin D, calcitonin, hormone replacement therapy, and bisphosphonates) and anabolics (such as parathyroid hormone [PTH]). Although the effects of corticosteroids on bone formation appear more important than those on bone resorption, antiresorptives appear effective by reducing steroid effects on bone remodeling and preserving microarchitecture.

Antiresorptive Agents

Hormone replacement therapy is often recommended for glucocorticoid-treated patients, but the supporting evidence is limited. There have been only two controlled trials in men. In a crossover study of 15 men receiving chronic steroids for asthma, testosterone 250 mg/month increased lumbar BMD by 5% after 12 months, which was significant compared with the calcium group.[34] Similarly, testosterone supplementation was superior to both nandrolone and placebo in a trial of 51 men, increasing lumbar BMD by 5.6% over 12 months.[35] In a randomized trial in postmenopausal women with rheumatoid arthritis, a small subgroup received chronic low-dose steroids plus estrogen and they increased lumbar BMD by 3.8% over 2 years compared with a 0.6% loss in the calcium-treated group.[36] None of these studies was powered for fracture.

These studies suggest an apparent benefit of calcium therapy for secondary prevention in patients receiving chronic low-dose corticosteroids, but most recent trials in patients starting corticosteroids in which calcium alone was used as the control therapy observed rapid rates of loss.[37-39] This suggests that calcium alone is probably insufficient to prevent rapid bone loss in patients starting high-dose corticosteroids.

Calcium is often used in combination with vitamin D in patients with corticosteroid-induced osteoporosis based on studies in the 1970s that measured only forearm BMD,[40] so their clinical relevance to vertebral fracture risk is unclear. Adachi and colleagues[41] compared combination calcium/vitamin D (1000 mg daily plus 50,000 U weekly, respectively) with placebo over 3 years in 62 patients starting corticosteroids (i.e., primary prevention). Bone loss at the lumbar spine was not significantly different between groups receiving calcium/vitamin D or placebo, and the amount of bone loss observed over 1 year with the calcium/vitamin D combination (4.9%) was similar to that seen in the calcium-treated control groups in other recent prevention studies.[37,39] However, a secondary prevention study by Buckley and associates[42] in 65 patients receiving chronic low-dose corticosteroids for rheumatoid arthritis observed an annual spinal loss of 2.0% in placebo-treated patients compared with a 0.7% gain in calcium/vitamin D_3–treated patients (1000 mg plus 500 IU/day, respectively). Other studies suggest an apparent benefit of calcium therapy for secondary prevention in patients receiving chronic low-dose corticosteroids,[34,36] but calcium alone is probably insufficient to prevent rapid bone loss in patients starting high-dose corticosteroids.[37-39]

Although the term *vitamin D* is sometimes used to encompass both the calciferols and active metabolites, they have quite distinct therapeutic effects. The most commonly used active hormonal forms of vitamin D are calcitriol (1,25-dihydroxy vitamin D) and alfacalcidol (1α-hydroxyvitamin D). A number of studies have examined their use in primary prevention of glucocorticoid-induced osteoporosis. One study compared the effect of calcium, calcitriol, or calcitonin in 103 patients starting corticosteroids.[37] Patients treated with calcium lost bone rapidly at the lumbar spine (−4.3% in 1 year), whereas patients treated with either calcitriol or calcitriol plus calcitonin lost at a much reduced rate (−1.3% and −0.2% per year, respectively). Results in both groups were significantly different from those in the calcium group. Another randomized double-blind controlled trial in 145 patients compared alfacalcidol with calcium.[43] After 12 months, the change in spinal BMD with alfacalcidol was +0.4% compared with −5.7% with calcium.

Another study has evaluated the efficacy of active vitamin D metabolites compared with simple vitamin D in patients on chronic corticosteroids.[44] Eighty-five patients on long-term corticosteroid therapy were randomized to either 1 µg alfacalcidol plus calcium 500 mg daily or 1000 IU vitamin D3 plus 500 mg calcium. Over 3 years, a small but significant increase was seen in lumbar spine BMD in the alfacalcidol group (+2.0%; $P < .0001$), with no significant changes at the femoral neck. Other studies have not revealed any benefit of active vitamin D metabolites compared with plain vitamin D.[45] Calcitonin has also been studied in patients starting corticosteroids and receiving chronic corticosteroids, with equivocal results. In two primary prevention studies, there was no statistically significant additional benefit of adding calcitonin to calcitriol or cholecalciferol.[37,46]

Several trials have examined the efficacy of bisphosphonates on corticosteroid-induced bone loss and vertebral fractures. Adachi and associates[41] studied 141 patients starting corticosteroids (i.e., primary prevention) who received prophylaxis with either cyclical etidronate or calcium. After 12 months, mean lumbar BMD change with etidronate was +0.6% compared with −3.2% in the calcium group. For postmenopausal women, there was a significant difference in the incidence of new vertebral fractures favoring etidronate (21.9% vs 3.2%). Saag and coworkers[47] reported the results of 477 corticosteroid-treated subjects who received prophylaxis with alendronate or calcium/vitamin D (800-1000 mg daily plus 250-500 IU daily, respectively). Patients were stratified according to whether they had received corticosteroids for less than 4 months, 4 to 12 months, or more than 12 months. Over 12 months of follow-up, the mean change in lumbar spine BMD in patients in the primary prevention group was +3.0% for alendronate 10 mg/day compared with −1% in the placebo group. In those who had received chronic corticosteroids for more than 12 months, the increase with alendronate was +2.8% compared with +0.2% for calcium. These data again suggest that supplementation with calcium/vitamin D is able to prevent further bone loss in patients taking chronic low-dose corticosteroids (secondary prevention). A post hoc analysis of incident vertebral fractures determined semiquantitatively significantly favored alendronate in postmenopausal women only (13% vs 4.4%). Cohen and coworkers[39] reported the results of a primary prevention trial in 224 corticosteroid-treated subjects who received prophylaxis with either residronate or calcium. Residronate 5 mg per day prevented spinal bone loss (+0.6%) as compared with calcium (−2.8%) over 12 months. Incident vertebral fracture rates were 17.3 % with calcium and 5.7 % for residronate 5 mg ($P = .072$). Vertebral fractures were only seen in postmenopausal women and men. Reid and associates[48] examined the effects of risedronate in 290 patients receiving chronic corticosteroid treatment (prednisone >7.5 mg/day for >6 months). Approximately one-third of patients had vertebral fractures at baseline. The control group, who was treated with calcium (1000 mg) plus vitamin D (400 IU) daily, showed a stable BMD over 12 months. However, treatment with risedronate in a dose of 5 mg significantly increased lumbar spine (+2.9%) and femoral neck (+1.8%) BMD. Treatment with risedronate 2.5 mg daily showed a similar though nonsignificant trend. Although not powered for fractures, 15% of patients in the control group versus 5% in the risedronate groups sustained new vertebral fractures, suggesting a 70% reduction in fracture rate. Boutsen and colleagues[49] performed a prevention study with intravenous pamidronate (90 mg for the first infusion, then 30 mg every 3 months plus calcium) for 12 months and found nearly a 4% increase in lumbar spine bone mass and a 3% increase in femoral neck bone mass, whereas the placebo group had a −6% change at the lumbar spine and a −4.1% change at the femoral neck.

Anabolic Agents

Lane and colleagues[50] performed a randomized controlled trial of hPTH (1-34) in estrogen-treated postmenopausal women with corticosteroid-induced osteoporosis (see Chapter 19). The patients treated with hPTH and estrogens had significant increases in bone mass (+35% by lumbar spine quantitative computed tomography, +11% by lumbar spine DXA, 1% hip) after 12 months, and essentially no changes were observed in the control group. All study patients were followed for an additional year after the hPTH (1-34) was discontinued, and total hip and femoral neck bone mass increased about 5% above baseline levels.[51] Treatment with PTH resulted in a dramatic increase in the biochemical markers of bone turnover. Bone formation, measured by osteocalcin, increased more than 150% above baseline levels within 1 month of the start of therapy and remained elevated for the treatment period. Bone resorption, measured with deoxypyridinoline cross-links, increased to the same levels as the bone formation marker, but this required 6 months of therapy.[50] The study was too small to determine whether hPTH (1-34) could reduce the incidence of new vertebral fractures.

CONCLUSION

Evidence from randomized controlled trials suggests that postmenopausal women receiving corticosteroids are at high risk of rapid bone loss and consequent vertebral fracture and should be actively considered for prophylactic measures. In men and premenopausal women receiving corticosteroids, the decision to intervene is less straightforward and depends on a number of factors, including the baseline BMD and anticipated dose and duration of corticosteroids. Based on the available evidence, the first choice for prevention would be a potent oral bisphosphonate such as alendronate or risedronate. In patients intolerant of oral bisphosphonates, intravenous bisphosphonates should be considered, or a vitamin D metabolite. Calcium alone appears unable to prevent rapid bone loss in patients starting corticosteroids, but calcium and vitamin D are appropriate adjunctive therapy. Testosterone should be considered if hypogonadism is present in men. Most clinical trial data are limited to 1 to 2 years, but it is likely that prophylactic therapy needs to be continued while patients continue taking significant doses of corticosteroid therapy. In patients receiving chronic low-dose corticosteroids (<7 mg/d of prednisone or its equivalent), treatment with calcium and vitamin D may be sufficient to prevent further bone loss, but if BMD is markedly low, a bisphosphonate should be used or PTH considered, because fracture risk is a function of multiple factors, including the degree of reduction in BMD and the duration of exposure to corticosteroids.

REFERENCES

1. Cushing H: The basophil adenomas of the pituitary body and their clinical manifestations. Bull Johns Hopkins Hosp 1932;50:137-95.
2. Sambrook PN, Lane NE: Corticosteroid osteoporosis. Balliere Best Pract Res Clin Rheumatol 2001;15:401-13.
3. Van Staa TP, Leufkens HGM, Abenhaim L, et al: Use of oral corticosteroids and risk of fractures. J Bone Miner Res 2000;15:993-1000.
4. Canalis E, Bilzekian JP, Angeli A, Giustina A: Perspectives on glucocorticoid induced osteoporosis. Bone 2004;34:593-98.
5. Weinstein RS: Glucocorticoid-induced osteoporosis. Rev Endocr Metab Disord 2001;2:65-73.
6. Morrison NA, Shine J, Verkest V, et al: 1,25 Dihydroxyvitamin D responsive element and glucocorticoid repression in the osteocalcin gene. Science 1989;246:1158-61.
7. Bressot C, Meunier PJ, Chapuy MC, et al: Histomorphometric profile, pathophysiology and reversibility of corticosteroid induced osteoporosis. Metab Bone Dis Rel Res 1979;1:303-11.
8. LoCascio V, Bonnucci E, Imbimbo B, et al: Bone loss in response to long-term glucocorticoid therapy. Bone Mineral 1992;8:39-51.
9. Klein RG, Arnaud SB, Gallagher JC, et al: Intestinal calcium absorption in exogenous hypercortisolism: role of 25-hydroxyvitamin D and corticosteroid dose. J Clin Invest 1977;60:253-59.
10. Hahn TJ, Halstead LR, Bran DT: Effects of short term glucocorticoid administration on intestinal calcium absorption and circulating vitamin D metabolite concentrations in man. J Clin Endocr Metab 1981;52:111-15.
11. Morris HA, Need AG, O'Loughlin PD, et al: Malabsorption of calcium in corticosteroid-induced osteoporosis, Calcif Tiss Int 1990;46:305-8.
12. Cosman F, Nieves J, Herbert J, et al: High-dose corticosteroids in multiple sclerosis patients exert direct effects on the kidney and skeleton. J Bone Miner Res 1994;9:1097-105.
13. Weinstein RS, Jilka RL, Parfitt AF, Manalagas SC: Inhibition of osteoblastogenesis and promotion of apoptosis of osteoblasts and osteocytes by corticosteroids. J Clin Invest 1998;102:272-82.
14. Sambrook PN, Hughes DR, Nelson AE, et al: Osteocyte viability with glucocorticoid therapy: relation to histomorphometry. Ann Rheum Dis 2003;62:1215-17.
15. Kotowicz MA, Hall S, Hunder GG, et al: Relationship of glucocorticoid dosage to serum bone Gla-protein concentration in patients with rheumatologic disorders. Arthritis Rheum 1990;33:1487-92.
16. Chappard D, Legrand E, Basle MF, et al: Altered trabecular architecture induced by corticosteroids: a bone histomorphometric study. J Bone Miner Res 1996;11:676-85.
17. Adinoff AD, Hollister JR: Steroid-induced fractures and bone loss in patients with asthma. N Engl J Med 1983;309:265-68.
18. Verstraeten A, Dequeker J: Vertebral and peripheral bone mineral content and fracture incidence in postmenopausal patients with rheumatoid arthritis. Ann Rheum Dis 1986;45:852-57.
19. Naganathan V, Jones G, Nash P, et al: Vertebral fracture risk with long term corticosteroids: prevalence, relationship to age, bone density and corticosteroid use. Arch Intern Med 2000;160:2917-22.
20. Gough AKS, Lilley J, Eyre S, et al: Generalised bone loss in patients with early rheumatoid arthritis occurs early and relates to disease activity. Lancet 1994;344:23-7.
21. Pearce G, Ryan PF, Delmas PD, et al: The deleterious effects of low-dose corticosteroids on bone density in patients with polymyalgia rheumatica. Br J Rheumatol 1998;37:292-99.
22. Van Staa TP, Laan RF, Barton IP, et al: Bone density threshold and other predictors of vertebral fracture in patients receiving oral glucocorticoid therapy. Arthritis Rheum 2003;48:3224-29.
23. Selby PL, Halsey JP, Adams KRH, et al: Corticosteroids do not alter the threshold for vertebral fractures. J Bone Miner Res 2000;15:952-56.
24. Sambrook PN, Kempler S, Birmingham J, et al: Corticosteroid effects on proximal femur bone loss. J Bone Miner Res 1990;5:1211-16.
25. Sambrook PN, Eisman JA, Champion GD, et al: Effect of low dose corticosteroids on bone mass in rheumatoid arthritis: a longitudinal study, Ann Rheum Dis 1989;48:535-38.
26. Pocock NA, Eisman JA, Dunstan CR, et al: Recovery from steroid-induced osteoporosis. Ann Intern Med 1987;107:319-23.
27. Laan RFJM, Van Riel PLCM, Van de Putte LBA: Low dose prednisone induces rapid reversible axial bone loss in patients with rheumatoid arthritis. Ann Intern Med 1993;119:963-68.
28. Priftis K, Everard ML, Milner AD: Unexpected side effects of inhaled steroids: a case report. Eur J Pediatr 1991;150:448-49.
29. Packe GE, Douglas JG, McDonald AF, et al: Bone density in asthmatic patients taking high dose inhaled beclomethasone and intermittent systemic corticosteroids. Thorax 1992;47:414-17.
30. Ebeling PR, Erbas B, Hopper JL, et al: Bone mineral density and bone turnover in asthmatics treated with long term inhaled or oral corticosteroids. J Bone Miner Res 1998;13:1283-89.
31. Wong CA, Walsh LJ, Smith CJP, et al: Inhaled corticosteroid use and bone mineral density in patients with asthma. Lancet 2000;355:1399-403.
32. Sambrook PN: Corticosteroid osteoporosis: practical implications of recent trials. J Bone Miner Res 2000;15:1645-49.
33. Cunnane G, Lane NE: Steroid-induced osteoporosis in systemic lupus erythematous. Rheum Dis Clin North Am 2000;26:211-29.
34. Reid IR, Wattie DJ, Evans MC, Stapleton JP: Testosterone therapy in glucocorticoid-treated men. Arch Intern Med 1996;156:1173-77.

35. Crawford BAL, Liu PY, Bleasel JF, Handelsman DJ: Randomised placebo-controlled trial of androgen effects on muscle and bone in men requiring long term systemic glucocorticoid treatment. J Clin Endocr Metab 2003;88:3167-76.
36. Hall GM, Daniels M, Doyle DV, Spector TD: The effect of hormone replacement therapy on bone mass in rheumatoid arthritis treated with and without steroids. Arthritis Rheum 1994;37:1499-505.
37. Sambrook PN, Birmingham J, Kelly PJ, et al: Prevention of corticosteroid osteoporosis: a comparison of calcium, calcitriol and calcitonin. N Engl J Med 1993;328:1747-52.
38. Adachi JD, Bensen WG, Brown J, et al: Intermittent etidronate therapy to prevent corticosteroid-induced osteoporosis. N Engl J Med 1997;337:382-87.
39. Cohen S, Levy RM, Keller M, et al: Resridronate therapy prevents corticosteroid-induced bone loss. Arthritis Rheum 1999;42:2309-18.
40. Hahn TJ, Hahn BH: Osteopenia in subjects with rheumatic diseases: principles of diagnosis and therapy. Semin Arthritis Rheum 1976;6:165-88.
41. Adachi J, Bensen W, Bianchi F, et al: Vitamin D and calcium in the prevention of corticosteroid-induced osteoporosis: a three year follow up study. J Rheumatol 1996;23:995-1000.
42. Buckley LM, Leib ES, Cartularo KS, et al: Calcium and vitamin D3 supplementation prevents bone loss in the spine secondary to low dose corticosteroids in patients with rheumatoid arthritis. Ann Intern Med 1996;125:961-68.
43. Reginster JY, Kuntz D, Verdicht W, et al: Prophylactic use of alfacalcidol in corticosteroid-induced osteoporosis. Osteoporos Int 1999;9:75-81.
44. Ringe JD, Coster A, Meng T, et al: Treatment of glucocorticoid-induced osteoporosis with alfacalcidol/calcium versus vitamin D/calcium. Calcif Tissue Int 1999;65:337-40.
45. Sambrook PN, Kotowicz M, Nash P, et al: Prevention and treatment of glucocorticoid induced osteoporosis: a comparison of calcitriol, vitamin D plus calcium and alendronate plus calcium. J Bone Miner Res 2003;18:919-24.
46. Healey J, Paget S, Williams-Russo P, et al: Randomised trial of salmon calcitonin to prevent bone loss in corticosteroid treated temporal arteritis and polymyalgia rheumatica. Calcif Tissue Int 1996;58:73-80.
47. Saag K, Emkey R, Schnitzler TJ, et al: Alendronate for the prevention and treatment of glucocorticoid induced osteoporosis. N Engl J Med 1998;339:292-99.
48. Reid DM, Hughes RA, Laan RFJM, et al: Efficacy and safety of daily risedronate in the treatment of corticosteroid induced osteoporosis in men and women: a randomised trial. J Bone Miner Res 2000;15:1006-13.
49. Boutsen Y, Jamart J, Esselinckx W, et al: Primary prevention of glucocorticoid-induced osteoporosis with intermittent intravenous pamidronate: a randomized trial. Calcif Tissue Int 1997;61:266-71.
50. Lane NE, Sanchez S, Modin GW, et al: Parathyroid hormone treatment can reverse corticosteroid-induced osteoporosis. J Clin Invest 1998;102:1627-33.
51. Lane NE, Pierini E, Modin G, et al: Bone mass continues to increase after parathyroid hormone treatment is stopped in glucocorticoid-induced osteoporosis. J Bone Miner Res 2000;15:944-51.

23 Osteoporosis after Solid Organ Transplantation

Naim M. Maalouf and Elizabeth Shane

SUMMARY

Post-transplantation bone loss and fractures cause substantial morbidity, particularly during the early post-transplant period and are influenced by a number of factors including the type of transplant and the immunosuppressive regimen used. Since the most rapid rates of bone loss and highest fracture incidence occur during the early posttransplant period, therapy should be considered before transplantation in patients with osteoporosis or immediately after transplantation in patients with normal BMD or osteopenia. Bisphosphonates should be considered first line therapy for prevention of bone loss during the first year after organ transplantation, but calcitriol can also be used as primary prevention or adjunctive therapy. Some controversy exists regarding management in the renal transplant population and the decision to use bisphosphonates in the long term renal transplant patient should be preceded by clinical evaluation to rule out other bone pathology.

Solid organ transplantation has become an established treatment option for several disease states, including acute and chronic liver failure, end-stage renal disease, end-stage pulmonary disease, and heart failure. The number of organs transplanted in the United States has increased steadily over the past few decades, and almost doubled since 1988, reaching nearly 25,000 in 2002 (Figure 23-1).[1] Thus, the total number of patients who have undergone solid organ transplantation in the United States now exceeds 300,000. With the increasing number of transplanted organs and the improved survival of transplant recipients, bone disease has emerged as a common complication of the transplantation process. Osteoporosis can be seen in up to one-half of transplant recipients, and vertebral fractures are found in almost one-third of the patients (Table 23-1).[2]

PATHOGENESIS OF TRANSPLANTATION-RELATED OSTEOPOROSIS

Many factors contribute to the pathogenesis of osteoporosis after organ transplantation. These include bone disease preceding transplantation, immunosuppressive medications, nutritional and lifestyle factors, and derangements of the parathyroid-calcium-vitamin D axis and the pituitary-gonadal axis (Figure 23-2). In this section, these factors are examined and discussed separately, although one should keep in mind that they are all intertwined in the context of organ transplantation.

Figure 23-1. Number of solid organs transplanted yearly in the United States since 1988. (Data from United Network for Organ Sharing.[1])

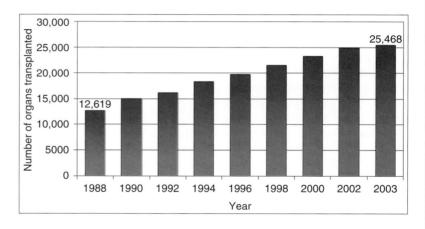

TABLE 23-1 PREVALENCE OF OSTEOPOROSIS* AND FRACTURES AFTER SOLID ORGAN TRANSPLANTATION		
	Prevalence after Transplantation, %	
Type of Transplant	Osteoporosis	Fracture
Kidney	11-56	Vertebral: 3-29 Peripheral: 11-22
Heart	25-50	Vertebral: 22-35
Liver	30-46	Vertebral: 29-47
Lung	57-73	42

*Defined as bone mineral density T-score < −2.5.
From Cohen A, Shane E: Osteoporosis after solid organ and bone marrow transplantation. Osteoporos Int 2003;14:617-30. © Springer 2003.

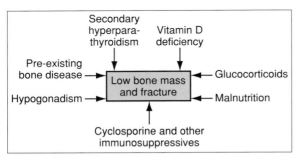

Figure 23-2. The multifactorial pathogenesis of osteoporosis after solid-organ transplantation. (Redrawn from Compston JE: Osteoporosis after liver transplantation. Liver Transplant 2003;9:321-30.)

Pretransplantation Bone Disease

Candidates for organ transplantation frequently suffer from fractures or osteoporosis, or both. Advanced age, poor nutrition, immobility, hypogonadism, cachexia, and lifestyle factors (such as smoking and alcohol abuse) frequently contribute to the poor skeletal health of patients with organ failure requiring transplantation. In addition, hepatic, pulmonary, cardiac, and renal failure have unique pathophysiologies that affect bone health before transplantation. These particular features are examined in this section.

Hepatic Osteodystrophy

Osteoporosis and fractures are relatively common findings in patients with chronic liver disease. Osteoporosis is found in 37% to 53% of cirrhotic patients referred for orthotopic liver transplantation.[3-5] Osteoporosis is seen more often in patients with primary biliary cirrhosis, in part because this condition mostly affects postmenopausal women, a patient population already at risk for osteoporosis.[6] A wide range of vertebral fracture rates (3-44%) has been reported among cirrhotic patients, and this is likely due to differences in the populations studied.[7] In some reports, bone histomorphometry studies have shown decreased bone volume,

accompanied by a reduction in parameters that reflect bone formation (osteoblast number, osteoblast surface area, bone formation rate)[8,9] and, in some reports, an increase in parameters reflecting bone resorption (osteoclast number, bone resorption surface).[9,10]

The decreased bone formation in patients with chronic liver disease has been ascribed to several factors, including excessive alcohol use, decreased hepatic synthesis of insulin-like growth factor-1 (IGF-1) levels, and hyperbilirubinemia. Alcohol use by itself has been implicated, even in the absence of chronic liver damage.[11] IGF-1, a trophic hormone produced in the liver in response to growth hormone, is known to stimulate both osteoblast proliferation and differentiation.[12,13] In a study of 32 consecutive patients with nonalcoholic liver cirrhosis, serum IGF-1 levels were lower than in control healthy subjects, and even lower levels were seen among cirrhotic patients who had osteoporosis.[14] In another study,[15] hyperbilirubinemia was found to reversibly impair osteoblast proliferation in vitro.

The increased bone resorption seen in some patients with advanced liver disease has been partly attributed to hypogonadism, a common finding in patients with cirrhosis. In a study comparing 39 male patients referred for liver transplantation with matched normal volunteers, more than one-half of the patients had decreased testosterone levels (Figure 23-3).[5] In addition, sex

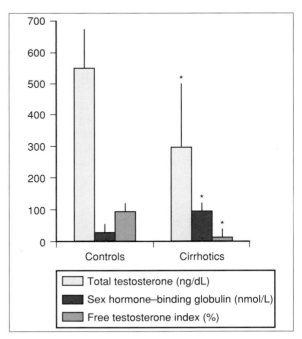

Figure 23-3. Plasma testosterone, sex hormone–binding globulin, and free testosterone in patients with cirrhosis and healthy age-matched control subjects. Data shown as mean and SD. * $P < .001$. (Redrawn from Monegal A, Navasa M, Guanabens N, et al: Osteoporosis and bone mineral metabolism disorders in cirrhotic patients referred for orthotopic liver transplantation. Calcif Tissue Int 1997;60:148-54. © Springer 1997.)

hormone–binding globulin was significantly increased, resulting in a marked reduction in the free testosterone index in cirrhotic patients compared with control subjects.[5] Basal levels of luteinizing hormone and follicle-stimulating hormone range from normal to moderately elevated,[16] implying defects both at the hypothalamic-pituitary level and at the gonadal level.

Additional factors contributing to osteoporosis in patients with liver cirrhosis include vitamin D deficiency, due to decreased hepatic synthesis of 25-hydroxy-vitamin D [25(OH)D] or to intestinal malabsorption, and glucocorticoid use (in the treatment of chronic autoimmune hepatitis).[17] Osteomalacia is a rare cause of reduced bone mineral density (BMD) in cases of hepatic osteodystrophy.[17]

Osteoporosis in End-Stage Pulmonary Disease

Patients with end-stage pulmonary disease commonly have osteoporosis,[18,19] and radiological evidence of vertebral fractures is seen in up to 29% of patients.[18,20] Risk factors for osteoporosis in patients with advanced lung disease include smoking, decreased ambulation, low body weight, and glucocorticoid use.[21] Cystic fibrosis is associated with additional risk factors, such as hypogonadism,[22] malnutrition, and pancreatic insufficiency, that may impair the absorption of calcium and vitamin D.[23,24] Pulmonary infections and the secondary release of inflammatory bone-resorbing cytokines have also been associated with increased bone resorption in patients with cystic fibrosis.[25] These patients typically have elevated levels of bone resorption markers, with normal levels of bone formation markers when compared with healthy control subjects.[26] In cystic fibrosis, the predominant finding on bone histomorphometry is reduced

cancellous bone area and osteoblast number, along with abnormalities in osteoclast number and activity.[27]

In a study of 70 patients with end-stage pulmonary disease awaiting lung transplantation, osteoporosis was present in 30% of patients at the lumbar spine and 49% at the femoral neck, and osteopenia was present in an additional one-third of the patients.[18] In the same study, vitamin D deficiency was more common among patients with cystic fibrosis than among patients with other lung diseases.[18]

Bone Disease in Congestive Heart Failure

Low BMD is frequently found in patients with congestive heart failure (CHF),[28,29] and 14% of patients with CHF awaiting transplantation had radiological evidence of vertebral compression fractures in one study.[29] In a report of 101 patients with severe CHF (New York Heart Association functional classes III and IV), referred for evaluation for cardiac transplantation, osteoporosis at the lumbar spine was seen in 7% and osteopenia in another 43% (Figure 23-4).[28]

In that same cohort, the mean serum 25(OH)D level was 21 ng/mL, and 17% had a frankly low 25(OH)D (<9 ng/mL). Low serum 25(OH)D levels in patients with severe CHF are probably due to a combination of factors, including insufficient synthesis in the skin (due to lack of sunlight exposure from decreased mobility), impaired vitamin D absorption due to bowel edema, and passive liver congestion impairing hepatic 25-hydroxylation of vitamin D. Low serum 25(OH)D levels are also associated with diminished exercise tolerance, as peak oxygen consumption during treadmill exercise testing was lower in patients with low 25(OH)D.[28]

Additional factors associated with CHF and its therapy that may contribute to bone loss include hypogonadism,

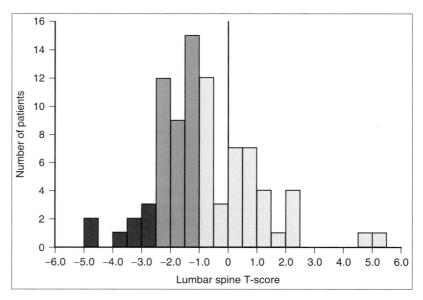

Figure 23-4. Frequency of distribution of lumbar spine bone mineral density in patients with severe congestive heart failure, expressed as T-score. Medium-shaded bars indicate osteopenia, dark-shaded bars indicate osteoporosis. (Redrawn from Shane E, Mancini D, Aaronson K, et al: Bone mass, vitamin D deficiency, and hyperparathyroidism in congestive heart failure. Am J Med 1997;103:197-97.)

long-term heparin administration and loop diuretic administration, mild renal insufficiency, and secondary hyperparathyroidism.[30]

Renal Osteodystrophy

Bone disease is found in virtually all patients with chronic kidney disease once glomerular filtration rate falls below 60 mL/min.[31,32] Compared with the general population, end-stage renal disease (ESRD) patients are 4.4-fold more likely to sustain a hip fracture, and the prevalence of vertebral fractures is as high as 21%.[33] Risk factors for fractures among patients with ESRD include older age, female sex, and duration of dialysis.[34,35]

The pathogenesis of renal osteodystrophy is complex, and several different mechanisms contribute to poor skeletal health. Based on histological features, renal osteodystrophy is classified as osteitis fibrosa, osteomalacia, adynamic disease, or mixed type (Table 23-2). Osteitis fibrosa, mainly caused by secondary hyperparathyroidism, is characterized by increased bone turnover and osteoclast activity resulting in increased resorption depth. The characteristic finding in osteomalacia is a mineralization defect with accumulation of unmineralized osteoid and low rates of bone turnover. Adynamic renal bone disease is characterized by decreased remodeling activity, and its pathogenesis remains poorly understood. Hypogonadism, β-microglobulin amyloidosis, and medications such as prednisone and cytotoxic drugs used in glomerulonephritis are all additional factors not shown in Table 23-2 that adversely affect skeletal health before renal transplantation.

Serum concentrations of parathyroid hormone (PTH) and bone-specific alkaline phosphatase, as well as BMD measurements, provide limited information on the degree and type of bone involvement. However, the gold standard in the diagnosis and classification of the skeletal lesions in renal osteodystrophy remains quantitative histomorphometry of transiliac crest bone biopsies after tetracycline labeling, an invasive procedure that is unfortunately of limited availability.[31] It should be stressed that measurement of BMD cannot be applied to the diagnosis of osteoporosis in patients with ESRD, as this technique does not distinguish among the various possible histological lesions that may be present and BMD may be low in any form of renal osteodystrophy.

Skeletal Effects of Immunosuppressive Drugs

Trends in the Use of Immunosuppressive Drugs

New trends in immunosuppressive drug use have arisen as novel molecules have become available. Since 1992, such trends have included the wider use of newer agents such as rapamycin and mycophenolate mofetil and an increase in the use of induction therapy with anti-

TABLE 23-2 CLASSIFICATION, DESCRIPTION, AND PATHOGENESIS OF RENAL OSTEODYSTROPHY		
Disorder	**Description**	**Pathogenesis**
Osteitis fibrosa	Increased remodeling frequency, increased osteoclast activity and resorption depth, marrow fibrosis	Secondary hyperparathyroidism
Osteomalacia	Defective mineralization, increased osteoid	Vitamin D deficiency, aluminum deposition, other unknown factors
A dynamic renal bone disease	Decreased remodeling, hypocellular bone surface	PTH oversuppression, other unknown factors

interleukin 2 receptor antibodies or antilymphocyte preparations. These trends have led to fewer episodes of rejection and lower cumulative glucocorticoid doses. Finally, a shift away from cyclosporine toward tacrolimus use has occurred in some transplantation programs.

Glucocorticoids

Glucocorticoids play a major role in the bone loss after transplantation. High doses (sometimes more than 1 mg/kg/day of prednisone) are usually prescribed immediately after transplantation, and the dose is then gradually tapered over the following few months. Additional doses may be given for the management of episodes of rejection.

The cause of glucocorticoid-induced osteoporosis is multifactorial (Figure 24-5). Early on, a phase of rapid bone loss is seen,[36] likely secondary to increased bone resorption due to a combination of renal calcium wasting,[37] decreased intestinal absorption of calcium,[38] and hypogonadotropic hypogonadism.[39,40] In addition, glucocorticoids directly promote osteoclastogenesis by increasing receptor activator of NF-κB ligand (RANKL) and decreasing osteoprotegerin.[41] With both acute and chronic use, bone formation is profoundly inhibited, as glucocorticoids reduce osteoblast proliferation, function (by inhibiting the expression of the genes for osteocalcin, type 1 collagen, and IGF-1),[41] and lifespan (by promoting osteoblast apoptosis).[42] In addition to their direct effects on the skeleton, glucocorticoids can induce a profound myopathy,[43] impairing balance and mobility, decreasing weight-bearing activity, and increasing the risk of falls and the potential for fractures.

Calcineurin Inhibitors

Cyclosporine A and tacrolimus (FK506) inhibit calcineurin, a T-cell phosphatase, and thus suppress T-cell

Figure 23-5. Factors involved in glucocorticoid-induced osteoporosis. Elevated RANKL/OPG ratio, hypogonadism, and secondary hyperparathyroidism contribute to the early and rapid phase of bone loss due to increased bone resorption. With acute and chronic use, bone formation is profoundly inhibited due to decreased proliferation, function, and lifespan of osteoblasts. OPG = osteoprotegerin; RANKL = receptor activator of NF-κB ligand.

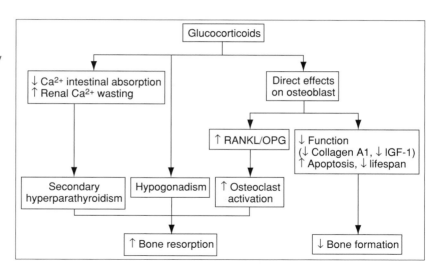

activation and production and release of interleukin-2 and other cytokines.[44] The isolated effects of calcineurin inhibitors on the human skeleton are somewhat unclear because, in the past, these drugs were rarely used alone (without glucocorticoids). Nowadays, more programs are using glucocorticoid-free regimens, so it may be possible to better address this issue.

In murine models, calcineurin inhibitors cause high turnover osteoporosis:[45] cyclosporine A stimulates both osteoclast and osteoblast activities in vivo, but resorption rates exceed formation rates, with a net loss in bone mass.[46,47]

T-lymphocytes are essential mediators of this bone loss, as T-cell–deficient rats (Rowett athymic nude rats) do not develop the expected cyclosporine A–mediated osteopenia.[48] Interestingly, and possibly related to the pathogenesis of bone disease, cyclosporine A–induced osteopenia is associated with testosterone deficiency[49] and is attenuated by parathyroidectomy.[50] A major side effect of cyclosporine A therapy is dose-related acute and chronic nephrotoxicity, often leading to secondary hyperparathyroidism,[51] which may also adversely affect skeletal health.

Tacrolimus, a fungal macrolide, also induces severe trabecular bone loss in rats,[45] although this bone loss may be less severe in humans than that induced by cyclosporine A.[52]

Other Immunosuppressive Agents

Other immunosuppressive agents could also affect bone metabolism, although the information available is limited: mycophenolate mofetil,[53] rapamycin,[54] and azathioprine[55] have shown no effects on bone volume in the rat model (Table 23-3).

TABLE 23-3 SKELETAL EFFECTS OF COMMONLY USED IMMUNOSUPPRESSIVE MEDICATIONS

Medication	Skeletal Effects
Glucocorticoids	Early: Increased resorption Late: Decreased bone formation and remodeling
Calcineurin Inhibitors	High turnover bone loss: Resorption greater than formation
Rapamycin	Rodents: Inhibits longitudinal growth, no osteoporosis
Azathioprine	Rodents: Increased osteoclast number, no change in bone volume
Mycophenolate Mofetil	No change in bone volume in rodents

Immobilization and Malnutrition after Transplantation

During the ever-longer times on the transplant waiting list, patients experience progressive disease-related decompensation, associated with reduced physical activity and malnutrition. In the absence of appropriate interventions, these complications can adversely affect skeletal health.[56]

Although the high-protein diet frequently recommended after transplantation is important for regain of muscle mass, it can also adversely affect bone metabolism. Protein catabolism generates large amounts of acid[57] that is partly buffered by the skeleton, leading to increased bone resorption and urinary excretion of calcium.[58] In addition, easing the restriction of sodium intake after transplantation could lead to sodium-induced urinary calcium losses and secondary increases in bone resorption.[59] Improvements in physical capacity and muscular strength after transplantation have been documented, although these levels remain lower than age-predicted levels in healthy populations.[60] Interestingly, severity of bone loss has been correlated with prolonged in-hospital stay after transplantation (and hence immobilization).[61]

Hypothalamic-Pituitary-Gonadal Axis after Transplantation

In many heart transplant recipients, testosterone levels fall immediately after transplantation but generally normalize within the first year (Figure 23-6).[62] Despite significant alterations in the hypothalamic-pituitary-gonadal axis and sex steroid metabolism before liver transplantation, physiological function resumes in the majority of patients after transplantation.[16] Specifically, serum gonadotropin and testosterone (total and free) levels increase in most liver transplant recipients, along with a decrease in estrogen and sex hormone–binding globulin levels 1 year after transplantation.[63] Although menstrual abnormalities are common in premenopausal women with chronic liver disease, transplantation leads to a restoration of normal menstrual function in 48% to 80% of cases, particularly in those who received transplantations for acute liver failure.[64,65] Renal transplantation corrects the hyperprolactinemia induced by uremia and is followed by restoration of the hypothalamic-pituitary-gonadal axis in many men and premenopausal women.[66,67] There is no published information on the gonadal function in lung transplant recipients.

Vitamin D and Parathyroid Hormone after Transplantation

Prospective studies in lung, heart, and liver transplant recipients indicate that serum 25(OH)D levels tend to gradually increase from the low levels seen before transplantation to normal levels, although this is likely related to the use of vitamin D supplements in most studies.[19,62,68]

A progressive increase in serum PTH concentration was noted in liver transplant recipients who were followed prospectively,[16,68] whereas no change was noted in the mildly elevated PTH levels after cardiac transplantation.[62] The mechanisms underlying the increased serum PTH levels are not well established but may be related to the decline in renal function seen in up to 20% of transplant recipients.[69]

In renal transplant recipients, serum PTH concentrations decrease progressively during the first 6 months after transplantation.[70] However, persistent hyperparathyroidism is detected in 25% to 43% of patients with a serum creatinine concentration of less than 1.5 mg/dL 1 year after grafting, probably due to the very slow involution of the hyperplastic parathyroid glands.[71,72] Pretransplant risk factors for persistent hyperparathyroidism in renal transplant recipients are longer time on dialysis and higher PTH levels.[73] Post-transplantation predictors include creatinine clearance (CrCl) of less than 70 mL/min, use of cyclosporine A, and low serum 25(OH)D levels.[74,75]

BONE LOSS AND FRACTURES AFTER TRANSPLANTATION

Bone Mineral Density after Transplantation

After solid organ transplantation, large decreases in bone density are observed in the first year. This decrease occurs mainly in the first 3 to 6 months[16,62,76,77] and is likely related to the large doses of glucocorticoids used immediately after grafting (Figure 23-7).[17,78] Early bone loss involves the lumbar spine (cancellous bone), a finding typical of glucocorticoid-induced bone loss. Rates of lumbar spine bone loss slow thereafter, with stabilization by 6 to 12 months, and even some recovery after liver, lung, and heart transplantation. One study reported continued increases in BMD up to 7 years following after transplantation.[68] Reports on BMD changes after renal transplantation differ somewhat. The rapid

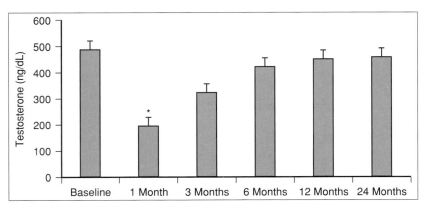

Figure 23-6. Serial testosterone levels in 55 men after heart transplantation. Data presented as mean ± SD. Normal range for serum testosterone: 300-1200 ng/dL. * *P* < .05 compared with baseline. (Redrawn from Shane E, Rivas M, McMahon DJ, et al: Bone loss and turnover after cardiac transplantation. J Clin Endocrinol Metab 1997;82:1497-506. ©1997, The Endocrine Society.)

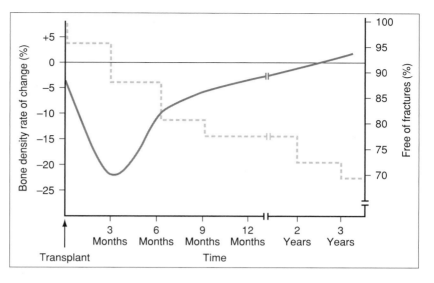

Figure 23-7. Annualized rate of loss of lumbar spine (solid line) and probability of remaining free of spine fractures (dashed line) after cardiac transplantation. Bone density changes are based on 70 patients followed after cardiac transplantation and treated with elemental calcium and vitamin D (data from Shane et al[62]). Fracture data based on 105 cardiac transplantation patients (data from Leidig-Bruckner et al[82]).

and significant early loss in bone density in the first 6 months[77] is followed by continued loss of approximately 1% yearly, up to 8 years after renal transplantation.[79]

Fractures after Transplantation

In heart and liver transplant recipients, the incidence of new fractures parallels the timing of the most rapid loss of BMD, with most fractures occurring within the first year after transplantation (see Figure 23-7).[80-82] After renal transplantation, the incidence of fracture remains elevated, consistent with the persistent decrease in bone density (Figure 23-8).[83] After lung, cardiac, and hepatic transplantation, fractures are more likely to occur at the spine and ribs,[76-81] whereas kidney transplant recipients experience relatively more fractures of the long bones and metatarsals.[84]

Risk factors for fractures after transplantation are summarized in Table 23-4 and include older age, prevalent fractures before transplantation, postmenopausal status, and lower body mass index. Additional risk factors in renal transplant recipients include the presence of diabetes mellitus and prolonged dialysis before transplantation.[85] The predictive roles of pretransplantation BMD[86] and of the cumulative glucocorticoid dose[79,83,87] are controversial. Serial measurements of bone density at the lumbar spine were not found to predict fracture risk after liver[88] or heart[81] transplantation.

The variation in fractures rates among various studies may be partly due to differences in the types and doses of immunosuppressive drugs and partly due to the differences in method of ascertainment (occurrence of symptomatic fractures versus analysis of prospectively obtained spine radiographs). However, fracture incidence may have declined in the past decade.[17,89] This is probably related to the considerable reduction in the dose and duration of glucocorticoid therapy, to earlier

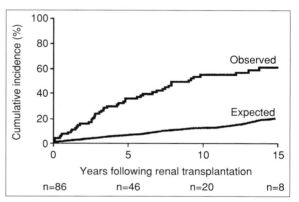

Figure 23-8. Observed versus expected cumulative incidence of any new fractures in renal transplant recipients. Data based on 86 Olmsted County, Minnesota, residents who underwent initial renal transplantation who were followed for 911 person-years. The cumulative incidence of any fracture at 15 years was 60% versus 20% expected (*P* < .001). (From Vautour LM, Melton LJ 3rd, Clarke BL, et al: Long-term fracture risk following renal transplantation: a population-based study. Osteoporos Int 2004;15:160-67. © Springer 2004.)

TABLE 23-4 FACTORS SHOWN TO BE PREDICTIVE OF INCREASED FRACTURE RISK IN SOLID ORGAN TRANSPLANTATION RECIPIENTS	
Organ	**Risk Factors**
Heart	Older age, postmenopausal status, ? Pretransplant BMD, ? steroid dose
Liver	Older age, postmenopausal status, pretransplantation fractures, low body mass index, ? pretransplant BMD, ? steroid dose, ? PBC
Kidney	Older age, postmenopausal status, time on dialysis, diabetes mellitus, ? pretransplant BMD, ? steroid dose

? Indicates risk factors that have been reported in some studies but refuted in other studies.
BMD = bone mineral density, PBC, primary biliary cirrhosis.

institution of preventive methods because of the wider recognition of transplantation-induced osteoporosis, and also to a trend to performing transplantation earlier in the course of the disease.[17]

Bone Histomorphometry after Transplantation

The only bone histomorphometric data on lung transplantation patients come from postmortem vertebral bone biopsy specimens from 11 post-transplant cystic fibrosis patients with a mean time from transplantation to death of 29 months.[27] There was severe osteopenia in both trabecular and cortical bone, with decreased osteoblastic and increased osteoclastic activity.[27] Data on bone biopsies in cardiac transplantation are also very scarce, with only one study describing findings in six patients evaluated at varying times after transplantation and manifesting markedly varied histomorphometric findings.[90] More information is available on liver transplant recipients.[91-94] Most of these studies demonstrate an increase in bone resorption at 3 months after transplantation, accompanied by a more robust increase in parameters of bone formation (osteoblast number and osteoid surface and volume) (Figure 23-9).[92] However, these data may only apply to liver transplant patients in whom osteoblast function is profoundly depressed prior to transplantation.

Although heterogeneous, alterations in markers of bone turnover follow the patterns seen on bone biopsy and are very similar in both liver and cardiac transplantation; an increase in resorption markers and a decrease in formation markers are noted early (up to 3 months).[16,78] This is followed by stabilization in resorption markers at an elevated level but an increase in bone formation markers.

Several publications have reported on the evolution of histologic bone findings in renal transplant recipients.[72] The findings vary widely, although the predominant lesion was characterized by low formation associated with a normal/high bone resorption.[95,96] Most studies of bone turnover markers in renal transplantation reflect a decrease in bone formation in the face of persistently elevated bone resorption.[97]

PREVENTION AND TREATMENT OF TRANSPLANTATION-RELATED OSTEOPOROSIS

Pretransplantation Measures
Identification and Correction of Risk Factors

All transplant candidates should be evaluated and treated prior to transplantation, because bone disease is common in these patients. Because waiting periods on the transplant list can be as long as 1 or 2 years, there is time to implement measures to improve skeletal health. Lifestyle factors such as immobilization, smoking, and alcohol abuse should be addressed. The use of medications that can negatively affect skeletal health (e.g., anticonvulsants, glucocorticoids, heparin, furosemide) should be assessed and minimized to the extent possible. Other factors that can be corrected include hypogonadism and negative calcium balance (due to malabsorption and/or vitamin D deficiency). Evaluation and treatment of renal osteodystrophy according to accepted guidelines[31] are recommended for all patients with ESRD.

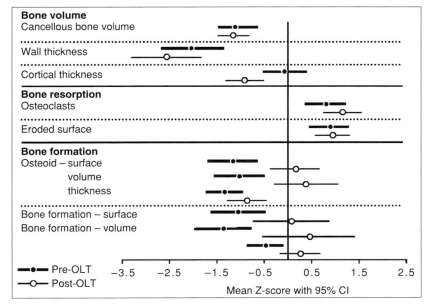

Figure 23-9. Findings on bone histomorphometry in 33 liver transplant recipients. Closed circles represent preorthotopic liver transplantation (OLT); open circles represent 3 months post-OLT. Bone histomorphometric parameters were expressed as Z-scores (sex-adjusted histomorphometric values), using normal female and male histomorphometric reference values of the Mayo Clinic Bone Histomorphometry Laboratory. (Redrawn from Guichelaar MM, Malinchoc M, Sibonga JD, et al: Bone histomorphometric changes after liver transplantation for chronic cholestatic liver disease. J Bone Miner Res 2003;18:2190-99, with permission of the American Society for Bone and Mineral Research.)

All patients should receive the recommended daily allowance for calcium (1000-1500 mg/day) and vitamin D (400-800 IU/day). It is unclear whether treatment of osteoporosis present before transplantation decreases the incidence of fractures after transplantation, because controlled studies regarding this issue have not been conducted. However, antiresorptive agents may help improve BMD in liver and heart transplant candidates and reduce fractures in other populations and thus their use can be supported on these bases. Bisphosphonates may increase the risk for adynamic bone disease in ESRD patients and are not approved for the treatment of these patients.[98]

Measurement of Bone Mineral Density

Lower BMD before transplantation has been cited as a risk factor for fractures after transplantation in some studies,[82] although this is not confirmed from other reports.[81,86] Nevertheless, BMD measurement is recommended by the American Gastroenterological Association,[7] the Kidney Disease Outcomes Quality Initiative Group,[99] and other authors.[2,17,100,101] In our view, it should be used to detect osteoporosis that exists before the transplant and can be helpful in selecting patients who would benefit from immediate initiation of antiresorptive or anabolic therapy. In patients with normal BMD, such therapy could be safely deferred until the time of transplantation. Again, however, interpretation of BMD measurements is difficult in the setting of renal bone disease, and the World Health Organization criteria for diagnosis of osteoporosis should not be used in these patients.

Prevention of Early Post-transplantation Bone Loss

Because rates of bone loss and fracture incidence are highest immediately after transplantation, preventive and therapeutic measures should be instituted at that time and without delay. In addition, the lack of reliable clinical predictors to identify individual patients who will experience osteoporotic fractures renders all transplant recipients candidates for preventive therapy. Prevention trials in post-transplantation osteoporosis are limited by their inclusion of small numbers of subjects, the absence of fracture data, the lack of randomization, and the fact that they are conducted in single centers in most studies, which may limit the generalization of results.

Exercise

The severity of post-transplantation bone loss was found to correlate with the duration of in-hospital stay in the first 3 post-transplantation months, suggesting a negative effect of prolonged immobilization.[61] The importance of physical activity in restoring BMD is demonstrated in three prospective, randomized, albeit very small studies conducted in heart[102,103] and lung[104] transplant recipients. The type of training consisted of supervised exercises of the lumbar extensor muscles (1 day/week) and upper and lower body (2 days/week), started 2 months after transplantation and continued for 6 months. These reports show that specific resistance training restored BMD toward pretransplantation levels more rapidly[102,104] and, in conjunction with alendronate, was more efficacious than alendronate alone (Figure 23-10).[103] Because resistance training has also been associated with somewhat higher BMD in other settings,[105] it may be helpful in other types of organ transplantation.

Calcium and Vitamin D

Replacement doses of calcium and vitamin D (up to 1000 IU) do not prevent clinically significant bone loss after transplantation, as demonstrated by the control arms of several trials studying the effects of different medications.[20,62,106] Nevertheless, trials that have demonstrated efficacy of other medications to prevent post-transplantation bone loss have all been conducted in the setting of calcium and vitamin D repletion, and it is our opinion that all transplant recipients should receive 1000 mg of elemental calcium and at least 400 IU of vitamin D daily.

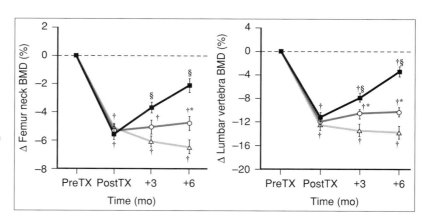

Figure 23-10. Effects of alendronate (10 mg/d) and resistance training initiated 2 months after cardiac transplantation on femoral neck and lumbar spine bone mineral density (BMD) in 25 transplant recipients followed for 6 months. Triangles represent control subjects (n = 9); circles represent alendronate (n = 8); and squares represent resistance training plus alendronate (n = 8). Data expressed as mean ± SEM. †$P < .05$ versus pretransplantation (PreTx) value; *$P < .05$ versus control; §$P < .05$ alendronate plus training versus alendronate alone or control. (Data from Braith et al.[103])

Vitamin D Metabolites

Calcium and calcidiol [25(OH)D] therapy was associated with an increase in BMD levels or prevention of further bone loss in heart transplant recipients[107] and renal transplant recipients.[108] The effects of calcitriol with calcium have been controversial. At doses averaging 0.25 μg daily, calcitriol did not significantly prevent lumbar spine bone loss in renal[109] and heart[110] transplant recipients. Studies of calcitriol therapy at doses greater than 0.5 μg daily have found different results. In a 2-year, randomized, double-blind study, calcitriol (0.5-0.75 μg daily) reduced proximal femur bone loss in heart and lung transplant recipients and reduced the occurrence of vertebral fractures and deformities, although not significantly.[111] However, there was no reduction of lumbar spine bone loss in that study. In another study, calcitriol (0.5 μg daily) reduced bone loss at the femoral neck and lumbar spine in a group of 75 heart transplant recipients compared with an untreated reference group.[89] At doses of 0.5 μg or higher, common side-effects of calcitriol therapy include hypercalcemia and hypercalciuria (seen in more than 50% of patients), which may develop at any time during therapy and which require close monitoring.[89,111]

Calcitonin

Calcitonin is ineffective in preventing early bone loss after transplantation.[2,10,112,113]

Bisphosphonates

Bisphosphonates are indicated for the prevention of glucocorticoid-induced osteoporosis, and their antiresorptive mechanism of action makes these drugs attractive in preventing the phase of rapid bone loss early after transplantation associated with increased bone resorption (see Figure 23-9). Several clinical trials have confirmed this benefit.

Compared with placebo, pamidronate (0.5 mg/kg), given as two intravenous infusions at the time of renal transplantation and 1 month later, prevented bone loss at the femoral neck and lumbar spine at 1 year[114] and protected the hip from bone loss during 4 years after transplantation (Figure 23-11).[115] Similar results have been reported with repeated intravenous doses of pamidronate in a controlled randomized study of 34 pulmonary transplant recipients[116] and in nonrandomized studies of heart,[117] lung,[106] and liver transplant recipients.[118] However, in a recent study of liver transplant recipients, a single dose of 60 mg IV pamidronate had no significant effect on fracture rate or BMD change after

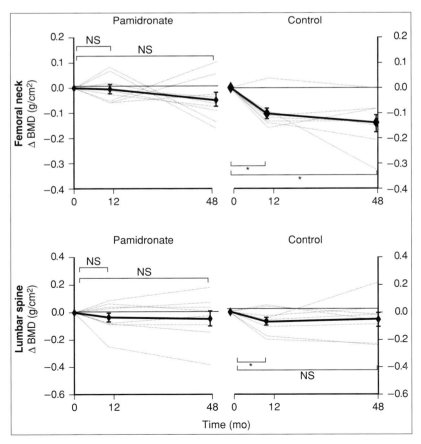

Figure 23-11. Changes in bone mineral density in renal transplant recipients treated at time of transplantation with two doses of pamidronate or placebo. * $P < .005$. NS = nonsignificant. (Redrawn from Fan SLS, Kumar S, Cunningham J: Long-term effects on bone mineral density of pamidronate given at the time of renal transplantation. Kidney Int 2003;63:2275-79, with permission of Blackwell Publishing.)

transplantation as compared with placebo.[119] This may be due to the administration of pamidronate as early as 3 months before transplantation in some patients. Alternatively, pamidronate might have prevented the increase in bone turnover that occurs in untreated patients after liver transplantation, as demonstrated by paired histomorphometry studies.[93] In a study of renal transplant recipients, repeated doses of intravenous pamidronate preserved vertebral BMD during treatment and 6 months after cessation of treatment. However, pamidronate treatment was associated with the development of adynamic bone histology (Figure 23-12), and no significant difference in the incidence of fractures was noted between the two groups in the study.[120]

Alendronate use (10 mg daily) significantly reduced bone loss at the femoral neck and lumbar spine in heart transplant recipients compared with an untreated reference group. However, alendronate was not significantly different than calcitriol (0.5 μg daily).[89] In renal transplant recipients, alendronate started immediately after grafting reduced bone loss in a nonrandomized study.[121]

Cyclical etidronate has been studied extensively but has fallen out of favor since the introduction of newer, more potent bisphosphonates. Two 4 mg IV doses of zoledronic acid given to 20 patients at 2 weeks and 3 months after renal transplantation led to higher bone mineral density values than placebo at 6 months but not at 3 years.[122] Another bisphosphonate not yet approved for the treatment of osteoporosis in the United States has also been studied. Ibandronate given intravenously with calcium had protective effects on BMD in liver[123] and kidney transplant recipients[124] as compared with calcium supplementation alone. However, no fracture data are available.

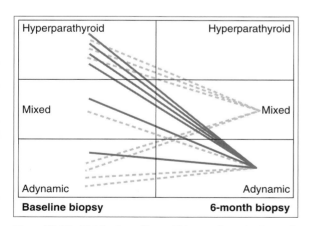

Figure 23-12. Distribution of bone histomorphometry in renal transplant recipients treated with 60 mg of pamidronate within 48 hours after transplantation followed by 30 mg at months 1, 2, 3, and 6 or placebo. Data based on six patients who received pamidronate and eight patients receiving placebo. (Data from Coco et al.[120])

In summary, oral and intravenous bisphosphonates, in conjunction with calcium and vitamin D, are effective in preventing post-transplantation bone loss when administration is started shortly after grafting. The optimal dose, timing, and frequency, particularly of intravenous bisphosphonate administration, remain to be determined. No reports to date demonstrate unequivocal protection from fractures. Their use after pediatric transplantation and in patients with poor renal function should be considered carefully. Finally, the risk of inducing or prolonging adynamic bone disease in renal transplant recipients, especially with repeated dosing, must be kept in perspective. However, we recommend their use after renal transplantation, at least for the first year when rates of bone loss are most rapid.

Treatment of Bone Loss in Long-Term Transplant Recipients

Despite the evidence for benefit of antiresorptive therapies instituted shortly after transplantation, many transplant recipients do not receive such therapies and have established osteoporosis and/or persistent ongoing bone loss. Several studies have examined treatment options for these patients.

Vitamin D Metabolites

One study has shown that calcitriol therapy (0.5 μg daily) is superior to calcium therapy alone in preserving lumbar spine bone mass in renal transplant recipients who were started on treatment approximately 3 years after grafting.[125] In another report of renal transplant recipients, on average 10 years after grafting, calcitriol (0.25 μg daily) and calcium did not significantly improve BMD compared with no treatment.[126] Similarly, calcitriol treatment did not result in additional improvement in lumbar spine BMD compared with calcium supplementation alone in two studies of cardiac transplantation recipients enrolled at 6 months[127] or 35 months[128] after grafting, although the interpretation of these two studies is confounded by the use of concomitant hormone therapy replacement in hypogonadal patients.

Calcitonin

Although ineffective in preventing early bone loss, calcitonin may have some benefit in the later post-transplant period in liver[129] and renal[130] transplant recipients and can be considered a safe alternative if other agents are contraindicated or poorly tolerated.

Bisphosphonates

Pamidronate (30 mg IV every 3 months for 2 years) was studied in 13 cardiac and 21 liver transplant recipients with osteoporosis, approximately 2 years after transplantation. Significant gains in lumbar spine and femoral neck BMD were noted compared with historical controls.[131] Therapy with 1 year of oral clodronate (1600 mg daily) initiated 6 months after transplantation in 64 cardiac transplant recipients with low BMD induced a significant increase in lumbar spine BMD at 1 year.[132] In renal transplant recipients with low bone mass, cyclical therapy with clodronate used at lower doses (800 mg daily) did not result in significant changes in spine BMD compared with calcium alone.[130]

Alendronate (10 mg daily) started approximately 5 years after renal transplantation grafting resulted in significant gains in BMD; again, the number of patients included was too small to show significant fracture prevention data.[133] In two other reports of long-term renal transplant recipients, alendronate resulted in significant increases in femoral neck and lumbar spine BMD.[134,135] In these two studies, the increase in bone mass was not different between alendronate and calcitriol.[134,135]

In another study of 58 long-term kidney transplant recipients more than 1 year after grafting, patients were divided into a group at high risk for bone loss or a low-risk group based on bone mineral density and markers of bone turnover.[136] The low-risk group was followed untreated and did not lose any further bone mass at the lumbar spine or femoral neck at 1 year. On the other hand, in the group with high bone turnover and osteoporosis or osteopenia, alendronate therapy (10 mg daily) decreased the rate of bone loss and increased bone mass over 1 year of treatment.[136] Although uncontrolled, this study may be helpful in guiding the treatment of long-term transplant recipients and in identifying those who may benefit from bisphosphonate therapy beyond the first post-transplantation year, when bone loss and fracture rates are highest.

Gonadal Hormone Replacement

Replacement of sex steroids is known to increase BMD in hypogonadal women and men with osteoporosis, although limited published information is available on transplant recipients. Transdermal estradiol was shown to improve lumbar spine and femoral neck BMD in an uncontrolled study of 18 postmenopausal liver transplant recipients followed for 2 years.[137] In another uncontrolled report, testosterone replacement, started 6 months after cardiac transplantation in hypogonadal men who were also receiving calcium and vitamin D, stabilized BMD at the lumbar spine within 24 months.[128] Risks associated with gonadal replacement[138,139] should be kept in perspective when considering this modality in transplant recipients.

Other Strategies for Prevention and Treatment of Bone Loss in Transplant Recipients

Parathyroid Hormone

Recombinant human PTH (1-34) is the only anabolic agent currently approved in the United States for the treatment of postmenopausal osteoporosis. It has been shown to improve BMD in patients with glucocorticoid-induced osteoporosis after 1 year of treatment,[140] and its effects appear to be sustained after its discontinuation in postmenopausal women receiving estrogen.[141] In the future, PTH may have a role in the treatment of transplantation osteoporosis, although its usefulness may be limited because of the secondary hyperparathyroidism that is commonly observed in long-term transplant recipients.

Glucocorticoid-Free Regimens

Glucocorticoids have been associated with several side effects in transplant recipients and are believed to play a major role in transplantation-related osteoporosis. This has led different investigators to evaluate immunosuppressive regimens that minimize exposure to glucocorticoids by tapering them more rapidly and eventually withdrawing them.[142] Glucocorticoid withdrawal accelerated the recovery of bone mass in 41 liver transplant recipients, compared with 28 patients from the same center in whom prednisone was continued (Figure 23-13).[143] Similar findings were reported in renal transplant recipients in whom prednisone was withdrawn 3 months after transplantation.[144] However, a meta-analysis evaluating the effects of prednisone withdrawal suggested that the occurrence of acute rejection and graft loss was greater than that

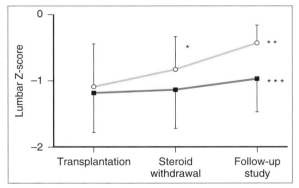

Figure 23-13. Serial bone mineral density measurements expressed as Z-scores (age- and sex-adjusted) of lumbar spine BMD in liver transplant recipients. Circles denote patients withdrawn from prednisone (n = 41); squares denote patients continued on prednisone (n = 28). Compared with baseline: *P < .01, **P < .001; between groups: *** P < .05. (Redrawn from Martinez G, Gomez R, Jodar E, et al: Long-term follow-up of bone mass after orthotopic liver transplantation: effect of steroid withdrawal from the immunosuppressive regimen. Osteoporos Int 2002;13:147-50. © Springer 2002.)

in control patients, dampening the enthusiasm for this practice.[145] Combining drug regimens using newer immunosuppressant agents with either glucocorticoid avoidance or more rapid dose-tapering needs further study and more long-term data before this can become a standard of care.

Calcineurin Inhibitor–Free Regimens

Minimizing the use of calcineurin inhibitors could potentially reduce the incidence of acute and chronic nephrotoxicity and minimize the occurrence of risk factors for cardiovascular disease such as hypertension and hyperlipidemia.[146] The results of protocols using calcineurin inhibitor–sparing regimens are inconclusive, and no specific data are available regarding the bone-sparing effects of such strategies.[142]

CONCLUSIONS

Fractures occur commonly after solid organ transplantation. Multiple interrelated factors contribute to the pathogenesis of osteoporosis in transplant recipients, including pretransplantation bone disease, immunosuppressive drugs, and lifestyle factors. Because bone loss and fracture incidence are greatest immediately after transplantation, early recognition of risk factors and rapid institution of preventive measures are needed to diminish the occurrence of fractures. Effective therapies incorporate pretransplant measures to treat preexisting bone disease and post-transplantation measures, including exercise, calcium and vitamin D repletion, and administration of antiresorptive agents initiated before or shortly after transplantation to counter the rapid bone loss induced by glucocorticoids. The optimal dose, timing, and frequency of administration of these therapies remain to be determined. At present, most controlled trials lack sufficient statistical power to demonstrate efficacy for fracture prevention.

In the past decade, the wider recognition of transplantation-related osteoporosis may have led to a decrease in the risk of fractures in the individual patient. Nonetheless, this progress may be offset by the rapid increase in the number of organs transplanted and the improved survival of transplant recipients, which ultimately puts a greater number of individuals at risk for transplantation-related osteoporosis. Even today, fracture rates remain unacceptably high in transplant recipients, necessitating continued vigilance on the part of organ transplantation programs to address a common complication of these procedures.

REFERENCES

1. United Network for Organ Sharing. Available at http://www.optn.org/data/annualReport.asp. Accessed December 3, 2004.
2. Cohen A, Shane E: Osteoporosis after solid organ and bone marrow transplantation. Osteoporos Int 2003;14:617-30.
3. Ninkovic M, Love SA, Tom B, et al: High prevalence of osteoporosis in patients with chronic liver disease prior to liver transplantation. Calcif Tis Int 2001;69:321-26.
4. Bjoro K, Brandsaeter B, Wiencke K, et al: Secondary osteoporosis in liver transplant recipients: a longitudinal study in patients with and without cholestatic liver disease. Scand J Gastroenterol 2003;38:320-27.
5. Monegal A, Navasa M, Guanabens N, et al: Osteoporosis and bone mineral metabolism disorders in cirrhotic patients referred for orthotopic liver transplantation. Calcif Tis Int 1997;60:148-54.
6. Floreani A, Newton JL, James OFW, et al: Osteoporosis is not a specific complication of primary biliary cirrhosis. Gut 2002;50:898.
7. American Gastroenterological Association medical position statement: Osteoporosis in hepatic disorders. Gastroenterology 2003;125:937-40.
8. Diamond TH, Stiel D, Lunzer M, et al: Hepatic osteodystrophy: static and dynamic bone histomorphometry and serum bone Gla-protein in 80 patients with chronic liver disease. Gastroenterology 1989;96:213-21.
9. Guichelaar MM, Malinchoc M, Sibonga J, et al: Bone metabolism in advanced cholestatic liver disease: analysis by bone histomorphometry. Hepatology 2002;36:895-903.
10. Cuthbert JA, Pak CY, Zerwekh JE, et al: Bone disease in primary biliary cirrhosis: increased bone resorption and turnover in the absence of osteoporosis or osteomalacia. Hepatology 1984;4:1-8.
11. Diez A, Puig J, Serrano S, et al: Alcohol-induced bone disease in the absence of severe chronic liver damage. J Bone Miner Res 1984;9:825-31.
12. Hock JM, Centrella M, Canalis E: Insulin-like growth factor 1 has independent effects on bone matrix formation and cell replication. Endocrinology 1988;122:254-60.
13. Hill PA, Tumber A, Meikle MC: Multiple extracellular signals promote osteoblast survival and apoptosis. Endocrinology 1997;138:3849-58.
14. Gallego-Rojo FJ, Gonzalez-Calvin JL, Munoz-Torres M, et al: Bone mineral density, serum insulin-like growth factor I, and bone turnover markers in viral cirrhosis. Hepatology 1998;28:695-99.
15. Janes CH, Dickson ER, Okazaki R, et al: Role of hyperbilirubinemia in the impairment of osteoblast proliferation associated with cholestatic jaundice. J Clin Invest 1995;95:2581-86.
16. Floreani A, Mega A, Tizian L, et al: Bone metabolism and gonad function in male patients undergoing liver transplantation: a two-year longitudinal study. Osteoporos Int 2001;12:749-54.
17. Compston JE: Osteoporosis after liver transplantation. Liver Transplantation 2003;9:321-30.
18. Shane E, Silverberg SJ, Donovan D, et al: Osteoporosis in lung transplantation candidates with end-stage pulmonary disease. Am J Med 1996;101:262-69.
19. Aris RM, Neuringer IP, Weiner MA, et al: Severe osteoporosis before and after lung transplantation. Chest 1996;109:1176-83.
20. Ferrari SL, Nicod LP, Hamacher J, et al: Osteoporosis in patients undergoing lung transplantation. Eur Respir J 1996;9:2378-82.
21. Gluck O, Colice G: Recognizing and treating glucocorticoid-induced osteoporosis in patients with pulmonary diseases. Chest 2004;125:1859-76.
22. Aris RM, Renner JB, Winders AD, et al: Increased rate of fractures and severe kyphosis: sequelae of living into adulthood with cystic fibrosis. Ann Intern Med 1998;128:186-93.
23. Stead RJ, Houlder S, Agnew J, et al: Vitamin D and parathyroid hormone and bone mineralisation in adults with cystic fibrosis. Thorax 1988;43:190-94.
24. Lark RK, Lester GE, Ontjes DA, et al: Diminished and erratic absorption of ergocalciferol in adult cystic fibrosis patients. Am J Clin Nutr 2001;73:602-6.
25. Ionescu AA, Nixon LS, Evans WD, et al: Bone density, body composition, and inflammatory status in cystic fibrosis. Am J Respir Crit Care Med 2000;162:789-94.

233

26. Aris RM, Ontjes DA, Buell HE, et al: Abnormal bone turnover in cystic fibrosis adults. Osteoporos Int 2002;13:151-57.

27. Haworth CS, Webb AK, Egan JJ, et al: Bone histomorphometry in adult patients with cystic fibrosis. Chest 2000;118:434-39.

28. Shane E, Mancini D, Aaronson K, et al: Bone mass, vitamin D deficiency, and hyperparathyroidism in congestive heart failure. Am J Med 1997;103:197-207.

29. Lee AH, Mull RL, Keenan GF, et al: Osteoporosis and bone morbidity in cardiac transplant recipients. Am J Med 1994;96:35-41.

30. Pisani B, Mullen GM: Prevention of osteoporosis in cardiac transplant recipients. Curr Opin Cardiol 2002;17:160-64.

31. Elder G: Pathophysiology and recent advances in the management of renal osteodystrophy. J Bone Miner Res 2002;17:2094-105.

32. Hruska KA, Teitelbaum SL: Renal osteodystrophy. N Engl J Med 1995;333:166-75.

33. Atsumi K, Kushida K, Yamazaki K, et al: Risk factors for vertebral fractures in renal osteodystrophy. Am J Kidney Dis 1999;33:287-93.

34. Alem AM, Sherrard DJ, Gillen DL, et al: Increased risk of hip fracture among patients with end-stage renal disease. Kidney Int 2000;58:396-99.

35. Stehman-Breen CO, Sherrard DJ, Alem AM, et al: Risk factors for hip fracture among patients with end-stage renal disease. Kidney Int 2000;58:2200-5.

36. Canalis E: Mechanisms of glucocorticoid action in bone: implications to glucocorticoid-induced osteoporosis. J Clin Endocrinol Metab 1996;81:3441-47.

37. Suzuki Y, Ichikawa Y, Saito E, et al: Importance of increased urinary calcium excretion in the development of secondary hyperparathyroidism of patients under glucocorticoid therapy. Metabolism 1983;32:151-56.

38. Kimberg DV, Baerg RD, Gershon E, et al: Effect of cortisone treatment on the active transport of calcium by the small intestine. J Clin Invest 1971;50:1309-21.

39. Sakakura M, Takebe K, Nakagawa S: Inhibition of luteinizing hormone secretion induced by synthetic LRH by long-term treatment with glucocorticoids in human subjects. J Clin Endocrinol Metab 1975;40:774-79.

40. Chrousos GP, Torpy DJ, Gold PW: Interactions between the hypothalamic-pituitary-adrenal axis and the female reproductive system: clinical implications. Ann Intern Med 1998;129:229-40.

41. Canalis E, Delany AM: Mechanisms of glucocorticoid action in bone. Ann N Y Acad Sci 2002;966:73-81.

42. Weinstein RS, Jilka RL, Parfitt MA, et al: Inhibition of osteoblastogenesis and promotion of apoptosis of osteoblasts and osteocytes by glucocorticoids: potential mechanisms of their deleterious effects on bone. J Clin Invest 1998;102:274-82.

43. Danneskiold-Samsoe B, Grimby G: The influence of prednisone on the muscle morphology and muscle enzymes in patients with rheumatoid arthritis. Clin Sci 1986;71:693-701.

44. Matsuda S, Koyasu S: Mechanisms of action of cyclosporine. Immunopharmacology 2000;47:119-25.

45. Epstein S: Post-transplantation bone disease: the role of immunosuppressive agents on the skeleton. J Bone Miner Res 1996;11:1-7.

46. Schlosberg M, Movsowitz C, Epstein S, et al: The effect of cyclosporin A administration and its withdrawal on bone mineral metabolism in the rat. Endocrinology 1989;124:2179-84.

47. Movsowitz C, Epstein S, Fallon M, et al: Cyclosporin-A in vivo produces severe osteopenia in the rat: effect of dose and duration of administration. Endocrinology 1988;123:2571-77.

48. Buchinsky FJ, Ma Y, Mann GN, et al: T lymphocytes play a critical role in the development of cyclosporin A-induced osteopenia. Endocrinology 1996;137:2278-85.

49. Bowman AR, Sass DA, Dissanayake IR, et al: The role of testosterone in cyclosporine-induced osteopenia. J Bone Miner Res 1997;12:607-15.

50. Epstein S, Dissanayake IR, Goodman GR, et al: Effect of the interaction of parathyroid hormone and cyclosporine A on bone mineral metabolism in the rat. Calcif Tis Int 2001;68:240-47.

51. Bennett WM, DeMattos A, Meyer MM, et al: Chronic cyclosporine nephropathy: the Achilles' heel of immunosuppressive therapy. Kidney Int 1996;50:1089-100.

52. Monegal A, Navasa M, Guanabens N, et al: Bone mass and mineral metabolism in liver transplant patients treated with FK506 or cyclosporine A. Calcif Tissue Int 2001;68:83-6.

53. Dissanayake IR, Goodman GR, Bowman AR, et al: Mycophenolate mofetil: a promising new immunosuppressant that does not cause bone loss in the rat. Transplantation 1998;65:275-78.

54. Joffe I, Katz I, Sehgal S, et al: Lack of change of cancellous bone volume with short-term use of the new immunosuppressant rapamycin in rats. Calcif Tis Int 1993;53:45-52.

55. Bryer HP, Isserow JA, Armstrong EC, et al: Azathioprine alone is bone sparing and does not alter cyclosporin A-induced osteopenia in the rat. J Bone Miner Res 1995;10:132-38.

56. Vintro AQ, Krasnoff JB, Painter P: Roles of nutrition and physical activity in musculoskeletal complications before and after liver transplantation. AACN Clin Issues 2002;13:333-47.

57. Sabry ZI, Shadarevian SB, Cowan JW, et al: Relationship of dietary intake of sulphur amino-acids to urinary excretion of inorganic sulphate in man. Nature 1965;206:931-33.

58. Reddy S, Wang C, Sakhaee K, et al: Effect of low-carbohydrate high-protein diets on acid-base balance, stone-forming propensity, and calcium metabolism. Am J Kidney Dis 2002;40:265-74.

59. Breslau NA, McGuire JL, Zerwekh JE, et al: The role of dietary sodium on renal excretion and intestinal absorption of calcium and on vitamin D metabolism. J Clin Endocrinol Metab 1982;55:369-73.

60. Painter P, Krasnoff J, Paul SM, et al: Physical activity and health-related quality of life in liver transplant recipients. Liver Transplantation 2001;7:213-19.

61. Kwan JT, Almond MK, Evans K, et al: Changes in total body bone mineral content and regional bone mineral density in renal patients following renal transplantation. Miner Electrolyte Metab 1992;18:166-68.

62. Shane E, Rivas M, McMahon DJ, et al: Bone loss and turnover after cardiac transplantation. J Clin Endocrinol Metab 1997;82:1497-506.

63. Madersbacher S, Ludvik G, Stulnig T, et al: The impact of liver transplantation on endocrine status in men. Clin Endocrinol 1996;44:461-66.

64. Laifer SA, Guido RS: Reproductive function and outcome of pregnancy after liver transplantation in women. Mayo Clin Proc 1995;70:388-94.

65. Mass K, Quint EH, Punch MR, et al: Gynecological and reproductive function after liver transplantation. Transplantation 1996;62:476-79.

66. Saha MT, Saha HH, Niskanen LK, et al: Time course of serum prolactin and sex hormones following successful renal transplantation. Nephron 2002;92:735-37.

67. Akbari F, Alavi M, Esteghamati A, et al: Effect of renal transplantation on sperm quality and sex hormone levels. BJU Int 2003;92:281-83.

68. Feller RB, McDonald JA, Sherbon KJ, et al: Evidence of continuing bone recovery at a mean of 7 years after liver transplantation. Liver Trans Surg 1999;5:407-13.

69. Ojo AO, Held PJ, Port FK, et al: Chronic renal failure after transplantation of a nonrenal organ. N Engl J Med 2003;349:931-40.

70. Julian B, Quarles L, Niemann K: Musculoskeletal complications after renal transplantation: pathogenesis and treatment. Am J Kidney Dis 1992;19:99-120.

71. Sperschneider H, Stein G: Bone disease after renal transplantation. Nephrol Dial Transplant 2003;18:874-77.

72. Torres A, Lorenzo V, Salido E: Calcium metabolism and skeletal problems after transplantation. J Am Soc Nephrol 2002;13:551-58.

73. Torres A, Rodriguez A, Concepcion M, et al: Parathyroid function in long-term renal transplant patients: importance of pre-transplant PTH concentrations. Nephrol Dial Transplant 1998;13:94-7.

74. Montalban C, De Francisco ALM, Marinoso ML, et al: Bone disease in long-term adult kidney transplant patients with normal renal function. Kidney Int 2003;63:129-32.

75. Reinhardt W, Bartelworth H, Jockenhovel F, et al: Sequential changes of biochemical bone parameters after kidney transplantation. Nephrol Dial Transplant 1998;13:434-40.

76. Shane E, Papadopoulos A, Staron RB, et al: Bone loss and fracture after lung transplantation. Transplantation 1999;68:220-27.

77. Julian BA, Laskow DA, Dubovsky J, et al: Rapid loss of vertebral mineral density after renal transplantation. N Engl J Med 1991;325:544-50.

78. Guo C-Y, Johnson A, Locke TJ, et al: Mechanisms of bone loss after cardiac transplantation. Bone 1998;22:267-71.

79. Pichette V, Bonnardeaux A, Prudhomme L, et al: Long-term bone loss in kidney transplant recipients: a cross-sectional and longitudinal study. Am J Kidney Dis 1996;28:105-14.

80. Ninkovic M, Skingle SJ, Bearcroft PW, et al: Incidence of vertebral fractures in the first three months after orthotopic liver transplantation. Eur J Gastroenterol Hepatol 2000;12:931-35.

81. Shane E, Rivas M, Staron RB, et al: Fracture after cardiac transplantation: a prospective longitudinal study. J Clin Endocrinol Metab 1996;81:1740-46.

82. Leidig-Bruckner G, Hosch S, Dodidou P, et al: Frequency and predictors of osteoporotic fractures after cardiac or liver transplantation: a follow-up study. Lancet 2001;357:342-47.

83. Vautour LM, Melton LJ 3rd, Clarke BL, et al: Long-term fracture risk following renal transplantation: a population-based study. Osteoporos Int 2004;15:160-67.

84. Ramsey-Goldman R, Dunn JE, Dunlop DD, et al: Increased risk of fracture in patients receiving solid organ transplants. J Bone Miner Res 1999;14:456-63.

85. Ball AM, Gillen DL, Sherrard D, et al: Risk of hip fracture among dialysis and renal transplant recipients. JAMA 2002;288:3014-18.

86. Grotz WH, Mundinger FA, Gugel B, et al: Bone fracture and osteodensitometry with dual energy X-ray absorptiometry in kidney transplant recipients. Transplantation 1994;58:912-15.

87. Wolpaw T, Deal CL, Fleming-Brooks S, et al: Factors influencing vertebral bone density after renal transplantation. Transplantation 1994;58:1186-89.

88. Hardinger KL, Ho B, Schnitzler MA, et al: Serial measurements of bone density at the lumbar spine do not predict fracture risk after liver transplantation. Liver Transplantation 2003;9:857-62.

89. Shane E, Addesso V, Namerow PB, et al: Alendronate versus calcitriol for the prevention of bone loss after cardiac transplantation. N Engl J Med 2004;350:767-76.

90. Glendenning P, Kent GN, Adler BD, et al: High prevalence of osteoporosis in cardiac transplant recipients and discordance between biochemical turnover markers and bone histomorphometry. Clin Endocrinol 1999;50:347-55.

91. Monegal A, Navasa M, Guanabens N, et al: Bone disease after liver transplantation: a long-term prospective study of bone mass changes, hormonal status and histomorphometric characteristics. Osteoporos Int 2001;12:484-92.

92. Guichelaar MM, Malinchoc M, Sibonga JD, et al: Bone histomorphometric changes after liver transplantation for chronic cholestatic liver disease. J Bone Miner Res 2003;18:2190-99.

93. Vedi S, Ninkovic M, Garrahan NJ, et al: Effects of a single infusion of pamidronate prior to liver transplantation: a bone histomorphometric study. Transplant Int 2002;15:290-95.

94. Vedi S, Greer S, Skingle SJ, et al: Mechanism of bone loss after liver transplantation: a histomorphometric analysis. J Bone Miner Res 1999;14:281-87.

95. Monier-Faugere M, Mawad H, Qi Q, et al: High prevalence of low bone turnover and occurrence of osteomalacia after kidney transplantation. J Am Soc Nephrol 2000;11:1093-99.

96. Carlini RG, Rojas E, Weisinger JR, et al: Bone disease in patients with long-term renal transplantation and normal renal function. Am J Kid Dis 2000;36:160-66.

97. Bellorin-Font E, Rojas E, Carlini RG, et al: Bone remodeling after renal transplantation. Kidney Int 2003;63:125-28.

98. Fan SL, Cunningham J: Bisphosphonates in renal osteodystrophy. Curr Opin Nephrol Hypertens 2001;10:581-88.

99. Kidney Disease Outcomes Quality Initiative (K/DOQI) Group: 2003 K/DOQI clinical practice guidelines for bone metabolism and disease in chronic kidney disease. Am J Kidney Dis 2003;42:suppl 3.

100. Dodd VA, Staron RB, Papadopoulos A, et al: Bone densitometry should be included in the evaluation of candidates for lung transplantation. J Transpl Coord 1999;9:119-23.

101. Crippin JS: Bone disease after liver transplantation. Liver Transplantation 2001;7:S27-S35.

102. Braith RW, Mills J, Welsch MA, et al: Resistance exercise training restores bone mineral density in heart transplant recipients. J Am Coll Cardiol 1996;28:1471-77.

103. Braith RW, Magyari PM, Fulton MN, et al: Resistance exercise training and alendronate reverse glucocorticoid-induced osteoporosis in heart transplant recipients. J Heart Lung Transplant 2003;22:1082-90.

104. Mitchell MJ, Baz MA, Fulton MN, et al: Resistance training prevents vertebral osteoporosis in lung transplant recipients. Transplantation 2003;76:557-62.

105. Menkes A, Mazel S, Redmond RA, et al: Strength training increases regional bone mineral density and bone remodeling in middle-aged and older men. J Appl Physiol 1993;74:2478-84.

106. Trombetti A, Gerbase MW, Spiliopoulos A, et al: Bone mineral density in lung-transplant recipients before and after graft: prevention of lumbar spine post-transplantation-accelerated bone loss by pamidronate. J Heart Lung Transplant 2000;19:736-43.

107. Meys E, Terreaux-Duvert F, Beaume-Six T, et al: Bone loss after cardiac transplantation: effects of calcium, calcidiol and monofluorophosphate. Osteoporos Int 1993;3:322-29.

108. Talalaj M, Gradowska L, Marcinowska-Suchowierska E, et al: Efficiency of preventive treatment of glucocorticoid-induced osteoporosis with 25-hydroxyvitamin D3 and calcium in kidney transplant patients. Transplant Proc 1996;28:3485-87.

109. Torres A, Garcia S, Gomez A, et al: Treatment with intermittent calcitriol and calcium reduces bone loss after renal transplantation. Kidney Int 2004;65:705-12.

110. Cremer J, Struber M, Wagenbreth I, et al: Progression of steroid-associated osteoporosis after heart transplantation. Ann Thorac Surg 1999;67:130-33.

111. Sambrook P, Henderson NK, Keogh A, et al: Effect of calcitriol on bone loss after cardiac or lung transplantation. J Bone Miner Res 2000;15:1818-24.

112. Garcia-Delgado I, Prieto S, Gil-Fraguas L, et al: Calcitonin, etidronate, and calcidiol treatment in bone loss after cardiac transplantation. Calcif Tissue Int 1997;60:155-59.

113. Hay JE, Malinchoc M, Dickson ER: A controlled trial of calcitonin therapy for the prevention of post-liver transplantation atraumatic fractures in patients with primary biliary cirrhosis and primary sclerosing cholangitis. J Hepatology 2001;34:292-98.

114. Fan SLS, Almond MK, Ball E, et al: Pamidronate therapy as prevention of bone loss following renal transplantation. Kidney Int 2000;57:684-90.

115. Fan SLS, Kumar S, Cunningham J: Long-term effects on bone mineral density of pamidronate given at the time of renal transplantation. Kidney Int 2003;63:2275-79.

116. Aris RM, Lester GE, Renner JB, et al: Efficacy of pamidronate for osteoporosis in patients with cystic fibrosis following lung transplantation. Am J Respir Crit Care Med 2000;162:941-46.

117. Krieg MA, Seydoux C, Sandini L, et al: Intravenous pamidronate as treatment for osteoporosis after heart transplantation: a prospective study. Osteoporos Int 2001;12:112-16.

118. Reeves HL, Francis RM, Manas DM, et al: Intravenous bisphosphonate prevents symptomatic osteoporotic vertebral collapse in patients after liver transplantation. Liver Transpl Surg 1998;4:404-9.

119. Ninkovic M, Love S, Tom BDM, et al: Lack of effect of intravenous pamidronate on fracture incidence and bone mineral density after orthotopic liver transplantation. J Hepatol 2002;37:93-100.

120. Coco M, Glicklich D, Faugere MC, et al: Prevention of bone loss in renal transplant recipients: a prospective, randomized trial of intravenous pamidronate. J Am Soc Nephrol 2003;14:2669-76.

121. Kovac D, Lindic J, Kandus A, et al: Prevention of bone loss in kidney graft recipients. Transplant Proc 2001;33:1144-45.

122. Schwarz C, Mitterbauer C, Heinze G, et al: Nonsustained effect of short-term bisphosphonate therapy on bone turnover three years after renal transplantation. Kidney Int 2004;65:304-9.

123. Hommann M, Abendroth K, Lehmann G, et al: Effect of transplantation on bone: osteoporosis after liver and multivisceral transplantation. Transplant Proc 2002;34:2296-98.

124. Grotz W, Nagel C, Poeschel D, et al: Effect of ibandronate on bone loss and renal function after kidney transplantation. J Am Soc Nephrol 2001;12:1530-37.

125. Ugur A, Guvener N, Isiklar I, et al: Efficiency of preventive treatment for osteoporosis after renal transplantation. Transplant Proc 2000;32:556-57.

126. Cueto-Manzano A, Konel S, Freemont A, et al: Effect of 1,25-dihydroxyvitamin D3 and calcium carbonate on bone loss

235

associated with long-term renal transplantation. Am J Kidney Dis 2000;35:227-36.

127. Stempfle HU, Werner C, Siebert U, et al: The role of tacrolimus (FK506)-based immunosuppression on bone mineral density and bone turnover after cardiac transplantation: a prospective, longitudinal, randomized, double-blind trial with calcitriol. Transplantation 2002;73:547-52.

128. Stempfle HU, Werner C, Echtler S, et al: Prevention of osteoporosis after cardiac transplantation: a prospective, longitudinal, randomized, double-blind trial with calcitriol. Transplantation 1999;68:523-30.

129. Valero MA, Loinaz C, Larrodera L, et al: Calcitonin and bisphosphonates treatment in bone loss after liver transplantation. Calcif Tissue Int 1995;57:15-19.

130. Grotz WH, Rump LC, Niessen A, et al: Treatment of osteopenia and osteoporosis after kidney transplantation. Transplantation 1998;66:1004-8.

131. Dodidou P, Bruckner T, Hosch S, et al: Better late than never? Experience with intravenous pamidronate treatment in patients with low bone mass or fractures following cardiac or liver transplantation. Osteoporosis Int 2003;14:82-9.

132. Ippoliti G, Pellegrini C, Campana C, et al: Clodronate treatment of established bone loss in cardiac recipients: a randomized study. Transplantation 2003;15:330-34.

133. Giannini S, Dangel A, Carraro G, et al: Alendronate prevents further bone loss in renal transplant recipients. J Bone Miner Res 2001;16:2111-17.

134. Koc M, Tuglular S, Arikan H, et al: Alendronate increases bone mineral density in long-term renal transplant recipients. Transplant Proc 2002;34:2111-13.

135. Jeffery JR, Leslie WD, Karpinski ME, et al: Prevalence and treatment of decreased bone density in renal transplant recipients: a randomized prospective trial of calcitriol versus alendronate. Transplantation 2003;76:1498-502.

136. Cruz DN, Brickel HM, Wysolmerski JJ, et al: Treatment of osteoporosis and osteopenia in long-term renal transplant patients with alendronate. Am J Transplantation 2002;2:62-7.

137. Isoniemi H, Appelberg J, Nilsson CG, et al: Transdermal oestrogen therapy protects postmenopausal liver transplant women from osteoporosis: a 2-year follow-up study. J Hepatol 2001;34:299-305.

138. Rossouw JE, Anderson GL, Prentice RL, et al: Writing Group for the Women's Health Initiative Investigators: Risks and benefits of estrogen plus progestin in healthy postmenopausal women: principal results from the Women's Health Initiative randomized controlled trial. JAMA 2002;288:321-33.

139. Rhoden EL, Morgentaler A: Risks of testosterone-replacement therapy and recommendations for monitoring. N Engl J Med 2004;350:482-92.

140. Lane NE, Sanchez S, Modin GW, et al: Parathyroid hormone treatment can reverse corticosteroid-induced osteoporosis: results of a randomized controlled clinical trial. J Clin Invest 1998;102:1627-33.

141. Lane NE, Sanchez S, Modin GW, et al: Bone mass continues to increase at the hip after parathyroid hormone treatment is discontinued in glucocorticoid-induced osteoporosis: results of a randomized controlled clinical trial. J Bone Miner Res 2000;15:944-51.

142. Marsh C: Calcineurin-sparing or steroid-sparing immunosuppression in renal transplantation. Curr Opin Organ Transplant 2002;7:145-56.

143. Martinez G, Gomez R, Jodar E, et al: Long-term follow-up of bone mass after orthotopic liver transplantation: effect of steroid withdrawal from the immunosuppressive regimen. Osteoporos Int 2002;13:147-50.

144. Nowacka-Cieciura E, Durlik M, Cieciura T, et al: Positive effect of steroid withdrawal on bone mineral density in renal allograft recipients. Transplantation Proc 2001;33:1273-77.

145. O'Shaughnessy EA, Dahl DC, Smith CL, et al: Risk factors for fractures in kidney transplantation. Transplantation 2002;74:362-66.

146. Taylor DO, Barr ML, Radovancevic B, et al: A randomized, multicenter comparison of tacrolimus and cyclosporine immunosuppressive regimens in cardiac transplantation: decreased hyperlipidemia and hypertension with tacrolimus. J Heart Lung Transplant 1999;18:336-45.

24 Epidemiology of Osteoporosis in Rheumatic Diseases

Luigi Sinigaglia and Massimo Varenna

SUMMARY

Local and generalized osteoporosis and related fractures are frequently encountered in rheumatoid arthritis, but also increasingly recognized in other rheumatic disease states, including systemic lupus erythematosus, ankylosing spondylitis, the spondyloarthritides and polymyalgia rheumatica. The causes are multifactorial, but they include the underlying inflammatory process, consequent reduced mobility, and secondary to therapy, especially corticosteroids. The clinical relevance of this issue is still underestimated and many patients do not undergo bone densitometry or receive medications for osteoporosis. This chapter outlines what is known about the epidemiology of osteoporosis in different rheumatic diseases with a special emphasis of risk factors and management.

Osteoporosis and related fragility fractures are frequently reported among rheumatic patients and contribute to a dramatic worsening of their quality of life. Bone has been recognized to be negatively affected by the disease process and often by the therapy itself in many rheumatic conditions such as rheumatoid arthritis, systemic lupus erythematosus, ankylosing spondylitis and spondyloarthritides, various connective tissue diseases, and polymyalgia rheumatica. The clinical relevance of this issue is still underestimated, and most patients do not routinely undergo bone densitometry or receive prescription medications for osteoporosis in everyday clinical practice.[1] This reflects an insufficient appreciation of this clinical challenge by most physicians and a general lack of consensus on appropriate screening and treatment for osteoporosis in rheumatic diseases. This chapter focuses on the burden of osteoporosis and fragility fractures in different rheumatic conditions and aims at emphasizing the importance of this complication for which, nowadays, effective preventive measures are available. Greater understanding of this problem will improve the quality of health care and the lives of rheumatic patients.

RHEUMATOID ARTHRITIS

Epidemiology of Osteoporosis in Rheumatoid Arthritis

Involvement of bone in rheumatoid arthritis (RA) was first described by Barwell in 1865.[2] Since then, it has been well known that both generalized and juxta-articular osteoporosis can occur in RA. The magnitude of generalized osteoporosis in RA is difficult to assess, and available data come from cross-sectional studies aimed at evaluating the prevalence of this complication. In comparing different studies, it is important to recognize potential problems in data interpretation due to variations in inclusion criteria and the diverse methods and sites of bone density measurements. In a large review published in 1996, based on analyses of 10 cross-sectional studies, including fewer than 100 patients each and performed by different techniques, including single- and dual-photon absorptiometry and quantitative computed tomography (QCT), the only conclusion reached was that patients with RA had lower bone mass than normal control subjects in the appendicular and axial skeleton.[3] More recently, the results of larger cross-sectional studies that used dual-energy x-ray absorptiometry (DXA) have become available, leading to more precise information. In a large cross-sectional study performed on 925 consecutive female patients with RA (73% of whom were postmenopausal) recruited in 21 Italian Rheumatology Centers, the frequency of osteoporosis assessed by DXA was as high as 28.8% at the lumbar spine and 36.2% at the femoral neck and increased linearly by Steinbrocker functional stage I to IV. Patients with vertebral or femoral osteoporosis had a significantly lower body mass index, a significantly longer disease duration, and a significantly higher grade of disability compared with nonosteoporotic subjects, even after adjusting for age.[4] Because these data reflect the prevalence of osteoporosis in a series of patients referred to rheumatological units, it is possible there was selection bias. Avoiding this problem, a large cross-sectional study was performed in Norway in 394 women with

RA aged 20 to 70 years, recruited from a validated RA register containing both mild and severe cases and suggested to be representative of the total RA population in the county.[5] In this study, the prevalence of osteoporosis in the whole sample was somewhat lower (16.8% at lumbar spine and 14.7% at femoral neck) but was as high as 31.5% and 28.6% for lumbar spine and femoral neck, respectively, in older age groups between 60 and 70 years of age. In this study, a twofold increased frequency of osteoporosis was observed in all age groups compared with the reference population.

Data on the prevalence of osteoporosis in men with RA are scanty. A study performed on 50 consecutive men with a median age of 67 years affected by long-standing RA reported a prevalence of femoral and lumbar osteoporosis of 29% and 19%, and the occurrence of reduced bone mineral density (BMD) was independent of blood testosterone concentrations.[6] In another study performed on 104 male RA patients, the overall prevalence was lower, between 10% and 13%, but increased to 42% when considering any site of measurement in older groups aged 60 to 69 years.[7] Another cross-sectional study that included 94 male patients with RA explored the overall frequency of reduced BMD (defined as a Z-score ≤1 standard deviation below the mean value in age-matched control subjects) and reported a twofold statistically significant increased frequency of patients with reduced bone mass for both the spine and the hip. In this study, multivariate analysis did not reveal consistent associations between reduced BMD and demographic or disease-related variables.[8]

As for primary osteoporosis, BMD in patients with RA is under multifactorial influence. Cross-sectional studies provide important information about the roles of time-invariant factors as determinants of osteoporosis in RA. The main studies conducted in this field using multivariate analysis models are in substantial agreement, indicating that age, body weight or body mass index, physical disability as measured by the Health Assessment Questionnaire (HAQ), and menopausal status are the most important independent statistically significant predictors of BMD or osteoporosis in women with RA either at the lumbar spine or proximal femur.[4,5] On the other hand, physical activity, as assessed by the Framingham activity index, correlated significantly with BMD in patients with RA and was found by multiple regression analysis to be a significant independent predictor of femoral bone density in 111 female patients.[9] These results have recently been confirmed by a study assessing the relationship between bone density and muscle function, indicating that after adjustment for confounding covariates, women with RA with reduced BMD of the femoral neck (e.g., T-score < −1) had a 20% lower quadriceps

strength than those with normal BMD.[10] In agreement with other studies indicating the relationship between BMD and surrogate measures of physical performance,[11-14] these data underline the importance of muscle strengthening training programs in the prevention of bone loss in patients with RA.

An even more intriguing question addressed by most cross-sectional studies relates to the roles of antirheumatic therapies as determinants of BMD and osteoporosis in patients with RA. In this respect, interpretation of studies in patients taking low-dose oral corticosteroids is difficult because of the number of factors involved that can influence BMD in these patients. In general, patients taking steroids are likely to have more severe disease and to be more disabled, which act as confounders. Two cross-sectional studies performed by dual-photon absorptiometry failed to demonstrate a statistically significant difference in terms of spinal or femoral BMD between RA women on corticosteroids and non-steroid–treated patients, concluding that low-dose prednisolone (mean daily dose between 6.6 and 8.5 mg) was not associated with an increased risk of osteoporosis.[15,16] Subsequent studies using QCT or DXA have given discrepant results. In a cross-sectional study of 74 patients with RA, patients taking oral corticosteroids had a 31% and 37% reduction in spinal trabecular and cortical BMD, respectively, compared with patients who did not undergo steroid treatment.[17] A DXA study performed on 195 postmenopausal patients with RA showed that current steroid usage led to a significant reduction in BMD and that both low and high cumulative dose groups were at risk for decreased BMD as compared with ex-user or nonuser counterparts.[18] Conversely, a recent cross-sectional study performed by DXA on 146 female patients with RA came to the conclusion that long disease duration, severity of disease, and decreased lean body mass but not corticosteroids were associated with generalized osteoporosis.[19] These results were confirmed by others using skeletal ultrasonography.[20] In another study performed on 120 postmenopausal elderly women, the subjects who were current users of steroids had the lowest BMD at the distal forearm and calcaneus and at the hip, but functional outcomes of RA largely accounted for these results.[21] On the other hand, two large cross-sectional studies found that current use of steroids is an independent predictor of reduced lumbar and femoral BMD[5] and of osteoporosis[4] and that a low-dose steroid regimen (current dose of 5.5 ± 4.5 mg in prednisone equivalent) was associated with a 50% increase of the risk for osteoporosis.[4] In the Norwegian study cohort, the prevalence of osteoporosis at the lumbar spine increased from 8.6% in never users to 10.1% in previous and to 26.6% in current steroid users.[5] These results are in agreement with data from a recent meta-analysis on the skeletal

in this population. Furthermore, in this study, almost 50% of fractures occurred in women with SLE who were younger than 50 years of age or premenopausal.[69]

In conclusion, the high prevalence of osteoporosis reported by most studies and the impressive increase in fracture rate in SLE patients represent an important challenge for clinicians. Strategies to counteract bone loss in SLE must be applied soon after disease onset and include effective treatment of the underlying disease, modification of any known risk factor for osteoporosis, use of corticosteroids at the lowest useful dosage, and the pharmacological treatment of osteoporosis in all patients with evidence of rapid bone loss.

ANKYLOSING SPONDYLITIS

Ankylosing spondylitis (AS) is the prototypical disease of a heterogeneous group of rheumatic disorders called spondyloarthropathies that share as a common feature a chronic inflammation of the axial skeleton. Despite extraosseous new bone formation being considered a hallmark of AS, osteoporosis is a well-recognized feature occurring even in early, mild forms of AS and leading to an increased rate of fractures. A radiographic bone loss has long been recognized in predensitometric studies[70,71] in which osteoporosis correlated with disease duration and older age. Studies performed on direct assessment of BMD by means of different bone densitometry techniques have been extensively reported on in the last decades and yield inconsistent results about the real prevalence of osteoporosis in AS patients, probably depending on the different tools used for evaluating bone mass, the cut-off point chosen to define osteoporosis, and some variables related to the disease itself such as the mean age of patients, the disease duration, and the anatomical evolution of AS.

Taken together, all studies performed by DXA at lumbar level revealed a decreased bone mass in early AS, in patients with normal spine mobility and normal or increased levels of exercise, before the radiological appearance of syndesmophytes, interapophyseal joint ankylosis, and ligamentous ossification.[72,73] In the same way, patients with a clinically mild disease without a radiographic anatomical evolution showed a reduced BMD despite a longer disease duration.[74] These results suggest that in AS, bone loss occurs rapidly, involves trabecular bone,[75] and does not result from spinal stiffness or immobility. Nevertheless, most studies demonstrate that cortical sites such as the femoral neck show a reduced BMD with decreases that appear to be inversely related to disease severity and duration.[73] However, femoral neck BMD reduction seems to be difficult to assess in early disease,[75] and the effects of hip involvement by AS represent a variable not evaluated in many studies. Femoral neck BMD in

men has been reported as around 10% lower than in control subjects,[72,76] with mean Z-scores of around −1.0.[73,74] Conversely, a finding widely shared in cases of advanced AS is a lumbar BMD that appears normal or even increased in comparison, not only with BMD of patients with early AS, but also with healthy control subjects.[77,78] This artifactual increase and the discrepancy between lumbar and femoral neck BMD is due to the anatomical progression of AS, with new bone formation that masks trabecular bone loss.

Therefore, although lumbar DXA is the best tool to identify and monitor patients with early or mild disease, alternative techniques have been proposed in later stages. QCT allows a selective measurement of vertebral trabecular bone and showed a striking reduction of bone mass also in patients with severe AS who did not have decreased lumbar BMD values as assessed by DXA.[75,79,80] QCT, on the other hand, shows a continued steady bone loss along with the anatomical disease progression.[80] However, the high costs and higher radiation dose of this technique are regarded as disadvantages. Lateral lumbar scanning by DXA that isolates the body of L3 vertebra from anterior and posterior syndesmophytes and the ankylosed posterior elements of the spine has also been demonstrated to be quite sensitive in detecting bone loss in cases of long-standing AS,[76,81] with a good correlation with femoral neck BMD. However, its value remains to be determined because of the lack of normative data, the higher precision error, and some technical difficulties that can arise in severely kyphotic patients (superposition of ribs or iliac crest).

Besides women included in mixed study groups,[73,79,82] two studies investigated BMD in female samples,[83,84] showing a lower reduction of bone mass, probably due to a less active disease as is frequently observed in female patients. Finally, patients with spinal involvement associated with other spondyloarthropathies have often been included as small subgroups in larger samples of AS patients. In general, these subjects show no differences in comparison with patients without associated bowel disease, psoriasis, and reactive arthritis, although a study of bone markers demonstrated some differences in bone metabolism among spondyloarthropathies.[85]

Taken together, the results of all these studies are consistent with a systemic process related to the disease itself that affects bone metabolism, not only by changes in mechanical stress related to spinal stiffness or immobility as proposed for advanced AS. The few longitudinal studies on BMD demonstrated a greater bone loss in patients with active disease and a correlation between serum inflammatory parameters, bone resorption markers, and decreases in BMD.[86,87] Because of these issues, it is not surprising that the literature offers inconsistent results about the association between osteoporosis and AS, with a prevalence ranging from 18.7%[88] to 42.8%.[80]

As a consequence of osteoporosis, vertebral compression fractures are frequently reported in patients with AS even if in clinical practice they are probably underdiagnosed and often attributed to exacerbations of the spondylotic process. It seems likely that different methods used to define vertebral fractures and differences in patient selection are responsible for the wide range of reported prevalence of vertebral fractures (Table 24-3), as some anatomical findings related to AS (spondylodiscitis or Romanus lesion) can give a spurious appearance of vertebral wedging. Despite the pathogenetic mechanisms that may involve the entire skeleton through a systemic inflammatory process, an increased rate of appendicular osteoporotic fractures has never been reported, and vertebral fractures seem to be the only clinical consequence of osteoporosis in AS patients. The early increase of vertebral fracture risk within 5 years of diagnosis of AS[89] is consistent with densitometric studies showing a significant bone loss in early disease. Nevertheless, neither lumbar BMD nor femoral BMD are good predictors of likelihood of fracture,[73,74] and this is probably related to the reported bias in lumbar DXA measurement in advanced stages and a lack of site specificity for femoral neck evaluation. The only study able to quantify the fracture risk in AS patients was published by Cooper and associates,[89] who, through a retrospective population-based study, showed an increased vertebral fracture risk as great as 7.6 (95% CI, 4.3-12.6) in comparison with the expected fracture incidence in the same community.

In general, vertebral fractures in patients with AS occur with increasing age, disease duration, and severity of disease,[73,74,89] showing the greatest prevalence two to three decades after diagnosis. It is likely that compression fractures contribute independently of the severity of the disease to spinal deformity and less

mobility of the spine and chest. As regards the site of vertebral fractures, midthoracic vertebrae and the dorsolumbar area are most commonly affected.[90]

In addition to compression fractures, transverse and transdiscal fractures may occur in advanced AS patients[91] also involving the cervical spine,[92] with a reported higher rate of neurological complications.[93] Alterations in the pattern of mechanical stresses within an ankylosed and rigid spine are considered responsible for this particular kind of vertebral fracture.

SYSTEMIC SCLEROSIS

Systemic sclerosis is a connective tissue disorder characterized by fibrosis, degenerative changes, and vascular lesions of the skin with internal organ involvement. Several studies have reported that systemic sclerosis is associated with osteoporosis by different possible pathogenetic mechanisms. Besides a chronic inflammation state, a reduced bone mass in systemic sclerosis patients could be related to decreased physical activity, low body mass index, earlier menopause, decreased vitamin D synthesis in the fibrotic skin, and involvement of the intestinal tract and kidneys that may impair calcium metabolism. Moreover, even if most patients are not usually exposed to corticosteroids, some manifestations of disease such as interstitial lung disease, arthritis, myositis, and acute pericarditis are commonly treated with corticosteroid therapy. In the same way, cyclophosphamide frequently prescribed to systemic sclerosis patients has been associated with premature ovarian failure.[96]

To date, a review of the literature does not allow definitive conclusions about an association between systemic sclerosis and decreased BMD, or whether the clinical features of systemic sclerosis such as disease duration, extent of cutaneous involvement, internal organ involvement, and subcutaneous calcinosis are directly related to osteoporosis risk. Most investigations

TABLE 24-3 PREVALENCE OF VERTEBRAL FRACTURES IN ANKYLOSING SPONDYLITIS					
Study	Number of Patients	Mean Age (y)	Sex Ratio (Male/Female)	Disease Duration (y)	Prevalence of Vertebral Fractures (%)
Hanson et al.[70]	50	Range, 29-75	40/10	ND	4
Donnelly et al.[73]	87	44	62/25	16	10.3
Mitra et al.[74]	66	44	66/0	9.8	16.7
Devogelaer et al.[79]	70	39 (male) and 35 (female)	60/10	15.4 (male) and 13.1 (female)	4.2
Toussirot et al.[82]	71	39	49/22	10.6	1.4
Cooper et al.[89]	158	33.8	121/37	ND	9.5
Ralston et al.[90]	111	41	98/13	17	18
Sivri et al.[94]	22	36	20/2	9.8	40.9
Baek et al.[95]	76	28	76/0	9.4	3.9

are retrospective, case-control studies involving small samples with an insufficient power to detect variables that have a real relationship with a reduced BMD. For example, Di Munno and coworkers[97] showed that patients with diffuse scleroderma and longer disease duration have lower BMD values with no correlation between BMD and body mass index. Instead, Da Silva and coworkers[98] found no differences between diffuse and limited disease. Frediani and coworkers[99] did not find any influence of disease duration on bone loss and Sampaio-Barros and coworkers[100] showed in 61 female systemic sclerosis patients that body mass index was the main variable influencing BMD. In the same way, internal organ involvement has been regarded as a factor influencing BMD values by some authors,[98] but has not been related to BMD values by others.[97] All these discrepancies could be considered to result from patient selection bias, since the most severe cases are more likely to be influenced by other risk factors for osteoporosis such as inactivity, poor nutritional state, chronic renal failure, and medications (corticosteroids and cyclophosphamide).

In an attempt to find an altered bone metabolism in systemic sclerosis patients, some studies have addressed this issue by studying bone markers. Most of them did not show changes in calcium metabolism or alterations in bone markers even in patients with subcutaneous calcinosis. The only bone marker that was reported to be increased was urinary pyridine cross-links.[101] However, it is still unclear whether this result is related to a systemic impairment of collagen turnover and fibrosis rather than an increased bone resorption.

Longitudinal studies will probably be able to confirm the association between systemic sclerosis and low bone mass, allowing clarification of whether the disease itself is actually associated with an increased osteoporosis risk.

PSORIATIC ARTHRITIS

In contrast to RA, studies of skeletal involvement in patients with psoriatic arthritis are scanty, probably because osteoporosis is a less frequently recognized feature in these subjects. Patients with axial involvement have been included in study groups of AS patients[73,87,88] without reported differences in comparison with other axial systemic sclerosis. With regard to oligo/polyarthritic subsets, psoriatic arthritis is believed to be associated with periarticular bone loss less severe than RA, as reported by radiological studies on patients with established disease.[102] Nevertheless, a recent study that used DXA to quantify periarticular BMD in patients with early disease showed no differences in periarticular bone loss in comparison with RA patients, even if in patients with psoriatic arthri-

tis there was no association between the degree of periarticular bone loss and the measures of joint inflammation.[103]

Few studies have investigated generalized osteoporosis in patients with psoriatic arthritis. Nolla and colleagues[104] found no differences in lumbar and femoral neck BMD in 52 patients with peripheral psoriatic arthritis compared with control subjects. Contrasting results have been found by Frediani and associates[105] studying 186 patients with nonaxial psoriatic arthritis. The prevalence of osteoporosis was 11% in young women, 47% in postmenopausal women, and 29% in men. Bone loss was more evident at the lumbar level in young women, whereas a reduced femoral neck BMD was detectable only in postmenopausal subjects. Besides well-recognized risk factors for osteoporosis such as age, years since menopause, and body mass index, the only variable specifically related to disease that was found to be predictive of osteoporosis risk was a disability index related to articular function (HAQ score).

POLYMYALGIA RHEUMATICA

Polymyalgia rheumatica is an inflammatory disease that affects an elderly population and is commonly treated with corticosteroids. Some studies on polymyalgia rheumatica patients have been designed to address the effects on bone metabolism exerted by low-dose corticosteroids, but the disease itself seems to alter bone turnover, causing bone loss very early in the disease, prior to treatment. Dolan and colleagues showed increased levels of resorption markers that correlated with pretreatment disease activity as measured by erythrocyte sedimentation rate and serum interleukin-6, suggesting an effect of systemic inflammation on bone turnover.[106] Patients with a higher acute-phase response at onset had reduced spine BMD before the treatment and a greater bone loss at 1 year. Moreover, by 24 months, as the steroid treatment was reduced or stopped, bone mass improved. Another longitudinal study showed different patterns of bone loss in polymyalgia rheumatica patients with a faster BMD decline in regions containing substantial amounts of trabecular bone and a slower and progressive bone loss at cortical sites.[107]

Considering these results, it seems difficult to distinguish the effects of corticosteroids from those of the disease. Even if the degree of inflammation at presentation suggests a role of the disease severity on the development of osteoporosis, it is likely that steroid treatment is the main determinant of bone loss in these patients, taking into account the short time that usually elapses between the onset of polymyalgia rheumatica and the start of steroid treatment.

REFERENCES

1. Solomon DH, Katz JN, Jacobs JP, et al: Management of gluco-corticoid induced osteoporosis in rheumatoid arthritis. Arthritis Rheum 2002;46:3136-42.
2. Barwell R: Diseases of joints. London: Hardwicke, 1865.
3. Deodhar AA, Woolf AD: Bone mass measurement and bone metabolism in rheumatoid arthritis: a review. Brit J Rheumatol 1996;35:309-22.
4. Sinigaglia L, Nervetti A, Mela Q, et al: A multicenter cross-sectional study on bone mineral density in rheumatoid arthritis. J Rheumatol 2000;27:2582-89.
5. Haugeberg G, Uhlig T, Falch JA, et al: Bone mineral density and frequency of osteoporosis in female patients with rheumatoid arthritis. Arthritis Rheum 2000;43:522-30.
6. Stafford L, Bleasel J, Giles A, et al: Androgen deficiency and bone mineral density in men with rheumatoid arthritis. J Rheumatol 2000;27:2786-90.
7. Tengstrand B, Hafstrom I: Bone mineral density in men with rheumatoid arthritis is associated with erosive disease and sul-fasalazine treatment but not with sex hormones. J Rheumatol 2002;29:2299-305.
8. Haugeberg G, Uhlig T, Falch JA, et al: Reduced bone mineral density in male rheumatoid arthritis patients. Arhritis Rheum 2000;43:2776-84.
9. Sambrook PN, Eisman JA, Champion GD, et al: Determinants of axial bone loss in rheumatoid arthritis. Arthritis Rheum 1987;30:721-27.
10. Madsen OR, Sorensen OH, Egsmose C: Bone quality and bone mass as assessed by quantitative ultrasound and dual energy x-ray absorptiometry in women with rheumatoid arthritis: relationship wit quadriceps strength. Ann Rheum Dis 2002;61:325-29.
11. Hakkinen A, Sokka T, Kotaniemi A, et al: A randomized two year study of the effects of dynamic strength training on muscle strength, disease activity, functional capacity and bone mineral density in early rheumatoid arthritis. Arthritis Rheum 2001;44:515-22.
12. Hansen M, Florescu A, Stoltenberg M, et al: Bone loss in rheumatoid arthritis: influence of disease activity, duration of the disease, functional capacity and corticoid treatment. Scand J Rheumatol 1996;25:367-76.
13. Als OS, Gotfredsen A, Riis B, et al: Are disease duration and degree of functional impairment determinants of bone loss in rheumatoid arthritis? Ann Rheum Dis 1985;44:406-11.
14. Shawe D, Hesp R, Gumpel JM, et al: Physical activity as a deter-minant of bone conservation in the radial diaphysis in rheuma-toid arthritis. Ann Rheum Dis 1993;52:579-81.
15. Sambrook PN, Eisman JA, Champion JD, et al: Osteoporosis in rheumatoid arthritis: safety of low-dose corticosteroids. Ann Rheum Dis 1986;45:950-3.
16. Leboff MS, Wade JP, Mackowiak S, et al: Low-dose prednisone does not affect calcium homeostasis or bone density in post-menopausal women with Rheumatoid Arthritis. J Rheumatol 1991;18:339-44.
17. Laan RFJM, Van Riel PLCM, Van Earning LJTH, et al: Vertebral osteoporosis in rheumatoid arthritis patients: effect of low-dose prednisolone therapy. Br J Rheumatol 1992;31:91-16.
18. Hall GM, Spector TD, Griffin AJ, et al: The effect of rheumatoid arthritis and steroid therapy on bone density in post-menopausal women. Arthritis Rheum 1993;36:1510-16.
19. Shibuya K, Hagino H, Morio Y, et al: Cross-sectional and longitu-dinal study of osteoporosis in patients with rheumatoid arthri-tis. Clin Rheumatol 2002;21:150-58.
20. Sambrook PN, Raj A, Hunter D, et al: Osteoporosis with low dose corticosteroids: contribution of underlying disease effects and discriminatory ability of ultrasound versus bone densitom-etry. J Rheumatol 2001;28:1063-67.
21. Lane NE, Pressman AR, Star VL, et al: Rheumatoid arthritis and bone mineral density in elderly women. J Bone Min Res 1995;20:257-63.
22. Van Staa TP, Leufkens HGM, Cooper C: The epidemiology of corticosteroid-induced osteoporosis: a meta-analysis. Oteoporos Int 2002;13:777-87.
23. Ton FN, Gunawardene C, Lee H, et al: Effects of low-dose pred-nisone on bone metabolism. J Bone Min Res 2005;20:464-70.
24. Haugeberg G, Orstavik RE, Uhlig T, et al: Bone loss in patients with rheumatoid arthritis. Arthritis Rheum 2002;46:1720-28.
25. Shenstone BD, Mahmoud A, Woodward R, et al: Longitudinal bone mineral density changes in early rheumatoid arthritis. Br J Rheumatol 1994;33:541-45.
26. Gough AKS, Lilley J, Eyre S, et al: Generalised bone loss in patients with early rheumatoid arthritis. Lancet 1994;344:23-7.
27. Kalla AA, Meyers OL, Chalton D, et al: Increased metacarpal bone mass following 18 months of slow-acting antirheumatic drugs for rheumatoid arthritis. Br J Rheumatol 1991;30:91-100.
28. Dolan AL, Moniz C, Abraha H, et al: Does active treatment of rheumatoid arthritis limit disease-associated bone loss? Rheumatology 2002;41:1047-51.
29. Quinn M: The effect of TNF blockade on bone loss in early rheumatoid arthritis. Arthritis Rheum 2002;46(suppl):S519.
30. Sambrook PN: The skeleton in rheumatoid arthritis: common mechanisms for bone erosion and osteoporosis? J Rheumatol 2000;27:2541-42.
31. Lodder MC, de Jong Z, Kostense PJ, et al: Bone mineral density in patients with rheumatoid arthritis: relation between disease severity and low bone mineral density. Ann Rheum Dis 2004;63:1576-80.
32. Forsblad d'Elia H, Larsen A, Waltbrand E, et al: Radiographic joint destruction in postmenopausal rheumatoid arthritis is strongly associated with generalised osteoporosis. Ann Rheum Dis 2003;62:617-23.
33. Forslind K, Keller C, Svensson B, et al: Reduced bone mineral density in early rheumatoid arthritis is associated with radiolog-ical joint damage at baseline and after two years in women. J Rheumatol 2003;30:2590-96.
34. Gough A, Sambrook PN, Devlin J, et al: Osteoclastic activation is the principal mechanism leading to secondary osteoporosis in rheumatoid arthritis. J Rheumatol 1998;25:1282-89.
35. Garnero P, Landewé R, Boers M, et al: Association of baseline levels of markers of bone and cartilage degradation with long-term progression of joint damage in patients with early rheumatoid arthritis. Arthritis Rheum 2002;46:2847-56.
36. Lodder MC, Haugeberg G, Lems WF, et al: Radiographic dam-age associated with low bone mineral density and vertebral deformities in rheumatoid arthritis: the Oslo-Truro-Amsterdam (OSTRA) Collaborative Study. Arthritis Rheum Arthritis Care Res 2003;49:209-15.
37. Hooyman JR, Melton LJ, Nelson AM, et al: Fractures after rheumatoid arthritis: a population-based study. Arthritis Rheum 1984;27:1353-61.
38. Peel NFA, Moore DJ, Barrington NA, et al: Risk of vertebral frac-ture and relationship to bone mineral density in steroid treated rheumatoid arthritis. Ann Rheum Dis 1995;54:801-6.
39. Orstavik RE, Haugeberg G, Mowinckel P, et al: Vertebral deformities in rheumatoid arthritis. Arch Intern Med 2004;164:420-5.
40. Cooper C, Coupland C, Mitchell M: Rheumatoid arthritis, cortico-steroid therapy and hip fracture. Ann Rheum Dis 1995;54:49-52.
41. Huusko TM, Korpela M, Karppi P, et al: Threefold increased risk of hip fractures with rheumatoid arthritis in central Finland. Ann Rheum Dis 2001;60:521-22.
42. Orstavik RE, Haugebergf G, Uhlig T, et al: Self reported non-ver-tebral fractures in rheumatoid arthritis and population based controls: incidence and relationship with bone mineral density and clinical variables. Ann Rheum Dis 2004;63:177-82.
43. Michel BA, Bloch D, Wolfe F, et al: Fractures in rheumatoid arthritis: an evaluation of associated risk factor. J Rheumatol 1993;20:1666-69.
44. Orstavik RE, Haugeberg G, Uhlig T, et al: Vertebral deformities in 229 female patients with rheumatoid arthritis: associations with clinical variables and bone mineral density. Arthritis Rheum Arthritis Care Res 2003;49:355-60.
45. Kaz Kaz H, Johnson D, Kerry S, et al: Fall-related risk factors and osteoporosis in women with rheumatoid arthritis. Rheumatology 2004;43:1267-71.

46. Jamison M, Neuberger GB, Miller PA: Correlates of falls and fear of falling among adults with rheumatoid arthritis. Arthritis Rheum Arthritis Care Res 2003;49:673-80.

47. Haugeberg G, Orstavik RE, Uhlig T, et al: Clinical decision rules in rheumatoid arthritis: do they identify patients at high risk for osteoporosis? Testing clinical criteria in a population based cohort of patients with rheumatoid arthritis recruited from the Oslo Rheumatoid Arthritis Register. Ann Rheum Dis 2002;61:1085-89.

48. Sinigaglia L, Varenna M, Binelli L, et al: Bone mass in systemic lupus erythematosus. Clin Exp Rheumatol 2000;18(suppl 2): S27-34.

49. Dhillon VB, Davies MC, Hall ML, et al: Assessment of the effect of oral corticosteroids on bone mineral density in systemic lupus erythematosus: a preliminary study with dual energy X ray absorptiometry. Ann Rheum Dis 1990;49:624-26.

50. Houssiau FA, Lefebvre C, Depresseux G, et al: Trabecular and cortical bone loss in systemic lupus erythematosus. Br J Rheumatol 1996;35:244-47.

51. Sels F, Dequeker J, Verwilghen J, et al: SLE and osteoporosis: dependence and/or independence on glucocorticoids. Lupus 1996;5:89-92.

52. Kalla AA, Fataar AB, Jessop SJ, et al: Loss of trabecular bone mineral density in systemic lupus erythematosus. Arthritis Rheum 1993;12:1726-34.

53. Formiga F, Moga I, Nolla JM, et al: Loss of bone mineral density in premenopausal women with systemic lupus erythematosus. Ann Rheum Dis 1995;54:274-6.

54. Li EK, Tam LS, Young RP, et al: Loss of bone mineral density in Chinese premenopausal women with systemic lupus erythematosus treated with corticosteroids. Br J Rheumatol 1998;37:405-10.

55. Pineau CA, Urowitz MB, Fortin D, et al: Osteoporosis in systemic lupus erythematosus: factors associated with referral for bone mineral density studies, prevalence of osteoporosis and factors associated with reduced bone density. Lupus 2004;13:436-41.

56. Pons F, Peris P, Guanabens N, et al: The effect of systemic lupus erythematosus and long-term steroid therapy on bone mass in premenopausal women. Br J Rheumatol 1995;34:742-6.

57. Kipen Y, Buchbinder R, Strauss BJG, et al: Prevalence of reduced bone mineral density in systemic lupus erythematosus and the role of glucocorticoids. J Rheumatol 1997;24:1922-9.

58. Sinigaglia L, Varenna M, Binelli L, et al: Determinants of bone mass in systemic lupus erythematosus: a cross-sectional study on premenopausal women. J Rheumatol 1999;26:1280-84.

59. Yee C-S, Crabtree N, Skan J, et al: Prevalence and predictors of fragility fractures in systemic lupus erythematosus. Ann Rheum Dis 2005;64:111-13.

60. Uaratanawong S, Deesomchoke U, Lertmaharit S, et al: Bone mineral density in premenopausal women with systemic lupus erythematosus. J Rheumatol 2003;30:2365-68.

61. Petri M: Musculoskeletal complications of systemic lupus erythematosus in the Hopkins Lupus Cohort: an update. Arthritis Care Res 1995;8:137-45.

62. Mok CC, Mak A, Ma KM: Bone mineral density in post-menopausal Chinese patients with systemic lupus erythematosus. Lupus 2005;14:106-12.

63. Formiga F, Nolla JM, Moga I, et al: Sequential study of bone mineral density in patients with systemic lupus erythematosus [letter]. Ann Rheum Dis 1996;55:857.

64. Hansen M, Halberg P, Kollerup G, et al: Bone metabolism in patients with systemic lupus erythematosus. Scand J Rheumatol 1998;27:197-206.

65. Kipen Y, Briganti E, Strauss B, et al: Three year follow up of bone mineral density change in premenopausal women with systemic lupus erythematosus. J Rheumatol 1999;26:310-17.

66. Trapani S, Civinini R, Ermini M, et al: Osteoporosis in juvenile systemic lupus erythematosus: a longitudinal study on the effects of steroids on bone mineral density. Rheumatol Int 1998;18:45-9.

67. Teichmann J, Lange U, Stracke H, et al: Bone metabolism and bone mineral density of systemic lupus erythematosus at the time of diagnosis. Rheumatol Int 1999;18:137-40.

68. Formiga F, Nolla JM, Mitjavila F, et al: Bone mineral density and hormonal status in men with systemic lupus erythematosus. Lupus 1996;5:623-26.

69. Ramsey-Goldman R, Dunn JE, Huang CF, et al: Frequency of fractures in women with systemic lupus erythematosus. Arthritis Rheum 1999;42:882-90.

70. Hanson CA, Shagrin JW, Duncan H: Vertebral osteoporosis in ankylosing spondylitis. Clin Orthop 1971;74:59-64.

71. Spencer DG, Park WM, Dick HM, et al: Radiological manifestations in 200 patients with ankylosing spondylitis: correlation with clinical features and HLA B27. J Rheumatol 1979;6:305-15.

72. Will R, Palmer R, Bhalla AK, et al: Osteoporosis in early ankylosing spondylitis: a primary event? Lancet 1989;2:1483-85.

73. Donnelly S, Doyle DV, Denton A, et al: Bone mineral density and vertebral compression fracture rates in ankylosing spondylitis. Ann Rheum Dis 1994;53:117-21.

74. Mitra D, Elvins DM, Speden DJ, Collins AJ: The prevalence of vertebral fractures in mild ankylosing spondylitis and their relationship to bone mineral density. Rheumatology 2000;39:85-9.

75. Lee LYS, Schlotzhauer T, Ott SM, et al: Skeletal status of men with early and late ankylosing spondylitis. Am J Med 1997;103:233-41.

76. Bronson WD, Walker SE, Hillman LS, et al: Bone mineral density and biochemical markers of bone metabolism in ankylosing spondylitis. J Rheumatol 1998;25:929-35.

77. Reid DM, Nicoll JJ, Kennedy NS, et al: Bone mass in ankylosing spondylitis. J Rheumatol 1986;13:932-35.

78. Mullaji AB, Upadhyay SS, Ho EK: Bone mineral density in ankylosing spondylitis. DEXA comparison of control subjects with mild and advanced cases. J Bone Joint Surg Br 1994;76:660-65.

79. Devogelaer J-P, Maldague B, Malghem J, Nagant de Deuxchaisnes C: Appendicular and vertebral bone mass in ankylosing spondylitis. Arthritis Rheum 1992;35:1062-67.

80. Lange U, Kluge A, Strunk J, et al: Ankylosing spondylitis and bone mineral density: what is the ideal tool for measurement? Rheumatol Int 2004;26:115-120.

81. Gilgil E, Kacar C, Tuncer T, Bütün B: The association of syndesmophytes with vertebral bone mineral density in patients with ankylosing spondylitis. J Rheumatol 2005;32:292-94.

82. Toussirot E, Michel F, Wendling D: Bone density, ultrasound measurements and body composition in early ankylosing spondylitis. Rheumatology 2001;40:882-88.

83. Juanola X, Mateo L, Nolla J-M, et al: Bone mineral density in women with ankylosing spondylitis. J Rheumatol 2000;27:1028-31.

84. Speden DJ, Calin AI, Ring FJ, Bhalla AK: Bone mineral density, calcaneal ultrasound, and bone turnover markers in women with ankylosing spondylitis. J Rheumatol 2002;29:516-21.

85. Grisar J, Bernecker PM, Aringer M, et al: Ankylosing spondylitis, psoriatic arthritis, and reactive arthritis show increased bone resorption, but differ with regard to bone formation. J Rheumatol 2002;29:1430-36.

86. Gratacos J, Collado A, Pons F, et al: Significant loss of bone mass in patients with early, active ankylosing spondylitis. Arthritis Rheum 1999;42:2319-24.

87. Maillefert JF, Aho LS, El Maghraoui A, et al: Changes in bone density in patients with ankylosing spondylitis: a two-year follow-up study. Osteoporos Int 2001;12:605-9.

88. El Maghraoui A, Borderie D, Cherruau B, et al: Osteoporosis, body composition, and bone turnover in ankylosing spondylitis. J Rheumatol 1999;26:2205-9.

89. Cooper C, Carbone L, Michet CJ, et al: Fracture risk in patients with ankylosing spondylitis: a population based study. J Rheumatol 1994;21:1877-82.

90. Ralston SH, Urquhart GDK, Brzeski M, Sturrock RD: Prevalence of vertebral compression fractures due to osteoporosis in ankylosing spondylitis. BMJ 1990;300:563-65.

91. Thorngren KG, Liedberg E, Aspelin P: Fractures of the thoracic and lumbar spine in ankylosing spondylitis. Arch Orthop Traumat Surg 1981;98:101-7.

92. Murray GC, Persellin RH: Cervical fracture complicating in ankylosing spondylitis: a report of eight cases and review of the literature. Am J Med 1981;70:1033-41.

93. Grisolia A, Bell R, Peltier L: Fractures and dislocations of the spine complicating ankylosing spondylitis J Bone Joint Surg Am 1967;49:339-44.

94. Sivri A, Killinc S, Gökce-Kutsal Y, Ariyürek M: Bone mineral density in ankylosing spondylitis. Clin Rheumatol 1996;15:51-4.

95. Baek HJ, Kang SW, Lee JY, et al: Osteopenia in men with mild and severe ankylosing spondylitis. Rheumatol Int 2005;26:30-4.

96. Mok CC, Lau CS, Wong RWS: Risk factors for ovarian failure in patients with systemic lupus erytematosus receiving cyclophosphamide therapy. Arthritis Rheum 1998;41:831-37.

97. Di Munno O, Mazzantini M, Massei P, et al: Reduced bone mass and normal calcium metabolism in systemic sclerosis with and without calcinosis. Clin Rheumatol 1995;14:407-12.

98. Da Silva HC, Szejnfeld VL, Assis LS, Sato EI: Study of bone density in systemic scleroderma. Rev Assoc Med Bras 1997;43:40-6.

99. Frediani B, Baldi F, Falsetti P, et al: Clinical determinants of bone mass and bone ultrasonometry in patients with systemic sclerosis. Clin Exp Rheum 2004;22:313-18.

100. Sampaio-Barros PD, Costa-Paiva L, Filardi S, et al: Prognostic factors of low bone mineral density in systemic sclerosis. Clin Exp Rheum 2005;23:180-84.

101. Istok R, Czirjak L, Lukac J, et al: Increased urinary pyridinoline cross-link compounds of collagen in patients with systemic sclerosis and Raynaud's phenomenon. Rheumatology (Oxford) 2001;40:140-46.

102. Wright V: Psoriatic arthritis: a comparative radiographic study of rheumatoid arthritis and arthritis associated with psoriasis. Ann Rheum Dis 1961;20:123-31.

103. Harrison BJ, Hutchinson CE, Adams J, et al: Assessing periarticular bone mineral density in patients with early psoriatic arthritis or rheumatoid arthritis. Ann Rheum Dis 2002;61:1007-11.

104. Nolla JM, Rozadilla A, Gomez-Vaquero C, et al: Bone mineral density in patients with peripheral psoriatic arthritis. Rev Rhum [Engl Ed] 1999;66:457-61.

105. Frediani B, Allegri A, Falsetti P, et al: Bone mineral density in patients with psoriatic arthritis. J Rheumatol 2001;28:138-43.

106. Dolan AL, Moniz C, Dasgupta B, et al: Effects of inflammation and treatment on bone turnover and bone mass in polymyalgia rheumatica. Arthritis Rheum 1997;40:2022-29.

107. Pearce G, Ryan PFJ, Delmas PD, et al: The deleterious effects of low-dose corticosteroids on bone density in patients with polymyalgia rheumatica. Br J Rheumatol 1998;37:292-99.

25

Pathogenesis of Inflammation-Induced Bone Loss

Mary Beth Humphrey and Mary C. Nakamura

SUMMARY

Inflammatory signals mediated by immune cells and cytokines have significant influence over osteoclast differentiation and funtion. Osteoclasts express a number of immune receptors and are regulated like related cells in the immune system, such as macrophages and dendritic cells. Inflammatory signals can also affect osteoblasts and other crucial cells in the bony microenvironment including synovial cells and chondrocytes, which may further contribute to the uncoupling of bone turnover. Osteopenia and juxta-articular erosion are consequences of chronic inflammatory autoimmune disease, however inflammatory signals appear to also play a role in postmenopausal osteoporosis.

Bony remodeling is an ongoing process throughout adult life that is tightly regulated by a balance of activity between osteoclasts that degrade bone and osteoblasts that lay down new bony matrix. Bony erosion and osteopenia result when the function of these two critical cell types is "uncoupled" and osteoclast activity is increased relative to new bone formation.[1] Osteoclasts are specialized as the only bone-resorbing cell type. Osteoclasts are differentiated from hematopoietic myeloid precursor cells under the regulation of specific cytokines, growth factors, and receptor signals.[2,3] It has become increasingly clear that inflammatory signals mediated by immune cells and cytokines also have significant influence over osteoclast differentiation and function. Inflammatory signals can have significant effects on osteoblasts and other crucial cells in the bony microenvironment, including synovial cells and chondrocytes, which may further contribute to the uncoupling of bone degradation and formation activities.[4-6] Thus, it has not been surprising that osteopenia and periarticular erosion are consequences in chronic inflammatory autoimmune disease; however, inflammatory signals likely also play a role in other types of bone loss such as postmenopausal osteoporosis.[7]

Recent studies have demonstrated that osteoclasts themselves express a number of immune receptors and are regulated like related cells in the innate immune system such as macrophages and dendritic cells.[8] Other cells in the innate immune system function as unique sensors to respond to stress, infectious or inflammatory changes in their microenvironment detected through soluble mediators and intercellular interactions. Although the innate inflammatory response is critical to fully develop an adaptive immune response, a consequence may be local tissue destruction at the same time.[9] Osteoclasts may function similarly, with resulting bone loss or erosion as a consequence of their activation as a part of the inflammatory response. As we begin to further understand the complexity of these interactions, it is likely that new points for therapeutic intervention in the process of bone remodeling will be identified that may be useful in autoimmune disease.

BONE LOSS IN AUTOIMMUNE DISEASE

Clinicians have long appreciated that patients with chronic inflammatory autoimmune diseases can suffer from both localized and generalized diffuse osteopenia and localized bony erosive disease in some cases.[4-6] Although at one time inflammation and bone loss were believed to be mediated by completely separate pathways, it is now clear that the immune system and skeletal system share a variety of regulatory mechanisms. Choi and colleagues[10] first used the term *osteoimmunology* to describe the study of the interrelationship between inflammation and bone remodeling. Osteoimmunology was first exemplified by studies demonstrating the critical regulation of osteoclastogenesis by cytokines produced by activated T cells: RANKL (receptor activator of nuclear factor-κB ligand) and interferon-γ (IFN-γ).[11] Although the degree of inflammation and the severity of bony erosive disease do not always completely correlate in human disease, inflammatory cytokines and receptors are critical factors in regulating the activity of osteoclasts that mediate disease.[12] Bony erosions are seen in several types of inflammatory arthritis—rheumatoid arthritis, psoriatic arthritis, and spondyloarthropathy—but each disease appears slightly different by histopathology, although each can result in bony destruction.[6,13,14] Thus, distinct diseases and different pathways of inflammation can lead to a similar pathological process resulting in excessive activation of osteoclasts near sites of inflammation.

RHEUMATOID ARTHRITIS

A significant consequence of rheumatoid arthritis (RA) is the development of periarticular osteopenia and focal erosions of the subchondral bone in joints with inflammatory synovitis and pannus formation. In cases of chronic synovitis and pannus formation, the synovial lining layer, which is normally one to three cells thick, becomes greatly hypertrophied (eight to 10 cells thick), with fibroblasts and macrophages as the primary cell populations in this layer.[15,16] Synovial cells are often categorized as type A (macrophage-like) and type B (fibroblast-like). The subintimal area of the synovium, which merges with the joint capsule, normally has few cells, as this is where the synovial blood vessels are located.[16] In RA, the subintimal layer has an intense cellular infiltrate with T and B lymphocytes, macrophages and mast cells, and some new blood vessel formation (angiogenesis).[16] The proportion and quantity of infiltrating inflammatory cells can vary considerably. In RA, the pannus or hypertrophied synovium directly invades and leads to erosion of the contiguous bone and cartilage. The hypertrophied rheumatoid synovium begins its invasion of bone at the sites of normal synovium attachment, which is anchored to both sides of the joint.[17,18] Erosions on either or both sides of the joint are often seen radiographically along with joint space narrowing indicative of reduction of the volume of cartilage.[19]

Bony erosion is generally mediated by osteoclasts, the only bone-resorbing cell type, and indeed osteoclast-like cells have been observed associated with localized bone erosion in RA.[20-22] Osteoclasts are essential for bony erosions in a transgenic mouse model for RA in which tumor necrosis factor (TNF)-α is overexpressed.[23] In the osteoclast-deficient *cfos-/-* mice, the TNF-α–mediated arthritis shows synovial inflammation but no bony erosions.[23] Osteoclast-like cells have been demonstrated in human RA tissue by histopathological studies by light microscopy showing multinucleated, tartrate-resistant acid phosphatase positive cells at the bone-pannus interface.[20] Electron microscopy has demonstrated resorption bays typical of osteoclastic activity in the subchondral bone of metacarpal heads in areas of pannus invasion.[22] Gravellese and associates[21] have demonstrated the pres-

ence of multinucleated cells in resorption lacunae at sites of subchondral bone pannus invasion. The osteoclast phenotype was also demonstrated by in situ hybridization showing the expression of genes associated with mature functional osteoclasts (calcitonin receptor, tartrate resistant acid phosphatase, cathepsin K).[21,24]

OSTEOCLAST DIFFERENTIATION AND RANK

Osteoclasts develop from monocyte/macrophage precursor cells under the influence of multiple cytokines, including macrophage colony-stimulating factor (M-CSF), interleukin (IL)-1, transforming growth factor (TGF)-β, IL-6, TNF-α, vitamin D_3, parathyroid hormone, and RANKL.[2,3] Although each of these factors regulates osteoclast development or function, either directly or indirectly, only RANKL signaling through its receptor RANK is absolutely required for osteoclastogenesis in vivo (Figure 25-1).[25] RANKL,[26] also known as TNF-related activation-induced cytokine (TRANCE),[27] osteoprotegerin ligand,[28] and osteoclast differentiation factor[29] is a type II transmembrane protein (carboxy-terminus outside the cell) that is present on the cell surface of osteoblasts, bone marrow stromal cells, fibroblasts, mammary epithelial cells, and activated T cells. RANKL binds to its receptor RANK, also termed TRANCE-receptor or osteoclast differentiation and activation receptor, which is found on dendritic cells, B cells, T cells, endothelial cells, fibroblasts, osteoclast precursors, and mature osteoclasts.[26] RANK is a member of the TNF receptor superfamily, and RANKL, like other TNF receptor ligands, is active as both a trimeric transmembrane protein and a soluble monomer after it is cleaved from the cell surface by the metalloprotease-disintegrin TNF-α converting enzyme.[31]

Another TNF family member, osteoprotegerin (OPG), inhibits osteoclastogenesis driven by RANK:RANKL signaling by binding to both membrane and soluble forms of RANKL, thus acting as a decoy receptor for RANKL.[28,29,32] OPG is produced by bone marrow stromal cells, T- and B-cells, dendritic cells, monocytes/macrophages, and megakaryocytes. The expression of RANKL and OPG is highly modulated by multiple osteotropic agents (Table 25-1), and the molecular balance of RANKL, RANK, and OPG profoundly affects bone remodeling.

The critical role of RANK signaling in normal bone maintenance was revealed in mice genetically deficient in RANK or RANKL that show severe osteopetrosis and abnormal tooth eruption secondary to the total absence of osteoclastogenesis.[25,33,34] Additionally, these mice lack lymph node development and have abnormal B- and T-cell development, indicating the critical role of RANK signaling in normal immune function.[25,33] Conversely, mice deficient in OPG or transgenic mice

Figure 25-1. Osteoclastogenesis. Osteoclasts are derived from bone marrow precursor cells in the myeloid lineage. Mononuclear precursor cells fuse to form multinucleated osteoclasts during differentiation. Macrophage colony-stimulating factor (M-CSF) and RANKL are essential stimuli for osteoclastogenesis at a number of steps. Mature osteoclasts are characterized by a multinucleated phenotype, with expression of tartrate resistant acid phosphatase, cathepsin K, $\alpha_v\beta_3$ integrin (vitronectin receptor) and calcitonin receptor.[2,3] (See Color Plates.)

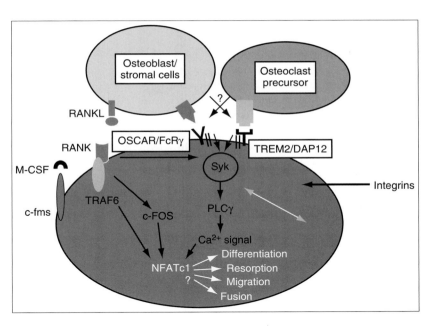

TABLE 25-1 MODULATORS OF RANKL AND OPG EXPRESSION			
	RANKL	**OPG**	**Studies**
Estradiol	No change	Increased	Hofbauer et al,[114] Saika et al,[182] Viereck et al[183]
Glucocorticoid	Increased	Decreased	Yasuda et al,[29] Brandstrom et al,[184] Vidal et al,[185] Gao et al[186]
Prostaglandin E2	Increased	Decreased	Brandstrom et al,[184] Suda et al,[187] Liu et al[188]
1,25 (OH)$_2$ vitamin D$_3$	Increased	Increased	Hofbauer et al,[52] Mukohyama et al,[189] Yasuda et al[190]
PTH	Increased	Decreased	Lee & Lorenzo,[191] Horwood et al[193]
PTHrP	Increased	Decreased	Thomas et al[194]
IGF-1	Increased	Decreased	Rubin et al[195]
IL-1	Increased	Increased	Nakashima et al,[196] Hofbauer et al,[197] Dai et al[198]
IL-6	Increased	No change	Palmqvist et al,[199] Kobayashi et al[200]
IL-11	Increased	No change	Nakashima et al,[196] Ahlen et al[201]
IL-17	Increased	Decreased	Nakashima et al[196]
IFN-γ	Increased	Increased	Nakashima et al[196]
TNF-α	Increased	Increased	Hofbauer et al,[52] Dai et al[198]
TGF-β	Decreased	Increased	Kobayashi et al,[200] Ishida et al,[202] Murakami et al,[203] Kaneda et al,[204] Quinn et al,[205] Thirunavukkarasu et al[206]
CD40L	Increased	Not tested	Anderson et al,[26] Yun et al[207]
BMP-2	Not tested	Increased	Hofbauer et al[52]

IFN = interferon; IL = interleukin; TGF = transforming growth factor; TNF = tumor necrosis factor.

expressing RANK-Fc have profound osteoporosis with increased osteoclastogenesis.[30,35] The importance of RANK signaling seen in mouse models is confirmed in human states of inherited skeletal disease, including familial expansile osteolysis or familial Paget disease, in which mutations in the RANK that lead to constitutive activation can drive abnormal bone remodeling and osteoclast activity.[36] Additionally, OPG gene mutations leading to loss of function result in idiopathic hyperphosphatasia or juvenile Paget disease[37-39] and OPG polymorphisms are associated with increased risk of osteoporotic fracture in women and men.[40]

Although RANKL directly activates the osteoclast and is required for normal osteoclast differentiation, it also regulates immune cell effector function and provides a survival signal to monocytes and dendritic cells.[26,27,42] These findings may be significant in terms of osteoclast recruitment during inflammatory states, given that recent studies suggest that immature dendritic cells may transdifferentiate into osteoclasts in vitro under the influence of RANKL and M-CSF.[43]

RANKL AND INFLAMMATORY ARTHRITIS

During states of acute or chronic inflammation such as rheumatoid arthritis, activated T-cells may act as a stimulus for osteoclastogenesis. This process is multifactorial, including T-cell production of RANKL as well as other proinflammatory cytokines such as TNF-α or IL-1.[44] Co-culture of activated T-cells with preosteoclasts can support osteoclastogenesis via T-cell production of RANKL in vitro, and injection of activated T-cells in RANKL-deficient mice can rescue osteoclastogenesis.[45] The importance of RANK and osteoclasts in inflammatory arthritis was demonstrated by the lack of development of bony erosions in RANK/TRANCE-deficient animals in a serum transfer model of inflammatory arthritis.[46] Blockade of RANKL via OPG treatment in transgenic mice expressing human TNF-α, or in adjuvant induced arthritis, also prevents erosive bone and cartilage disease, further supporting the role of proinflammatory cytokines driving RANKL in vivo.[45,47,48] TNF-α and other inflammatory cytokines are produced by activated macrophages and activated T-cells in the RA inflamed synovium.[12,49-51] TNF-α is a strong stimulus for the upregulation of RANKL expression by osteoblast lining cells.[52] Human studies reveal that RANKL and OPG levels are markedly elevated in patients with rheumatoid arthritis and that treatment with anti-TNF-α leads to normalization.[53] The success of TNF-α blockade therapy in many patients with RA has demonstrated the importance of this cytokine on inflammatory synovitis. TNF-α blockade has also been demonstrated to inhibit bony erosion, although whether this outcome is due to the diminished inflammatory synovitis, the decrease in osteoclast precursors, or direct effects on osteoclast differentiation and function is not completely delineated.[54,55] Many other cytokines are also known to regulate both RANKL and OPG levels (see Table 25-1), which directly stimulate or block osteoclast formation. Some of these cytokines may be of greater influence in the population of RA patients who do not respond to anti-TNF-α therapy.

OSTEOPENIA AND OSTEOPOROSIS IN RHEUMATOID ARTHRITIS

In the area of joints affected by chronic inflammatory synovitis, periarticular osteopenia is a radiographic feature common in RA. Histological studies of bone in these areas demonstrate aggregates of inflammatory cells (macrophages and lymphocytes) in the bone marrow, an increase in osteoid surface area, and an increase in resorption surfaces populated by osteoclasts.[56,57] Thus, an increase in bony remodeling by osteoclasts is observed without a corresponding increase in osteoblast activity to form new bone.[56,57] These areas lack direct synovial interaction with the bone surface but are likely subject to the effects of inflammatory mediators produced locally by inflamed synovial tissue. Although local bone loss in distinct areas of inflammation is prominent in RA, diffuse bone loss resulting in generalized osteoporosis is also common.[58,59] Osteoporosis is observed in the vertebral column and peripherally, predisposing to increased risk of both vertebral and hip fractures.[60,61] Multiple factors may contribute to the generalized bone loss, including lack of activity, glucocorticoid use, use of immunosuppressive drugs, and estrogen loss.[62] The role of systemic cytokines such as IL-1, TNF-α, and IL-6 has not been examined in the setting of generalized bone loss in RA. Interestingly, one histomorphometric evaluation of bone in the absence of corticosteroid use suggested that the primary defect is a decrease in bone formation rather than increased bony resorption.[63] In contrast, studies examining urinary biochemical markers of bone turnover suggest that bone resorption is increased, which is associated with disease activity.[57,64] The discrepant findings may be due to differences in patients, treatments, stage of disease, or other variables, but they highlight the truly multifactorial nature of generalized bone loss in RA. It may be that in the more localized areas of bone loss with marked synovitis and associated inflammation, the direct effects of inflammatory mediators more easily predominate.

SPONDYLOARTHROPATHY

Spondyloarthropathies represent a distinct type of inflammatory arthritis with the common clinical feature being inflammation in the sacroiliac joints. Both acute and chronic inflammations of other parts of the spine and enthesitis or chronic inflammation at the sites of tendon insertion into bone are generally seen in patients with ankylosing spondylitis with some asymmetric peripheral joint synovitis as well.[65] Reactive arthritis commonly demonstrates more prominent peripheral joint synovitis and occurs after extra-articular bacterial infections of the urogenital and gastrointestinal tracts.[66] These diseases also share the well-recognized association with the class I MHC (major histocompatibility complex) HLA B27 allele.[66,67] Although potential roles for HLA-B27 in inflammatory spondyloarthropathy in the immune response have been extensively examined,[13,67] the exact mechanism leading to the susceptibility for these disorders remains undefined.

Spondyloarthropathies are distinct from rheumatoid arthritis, given the presence of inflammatory enthesopathy and the resultant progressive ossification of the spine, and recent studies have demonstrated that the peripheral synovitis also demonstrates distinct histopathological changes compared with RA.[68,69] Baeten and coworkers[68] demonstrated that the synovitis in peripheral joints is characterized by extensive hypervascularity and the presence of specific macrophage and T-cell subsets. CD163+ macrophages and local production of soluble CD163 were associated with the degree of inflammation in synovial tissue from spondyloarthropathy patients and not in RA patients. CD163 is a transmembrane scavenger receptor expressed on a subset of activated macrophages. Interestingly, the same subsets of macrophages and T-cells seen in synovial tissue were also identified in the gut mucosa in patients with Crohn disease and spondyloarthropathy, even without evidence of histological bowel wall inflammation.[70] This latter finding suggests that early immune alteration of the gut may play a role in development of the disease. CD163+ macrophages have been demonstrated to release greater amounts of IL-1 and TNF-α in vitro after lipopolysaccharide stimulation than CD163– macrophages.[71] Baeten and coworkers[72] propose that neovascularization and recirculation of specific inflammatory cells between the gut and synovium may be critical in the development of spondyloarthropathies. Macrophage-derived cytokines such as TNF-α, INF-γ, and IL-10 are prominent in these chronic disease states,[73] and the described clinical benefit of TNF-α blockade in these disorders clearly supports a significant role for that cytokine in these diseases.[74] An unresolved issue remains how antecedent infection induces inflammation and erosion in the sacroiliac joints in the absence of viable organisms. Interestingly, a recent study demonstrated that synovial fibroblasts infected with *Salmonella typhimurium* could mediate osteoclast differentiation and activation through regulation of RANKL expression on the fibroblasts.[75]

A few studies have examined the histopathology of the peripheral enthesopathy in spondyloarthropathy patients.[76-78] Ball[76] reported that the affected entheses showed multiple microfoci at different stages of the inflammatory process with zones of healthy tissue. He proposed that the initial inflammatory lesion appeared to be an erosion in the adjacent subchondral bone. The microfoci of inflammation contained lymphocytes and plasma cells, in addition to scattered neutrophils. The marrow spaces adjacent to the entheseal lesion were abnormal, with central bone marrow edema, little hematopoietic tissue, and fibrosis appearing like subacute osteomyelitis.[76,78,79] The erosive lesions appeared to heal by reactive formation of new bone within the fibrous connective tissue. The new bone filled the initial bony defect, forming a bridge to the ligament and creating a new enthesis in effect.[76] The factors leading to targeting of the entheses in this process remain undefined, but several have been proposed, including mechanical loading leading to microtrauma, locally triggered inflammation secondary to bacterial products, autoimmune response to entheseal fibrocartilage, or a primary bone marrow disorder leading to the development of localized sterile osteomyelitis.[80,81]

In cases of ankylosing spondylitis, diffuse bone loss predominates at the spine, the area of predominant inflammatory symptoms.[82] Diffuse osteoporosis resulting in loss of bone strength in the area of ligamentous calcification is now recognized as a significant feature in progressive disease. Vertebral fracture rates in ankylosing spondylitis have ranged from 4% to 18% in a number of studies,[83-86] whereas peripheral fracture rates were similar to the rate in the population at large.[86] In the ankylosing spondylitis patient, vertebral fractures can lead to significant morbidity and mortality due to neurological complications.[87-90] Similar to RA, the diffuse bone loss in patients with ankylosing spondylitis is likely multifactorial, with many of the same contributing factors, but loss of mobility due to ankylosis may be of greater significance. Several studies have demonstrated increased urinary markers of bone turnover corresponding with serum markers of inflammation (erythrocyte sedimentation rate, C-reactive protein) and levels of proinflammatory cytokines.[91] The diffuse loss of vertebral bone associated with the excessive mineralization of the surrounding ligaments remains an unexplained paradox, yet it is clear that both processes progress in the presence of continuing inflammation.[84,92,93] Consistent with this, TNF-α blockade has been demonstrated to be effective in relieving symptoms and increasing bone density in ankylosing spondylitis patients.[94]

PSORIATIC ARTHRITIS

Psoriatic arthritis is characterized by the presence of both inflammatory skin and bone diseases and can phenotypically appear with a joint distribution pattern similar to either rheumatoid arthritis or spondyloarthropathy.[95] Interestingly, histopathological studies of inflamed synovium have demonstrated that psoriatic arthritis synovitis shares features of synovitis associated with spondyloarthropathies rather than RA.[68,96] The most prominent histopathological findings in the psoriatic arthritis synovium were vascular changes showing endothelial cell swelling, inflammatory cell infiltration, and marked thickening of the vessel wall.[68,97,98] Synovial biopsies examined by blinded observers demonstrated that tissue from psoriatic arthritis patients had less thickness of the synovial lining layer and more hypervascularity than tissue from RA patients.[68] Although RA synovial tissue showed more lymphoid aggregates and CD1a+ cells, a marker for monocytoid dendritic cells, psoriatic arthritis tissue showed greater macrophage and neutrophil infiltration.[68] Immunohistochemical analysis of psoriatic arthritis synovium demonstrates RANK-positive perivascular mononuclear cells and osteoclasts as well as high RANKL expression and high TNF-α expression in the synovial lining layer.[99,100] OPG expression was observed to be confined to the endothelium; therefore, the local RANKL/OPG ratio to which osteoclast precursors would be exposed was particularly high.[99]

The cytokine IL-18, a member of the IL-1 superfamily, has been found in increased levels in serum and synovial tissue in patients with psoriatic arthritis and may play multiple roles in mediating disease.[101] IL-18 is produced primarily by macrophages and is induced by IL-1 and TNF-α. IL-18 can also stimulate angiogenesis, upregulate chemokine expression on synovial fibroblasts, and recruit mononuclear cells.[102]

Psoriatic arthritis is also known for particularly aggressive bony erosions with dramatic joint space loss, acrolysis, and "pencil-in-cup" erosions on radiographs, along with aggressive new bone formation and ankylosis.[103] Recent studies showed that psoriatic arthritis patients with bony erosive disease demonstrated an increase in circulating osteoclast precursor frequency (CD11b+, CD14+, CD51/CD61+, RANK+ cells) as compared with normal control subjects.[99] It was also found that peripheral blood mononuclear cells from psoriatic arthritis patients readily formed osteoclasts in vitro without exogenous addition of RANKL and M-CSF, although osteoclastogenesis could be inhibited by OPG or anti-TNF-α.[99] Studies in mice have also shown that TNF-α increases osteoclast precursor frequency, which is reversible with anti-TNF-α therapy.[104,105] In vivo in the psoriatic arthritis patient, osteoclast precursor frequency was observed to decrease after anti-TNF-α therapy.[99] Thus, in psoriatic arthritis an increase in circulating osteoclast precursors induced by TNF-α, followed by recruitment to localized synovium rich in RANKL and TNF-α, facilitates osteoclastogenesis, likely promoting aggressive erosions in subchondral bone.[99]

ESTROGEN DEFICIENCY–DRIVEN INFLAMMATORY BONE LOSS

The protective effects of sex steroids including estrogen on bone are well known. Estrogen receptors are present on bone cells including osteoblasts, osteoclasts, stromal cells, and chondrocytes.[106-109] Estrogen acts to inhibit bone remodeling by multiple mechanisms, including the upregulation of OPG, the decoy receptor for RANKL, and the downregulation of osteoclast-inducing molecules such as M-CSF, RANK, IL-1, IL-6, and TNF-α.[7,110-117] Estrogen also promotes osteoclast apoptosis via the production of TGF-β[118] and prevents osteoblast and osteocyte apoptosis,[119] thus promoting bone formation. Whether it is caused by age-related menopause or surgical ovariectomy, estrogen deficiency drives rapid and prolonged bone loss via recruitment and activation of osteoclasts. Recent studies have provided an additional intriguing link between abnormal bone remodeling in states of estrogen deficiency and activation of the immune system.

Estrogen deficiency in both mice and humans leads to sustained increases in pro-osteoclastic cytokines TNF-α and IL-1.[120,121] Estrogen-deficient bone loss in mice is TNF-α-dependent and requires activated T-cells. In vitro, T-cell cultures from ovariectomized mice have a fourfold increase in TNF-α compared with sham-operated or estrogen-treated ovariectomized mice, and furthermore treatment of ovariectomized mice with blocking antibodies to TNF-α prevents ovariectomy-induced bone loss.[122] Athymic mice (T-cell deficient) fail to exhibit elevations of IL-1 and TNF-α levels and are resistant to ovariectomy-induced bone loss.[122] Estrogen deficiency increases the pool of activated TNF-α-producing T-cells in bone marrow without altering the production of TNF-α per cell.[123] TNF-α signaling is critical, as mice deficient in TNF-α or the p55 TNF-α receptor are protected from ovariectomy-induced bone loss.[123] These activated T-cells express high levels of RANKL and can support osteoclastogenesis in co-culture in vitro.[124]

Estrogen deficiency subsequently has been shown to drive T-cell activation via enhanced antigen presentation by macrophages.[125] Enhanced antigen presentation results from IFN-γ induced upregulation of a transcription factor, class II transactivator, which leads to increased expression of MHC class II molecules on macrophages.[125] Recent studies have also shown that estrogen induces TGF-β and suppresses IFN-γ synthesis, resulting in attenuated T-cell antigen presentation and activation.[126] Consistent with these results, mice with a T-cell–specific blockade in TGF-β signaling fail to respond to estrogen treatment and cannot reverse ovariectomy-induced bone loss.[126] Additionally, TGF-β levels in bone marrow decrease after ovariectomy and overexpression of TGF-β during ovariectomy prevents estrogen-deficient bone loss in vivo.[126] The immune modulatory effects of TGF-β are wide and include inhibition of T-cell proliferation, differentiation and activation, promotion of suppressor T-cells or regulatory T-cells, and inhibition of dendritic cell maturation.[127] Estrogen deficiency related decreases in TGF-β may lead to decreases in T regulatory cells, allowing the proliferation of effector T-cells and immune activation.

These studies have shown convincing evidence that ovariectomy-induced bone loss in mice is secondary to enhanced immune function from T-cell activation and cytokine production. Whether similar mechanisms play a role in estrogen-deficient bone loss in humans has not been fully determined. Several cytokines, including IL-1, TNF-α, IL-6, and granulocyte-macrophage colony-stimulating factor, are increased in the bone marrow of early postmenopausal women compared with those in premenopause or late postmenopause.[128] However, TGF-β levels have not been shown to correlate with age or menopausal status in human bone samples.[129,130] Recent studies have shown that postmenopausal women have increased expression of RANKL on bone marrow stromal cells, T-cells, and B-cells compared with premenopausal or estrogen-treated postmenopausal women.[131] Additionally, peripheral monocyte culture samples from osteoporotic women form more osteoclasts, have higher bone-resorbing activity, and produce significantly more TNF-α and RANKL than culture samples from nonosteoporotic control subjects.[132] Serum levels of RANKL do not differ according to estrogen status in women; however, clinical trials of RANKL blockade via therapeutic injection of OPG or anti-RANKL antibodies have shown promise in sustained suppression of both bone resorption and formation markers consistent with decreased bone remodeling in postmenopausal osteoporosis.[133,134] The importance of T-cell activation driving estrogen-deficient bone loss has yet to be studied in humans.

T-CELLS, CYTOKINES, AND SOLUBLE MEDIATORS OF INFLAMMATION

RANKL, or TRANCE, was cloned as a molecule on activated T-cells that functioned to promote dendritic cell survival and activation and RANKL has been shown to be required for normal lymphocyte and lymph node development.[26,27,135] Thus, RANK/RANKL signals are uniquely positioned to regulate interactions between T cells, dendritic cells, macrophages, and osteoclasts. Both T-cell receptor specific activation and more nonspecific stimuli such as concanavalin A can upregulate RANKL on T-cells.[31,136] RANKL can be cleaved from T-cells by a TNF-α converting enzyme or matrix metalloproteinase resulting in functionally active soluble RANKL.[31] Whether T cells can under some circumstances directly stimulate osteoclast formation in inflammatory arthritis is not clear; however, T-cells clearly influence expression of macrophage cytokines such as IL-15, IL-1, and TNF-α which act directly on osteoclasts and osteoclast precursors.[137] T-cell produced cytokines such as IL-17, IL-1, and TNF-α also stimulate osteoblasts to increase RANKL expression, which promotes osteoclastogenesis.[138]

All activated T-cells express RANKL; therefore, it was postulated that other inhibitory factors must exist that inhibit osteoclast formation in circulation. In fact, co-culture of anti-CD3 activated splenic T cells with osteoclast precursors strongly inhibited osteoclastogenesis.[11] Studies by Takayanagi and associates identified IFN-γ as the critical inhibitory factor produced by activated T-cells, which inhibits osteoclastogenesis by interfering with RANK signals.[11] RANKL also stimulates its own feedback system to downregulate osteoclastogenesis as it induces the IFN-β gene in osteoclast precursor cells. IFN-β inhibits osteoclast differentiation by interfering with the RANKL-induced expression of c-Fos, an essential transcription factor for the formation of osteoclasts.[139] Thus, cytokines such as IFN-β and IFN-γ that are critical in the formation of the normal immune response are also important regulators of osteoclast differentiation and bone homeostasis (Figure 25-2).

Cells surrounding osteogenic cells also influence bone remodeling through cytokine secretion. Synovial fibroblasts can contribute to osteoclast formation through expression of RANKL,[24] secreting cathepsins, chemokines, and the proinflammatory cytokine IL-1, which can be produced at high levels.[140] Although an effect of TNF-α is the stimulation of IL-1 production, the effects of TNF-α blockade and IL-1 blockade in clinical RA models suggest that TNF-α effects are not all mediated through IL-1.[47,141,142] Recombinant soluble IL-1RA, which competes with IL-1 binding for the IL1-R1 receptor, thus blocking IL-1 signals, is currently used in the treatment of RA.[143] Blockade of IL-1 has demonstrated clinical benefit in RA and radiographic progression of bony erosion was retarded, confirming a role for IL-1 in osteoclast activation.[141] Combined therapy blocking TNF-α and IL-1 has been demonstrated to be useful in a murine arthritis model overexpressing TNF-α.[47] IL-1 and TNF-α have effects on osteoclasts, osteoblasts, and stromal cells. IL-1 directly activates osteoclasts and can delay osteoclast apoptosis.[144] TNF-α augments RANKL induced osteoclast differentiation.[145] Both IL-1 and TNF-α can induce apoptosis of osteoblasts, which leads to decreased bone formation.[146] IL-1 and TNF-α also cause dysregulation of chondrocyte function and induce

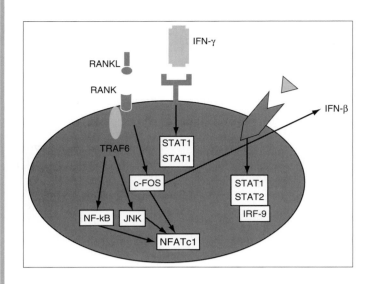

Figure 25-2. Regulation of osteoclastogenesis by interferon (IFN)-γ and IFN-β. Activated synovial cells express RANKL. If IFN-γ is also expressed during inflammation, IFN-γ will inhibit osteoclastogenesis by downregulating TRAF6 expression, which is required for RANK signaling. RANK signals also induce IFN-β, which also downregulates RANK signaling by inhibiting the expression of c-Fos. Thus, inflammatory signals are significant regulators of osteoclastogenesis and are important in the regulation of bone remodeling. [10,11,138] (See Color Plates.)

chondrocytes to release matrix metalloproteinases and cathepsins that directly degrade the cartilage matrix.[147] Other osteoclast stimulating factors include IL-6, M-CSF, macrophage inflammatory protein (MIP)1-α, IL-17, IL-11, IL-15, and parathyroid hormone related peptide (PTHrP) which promote osteoclastogenesis in the presence of RANKL.[148] Thus, during inflammation, cytokines can have synergistic effects in promoting osteoclastogenesis and bone resorption, in part due to an effective increase in RANKL brought on by changes in RANKL and OPG production by cells surrounding osteoclast precursors (see Table 25-1). The finding of abnormal bone density in recent studies of mice deficient in signaling molecules used in cytokine receptor signaling suggests that these signals play a role in normal bone remodeling and homeostasis as well.[149-151] Like other immune cells, osteoclasts are regulated by a complex network of signals from cytokines and surrounding cells, which are integrated through cell surface receptors. Recent studies revealed the involvement of a relatively new group of immune receptors that provide critical signals that are required in addition to RANK signals for osteoclastogenesis.[152,153]

ITAM-ASSOCIATED RECEPTORS IN OSTEOCLAST DIFFERENTIATION

Osteoclasts are related to innate immune cells in the myeloid lineage including monocytes, macrophages, mast cells, and dendritic cells.[2,3] The differentiation and function of these innate immune cells are highly regulated by a variety of innate immune receptors that until recently had not been examined on osteoclasts. Osteoclast differentiation and function had clearly been shown to require activation of specific cell surface

receptors, with an absolute requirement for stimulation of RANK and c-fms (receptor for M-CSF)[2]; however, it was suspected that other regulatory mechanisms were involved given the lack of osteoclast formation by all cells expressing RANK and c-fms. A group of receptors categorized as ITAM (immunotyrosine-based activating motif) signaling receptors were known to play a role in the differentiation of related myeloid cells, and it was recently demonstrated that there is a critical role for the ITAM-containing adapter proteins DAP12 and the FcRγ chain (Fc Receptor γ chain) in osteoclast differentiation.[152-154] Mice deficient in both the DAP12 and FcRγ ITAM-bearing adapters are significantly osteopetrotic and show a severe defect in osteoclast development, which demonstrates the requirement for ITAM signals in bone.[152,153]

Humans with a genetic deficiency in DAP12 have a rare recessively inherited human disease involving bony abnormalities, polycystic lipomembranous osteodysplasia with sclerosing leukoencephalopathy, also known as Nasu-Hakola disease.[155] This condition is characterized by multiple bony cysts, osteopenia, dementia, and premature death by age 50. Affected individuals develop large bony cysts in the spongy bone and typically present in their teens or early 20s with arthritis or pathological fractures.[156,157] Patients also have generalized cortical bone demineralization with early-onset osteoporosis. The differences in the human and murine DAP12[-/-] phenotypes have not been explained, although both demonstrate the same in vitro defect in osteoclast differentiation.[158-160]

DAP12 and FcRγ are transmembrane adapter proteins that associate with different types of transmembrane receptors in different cell types.[161] The ability to induce DAP12 or FcRγ surface expression is a defining

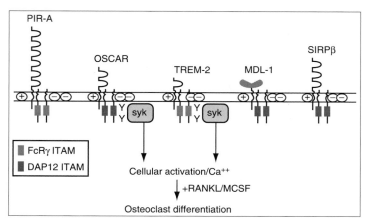

Figure 25-3. ITAM-associated receptors expressed on osteoclasts. Immunoreceptors on osteoclasts can be associated with either the DAP12 or the FcRγ ITAM-signaling chains. Receptors identified on osteoclasts or preosteoclasts by reverse-transcriptase polymerase chain reaction and/or surface antibody staining include OSCAR and PIR-A, which both contain extracellular immunoglobulin domains and are associated with the FcRγ chain (red ITAM domains). DAP12-associated receptors (shaded ITAM domains) include TREM-2 and SIRP-β with extracellular immunoglobulin domains and MDL-1 with an extracellular C-type lectin domain. The receptors pair in the membrane with either DAP12 or FcRγ via complementary charged amino acid residues in the transmembrane domains of each protein. Upon stimulation of the extracellular domain of the receptor, DAP12 or FcRγ are tyrosine phosphorylated on residues in the ITAM motif and the syk tyrosine kinase is recruited to the phosphotyrosines. Activation of the syk tyrosine kinase leads to initiation of intracellular signaling cascades.[152,154,160,169] (See Color Plates.)

characteristic of these ITAM-associated receptors.[161] The DAP12 associated receptors in myeloid cells include two types of immunoglobulin domain receptors (members of the TREM family and SIRP-β) and a C-type lectin receptor, MDL-1 (Figure 25-3). The TREM receptors (triggering receptors expressed on myeloid cells), TREM1, -2, and -3, are single immunoglobulin-domain type I transmembrane receptors,[162-165] whereas SIRP-β (signal regulatory protein-β) contains three immunoglobulin domains in the extracellular region.[166] MDL-1 (myeloid DAP12-associated lectin) and NKG2D are type II integral membrane proteins with extracellular lectin domains.[167,168]

Osteoclasts have been demonstrated by reverse-transcriptase polymerase chain reaction to express transcripts for DAP12, TREM-2, TREM-3, and MDL-1, but not TREM-1.[160] ITAM adapter proteins demonstrated to be present in preosteoclasts by protein analysis include the receptor proteins SIRP-β, PIR-A, TREM-2, OSCAR, and FcRIII.[152] Mouse OSCAR, which pairs with the FcRγ chain, was previously demonstrated to be present on osteoclasts in a cell-specific manner by mAb surface binding, although human OSCAR is more widely distributed on other myeloid cells.[169,170] Receptors identified in osteoclasts are shown in Figure 25-3. Additional studies are needed to complete our knowledge of the repertoire of immunoreceptors involved in osteoclast regulation.

ITAM-dependent signaling receptors in leukocytes are critical regulators controlling proliferation, sur-vival, and differentiation to mature immune effector cells. Osteoclasts are likely similar to other innate immune cells that are highly regulated by arrays of receptors that allow them to sense and respond to local microenvironmental changes. The ITAM motif is utilized by the T-cell receptor and the B-cell receptor and mediates intracellular signals through syk family tyrosine kinases with involvement of src family kinases, to activate a multitude of effector functions. Studies by Koga and associates have demonstrated that ITAM-associated receptors are required during osteoclastogenesis for induction of the critical transcription factor NFATc1.[152,171] NFATc1 has been proposed as a transcription factor that functions as a master regulator in osteoclastogenesis. In $DAP12^{-/-}FcR\gamma^{-/-}$ osteoclast precursors defective in osteoclastogenesis, no NFATc1 is induced and reintroduction of NFATc1 into $DAP12^{-/-}FcR\gamma^{-/-}$ cells can rescue osteoclast differentiation.[152] The model proposed by Takayanagi suggests that ITAM-signaling receptors function as critical co-stimulators for osteoclast differentiation with RANKL and M-CSF (Figure 25-4). Thus, during osteoclastogenesis, ITAM signals provide critical costimuli to RANKL/TRANCE signals, which parallels the requirement for co-stimulation seen in other immune cell types.[8,152]

In the bone, we are only beginning to dissect the functions of DAP12 and FcRγ and their associated receptors, as we have not yet identified all the receptors present or the ligands with which they interact. Clearly, specific ligands in the bone microenvironment need to be identi-

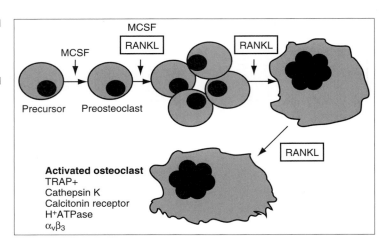

Figure 25-4. Model for role of ITAM-associated immune receptors in osteoclastogenesis. Signals mediated by RANK cooperate with signals from ITAM-bearing adapter chains to stimulate osteoclast differentiation and activation. Upon stimulation of their associated receptor, ITAM adapters are tyrosine phosphorylated and recruit syk kinase, which leads to activation of PLC-γ and calcium signaling. ITAM adapter mediated signals are required for activation of the critical osteoclastogenic transcription factor NFATc1. Immunoreceptors that associate with DAP12 may have ligands expressed on other osteoclast precursor cells, whereas FcRγ-associated immunoreceptors are predicted to interact with ligands on osteoblast or stromal cells.[8,152,153] (Modified from Koga et al.[152] and Takayanagi.[8]) (See Color Plates.)

fied to better understand the regulation of osteoclasts during bony remodeling. Because the ITAM signaling pathway is required for osteoclastogenesis, these receptors and/or their signaling intermediates may be useful as potential targets for therapeutics to regulate bony remodeling. It is interesting that several current immunosuppressive agents, including cyclosporine and leuflunomide, used in rheumatoid arthritis, are known to inhibit this pathway and some of their effects may be due to inhibition of osteoclast development.[172,173] Osteoclasts are highly influenced by ever-changing local stimuli from their surrounding cellular and matrix environments, and we need to better determine how they use receptors to sense such changes.

POTENTIAL THERAPIES

Osteoclasts have been implicated as playing a critical role in mediating both localized bony erosion and diffuse bone loss in a number of inflammatory bone diseases.[174] Indeed, bisphosphonate therapy directed at osteoclasts has been demonstrated to be effective in murine models of inflammatory arthritis and is being evaluated in patients with erosive arthritis.[175-177] Thus, blockade of osteoclast differentiation has become an attractive point for therapeutic intervention to prevent the morbidity and mortality of these diseases. The therapeutic potential of blocking the RANK/RANKL signaling pathway is currently under intense study for human bone diseases, including osteoporosis and skeletal metastases.[178] Currently, studies are underway to determine the effects of RANKL blockade with OPG, OPG-like proteins, or anti-RANKL antibodies. A single dose of OPG in postmenopausal women resulted in sustained suppression of both bone resorption and formation markers consistent with decreased bone remodeling.[134] An initial anti-RANKL antibody study in postmenopausal women also shows a sustained suppression in markers of bone turnover for up to 6 months without apparent adverse effects.[133] Treatment of patients with multiple myeloma and patients with metastatic breast cancer with OPG showed decreases in bone resorptive markers comparable with pamidronate.[179] These small short-term studies show promise for treatment of a variety of disease states with abnormally high bone turnover, including erosive inflammatory arthritis.[180] Longer studies to determine the role of these agents in preventing decreases in bone mineral density secondary to inflammation, glucocorticoids, malignancy, or estrogen deficiency are needed to fully evaluate RANKL blockade as a novel therapeutic agent in human bone disease.

Current interventions focused on cytokine blockade have been successful in treating many patients with inflammatory arthritis, but other patients remain with poorly controlled disease unresponsive to these agents. Combination therapy blocking multiple cytokines simultaneously will likely be limited by immunosuppressive effects, particularly with regard to the response to infection.[181] The identification of other regulatory pathways in osteoclasts involving innate immune receptors may be potential targets, although a better understanding of the exact roles these receptors play in bony remodeling is essential. The immune and skeletal systems appear to be so closely linked that complete inhibition of any of these pathways may not be desirable and modulation is likely a better goal to avoid detrimental immunosuppressive effects. Future therapies for inflammatory bone disease will likely continue to include efforts to eliminate both inflammation and osteoclast activation, as both processes contribute to symptoms and disability.

REFERENCES

1. Katagiri T, Takahashi N: Regulatory mechanisms of osteoblast and osteoclast differentiation. Oral Dis 2002;8:147-59.
2. Boyle WJ, Simonet WS, Lacey DL: Osteoclast differentiation and activation. Nature 2003;423:337-42.
3. Teitelbaum SL, Ross FP: Genetic regulation of osteoclast development and function. Nat Rev Genet 2003;4:638-49.
4. Goldring SR: Inflammatory mediators as essential elements in bone remodeling. Calcif Tissue Int 2003;73:97-100.
5. Haynes DR: Bone lysis and inflammation. Inflamm Res 2004;53:596-600.
6. Goldring SR, Gravallese EM: Mechanisms of bone loss in inflammatory arthritis: diagnosis and therapeutic implications. Arthritis Res 2000;2:33-7.
7. Pacifici R: Estrogen, cytokines, and pathogenesis of post-menopausal osteoporosis. J Bone Miner Res 1996;11:1043-51.
8. Takayanagi H: Mechanistic insight into osteoclast differentiation in osteoimmunology. J Mol Med 2005;83:170-79.
9. Taylor PR, Martinez-Pomares L, Stacey M, et al: Macrophage receptors and immune recognition. Annu Rev Immunol 2005;23:901-44.
10. Arron JR, Choi Y: Bone versus immune system. Nature 2000;408:535-36.
11. Takayanagi H, Ogasawara K, Hida S, et al: T-cell-mediated regulation of osteoclastogenesis by signalling cross-talk between RANKL and IFN-gamma. Nature 2000;408:600-5.
12. Gravallese EM, Goldring SR: Cellular mechanisms and the role of cytokines in bone erosions in rheumatoid arthritis. Arthritis Rheum 2000;43:2143-51.
13. Kim TH, Uhm WS, Inman RD: Pathogenesis of ankylosing spondylitis and reactive arthritis. Curr Opin Rheumatol 2005;17:400-5.
14. Ritchlin CT: Pathogenesis of psoriatic arthritis. Curr Opin Rheumatol 2005;17:406-12.
15. Bresnihan B, Tak PP: Synovial tissue analysis in rheumatoid arthritis. Bailliere Best Pract Res Clin Rheumatol 1999;13:645-59.
16. Tarner IH, Harle P, Muller-Ladner U, et al: The different stages of synovitis: acute vs chronic, early vs late and non-erosive vs erosive. Best Pract Res Clin Rheumatol 2005;19:19-35.
17. Goldring SR, Gravallese EM: Pathogenesis of bone erosions in rheumatoid arthritis. Curr Opin Rheumatol 2000;12:195-99.
18. Tak PP, Bresnihan B: The pathogenesis and prevention of joint damage in rheumatoid arthritis: advances from synovial biopsy and tissue analysis. Arthritis Rheum 2000;43:2619-33.
19. Evangelisto A, Wakefield R, Emery P: Imaging in early arthritis. Best Pract Res Clin Rheumatol 2004;18:927-43.
20. Bromley M, Woolley DE: Chondroclasts and osteoclasts at subchondral sites of erosion in the rheumatoid joint. Arthritis Rheum 1984;27:968-75.
21. Gravallese EM, Harada Y, Wang JT, et al: Identification of cell types responsible for bone resorption in rheumatoid arthritis and juvenile rheumatoid arthritis. Am J Pathol 1998;152:943-51.
22. Leisen JC, Duncan H, Riddle JM, Pitchford WC: The erosive front: a topographic study of the junction between the pannus and the subchondral plate in the macerated rheumatoid metacarpal head. J Rheumatol 1988;15:17-22.
23. Redlich K, Hayer S, Ricci R, et al: Osteoclasts are essential for TNF-alpha-mediated joint destruction. J Clin Invest 2002;110:1419-27.
24. Gravallese EM, Manning C, Tsay A, et al: Synovial tissue in rheumatoid arthritis is a source of osteoclast differentiation factor. Arthritis Rheum 2000;43:250-58.
25. Dougall WC, Glaccum M, Charrier K, et al: RANK is essential for osteoclast and lymph node development. Genes Dev 1999;13:2412-24.
26. Anderson D, Maraskovsky E, Billingsley WL, et al: A homologue of the TNF receptor and its ligand enhance T-cell growth and dendritic-cell function. Nature 1997;390:175-79.
27. Wong BR, Josien R, Lee SY, et al: TRANCE (tumor necrosis factor [TNF]-related activation-induced cytokine), a new TNF family member predominantly expressed in T cells, is a dendritic cell-specific survival factor. J Exp Med 1997;186:2075-80.
28. Lacey DL, Timms E, Tan HL, et al: Osteoprotegerin ligand is a cytokine that regulates osteoclast differentiation and activation. Cell 1998;93:165-76.
29. Yasuda H, Shima N, Nakagawa N, et al: Osteoclast differentiation factor is a ligand for osteoprotegerin/osteoclastogenesis-inhibitory factor and is identical to TRANCE/RANKL. Proc Natl Acad Sci U S A 1998;95:3597-602.
30. Hsu H, Lacey DL, Dunstan CR, et al: Tumor necrosis factor receptor family member RANK mediates osteoclast differentiation and activation induced by osteoprotegerin ligand. Proc Natl Acad Sci U S A 1999;96:3540-5.
31. Lum L, Wong BR, Josien R, et al: Evidence for a role of a tumor necrosis factor-alpha (TNF-alpha)-converting enzyme-like protease in shedding of TRANCE, a TNF family member involved in osteoclastogenesis and dendritic cell survival. J Biol Chem 1999;274:13613-18.
32. Simonet WS, Lacey DL, Dunstan CR, et al: Osteoprotegerin: a novel secreted protein involved in the regulation of bone density. Cell 1997;89:309-19.
33. Kong YY, Yoshida H, Sarosi I, et al: OPGL is a key regulator of osteoclastogenesis, lymphocyte development and lymph-node organogenesis. Nature 1999;397:315-23.
34. Li J, Sarosi I, Yan XQ, et al: RANK is the intrinsic hematopoietic cell surface receptor that controls osteoclastogenesis and regulation of bone mass and calcium metabolism. Proc Natl Acad Sci U S A 2000;97:1566-71.
35. Bucay N, Sarosi I, Dunstan CR, et al: Osteoprotegerin-deficient mice develop early onset osteoporosis and arterial calcification. Genes Dev 1998;12:1260-68.
36. Hughes AE, Ralston SH, Marken J, et al: Mutations in TNFRSF11A, affecting the signal peptide of RANK, cause familial expansile osteolysis. Nat Genet 2000;24:45-8.
37. Whyte MP, Obrecht SE, Finnegan PM, et al: Osteoprotegerin deficiency and juvenile Paget's disease. N Engl J Med 2002;347:175-84.
38. Whyte MP, Mumm S: Heritable disorders of the RANKL/OPG/RANK signaling pathway. J Musculoskelet Neuronal Interact 2004;4:254-67.
39. Cundy T, Hegde M, Naot D, et al: A mutation in the gene TNFRSF11B encoding osteoprotegerin causes an idiopathic hyperphosphatasia phenotype. Hum Mol Genet 2002;11:2119-27.
40. Arko B, Prezelj J, Komel R, et al: Sequence variations in the osteoprotegerin gene promoter in patients with post-menopausal osteoporosis. J Clin Endocrinol Metab 2002;87:4080-4.
41. Langdahl BL, Carstens M, Stenkjaer L, Eriksen EF: Polymorphisms in the osteoprotegerin gene are associated with osteoporotic fractures. J Bone Miner Res 2002;17:1245-55.
42. Seshasayee D, Wang H, Lee WP, et al: A novel in vivo role for osteoprotegerin ligand in activation of monocyte effector function and inflammatory response. J Biol Chem 2004;279:30202-9.
43. Rivollier A, Mazzorana M, Tebib J, et al: Immature dendritic cell transdifferentiation into osteoclasts: a novel pathway sustained by the rheumatoid arthritis microenvironment. Blood 2004;104:4029-37.
44. Kotake S, Udagawa N, Hakoda M, et al: Activated human T cells directly induce osteoclastogenesis from human monocytes: possible role of T cells in bone destruction in rheumatoid arthritis patients. Arthritis Rheum 2001;44:1003-12.
45. Kong YY, Feige U, Sarosi I, et al: Activated T cells regulate bone loss and joint destruction in adjuvant arthritis through osteoprotegerin ligand. Nature 1999;402:304-9.
46. Pettit AR, Ji H, von Stechow D, et al: TRANCE/RANKL knockout mice are protected from bone erosion in a serum transfer model of arthritis. Am J Pathol 2001;159:1689-99.
47. Zwerina J, Hayer S, Tohidast-Akrad M, et al: Single and combined inhibition of tumor necrosis factor, interleukin-1, and RANKL pathways in tumor necrosis factor-induced arthritis: effects on synovial inflammation, bone erosion, and cartilage destruction. Arthritis Rheum 2004;50:277-90.

48. Keffer J, Probert L, Cazlaris H, et al: Transgenic mice expressing human tumour necrosis factor: a predictive genetic model of arthritis. EMBO J 1991;10:4025-31.

49. Feldmann M, Maini RN: The role of cytokines in the pathogenesis of rheumatoid arthritis. Rheumatology (Oxford) 1999;38(Suppl 2):3-7.

50. Chu CQ, Field M, Allard S, et al: Detection of cytokines at the cartilage/pannus junction in patients with rheumatoid arthritis: implications for the role of cytokines in cartilage destruction and repair. Br J Rheumatol 1992;31:653-61.

51. Deleuran BW, Chu CQ, Field M, et al: Localization of tumor necrosis factor receptors in the synovial tissue and cartilage-pannus junction in patients with rheumatoid arthritis. Implications for local actions of tumor necrosis factor alpha. Arthritis Rheum 1992;35:1170-8.

52. Hofbauer LC, Dunstan CR, Spelsberg TC, et al: Osteoprotegerin production by human osteoblast lineage cells is stimulated by vitamin D, bone morphogenetic protein-2, and cytokines. Biochem Biophys Res Commun 1998;250:776-81.

53. Ziolkowska M, Kurowska M, Radzikowska A, et al: High levels of osteoprotegerin and soluble receptor activator of nuclear factor kappa B ligand in serum of rheumatoid arthritis patients and their normalization after anti-tumor necrosis factor alpha treatment. Arthritis Rheum 2002;46:1744-53.

54. Breedveld FC, Emery P, Keystone E, et al: Infliximab in active early rheumatoid arthritis. Ann Rheum Dis 2004;63:149-55.

55. Genovese MC, Bathon JM, Martin RW, et al: Etanercept versus methotrexate in patients with early rheumatoid arthritis: two-year radiographic and clinical outcomes. Arthritis Rheum 2002;46:1443-50.

56. Shimizu S, Shiozawa S, Shiozawa K, et al: Quantitative histologic studies on the pathogenesis of periarticular osteoporosis in rheumatoid arthritis. Arthritis Rheum 1985;28:25-31.

57. Gough A, Sambrook P, Devlin J, et al: Osteoclastic activation is the principal mechanism leading to secondary osteoporosis in rheumatoid arthritis. J Rheumatol 1998;25:1282-89.

58. Sambrook P, Nguyen T: Vertebral osteoporosis in rheumatoid arthritis patients: effect of low dose prednisone therapy. Br J Rheumatol 1992;31:573-74.

59. Gough AK, Lilley J, Eyre S, et al: Generalised bone loss in patients with early rheumatoid arthritis. Lancet 1994;344:23-7.

60. Spector TD, Hall GM, McCloskey EV, Kanis JA: Risk of vertebral fracture in women with rheumatoid arthritis. BMJ 1993;306:558.

61. Hooyman JR, Melton LJ 3rd, Nelson AM, et al: Fractures after rheumatoid arthritis: a population-based study. Arthritis Rheum 1984;27:1353-61.

62. Sambrook PN, Eisman JA, Champion GD, et al: Determinants of axial bone loss in rheumatoid arthritis. Arthritis Rheum 1987;30:721-28.

63. Mellish RW, O'Sullivan MM, Garrahan NJ, Compston JE: Iliac crest trabecular bone mass and structure in patients with non-steroid treated rheumatoid arthritis. Ann Rheum Dis 1987;46:830-36.

64. Sinigaglia L, Varenna M, Binelli L, et al: Urinary and synovial pyridinium crosslink concentrations in patients with rheumatoid arthritis and osteoarthritis. Ann Rheum Dis 1995;54:144-47.

65. Sieper J, Braun J, Rudwaleit M, et al: Ankylosing spondylitis: an overview. Ann Rheum Dis 2002;61(Suppl 3):iii8-18.

66. Toivanen A, Toivanen P: Reactive arthritis. Best Pract Res Clin Rheumatol 2004;18:689-703.

67. Ramos M, Lopez de Castro JA: HLA-B27 and the pathogenesis of spondyloarthritis. Tissue Antigens 2002;60:191-205.

68. Baeten D, Kruithof E, De Rycke L, et al: Infiltration of the synovial membrane with macrophage subsets and polymorphonuclear cells reflects global disease activity in spondyloarthropathy. Arthritis Res Ther 2005;7:R359-69.

69. Baeten D, Kruithof E, De Rycke L, et al: Diagnostic classification of spondylarthropathy and rheumatoid arthritis by synovial histopathology: a prospective study in 154 consecutive patients. Arthritis Rheum 2004;50:2931-41.

70. Demetter P, De Vos M, Van Huysse JA, et al: Colon mucosa of patients both with spondyloarthritis and Crohn's disease is enriched with macrophages expressing the scavenger receptor CD163. Ann Rheum Dis 2005;64:321-4.

71. Baeten D, Demetter P, Cuvelier CA, et al: Macrophages expressing the scavenger receptor CD163: a link between immune alterations of the gut and synovial inflammation in spondyloarthropathy. J Pathol 2002;196:343-50.

72. De Keyser F, Baeten D, Van den Bosch F, et al: Gut inflammation and spondyloarthropathies. Curr Rheumatol Rep 2002;4:525-32.

73. Butrimiene I, Jarmalaite S, Ranceva J, et al: Different cytokine profiles in patients with chronic and acute reactive arthritis. Rheumatology (Oxford) 2004;43:1300-4.

74. De Keyser F, Baeten D, Van den Bosch F, et al: Infliximab in patients who have spondyloarthropathy: clinical efficacy, safety, and biological immunomodulation. Rheum Dis Clin North Am 2003;29:463-79.

75. Zhang X, Aubin JE, Kim TH, et al: Synovial fibroblasts infected with Salmonella enterica serovar typhimurium mediate osteoclast differentiation and activation. Infect Immun 2004;72:7183-89.

76. Ball J: Enthesopathy of rheumatoid and ankylosing spondylitis. Ann Rheum Dis 1971;30:213-23.

77. Laloux L, Voisin MC, Allain J, et al: Immunohistological study of entheses in spondyloarthropathies: comparison in rheumatoid arthritis and osteoarthritis. Ann Rheum Dis 2001;60:316-21.

78. McGonagle D, Marzo-Ortega H, O'Connor P, et al: Histological assessment of the early enthesitis lesion in spondyloarthropathy. Ann Rheum Dis 2002;61:534-37.

79. Ball J: The enthesopathy of ankylosing spondylitis. Br J Rheumatol 1983;22(4 Suppl 2):25-8.

80. Claudepierre P, Voisin MC: The entheses: histology, pathology, and pathophysiology. Joint Bone Spine 2005;72:32-7.

81. McGonagle D, Emery P: Enthesitis, osteitis, microbes, biomechanics, and immune reactivity in ankylosing spondylitis. J Rheumatol 2000;27:2302-4.

82. El Maghraoui A: Osteoporosis and ankylosing spondylitis. Joint Bone Spine 2004;71:291-95.

83. Hansen CA, Shagrin JW, Duncan H: Vertebral osteoporosis in ankylosing spondylitis. Clin Orthop 1971;74:59-64.

84. Ralston SH, Urquhart GD, Brzeski M, Sturrock RD: Prevalence of vertebral compression fractures due to osteoporosis in ankylosing spondylitis. BMJ 1990;300:563-5.

85. Donnelly S, Doyle DV, Denton A, et al: Bone mineral density and vertebral compression fracture rates in ankylosing spondylitis. Ann Rheum Dis 1994;53:117-21.

86. Cooper C, Carbone L, Michet CJ, et al: Fracture risk in patients with ankylosing spondylitis: a population based study. J Rheumatol 1994;21:1877-82.

87. Fox MW, Onofrio BM, Kilgore JE: Neurological complications of ankylosing spondylitis. J Neurosurg 1993;78:871-78.

88. Tico N, Ramon S, Garcia-Ortun F, et al: Traumatic spinal cord injury complicating ankylosing spondylitis. Spinal Cord 1998;36:349-52.

89. Olerud C, Frost A, Bring J: Spinal fractures in patients with ankylosing spondylitis. Eur Spine J 1996;5:51-5.

90. Lehtinen K: Mortality and causes of death in 398 patients admitted to hospital with ankylosing spondylitis. Ann Rheum Dis 1993;52:174-6.

91. El Maghraoui A, Borderie D, Cherruau B, et al: Osteoporosis, body composition, and bone turnover in ankylosing spondylitis. J Rheumatol 1999;26:2205-9.

92. Meirelles ES, Borelli A, Camargo OP: Influence of disease activity and chronicity on ankylosing spondylitis bone mass loss. Clin Rheumatol 1999;18:364-68.

93. Karberg K, Zochling J, Sieper J, et al: Bone loss is detected more frequently in patients with ankylosing spondylitis with syndesmophytes. J Rheumatol 2005;32:1290-98.

94. Demis E, Roux C, Breban M, Dougados M: Infliximab in spondylarthropathy: influence on bone density. Clin Exp Rheumatol 2002;20(6 Suppl 28):S185-6.

95. Helliwell PS, Taylor WJ: Classification and diagnostic criteria for psoriatic arthritis. Ann Rheum Dis 2005;64(Suppl 2):ii3-8.

96. Kruithof E, Baeten D, De Rycke L, et al: Synovial histopathology of psoriatic arthritis, both oligo- and polyarticular, resembles spondyloarthropathy more than it does rheumatoid arthritis. Arthritis Res Ther 2005;7:R569-80.

97. Espinoza LR, Vasey FB, Espinoza CG, et al: Vascular changes in psoriatic synovium: a light and electron microscopic study. Arthritis Rheum 1982;25:677-84.

98. Reece RJ, Canete JD, Parsons WJ, et al: Distinct vascular patterns of early synovitis in psoriatic, reactive, and rheumatoid arthritis. Arthritis Rheum 1999;42:1481-84.

99. Ritchlin CT, Haas-Smith SA, Li P, et al: Mechanisms of TNF-alpha- and RANKL-mediated osteoclastogenesis and bone resorption in psoriatic arthritis. J Clin Invest 2003;111:821-31.

100. Danning CL, Illei GG, Hitchon C, et al: Macrophage-derived cytokine and nuclear factor kappaB p65 expression in synovial membrane and skin of patients with psoriatic arthritis. Arthritis Rheum 2000;43:1244-56.

101. Rooney T, Murphy E, Benito M, et al: Synovial tissue interleukin-18 expression and the response to treatment in patients with inflammatory arthritis. Ann Rheum Dis 2004;63:1393-8.

102. Reddy P: Interleukin-18: recent advances. Curr Opin Hematol 2004;11:405-10.

103. Resnick D, Niwayama G: Psoriatic arthritis. In: Resnick D, Niwayama G, eds: Diagnosis of bone and joint disorders. Philadelphia: W.B. Saunders, 1981:320-28.

104. Li P, Schwarz EM, O'Keefe RJ, et al: RANK signaling is not required for TNF alpha-mediated increase in CD11(hi) osteoclast precursors but is essential for mature osteoclast formation in TNFalpha-mediated inflammatory arthritis. J Bone Miner Res 2004;19:207-13.

105. Li P, Schwarz EM, O'Keefe RJ, et al: Systemic tumor necrosis factor alpha mediates an increase in peripheral CD11b high osteoclast precursors in tumor necrosis factor alpha-transgenic mice. Arthritis Rheum 2004;50:265-76.

106. Bellido T, Girasole G, Passeri G, et al: Demonstration of estrogen and vitamin D receptors in bone marrow-derived stromal cells: up-regulation of the estrogen receptor by 1,25-dihydroxyvitamin-D3. Endocrinology 1993;133:553-62.

107. Benz DJ, Haussler HM, Komm BS: Estrogen binding and estrogenic responses in normal human osteoblast-like cells. J Bone Miner Res 1991;6:531-41.

108. Komm BS, Terpening CM, Benz DJ, et al: Estrogen binding, receptor mRNA, and biologic response in osteoblast-like osteosarcoma cells. Science 1988;241:81-4.

109. Eriksen EF, Colvard DS, Berg NJ, et al: Evidence of estrogen receptors in normal human osteoblast-like cells. Science 1988;241:84-6.

110. Manolagas SC, Jilka RL: Bone marrow, cytokines, and bone remodeling: emerging insights into the pathophysiology of osteoporosis. N Engl J Med 1995;332:305-11.

111. Sarma U, Edwards M, Motoyoshi K, Flanagan AM: Inhibition of bone resorption by 17beta-estradiol in human bone marrow cultures. J Cell Physiol 1998;175:99-108.

112. Shevde NK, Bendixen AC, Dienger KM, Pike JW: Estrogens suppress RANK ligand-induced osteoclast differentiation via a stromal cell independent mechanism involving c-Jun repression. Proc Natl Acad Sci U S A 2000;97:7829-34.

113. Lea CK, Sarma U, Flanagan AM: Macrophage colony stimulating-factor transcripts are differentially regulated in rat bone-marrow by gender hormones. Endocrinology 1999;140:273-79.

114. Hofbauer LC, Khosla S, Dunstan CR, et al: Estrogen stimulates gene expression and protein production of osteoprotegerin in human osteoblastic cells. Endocrinology 1999;140:4367-70.

115. Ammann P, Rizzoli R, Bonjour JP, et al: Transgenic mice expressing soluble tumor necrosis factor-receptor are protected against bone loss caused by estrogen deficiency. J Clin Invest 1997;99:1699-703.

116. Lorenzo JA, Naprta A, Rao Y, et al: Mice lacking the type I interleukin-1 receptor do not lose bone mass after ovariectomy. Endocrinology 1998;139:3022-5.

117. Poli V, Balena R, Fattori E, et al: Interleukin-6 deficient mice are protected from bone loss caused by estrogen depletion. EMBO J 1994;13:1189-96.

118. Manolagas SC: Birth and death of bone cells: basic regulatory mechanisms and implications for the pathogenesis and treatment of osteoporosis. Endocr Rev 2000;21:115-37.

119. Jilka RL, Weinstein RS, Bellido T, et al: Osteoblast programmed cell death (apoptosis): modulation by growth factors and cytokines. J Bone Miner Res 1998;13:793-802.

120. Miyaura C, Kusano K, Masuzawa T, et al: Endogenous bone-resorbing factors in estrogen deficiency: cooperative effects of IL-1 and IL-6. J Bone Miner Res 1995;10:1365-73.

121. Pacifici R, Brown C, Puscheck E, et al: Effect of surgical menopause and estrogen replacement on cytokine release from human blood mononuclear cells. Proc Natl Acad Sci U S A 1991;88:5134-38.

122. Cenci S, Weitzmann MN, Roggia C, et al: Estrogen deficiency induces bone loss by enhancing T-cell production of TNF-alpha. J Clin Invest 2000;106:1229-37.

123. Roggia C, Gao Y, Cenci S, et al: Up-regulation of TNF-producing T cells in the bone marrow: a key mechanism by which estrogen deficiency induces bone loss in vivo. Proc Natl Acad Sci U S A 2001;98:13960-5.

124. Horwood NJ, Kartsogiannis V, Quinn JM, et al: Activated T lymphocytes support osteoclast formation in vitro. Biochem Biophys Res Commun 1999;265:144-50.

125. Cenci S, Toraldo G, Weitzmann MN, et al: Estrogen deficiency induces bone loss by increasing T cell proliferation and life-span through IFN-gamma-induced class II transactivator. Proc Natl Acad Sci U S A 2003;100:10405-10.

126. Gao Y, Qian WP, Dark K, et al: Estrogen prevents bone loss through transforming growth factor beta signaling in T cells. Proc Natl Acad Sci U S A 2004;101:16618-23.

127. Gorelik L, Flavell RA: Transforming growth factor-beta in T-cell biology. Nat Rev Immunol 2002;2:46-53.

128. Bismar H, Diel I, Ziegler R, Pfeilschifter J: Increased cytokine secretion by human bone marrow cells after menopause or discontinuation of estrogen replacement. J Clin Endocrinol Metab 1995;80:3351-5.

129. Pfeilschifter J, Diel I, Scheppach B, et al: Concentration of transforming growth factor beta in human bone tissue: relationship to age, menopause, bone turnover, and bone volume. J Bone Miner Res 1998;13:716-30.

130. Bismar H, Kloppinger T, Schuster EM, et al: Transforming growth factor beta (TGF-beta) levels in the conditioned media of human bone cells: relationship to donor age, bone volume, and concentration of TGF-beta in human bone matrix in vivo. Bone 1999;24:565-69.

131. Eghbali-Fatourechi G, Khosla S, Sanyal A, et al: Role of RANK ligand in mediating increased bone resorption in early postmenopausal women. J Clin Invest 2003;111:1221-30.

132. D'Amelio P, Grimaldi A, Pescarmona GP, et al: Spontaneous osteoclast formation from peripheral blood mononuclear cells in postmenopausal osteoporosis. FASEB J 2005;19:410-12.

133. Bekker PJ, Holloway DL, Rasmussen AS, et al: A single-dose placebo-controlled study of AMG 162, a fully human monoclonal antibody to RANKL, in postmenopausal women. J Bone Miner Res 2004;19:1059-66.

134. Bekker PJ, Holloway D, Nakanishi A, et al: The effect of a single dose of osteoprotegerin in postmenopausal women. J Bone Miner Res 2001;16:348-60.

135. Josien R, Wong BR, Li HL, et al: TRANCE, a TNF family member, is differentially expressed on T cell subsets and induces cytokine production in dendritic cells. J Immunol 1999;162:2562-68.

136. Wang R, Zhang L, Zhang X, et al: Regulation of activation-induced receptor activator of NF-kappaB ligand (RANKL) expression in T cells. Eur J Immunol 2002;32:1090-98.

137. McInnes IB, Leung BP, Sturrock RD, et al: Interleukin-15 mediates T cell-dependent regulation of tumor necrosis factor-alpha production in rheumatoid arthritis. Nat Med 1997;3:189-95.

138. Kotake S, Udagawa N, Takahashi N, et al: IL-17 in synovial fluids from patients with rheumatoid arthritis is a potent stimulator of osteoclastogenesis. J Clin Invest 1999;103:1345-52.

139. Takayanagi H, Kim S, Matsuo K, et al: RANKL maintains bone homeostasis through c-Fos-dependent induction of interferon-beta. Nature 2002;416:744-49.

140. Kontoyiannis D, Kollias G: Fibroblast biology. Synovial fibroblasts in rheumatoid arthritis: leading role or chorus line? Arthritis Res 2000;2:342-43.

141. Dayer JM: Interleukin 1 or tumor necrosis factor-alpha: which is the real target in rheumatoid arthritis? J Rheumatol Suppl 2002;65:10-5.

142. Joosten LA, Helsen MM, Saxne T, et al: IL-1 alpha beta blockade prevents cartilage and bone destruction in murine type II collagen-induced arthritis, whereas TNF-alpha blockade only ameliorates joint inflammation. J Immunol 1999;163:5049-55.

261

143. Jiang Y, Genant HK, Watt I, et al: A multicenter, double-blind, dose-ranging, randomized, placebo-controlled study of recombinant human interleukin-1 receptor antagonist in patients with rheumatoid arthritis: radiologic progression and correlation of Genant and Larsen scores. Arthritis Rheum 2000;43:1001-9.

144. Jimi E, Nakamura I, Duong LT, et al: Interleukin 1 induces multinucleation and bone-resorbing activity of osteoclasts in the absence of osteoblasts/stromal cells. Exp Cell Res 1999; 247:84-93.

145. Lam J, Takeshita S, Barker JE, et al: TNF-alpha induces osteoclastogenesis by direct stimulation of macrophages exposed to permissive levels of RANK ligand. J Clin Invest 2000;106:1481-88.

146. Tsuboi M, Kawakami A, Nakashima T, et al: Tumor necrosis factor-alpha and interleukin-1beta increase the Fas-mediated apoptosis of human osteoblasts. J Lab Clin Med 1999;134:222-31.

147. Goldring SR, Goldring MB: The role of cytokines in cartilage matrix degeneration in osteoarthritis. Clin Orthop Relat Res 2004;427(Suppl):S27-36.

148. Goldring SR: Pathogenesis of bone and cartilage destruction in rheumatoid arthritis. Rheumatology (Oxford) 2003;42 (Suppl 2):ii11-6.

149. Kim S, Koga T, Isobe M, et al: Stat1 functions as a cytoplasmic attenuator of Runx2 in the transcriptional program of osteoblast differentiation. Genes Dev 2003;17:1979-91.

150. Ohishi M, Matsumura Y, Aki D, et al: Suppressors of cytokine signaling-1 and -3 regulate osteoclastogenesis in the presence of inflammatory cytokines. J Immunol 2005;174:3024-31.

151. Sims NA, Jenkins BJ, Nakamura A, et al: Interleukin-11 receptor signaling is required for normal bone remodeling. J Bone Miner Res 2005;20:1093-102.

152. Koga T, Inui M, Inoue K, et al: Costimulatory signals mediated by the ITAM motif cooperate with RANKL for bone homeostasis. Nature 2004;428:758-63.

153. Mocsai A, Humphrey MB, Van Ziffle JA, et al: The immunomodulatory adapter proteins DAP12 and Fc receptor gamma-chain (FcRgamma) regulate development of functional osteoclasts through the Syk tyrosine kinase. Proc Natl Acad Sci U S A 2004;101:6158-63.

154. Isakov N: ITAMs: immunoregulatory scaffolds that link immunoreceptors to their intracellular signaling pathways. Receptors Channels 1998;5:243-53.

155. Paloneva J, Kestila M, Wu J, et al: Loss-of-function mutations in TYROBP (DAP12) result in a presenile dementia with bone cysts. Nat Genet 2000;25:357-61.

156. Verloes A, Maquet P, Sadzot B, et al: Nasu-Hakola syndrome: polycystic lipomembranous osteodysplasia with sclerosing leukoencephalopathy and presenile dementia. J Med Genet 1997;34:753-7.

157. Chaabane M, Larnaout A, Sebai R, et al: Nasu-Hakola disease in two Tunisian siblings: new radiological findings. Neuroradiology 2000;42:375-78.

158. Paloneva J, Mandelin J, Kiialainen A, et al: DAP12/TREM2 deficiency results in impaired osteoclast differentiation and osteoporotic features. J Exp Med 2003;198:669-75.

159. Kaifu T, Nakahara J, Inui M, et al: Osteopetrosis and thalamic hypomyelinosis with synaptic degeneration in DAP12-deficient mice. J Clin Invest 2003;111:323-32.

160. Humphrey MB, Ogasawara K, Yao W, et al: The signaling adapter protein DAP12 regulates multinucleation during osteoclast development. J Bone Miner Res 2004;19:224-34.

161. Lanier LL, Bakker AB: The ITAM-bearing transmembrane adaptor DAP12 in lymphoid and myeloid cell function. Immunol Today 2000;21:611-14.

162. Bouchon A, Hernandez-Munain C, Cella M, Colonna M: A DAP12-mediated pathway regulates expression of CC chemokine receptor 7 and maturation of human dendritic cells. J Exp Med 2001;194:1111-22.

163. Bouchon A, Dietrich J, Colonna M: Cutting edge: inflammatory responses can be triggered by TREM-1, a novel receptor expressed on neutrophils and monocytes. J Immunol 2000;164:4991-95.

164. Daws MR, Lanier LL, Seaman WE, Ryan JC: Cloning and characterization of a novel mouse myeloid DAP12-associated receptor family. Eur J Immunol 2001;31:783-91.

165. Chung DH, Seaman WE, Daws MR: Characterization of TREM-3, an activating receptor on mouse macrophages: definition of a family of single Ig domain receptors on mouse chromosome 17. Eur J Immunol 2002;32:59-66.

166. Dietrich J, Cella M, Seiffert M, et al: Cutting edge: signal-regulatory protein beta 1 is a DAP12-associated activating receptor expressed in myeloid cells. J Immunol 2000;164:9-12.

167. Bakker AB, Baker E, Sutherland GR, et al: Myeloid DAP12-associating lectin (MDL)-1 is a cell surface receptor involved in the activation of myeloid cells. Proc Natl Acad Sci U S A 1999;96:9792-6.

168. Diefenbach A, Tomasello E, Lucas M, et al: Selective associations with signaling proteins determine stimulatory versus costimulatory activity of NKG2D. Nat Immunol 2002;3:1142-49.

169. Kim N, Takami M, Rho J, et al: A novel member of the leukocyte receptor complex regulates osteoclast differentiation. J Exp Med 2002;195:201-9.

170. Merck E, Gaillard C, Gorman DM, et al: OSCAR is an FcRgamma-associated receptor that is expressed by myeloid cells and is involved in antigen presentation and activation of human dendritic cells. Blood 2004;104:1386-95.

171. Takayanagi H, Kim S, Koga T, et al: Induction and activation of the transcription factor NFATc1 (NFAT2) integrate RANKL signaling in terminal differentiation of osteoclasts. Dev Cell 2002;3:889-901.

172. Urushibara M, Takayanagi H, Koga T, et al: The antirheumatic drug leflunomide inhibits osteoclastogenesis by interfering with receptor activator of NF-kappa B ligand-stimulated induction of nuclear factor of activated T cells c1. Arthritis Rheum 2004;50:794-804.

173. Hirotani H, Tuohy NA, Woo JT, et al: The calcineurin/nuclear factor of activated T cells signaling pathway regulates osteoclastogenesis in RAW264.7 cells. J Biol Chem 2004;279: 13984-92.

174. Walsh NC, Gravallese EM: Bone loss in inflammatory arthritis: mechanisms and treatment strategies. Curr Opin Rheumatol 2004;16:419-27.

175. Shmerling RH, Goldring SR: Intermittent infusions of zoledronic acid are as effective as daily bisphosphonates in increasing bone mineral density in post-menopausal women. Clin Exp Rheumatol 2003;21:151-52.

176. Herrak P, Gortz B, Hayer S, et al: Zoledronic acid protects against local and systemic bone loss in tumor necrosis factor-mediated arthritis. Arthritis Rheum 2004;50:2327-37.

177. Goldring SR, Gravallese EM: Bisphosphonates: environmental protection for the joint? Arthritis Rheum 2004;50:2044-47.

178. Hofbauer LC, Schoppet M: Clinical implications of the osteoprotegerin/RANKL/RANK system for bone and vascular diseases. JAMA 2004;292:490-95.

179. Body JJ, Greipp P, Coleman RE, et al: A phase I study of AMGN-0007, a recombinant osteoprotegerin construct, in patients with multiple myeloma or breast carcinoma related bone metastases. Cancer 2003;97(3 Suppl):887-92.

180. Nakashima T, Wada T, Penninger JM: RANKL and RANK as novel therapeutic targets for arthritis. Curr Opin Rheumatol 2003;15:280-87.

181. Dinarello CA. Anti-cytokine therapeutics and infections. Vaccine 2003;21(Suppl 2):S24-34.

182. Saika M, Inoue D, Kido S, Matsumoto T: 17 beta-estradiol stimulates expression of osteoprotegerin by a mouse stromal cell line, ST-2, via estrogen receptor-alpha. Endocrinology 2001;142:2205-12.

183. Viereck V, Grundker C, Blaschke S, et al: Raloxifene concurrently stimulates osteoprotegerin and inhibits interleukin-6 production by human trabecular osteoblasts. J Clin Endocrinol Metab 2003;88:4206-13.

184. Brandstrom H, Bjorkman T, Ljunggren O: Regulation of osteoprotegerin secretion from primary cultures of human bone marrow stromal cells. Biochem Biophys Res Commun 2001;280:831-5.

185. Vidal NO, Brandstrom H, Jonsson KB, Ohlsson C: Osteoprotegerin mRNA is expressed in primary human osteoblast-like cells: down-regulation by glucocorticoids. J Endocrinol 1998;159:191-95.

186. Gao YH, Shinki T, Yuasa T, et al: Potential role of cbfa1, an essential transcriptional factor for osteoblast differentiation, in

osteoclastogenesis: regulation of mRNA expression of osteoclast differentiation factor (ODF). Biochem Biophys Res Commun 1998;252:697-702.

187. Suda K, Udagawa N, Sato N, et al: Suppression of osteoprotegerin expression by prostaglandin E2 is crucially involved in lipopolysaccharide-induced osteoclast formation. J Immunol 2004;172:2504-10.

188. Liu XH, Kirschenbaum A, Yao S, Levine AC: Cross-talk between the interleukin-6 and prostaglandin E(2) signaling systems results in enhancement of osteoclastogenesis through effects on the osteoprotegerin/receptor activator of nuclear factor-(kappa)B (RANK) ligand/RANK system. Endocrinology 2005;146:1991-98.

189. Mukohyama H, Ransjo M, Taniguchi H, et al: The inhibitory effects of vasoactive intestinal peptide and pituitary adenylate cyclase-activating polypeptide on osteoclast formation are associated with upregulation of osteoprotegerin and downregulation of RANKL and RANK. Biochem Biophys Res Commun 2000;271:158-63.

190. Yasuda H, Shima N, Nakagawa N, et al: Identity of osteoclastogenesis inhibitory factor (OCIF) and osteoprotegerin (OPG): a mechanism by which OPG/OCIF inhibits osteoclastogenesis in vitro. Endocrinology 1998;139:1329-37.

191. Lee SK, Lorenzo JA: Parathyroid hormone stimulates TRANCE and inhibits osteoprotegerin messenger ribonucleic acid expression in murine bone marrow cultures: correlation with osteoclast-like cell formation. Endocrinology 1999;140:3552-61.

192. Huang JC, Sakata T, Pfleger LL, et al: PTH differentially regulates expression of RANKL and OPG. J Bone Miner Res 2004;19:235-44.

193. Horwood NJ, Elliott J, Martin TJ, Gillespie MT: Osteotropic agents regulate the expression of osteoclast differentiation factor and osteoprotegerin in osteoblastic stromal cells. Endocrinology 1998;139:4743-46.

194. Thomas RJ, Guise TA, Yin JJ, et al: Breast cancer cells interact with osteoblasts to support osteoclast formation. Endocrinology 1999;140:4451-58.

195. Rubin J, Ackert-Bicknell CL, Zhu L, et al: IGF-I regulates osteoprotegerin (OPG) and receptor activator of nuclear factor-kappa B ligand in vitro and OPG in vivo. J Clin Endocrinol Metab 2002;87:4273-79.

196. Nakashima T, Kobayashi Y, Yamasaki S, et al: Protein expression and functional difference of membrane-bound and soluble receptor activator of NF-kappa B ligand: modulation of the expression by osteotropic factors and cytokines. Biochem Biophys Res Commun 2000;275:768-75.

197. Hofbauer LC, Lacey DL, Dunstan CR, et al: Interleukin-1beta and tumor necrosis factor-alpha, but not interleukin-6, stimulate osteoprotegerin ligand gene expression in human osteoblastic cells. Bone 1999;25:255-9.

198. Dai SM, Nishioka K, Yudoh K: Interleukin (IL) 18 stimulates osteoclast formation through synovial T cells in rheumatoid arthritis: comparison with IL1 beta and tumour necrosis factor alpha. Ann Rheum Dis 2004;63:1379-86.

199. Palmqvist P, Persson E, Conaway HH, Lerner UH: IL-6, leukemia inhibitory factor, and oncostatin M stimulate bone resorption and regulate the expression of receptor activator of NF-kappa B ligand, osteoprotegerin, and receptor activator of NF-kappa B in mouse calvariae. J Immunol 2002;169:3353-62.

200. Kobayashi Y, Hashimoto F, Miyamoto H, et al: Force-induced osteoclast apoptosis in vivo is accompanied by elevation in transforming growth factor beta and osteoprotegerin expression. J Bone Miner Res 2000;15:1924-34.

201. Ahlen J, Andersson S, Mukohyama H, et al: Characterization of the bone-resorptive effect of interleukin-11 in cultured mouse calvarial bones. Bone 2002;31:242-51.

202. Ishida A, Fujita N, Kitazawa R, Tsuruo T: Transforming growth factor-beta induces expression of receptor activator of NF-kappa B ligand in vascular endothelial cells derived from bone. J Biol Chem 2002;277:26217-24.

203. Murakami T, Yamamoto M, Ono K, et al: Transforming growth factor-beta1 increases mRNA levels of osteoclastogenesis inhibitory factor in osteoblastic/stromal cells and inhibits the survival of murine osteoclast-like cells. Biochem Biophys Res Commun 1998;252:747-52.

204. Kaneda T, Nojima T, Nakagawa M, et al: Endogenous production of TGF-beta is essential for osteoclastogenesis induced by a combination of receptor activator of NF-kappa B ligand and macrophage-colony-stimulating factor. J Immunol 2000;165:4254-63.

205. Quinn JM, Itoh K, Udagawa N, et al: Transforming growth factor beta affects osteoclast differentiation via direct and indirect actions. J Bone Miner Res 2001;16:1787-94.

206. Thirunavukkarasu K, Miles RR, Halladay DL, et al: Stimulation of osteoprotegerin (OPG) gene expression by transforming growth factor-beta (TGF-beta). Mapping of the OPG promoter region that mediates TGF-beta effects. J Biol Chem 2001;276:36241-50.

207. Yun TJ, Chaudhary PM, Shu GL, et al: OPG/FDCR-1, a TNF receptor family member, is expressed in lymphoid cells and is up-regulated by ligating CD40. J Immunol 1998;161:6113-21.

26

The Prevention and Treatment of Inflammation-Induced Bone Loss: Can It Be Done?

Evange Romas

SUMMARY

The inflammatory process in rheumatoid arthritis elicits intense bone loss manifested as articular bone erosions, juxta-articular osteopenia, and systemic osteoporosis. Animal studies have transformed our perception of this bone loss and highlighted the pathogenic role of osteoclasts. The tumor necrosis factor (TNF) family of cytokines, especially TNF-α and RANKL, and their respective receptors p55 and RANK, are pivotal for inducing bone destruction. Targeted TNF or RANKL antagonism reliably prevents inflammatory induced bone loss, and direct osteoclast inhibition with potent bisphosphonates is an emerging therapeutic tool. As a primary strategy, the concept of downregulating osteoclasts to prevent inflammatory bone loss is well established. However, the precise role of anabolic therapy to augment repair of bone damage requires further investigation.

A critical feature of rheumatoid arthritis (RA) is its propensity to destroy cartilage and bone.[1] The presence of bone erosions is synonymous with irreversible joint damage and associated with pain, reduced physical and emotional functioning, and increased risk of mortality.[2] Joint destruction is associated with generalized osteoporosis and fracture susceptibility, because both phenomena reflect high inflammatory disease activity.[3,4]

Osteoclasts are uniquely capable of bone degradation, and the concept that osteoclasts drive bone loss in RA is now widely accepted.[5] Osteoclasts are consistently detected at erosion sites in all animal models of destructive arthritis as well as human RA.[6] Synovial inflammation generates tumor necrosis factor (TNF)-α, macrophage colony-stimulating factor (M-CSF), and receptor activator of nuclear factor-κB ligand (RANKL), cytokines that fuel osteoclastogenesis and arthritic bone destruction. The targeted removal of osteoclasts by TNF-blockers or RANKL antagonism or genetic manipulation in animal models potently blocks this bone destruction.[7-12]

The importance of osteoclast-mediated joint destruction has prompted renewed interest in bisphonates to address inflammatory bone loss in RA. Accordingly, targeting osteoclasts in autoimmune or TNF-dependent models of RA with powerful third-generation bisphosphonates recapitulates bone protection.[13,14] Downregulation of osteoclasts has emerged as a powerful strategy for the prevention of inflammatory-induced bone loss. Intriguingly, this avenue of bone protection is not necessarily contingent on suppression of synovial inflammation.

Bone loss manifest as focal bone erosion and juxta-articular osteoporosis is a consequence of a distorted bone turnover in the context of chronic inflammation. Osteoblasts as well as osteoclasts are detected near active bone erosions, and it is likely that defects of both cell types contribute to the bone loss. In fact, osteoblasts are suppressed by exposure to inflammatory cytokines such as TNF.[15] The precise role of reduced osteoblast function in inflammatory bone loss is uncertain.

The prevention of structural joint damage is now a central tenet of contemporary antirheumatic drug therapy.[16] A concerted approach to address inflammatory bone loss requires consideration of several possible strategies: 1) intensive interference with inflammatory synovial processes that stimulate bone erosion, above all, TNF overproduction; 2) blockade of pathogenic osteoclasts; and 3) stimulation of osteoblast recruitment and/or function to promote skeletal repair.

BONE LOSS IN RHEUMATOID ARTHRITIS

Three distinct types of bone loss are delineated in RA: 1) focal articular bone erosion, 2) juxta-articular osteopenia adjacent to arthritis, and 3) systemic osteoporosis at sites distant from inflamed joints. Although initially conceptualized as separate phenomena, an early hint for a shared pathogenesis involving osteoclasts was that radiographic erosion was found to be strongly associated with systemic osteoporosis.[17]

Bone erosions are a radiological hallmark of RA and accompany severe arthritis along with the presence of rheumatoid factor and antibodies to cyclic citrullinated peptides.[18,19] They occur early in the disease, and after 6 months, 70% of patients have bone erosions detected by magnetic resonance imaging.[20] Magnetic resonance imaging detects increased water content in the bone marrow adjacent to inflamed joints, both in the absence and in the presence of erosion. The histological correlate of this "bone edema" is uncertain, although aspiration has yielded CD34+ bone marrow cells, which are potential osteoclast precursors.[21]

Juxta-articular osteopenia adjacent to inflamed joints is one of the first radiographic signs of RA, maximal in early disease, correlated positively with disease activity and negatively with disease duration. Biopsies of juxta-articular bone have revealed numerous osteoclasts as well as increased osteoid and resorptive surfaces consistent with high bone turnover and negative bone balance.

Generalized osteoporosis is prevalent in RA and associated with increased fracture rates. Unlike postmenopausal osteoporosis, osteoporosis is characterized by relatively preserved axial (lumbar spine) bone and marked loss at appendicular sites (hip and radius) in RA. The central determinant of systemic bone loss is the underlying inflammatory disease process. Thus, progressive bone loss in early RA before steroid therapy is clearly correlated to measures of inflammatory disease activity (serum C-reactive protein) as well as increased biomarkers reflecting osteoclastic activity.[22]

OSTEOCLASTOGENESIS IN INFLAMMATORY ARTHRITIS

The receptor activator of nuclear factor-κB ligand is a TNF family cytokine that is essential for the induction of osteoclastogenesis as shown by targeted disruption of the gene in mice, resulting in defective lymph node organogenesis and lymphocyte differentiation and osteopetrosis caused by a complete absence of osteoclasts.[23] The discovery of the RANKL/RANK/OPG (osteoprotegerin) system therefore divulged the molecular basis of osteoclastogenesis and explicitly revealed a nexus between the immune and bone systems relevant to RA.[23,24]

After the discovery that osteoclastogenesis and bone turnover were regulated by expression of RANKL/RANK and its soluble decoy receptor, OPG, their expression was investigated in arthritis. These studies revealed that RANKL mRNA was detected by reverse-transcriptase polymerase chain reaction in synovium from patients with RA but not in healthy synovium.[25] RANKL was detected in synovial fibroblasts and activated T cells from peripheral blood as well as synovial tissue.[26,27] In our own in situ hybridization studies, CD3+ T cells, osteoblasts, and fibroblast-like synoviocytes in RA synovium all stained intensely for RANKL.[27] Similarly, in collagen-induced arthritis, RANKL and OPG were detected at the erosion sites.[12]

Osteoclastic erosion was also defined in psoriatic arthritis, which like RA is characterized by synovitis and focal bone destruction.[28] The severity of bone erosion was correlated to circulating mononuclear osteoclast precursors, revealing a novel mechanism for enhanced osteoclastogenesis in psoriatic arthritis. Circulating osteoclast precursors were also elevated in human TNF-α transgenic (hTNF Tg) mice and fell after anti-TNF therapy.[29]

In vitro studies showed that osteoblasts and T-cells expressed RANKL and supported osteoclast differentiation when co-cultured with myeloid precursors.[24,27,30] Co-cultures of synovial fibroblasts and monocytes also generated osteoclasts in vitro.[26] Thus, multiple cell types present in inflamed joint tissues, such as activated T-cells, fibroblasts, and osteoblastic-stromal cells, express RANKL.

The transcriptional program leading to osteoclastogenesis has been dissected in detail. Osteoclast differentiation depends on cooperation of RANKL and immunoreceptor tyrosine-based activation motif (ITAM) signals in osteoclast precursors.[31] The phosphorylation of ITAM stimulated by immunoreceptors and RANKL-RANK interaction results in the recruitment of syk family kinases, leading to the activation of phospholipase Cγ and calcium signaling, which is critical for NFATc1 induction, a master transcription factor for osteoclast development.[32] NFATc1 induction is also dependent on c-Fos and TRAF6, which are activated by RANKL.[33,34] Immunoreceptors associated with FcRγ are activated exclusively by ligands expressed by osteoblasts, whereas those associated with DAP12 are activated by ligands expressed on osteoclast precursor cells themselves.[35]

Although T-cells express RANKL, they also produce osteoclast inhibitors, such as interferon-γ and interleukin (IL)-4.[36-38] Interferon-β production induced by RANKL autoregulates osteoclastogenesis.[39] Thus, the role of T-cells in osteoclastogenesis is complex and depends on the suite of prevailing cytokines.[40] Under some conditions, T-cells may not drive osteoclastogenesis even if RANKL is expressed. In the presence of high levels of TNF, sub-osteoclastogenic ("permissive") amounts of RANKL may be sufficient for TNF to drive RANKL-mediated osteoclastogenesis.[41] In essence, although there is evidence for a direct contribution of T-cell–derived RANKL, expression of RANKL by fibroblast-like synoviocytes or osteoblasts (induced by IL-6 type cytokines, IL-17, and possibly parathyroid hormone related peptide [PTHrP]) may be quantitatively more important for osteoclastogenesis.[42-44]

Osteoclast formation in arthritis models is a swift and dynamic process leading to rapid attack on juxta-articular bone, a prerequisite for early-onset structural damage.[45] Since osteoclasts have a finite lifespan, continuous replenishment of the local osteoclast pool is probably necessary to achieve progressive bone damage.[46] From the perspective of bone erosions in RA, major targets of RANKL are RANK-positive osteoclast percursors, primarily monocytes that populate inflamed synovium, as well as myeloid lineage cells resident in bone marrow. Direct cell-to-cell contact between stromal cells and osteoclast percursors efficiently presents the molecular signals (i.e., RANKL + M-CSF) necessary for osteoclast differentiation.[47] In synovium, the main stromal osteoclast support cells are fibroblast-like synoviocytes, whereas the main osteoclast support cells in subchondral bone are osteoblasts (Figure 26-1).

Figure 26-1. (A) Cellular and molecular interactions in the synovial compartment facilitate osteoclast differentiation and focal bone erosion at the synovial/bone interface. The main stromal support cell is the activated fibroblast-like synoviocytes, which express membrane-bound macrophage colony-stimulating factor (M-CSF) (not shown) and RANKL. These processes lead to an imbalance in bone resorption relative to bone formation, exhibited as "extrinsic" focal bone erosion. (B) Cellular and molecular interactions in the subchondral bone marrow compartment facilitate osteoclast differentiation and subchondral bone erosion. The main stromal support cell is the stromal-osteoblasts which express membrane-bound M-CSF (not shown) and RANKL. These processes lead to an imbalance in bone resorption relative to formation, exhibited as subchondral bone erosion and juxta-articular osteoporosis. (See Color Plates.)

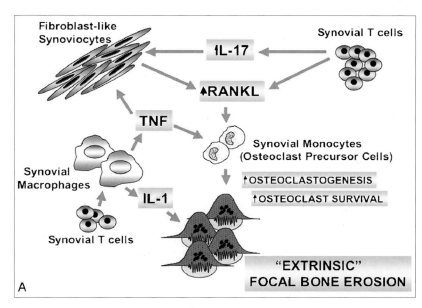

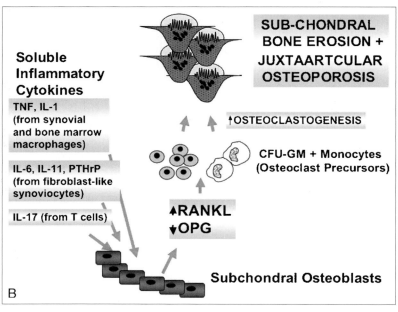

ROLE OF TUMOR NECROSIS FACTOR IN ARTHRITIC BONE DESTRUCTION

The inflamed synovium is a prodigious source of inflammatory cytokines such as TNF-α, IL-1, IL-6, and IL-17.[48] All of these cytokines increase stromal cell expression of RANKL and/or reduce OPG expression. Through pleiotropic activities on multiple cells, TNF-α is the dominant cytokine for arthritic bone destruction. In fact, the pre-eminence of TNF production is probably responsible for endowing the rheumatoid synovium with its proclivity for bone destruction.

Unlike more benign arthropathies, RA is characterized by greater synovial TNF induction and higher levels of TNF in the synovial fluids,[49] which preferentially promotes osteoclastogenesis through the p55 receptor on osteoclast progenitors.[50] TNF production is stimulated by T-cell–derived interferon-γ and direct cell-to-cell contact with T cells.[51,52] The immunogenetic susceptibility to RA conferred by the presence of the "shared epitope" is associated with rheumatoid factor and anti-cyclic citrullinated peptide production, and the resultant immune complexes in the joints amplify monocyte/macrophage TNF production.[53]

Activities of TNF that promote osteoclastogenesis are as follows:

1. TNF directly promotes osteoclast differentiation of monocytes and macrophages exposed to permissive levels of RANKL.[8]
2. TNF stimulates stromal-osteoblast RANKL production (through a mechanism involving IL-1 and IL-17).[54]
3. TNF stimulates RANKL production by T- and B-cells.
4. TNF stimulates stromal-osteoblast production of M-CSF.
5. TNF enhances stromal cell expression of RANKL.[48]

Remarkably, the TNF blockers in clinical use tend to interfere with destructive events in RA more readily than inflammatory synovitis. In fact, TNF antagonism may arrest joint destruction in some patients despite little improvement in inflammation.[55] This phenomenon may imply that TNF is a principal driver for bone loss, whereas other cytokines are responsible for symptoms. Alternatively, TNF levels may be reduced to subthreshold levels such that osteoclast propagation is suppressed, while sufficient TNF is available to mediate synovial proliferation.

Besides TNF, the other key inflammatory cytokines include IL-1 and IL-6. The pathogenic involvement of these cytokines is supported by the occurrence of erosive arthritis in mice lacking the IL-1 receptor antagonist and inhibitory effects of IL-6 receptor antibodies in experimental arthritis.[56,57] Overall, IL-1 antagonism is not as efficacious as TNF blockade in preventing radiographic bone erosions in RA.[58] This may reflect suboptimal dosing of IL-1ra, but more likely (although this premise is controversial) it implies a lesser role for IL-1.[59] With respect to osteoclast biology, it appears that, through p55 receptors, TNF drives osteoclast differentiation, whereas IL-1 is more important for extending the lifespan of nascent osteoclasts.[10] Evidently, a destructive synergy exists between TNF, IL-17, IL-1, and the IL-6 type cytokines that induces RANK-mediated bone loss (see Figure 26-1).

In contradistinction to TNF blockers, although traditional disease-modifying drugs significantly retard erosion, bone loss continues in many or most patients. This implies continuing TNF production sufficient to stimulate osteoclastic erosions. In fact, methotrexate therapy preferentially reduces endogenous IL-1, and this may explain the greater clinical benefits (for radiological progression) of adding TNF blockers to methotrexate.[60-62]

INFLAMMATORY BONE LOSS: TARGETING RANK-MEDIATED OSTEOCLASTOGENESIS

Proof of the role of osteoclasts in inflammatory bone loss came from models of arthritis and especially by employing genetically altered mice (Table 26-1). In initial studies, OPG prevented articular bone destruction in both adjuvant and collagen-induced arthritis.[12,24] Similarly, mutant mice that completely lacked osteoclasts (RANKL-deficient or *c-fos*-deficient mice), were protected from bone destruction induced by serum transfer or crossing with hTNF Tg mutants.[8,11] TNF-mediated bone loss (hTNF Tg mice) was reduced by OPG, RANK:Fc, or crossing with RANK–/– mutants.[7,9,63]

In all models, drastically reduced osteoclast numbers were associated with bone protection, yet synovial inflammation was not reduced by RANKL antagonism (see Table 26-1). Notably, cartilage protection in these models was minimal or absent, signifying that divergent cellular mechanisms are responsible for bone or cartilage loss,[48,64] and cartilage damage was mostly independent of RANK-mediated osteoclastogenesis. These findings are consistent with recent descriptions of the critical role for ADAMTS-5 in arthritic cartilage degradation.[65,66]

BISPHOSPHONATES FOR INFLAMMATION-INDUCED BONE LOSS

The bisphosphonates are analogues of inorganic pyrophosphate in which an oxygen atom has been replaced with a carbon atom. The phosphate-carbon-

TABLE 26-1 TARGETING OSTEOCLASTOGENESIS IN ANIMAL MODELS OF INFLAMMATORY ARTHRITIS

Arthritis Model	Intervention	Effect on Bone Destruction	Effect on Synovial Inflammation	Study
Adjuvant arthritis in rats	OPG 1 mg/kg/day	↓↓↓	—	Kong et al[24]
CIA in rats	Fc-OPG 3 mg/kg/day	↓↓ (60%)	—	Romas et al[12]
CIA in rats	Single dose ZA 100 μg/kg	↓↓↓ (80%)	↑ (transient)	Sims et al[14]
K/BxN serum transfer in RANKL–/– mice	None	↓↓↓	—	Pettit et al[11]
hTNF Tg mice	OPG	↓↓↓	—	Redlich et al[7]
hTNF Tg mice	Infliximab	↓↓↓ (80%)	↓↓ (50%)	Redlich et al[7]
hTNF Tg mice	Infliximab + OPG	↓↓↓ (85%)	↓↓↓ (80%)	Redlich et al[7]
hTNF Tg mice	Repeated ZA dosing	↓↓↓ (95%)	—	Herrak et al[13]
hTNF Tg mice	RANK:Fc 10 mg/kg alternate days	↓↓↓	—	Li et al[63]
hTNF Tg x c-fos–/– mice	None	↓↓↓	—	Redlich et al[8]
hTNF Tg x RANK–/– mice	None	↓↓↓	↓	Redlich et al[8]

CIA = collagen-induced arthritis; hTNF Tg = human TNF-α transgenic; OPG = osteoprotegerin; X = hybrid or cross; ZA = zoledronic acid.

phosphate moiety confers their high-affinity binding property to hydroxyapatite mineral where the drugs preferentially interfere with osteoclastic bone resorption. Their properties have been extensively reviewed.[67,68] The more potent amino-bisphosphonates pamidronate, alendronate, risedronate, and zoledronate exert their inhibitory effects on osteoclast function by inhibiting farnesyl pyrophosphate synthase, an enzyme in the mevalonate pathway necessary for lipid modification (prenylation) of small guanosine triphosphate binding proteins. This process alters cytoskeletal organization and intracellular trafficking, resulting in inhibition of osteoclast function. The non-amino-bisphosphonates such as etidronate and clodronate are metabolized to nonhydrolyzable analogues of adenosine triphosphate and act as inhibitors of ATP-dependent enzymes, leading to enhanced osteoclast apoptosis.

Based on the insights gained from targeting RANKL in arthritis, invoking bisphosphonates for bone protection is timely and rational; however, the use of bisphosphonates in treating arthritis is certainly not a novel idea. Early-generation bisphosphonates were extensively tested in experimental arthritis models, primarily as anti-inflammatory drugs targeting macrophages. The amino-bisphosphonates were generally avoided because of their reputed proinflammatory effects. These studies showed reduced biomarkers of bone resorption and variable joint protection; however, any effects on focal bone erosion were poorly documented.[69-72]

We reported the effect of zoledronic acid (ZA), a highly potent bisphosphonate in the effector phase of collagen-induced arthritis.[14] A single pulse of ZA prevented radiological bone erosions (Figure 26-2). At the highest dose tested (100 μg/kg), histological erosion scores were reduced by 80%. Juxta-articular bone loss was abrogated, trabecular bone mass increased above control levels after 2 weeks, and the elevated bone resorption biomarker CTX-I was normalized. In contrast, ZA had no useful effects on synovial inflammation or cartilage damage. Higher dose ZA (50-100 μg/kg) was mildly proinflammatory; yet, despite the continuing synovitis, ZA protected arthritic bone. A similar study using repetitive dosing of ZA in the hTNF Tg mice showed comparable reduction in bone erosions and prevention of systemic osteoporosis.[13] Osteoclast numbers in both studies were drastically reduced. From our own histomorphometric analysis of collagen-induced arthritis, we concluded that ZA exerts bone protection by downregulating osteoclast numbers and reducing osteoclast activity.[14] In contrast, calcitonin, a much weaker antiresorptive agent that does not downregulate osteoclast numbers, failed to modulate bone erosions in hTNF Tg mice.[13]

At present, it is uncertain whether bisphosphonates could inhibit radiological bone erosion in cases of human RA. Only a few randomized clinical trials exploring erosion protection have been published, and nearly all involved weaker first- and second-generation agents.[73-81] Because of small patient numbers, varying selection criteria and trial designs, and short follow-up

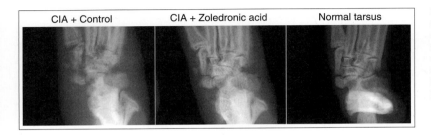

CIA + Control   CIA + Zoledronic acid   Normal tarsus

Figure 26-2. Radiological bone erosions are prevented by zoledronic acid treatment. Collagen-induced arthritis treated without (left panel) or with (middle panel) a single pulse of zoledronic acid, 100 µg/kg. A non-inflamed tarsus is shown on the right panel

periods, interpretation of these trials is problematic. However, several conclusions are possible:

1. Clodronate, etidronate, and pamidronate possess trivial anti-inflammatory activity.
2. Etidronate and pamidronate reduced biomarkers of bone resorption and pamidronate stabilized progressive bone loss in the axial and appendicular skeleton.
3. Etidronate and low-dose oral pamidronate did not reduce erosions, but high-dose pamidronate blunted bone erosion but not joint space narrowing (i.e., cartilage loss).
4. ZA prevented generalized bone loss in early RA and reduced new MRI bone lesions at the carpus by up to 60%. There are no data for any effect on radiographic erosions.

Surprisingly, the most potent third-generation bisphosphonates, which exhibit the most profound inhibitory effects on osteoclasts, have not been assessed in sufficiently powered randomized trials with radiological erosion as a primary endpoint. Owing to the high costs and uncertain long-term safety of TNF antagonists, investigator-led studies of third-generation bisphosphonates to prevent inflammatory-induced bone loss are both necessary and desirable.

INFLAMMATORY BONE LOSS: TARGETING OSTEOBLASTS

It is unknown whether established RA bone erosions can be properly reconstituted, although reports of erosion "repair" after anti-inflammatory therapy are a testament to this possibility.[82] Osteoclastic activity cannot be viewed separately from osteoblasts, because these two cell populations are linked through physiological coupling. Osteoblasts are present in arthritic bone erosions, but the detailed kinetics and fate of osteoblasts relative to osteoclasts at these sites are not elucidated.[83] In view of the coupling of osteoblasts to osteoclasts, it is likely that osteoblasts at erosion sites are a response to osteoclastic activity, not reactive to inflammatory synovitis, although this question has not been resolved. Clearly, the osteoblastic response in active erosions is feeble,

resulting in net bone loss. Cytokines such as TNF downregulate osteoblasts in part by interfering with the master transcription factor Runx-2.[15,84,85] Fundamentally, osteoblastic suppression may be additive to bone-damaging effects of TNF-induced osteoclastogenesis.

At present, parathyroid hormone (PTH) is the only useful bone anabolic agent available, and its use has been extensively documented in animals and humans with osteoporosis due to estrogen deficiency.[86] The effects of PTH are determined by the dynamics of its presentation to osteoblasts. At a constant level, PTH downregulates OPG, increasing osteoclastogenesis, while pulsed administration stimulates osteoblastogenesis, increases bone remodeling, and leads to gains in bone mass. Pulsed PTH therapy was tested in animal models of inflammatory bone loss. Short-term PTH alone had no measurable effects on bone destruction in hTNF Tg mice, yet in the context of anti-TNF or anti-RANKL therapy, mice treated with PTH exhibited greater bone protection and repair of articular erosions.[87] Similar effects were reported in immune-mediated models of arthritis.[88] It is important to note that concomitant osteoclast inhibition may blunt the effect of PTH, as reported with alendronate.[89,90] Therefore, it remains to be seen if these results can be reproduced in treatment settings that mandate profound osteoclast inhibition.

CONCLUSION

The revelation of molecular mechanisms that link immune and bone cells and govern osteoclast recruitment has transformed our conception of pathogenic events in RA. Inflammatory synovitis induces profound bone loss, and osteoclasts are the instrument of this destruction. TNF blockers have an established role in the prevention of inflammatory bone loss, and the importance of T cells in perpetuating synovitis and bone destruction in RA is emerging from successful clinical trials of T cell co-stimulation blockade with CTLA-immunoglobulin fusion protein (abatacept).[91] TNF-antagonism reliably arrests radiological progression in RA, and proof-of-concept studies show that RANKL inhibition prevents inflammatory bone loss.

INDEX

Note: Page numbers followed by f indicate figures; those followed by t indicate tables.